IMPROVING QUALITY

A Guide to Effective Programs

Second Edition

Claire Gavin Meisenheimer, PhD, RN, CNAA
Health Care Consultant
Professor
University of Wisconsin Oshkosh
Oshkosh, Wisconsin

AN ASPEN PUBLICATION®
Aspen Publishers, Inc.
Gaithersburg, Maryland
1997

The authors have made every effort to ensure the accuracy of the information herein. However, appropriate information sources should be consulted, especially for new or unfamiliar procedures. It is the responsibility of every practitioner to evaluate the appropriateness of a particular opinion in the context of actual clinical situations and with due considerations to new developments. Authors, editors, and the publisher cannot be held responsible for any typographical or other errors found in this book.

Library of Congress Cataloging in Publication Data
Improving quality : a guide to effective programs / [edited by]
Claire Meisenheimer.—2nd ed.
p.   cm.
Includes bibliographical references and index.
ISBN 0-8342-0910-1 (casebound)
1. Nursing—Quality control.   I. Meisenheimer, Claire Gavin.
RT85.5.I47   1997
362.1'73' 0685—dc21   97-5136
CIP

Orders: (800) 638-8437
Customer Service: (800) 234-1660

About Aspen Publishers • For more than 35 years, Aspen has been a leading professional publisher in a variety of disciplines. Aspen's vast information resources are available in both print and electronic formats. We are committed to providing the highest quality information available in the most appropriate format for our customers. Visit Aspen's Internet site for more information resources, directories, articles, and a searchable version of Aspen's full catalog, including the most recent publications: **http://www.aspenpub.com**
Aspen Publishers, Inc. • The hallmark of quality in publishing
Member of the worldwide Wolters Kluwer group.

Editorial Resources: Brian MacDonald
Library of Congress Catalog Card Number: 97-5136
ISBN: 0-8342-0910-1

Printed in the United States of America
1   2   3   4   5

With great appreciation and affection:

To Elliott, my special husband and friend of 38 years

To my wonderful children: Holly, Scott, and Wendy

To my precious twin granddaughters: Britny and Samantha

and

In memory of Delia Pageau Gavin, my mother,

who taught us all the meaning of quality.

Thank you for all your support.

Table of Contents

Contributors

Tonia Dandry Aiken, RN, BSN, JD
Past President
The American Association of Nurse Attorneys
President
RN Development, Inc.
Metairie, Lousiana

Julia W. Aucoin, MN, RN, C
Faculty
North Carolina Central University
Vice President
RN Development, Inc.
Metairie, Louisiana

Adrianne E. Avillion, DEd, RN, CRRN, CNA
President
AEA Consulting
York, Pennsylvania

Barbara J. Brown, EdD, RN, FAAN, FNAP
Health Care Administrative Consultant
Editor, *Nursing Administration Quarterly*
Fraser, Colorado

Judith M. Bulau, MSN, RN, PHN
Health Care Consultant
Minneapolis, Minnesota

Margaret J. Bull, PhD, RN, FAAN
Associate Professor
University of Minnesota School of Nursing
Minneapolis, Minnesota

Kathryn L. Clark, MS, RN
Clinical Programs Manager
Columbia Practice Management
President and Owner
ETC: An Education, Training, and Consultation
    Business
Oklahoma City, Oklahoma

Mary E. Cohan, MD
Assistant Professor of Medicine, Division of
    Geriatrics
Medical College of Wisconsin
Milwaukee, Wisconsin

Judy Crouch-Smolarek, MSN, RN
Director of Nursing and Health Officer
Neenah Public Health Department
Neenah, Wisconsin

Nancy E. Donaldson, DNSc, RN
Principal
Donaldson and Associates
Newport Beach, California

Willa L. Fields, RN, DNSc
Systemwide Director of Quality Measurement
Sharp HealthCare
San Diego, California

Joann Genovich-Richards, PhD, MBA, MSN, RN
Vice President
Rockburn Institute
Elkridge, Maryland

Debra Gillett, RN, BSN
Consultant
Griffin Management, Inc.
Scottsdale, Arizona

Dale Glaser, PhD, MS, MA
Methods Analyst
Sharp HealthCare
Adjunct Faculty
San Diego State University
University of San Diego
United States International University
San Diego, California

Linda Gonia, MHA, RN
QA Coordinator
Family Health Plan
Bluemound Health Center
Milwaukee, Wisconsin

Kathleen M. Griffin, PhD
President and CEO
Griffin Management, Inc.
Scottsdale, Arizona

Maria Hill, MS, RN
Senior Consultant
The Center for Case Management, Inc.
South Natick, Massachusetts

Roxana Huebscher, PhD, RN, FNP–C
Associate Professor, College of Nursing
University of Wisconsin Oshkosh
Oshkosh, Wisconsin

Marsha Magnusen Hughes, MSN, MSE
Director/Hospice Hope/Home Oxygen/DME
St. Agnes Hospital
Fond du Lac, Wisconsin

Patricia Kelly-Heidenthal, MSN, RN
Associate Professor, Department of Nursing
Purdue University Calumet
Hammond, Indiana

Susan K. Kratz, BSN, RN
Public Health Nurse Consultant
Department of Family Services, Division
   of Health, Bureau of Public Health
Green Bay, Wisconsin

Elizabeth R. Larson, MSN, RN
Associate Professor Emeritus
College of Nursing
University of Wisconsin Oshkosh
Oshkosh, Wisconsin

Shirley Ann Larson, BSN, MSN, RN
Clinical Assessment and Risk Evaluation
   Coordinator
Clement J. Zablocki VA Medical Center, CARE
   Section
Milwaukee, Wisconsin

Karen Ann Lentz, BSN, RN, CPUR
Clinical Assessment and Risk Evaluation
   Coordinator
Clement J. Zablocki VA Medical Center
Milwaukee, Wisconsin

Ellen M. Lewis, MSN, RN
Program Administrator—Nursing and Allied
   Health
Associate Clinical Professor
College of Medicine, University of California,
   Irvine
Irvine, California

Anna Marie Lieske, MS, RN
Chief, CARE Section
Clement J. Zablocki VA Medical Center
Milwaukee, Wisconsin

Sandra M. Mareno
Quality Advisor
Villa Clement Medical Center
Milwaukee, Wisconsin

Lori C. Marshall, MSN, RN
Education Specialist
Children's Hospital of Orange County,
  Education Department
Orange, California

Angella D. Mattheis, BSN
Community Relations/Quality Assurance
  Coordinator
St. Agnes Hospital Home Delivered Services
Hospice Hope, Homecare, Home Oxygen/
  Home Medical Equipment
Fond du Lac, Wisconsin

Claire G. Meisenheimer, PhD, RN, CNAA
Health Care Consultant
Professor, Graduate Program
Coordinator, Nursing Administration Emphasis
University of Wisconsin Oshkosh
Oshkosh, Wisconsin

**Allen Nottingham, MS, RN, Doctoral
  Candidate**
Coordinator, Remote Cardiac Services
Columbia Presbyterian Hospital
Oklahoma City, Oklahoma
Assistant Professor
Department of Nursing
University of Central Oklahoma
Edmond, Oklahoma

Lenard L. Parisi, RN, MA, CPHQ
Director, Quality Assessment and Improvement
Mount Sinai Medical Center Home Health
  Agency
New York, New York

Cindy Parsons, ARNP, MS, CS
Patient Services Manager, Psychiatry
Tampa General Healthcare
Tampa, Florida

Ted Pfeiffer, MBA
Associate
APM, Inc.
Chicago, Illinois

Traci L. Raether, MSN, RN
Quality Resources Director
Evergreen Retirement Community, Inc.
Oshkosh, Wisconsin

Katrina Sargent-Deziel, RN
Primary Nurse, Case Manager
Hospice of Cape Cod
Yarmouthport, Massachusetts

June A. Schmele, PhD, RN
Associate Professor, College of Nursing
Adjunct Associate Professor
Department of Health Administration and Policy
College of Public Health
University of Oklahoma
Oklahoma City, Oklahoma

Roy L. Simpson, RN, C, FNAP, FAAN
Executive Director, Nursing Affairs
HBO & Company
Atlanta, Georgia

Carolyn H. Smeltzer, EdD, MSN, RN, FAAN
Partner
Coopers and Lybrand
Chicago, Illinois

**George Byron Smith, RN, C, MSN, CCM,
  CNAA**
Clinical Care Manager
Tampa General Hospital—University Psychiatric
  Center
Tampa, Florida

Ann Marie Vonglis, MSN, CNA, RN
Manager, Staff Development
Coordinator, Nursing Quality Management
Western Medical Center/Santa Ana
Santa Ana, California

Diane R. Weber, MHA, BSN
Director, Quality Services
University Health System Consortium, Inc.
Oak Brook, Illinois

Marjorie D. Weiss, PhD, NP
President and CEO
Occupational Health Systems of Wisconsin
Appleton, Wisconsin
Former Director, The Partnership Project
United Health Group
Appleton, Wisconsin

Mary Ellen Wurzbach, RN, MSN, FNP, PhD
Associate Professor, College of Nursing
University of Wisconsin Oshkosh
Oshkosh, Wisconsin

Barbara J. Youngberg, BSN, MSW, JD
Vice President
Insurance, Risk & Quality Management
University Health System Consortium, Inc.
Oak Brook, Illinois

Foreword

If it sounds too good, it usually isn't. The competition among health care providers has led consumers to question the "goodness" of health care. Moreover, the health care revolution has placed tremendous burdens on providers who are sincerely attempting to provide quality care in a dynamic, changing health care environment with diminishing resources.

Consumer needs and expectations vary greatly in terms of the consumers' access to quality care, their choice of health care provider determined by their level of trust and relationship with that provider, their educational preparation and previous experiences, the level of accountability expected of their providers, and their ability to determine health care quality. *Improving Quality: A Guide to Effective Programs* serves as a universal resource for providers in all types of health care organizations, as well as students and faculty offering the principles and practices of quality improvement in their educational institutions.

Incorporating TQM into the organization's vision, mission statements, and guiding principles and practices affords management an opportunity to create a detailed and workable strategic plan of action for the delivery and continuous improvement of quality care. The scope of quality assessment ranges from a narrow focus on issues such as availability, acceptability, accessibility, affordability, and appropriateness of the whole patient system.

Managed care and case management; flexible, focused, and useful information systems; patient outcomes research; and overall clinical and administrative processes are significant additions to this guide. The linking of accountability with specific performance standards that reflect the varied expectations of customers and suppliers, clarifying roles and relationships, and conducting performance evaluations to ensure competence and continuous improvement are major cornerstones on which to establish the framework of quality improvement.

The market understands and appreciates various "good housekeeping seal-of-approval awards." In 1994, the University of Michigan Health Systems received the State of Michigan Quality Leadership Award, a state quality award based on the Malcolm Baldrige National Quality Award criteria; in 1990, they were recognized by the Healthcare Forum (San Francisco) and Witt Associates, Inc. (Chicago), the only nationwide award for quality given to health care organizations in the United States. In 1997, the Joint Commission will formally announce the Codman Awards to focus attention on the importance of using performance data to drive quality improvement activities in each field in which the Joint Commission provides accreditation services—ambulatory care, behavioral health care, health care networks, home care, hospitals, laboratories, and long-term care. Organizations will be rewarded for "developing practical, cost-effective measurement approaches that demonstrably make a difference" (Joint Commission, 1996).

The current health care system is a work in progress. As we move into the 21st century, quality improvement programs will provide a vehicle for multiple collaboration efforts in all arenas of professional practice. The power of health care providers will be exhibited by their ability to create environments in which desired outcomes are achieved. Competition is driving our entire economic system, resulting in improved customer service and quality products. The same market forces evidenced in fierce competition and cost-reduction measures are now driving the health care system as well. Since 1987, businesses have recognized organizational performance with the prestigious Malcolm Baldrige National Quality Award[*].

The revolution in health care challenges all providers to create new environments for care that empower the consumer to express, decide, and act on their own health care needs and requirements. Consumer satisfaction is the hallmark of excellence; health care professionals have an enormous task to provide that excellence in health care.

Barbara J. Brown, EdD, RN, FAAN, FNAP, CNAA

Editor, *Nursing Administration Quarterly*

Consultant, Health Care Administration

Adjunct Associate Clinical Professor
Vanderbilt University
School of Nursing
Nashville, Tennessee
University of Washington,
School of Nursing
Seattle, Washington
University of Colorado,
School of Nursing
Boulder, Colorado
Professor, Health Care Administration
College of St. Francis
Joliet, Illinois

---

[*] The Malcolm Baldrige National Quality Award, originated in 1987 as Public Law 100-107, introduced pilot activities in 1994 and 1995. The Malcolm Baldrige National Quality Award Healthcare Pilot Criteria 1995 Booklet emphasizes the following criteria categories:

- Patient healthcare results
- Patient satisfaction
- Other stakeholder satisfaction
- Administrative and business results, including financial indicators
- Community health and public responsibilities
- Human resource performance development
- Organizational performance relative to competitors and similar health care organizations

REFERENCES

Berman, S. (1995). Using Malcolm Baldrige Quality Award criteria for improvement: An interview with Ellen Gaucher. *Journal of Quality Improvement, 21*(2), 249–256.

Jensen, L. (1996). Improving healthcare quality: application of the Baldrige process. *Journal of Nursing Administration, 28*(7/8), 51–54.

Joint Commission on Accreditation of Healthcare Organizations. (1996). Joint Commission announces creation of performance improvement awards. *Joint Commission Perspectives: Official Joint Commission Newsletter, 16*(4), 1, 4.

Preface

Becoming a global society is changing the way we think and behave: reengineering our organizations with a common culture, vision, and incentives; inspiring, deploying, and enabling our human resources; and creating measures that reward value-adding work across the continuum are all providing challenges and opportunities. Driven by concern for profitability and survival in the private business sector and political pressure at the state and federal levels, cataclysmic activity within the American health care system is reshaping health care delivery. Various modes of consolidation, integration, networks, and relationships among providers, some of whom refused to speak to one another previously, are accelerating at unprecedented rates.

Our current health care "non-system" is quickly being transformed into a managed care system characterized by global capitation and risk-sharing, with an emphasis on primary care and prevention. While the patient has historically been considered ahead of profits, health care has never been divorced from economics. However, the pendulum has now swung toward an almost mystical idealism of the "market." "The private sector revolution has succeeded in restricting the flow of resources into health care in a way the government could not have done and survived politically" (Health Trends Report, 1997, p. 15).

The "major bullets" of the past, including "downsizing and rightsizing"—which in many cases have proven to be dumb decisions—"diversification," "corporate restructuring/redesign," "horizontal vs vertical," and more recently, "virtual integration," have given way to "patient/customer focused care," "reengineering," and "managed care," with case management, practice guidelines, variance tracking, disease state management, and outcomes management tools and techniques. The independent status of hospitals continues to decline and hospitals that don't get picked into the network are dead. With all this competition, a major question becomes: Who is the customer? The patient? The employer? The payer?

Simultaneously, the market is signaling that **accountability** will largely determine the credibility of the new system. **Value** is still a fundamental core issue today. New business strategies to make changes that bring together the right balance of the triad—quality, cost, and access/utilization—will require a data infrastructure that will produce accurate, comprehensive, timely, and readily accessible information within an integrated delivery system approach to care. While the link between quality and cost has been weak in measuring market success, the consumer—patients, employers, and payers of care—are now demanding to know what value they are receiving for their health care dollars.

In this new era of accountability, all consumers expect standards with outcome measures, target benchmarks, report cards, and competing on quality. Excellence is demanded and is being measured by extensive organizational, national and the beginnings of international data sets that demonstrate clinical and financial effectiveness. Sensitive data—report cards—describing practitioners and the delivery of good and bad health care outcomes will differentiate one organization from another. Organizations will be recognized for their quality efforts rather than their rationing of care for the sake of cost. Discounting provider charges and other artificial cost-cutting measures may reduce costs in the short term; the long-term impact of managed care on health cost growth is still unclear.

To excel in the marketplace, learning organizations are creating an organizational culture that values learning and sharing. They recognize that health care is being dominated by regional and state-wide relationships and nationally owned organizations are becoming a dominant entity. This globalization fosters interdependency that pushes the boundaries, using systems thinking and collaboration between individuals and groups. Lipman-Blumen (1996) described this new model of leadership as "connective leadership" emphasizing connecting, entrusting and empowering rather than controlling, directing or competing. She promotes establishing alliances, cultivating relationships, looking for new opportunities, and the use of a business approach that builds cultures, networks, information, and intellectual exchanges intended to get the real work of patient care accomplished. Successful health care organizations are learning to adopt this business mentality by creating a paradigm shift to total quality management.

Total quality management is an industrial model developed in the United States and successfully implemented in Japan following World War II; the writings of gurus—Deming, Juran, Crosby, Shewhart, Donabedian, Peters, and others—have received great attention. The TQM philosophy provides a managerial approach encompassing meeting the customers' requirements, error-free performance (doing it

right the first time), and the concept of continuous quality improvement (CQI) (known in Japan as **kaizen**—doing things better, little by little, all the time) using a series of problem solving tools and techniques related to statistical process control.

Traditionally, quality assurance/assessment has been perceived as a fragmented, oversight mechanism to enhance public accountability through various monitoring and evaluation reviews. While quality improvement and quality assurance/assessment are **not** synonymous, they do have a symbiotic relationship. Continuous and relentless improvement is based on assessing (1) structure, including the competence of professionals practicing in a resource-relevant culture, (2) process—the activities and behaviors (composite performance of key functions) employed, based on current knowledge; and (3) acceptable clinical and administrative outcomes. Building on a comprehensive, integrated, and coordinated quality improvement program, CQI acknowledges the humanity and complexity of health care organizations. CQI consists of a wide array of clinical, managerial, and organizational activities designed to remove waste and unpredictability, and to achieve previously unprecedented levels of performance. Outcomes are measured in terms of the needs and expectations of customers—that is, whoever is the recipient of the processes. TQM, embedded in the corporate culture, becomes a way of life; it provides an increasingly understood common language and set of tools. Cutting-edge systems are leveraging TQM and CQI into a force for strategic planning and reengineering.

In the context of TQM/CQI, the quest for quality is a challenging journey beginning with awareness and a commitment. The second edition of *Improving Quality: A Guide to Effective Programs* has been redesigned and enhanced to provide readers an opportunity to assess their understanding of quality care processes and to review their existing QI programs using TQM/CQI principles and practices to meet their organization's internal, professional accountabilities and the external needs and expectations of accrediting and licensing groups and various purchasers of services. Appropriate audiences include all health professionals committed to improving quality of care: boards of directors and administrators responsible for policy development and creating supportive environments in which continuous improvement is a way of life; practitioners seeking to blend their professional models with business models of practice; quality improvement directors responsible for coordinating and facilitating assessment and evaluation activities; resource management departments and continuing education persons responsible for education and training of employees and members of the community; faculty of both undergraduate and graduate programs responsible for teaching the tenets of quality, the techniques necessary for developing and monitoring practice guidelines, tracking outcomes, and the strategies for integrating risk management, utilization review and quality improvement; researchers concerned with accurate, valid, and reliable data to support changing practice; and consultants wishing to assist in reviewing and developing educational processes in organizations.

The content for this book is organized to allow multiple entry points. Depending on the reader's interest or concerns, an individual chapter or chapters will provide the information needed, using practical examples of quality improvement plans, forms, tools, and techniques to continuously improve quality. *Improving Quality: A Guide to Effective Programs* is divided into 5 parts.

Part I: Understanding the Foundation for Quality Improvement

- Chapter 1: "Lessons From the Past: Vision for the Future of Quality Care" documents the historical origins and evolution of quality assurance; knowing one's origins allows for the transformation to the present and planning for the future.
- Creating an environment in which the transition to a TQM/CQI system, reflected

not only in vision or mission statements, but also in behaviors, is described in Chapter 2: "Quality Outcomes Management: Executive Role Imperative." Applying the leadership role in managing quality outcomes using a Plan-Do-Check-Act framework details an effective model for improving performance.

Part II: Quality Improvement Process: Components of a Program

Total Quality Management (TQM), considered a corporate initiative, must be customer-driven from the top down, with a strategic plan reflecting an emphasis on quality with appropriate resource allocation. Part II: Chapters 3 through 7 will guide readers through the structuring of a Quality Improvement program.

- Because standards are dynamic due to changing social values, resources, rampant changes in technology, and research enhancing current knowledge regarding effectiveness of treatments and procedures, standards chosen to improve performance must include professional standards and external accrediting and regulatory requirements. Chapter 3: "Standards: The Basis of a Quality Improvement Program" provides an overview of various standards; Chapters in Part V will discuss standards applicable to various clinical sites.
- Because extant quality systems are at different levels of evolution, Chapter 4: "Building a Quality Improvement Program around Patient Care" is extremely useful in providing readers tools to assess an organization's readiness to change and exhibits to facilitate the transition.
- In the short term, organizations may assess measures that make them look good; as indicator selection becomes more sophisticated, using such classifications as functional status and clinical performance, Chapter 5: "Selecting Quality Initiatives and Methodologies" will prove helpful to readers as they need to develop relevant and useful indicators and appropriate data

collection methodologies. Asking the right questions in the right manner is key to collecting valid and reliable data.

- Converting data to information, presenting clear and concise reports with creative visual methods, and developing reporting mechanisms that ensure confidentiality of sensitive data (e.g., report cards), are the major foci of Chapter 6: "Communicating Quality Outcomes."
- The final step before the process can repeat itself is evaluation, that is, measuring the effectiveness of the quality improvement program, the actual impact on the system and patient care, and the resultant professional and organizational changes. Managing the change process, as discussed in Chapter 7: "Evaluating Quality Improvement: Effectiveness and Cost," will increase productivity and an organization's competitive edge in the marketplace.

Part III: Processes Integral to Improving Quality

- Relationships are at the heart of every service organization. Only by exceeding expectations and providing value added services will health care organizations achieve accountability to patients (customers, consumers). As partners, patients know whether symptoms are relieved, if quality of life has been extended, if functional health status is restored, and whether they have been treated with compassion and courtesy. Chapter 8: "The Customer: Perspectives and Expectations of Quality," describes the customer-supplier relationship and a variety of forces impacting consumer satisfaction surveys—a major source of critical data.
- Historically, quality assurance/assessment, risk management, and utilization review have been perceived as separate functions, with different individuals or departments responsible for monitoring the various activities. Chapter 9: "Integrating Risk Management, Utilization Management,

and Quality Management: Maximizing Benefit through Integration" identifies opportunities to integrate numerous clinical and administrative functions to benefit patient care.

- While federal and state legislative mandates are proliferating, it must be noted that, when based on political motivation, they diminish the importance of clinical scientific judgment as the basis for quality patient care. As a litigious society with sophisticated consumers, the potential for professional liability and malpractice has increased due to decreased lengths of stay, increased acuity levels, inadequate training and shortage of experienced workers in some practice sites (home care, long-term care), stricter reimbursement policies by payors, managed care, etc. A new chapter, Chapter 10: "Legal Implications Inherent in Improving Quality," addresses standards of care and standards of practice used to determine negligence or malpractice and various laws applicable to quality care.
- Aside from private and public insurance issues, a number of medical ethics issues have arisen, such as organ transplantation, physician-assisted suicide, rationing, and scarce resources. Another new chapter, Chapter 11: "Improving Quality Care: An Ethical Imperative in a Time of Change," describes the relationship between quality improvement and bioethics, and provides readers with tools to assess an organization's readiness to develop a bioethics committee to oversee various points of debate.
- Chapter 12: "Linking Quality Improvement, Outcome Research, and Program Evaluation" will be of interest to faculty in educational institutions, as well as professionals in clinical agencies; appreciating the processes as analogous, but distinct, in application to patient care is important, as data is generated with differing methodologies intended to improve patient care.

- Our capacity to improve care is directly related to our ability to gather comprehensive, valid, reliable, and timely data, and interpret and use it appropriately. The sheer amount of data collected in the process of meeting economic, social, and political demands for accountability have made the automation of quality and resource management imperative. Guidelines for choosing an integrated quality information system that manages data on suppliers (vendors), key process characteristics, outcomes of care, cost elements, and satisfaction of patients/families, payers, employees, physicians, and community organizations are provided in Chapter 13: "Basic Tools for a Quality Improvement-Based Approach to Information System Selection and Implementation."
- Chapter 14: "Managing Quality Through Outcome-Based Practice: CareMaps, Case Management and Variance Analysis," is a new and critical addition to this book. The author has described the development of a variance management system as well as CareMaps and Case Management as collaborative strategies for achieving positive patient oucomes in a cost-effective manner.

Part IV: Developing the Professional to Manage Quality

The transition to a TQM/CQI system, reflected not only in mission statements but also in behaviors, will take several years as organizations actively work toward creating employee commitment to continuously strive to improve services while meeting customers' needs. Education and retraining, destroying barriers between groups, and instituting pride of workmanship and ownership, eliminating numerical quotas and exhortations, and ending the practice of awarding business on price tag alone take time and effort, as they require individuals to change their value systems. Part IV was designed to address the human resources imperative to implement successful quality improvement programs.

The reality of our health care situation is that TQM/CQI and the professional model must work in concert if the quality of health care is to improve. The highly trained professional assimilates the flood of technical information that medical research has developed; thus, paradoxically, multidisciplinary or cross-functional "team" participation may be perceived as a threat to professional autonomy while at the same time contributing to individual and group autonomy. Integrated quality programs will always require professional clinical judgment as well as the consumer's perception of care, some areas of which may not be precisely quantifiable. Orchestrating the independent actions of professionals and project-oriented teams, managers' current leadership roles at the top, middle, and bottom of the hierarchy will alter as they model, teach, facilitate, and empower teams to collect, analyze, and solve problems impacting them.

- Chapter 15: "Quality Improvement Teams and Teamwork" and Chapter 16: "Using Statistical Process Control Tools in the Quality Process," are two new chapters addressing the development of "teams" and a variety of statistical process control (SPC) tools to facilitate a team's decision-making process.
- Chapter 17: "Preparing the Undergraduate Student and Faculty to Use Quality Improvement in Practice" and Chapter 18: "Graduate Preparation for Managing Quality in Practice in the 21st Century" were written by experts in universities and clinical practice to assist faculty, staff development, and continuing education programmers to provide students with theoretical content regarding quality and involve them in meaningful, "real-world" experiences to instill the value of that accountability by assessing and continually improving performance is part of professional practice.
- Chapter 19: "A Continuous Quality Improvement Program: Developing the Em-

ployee" describes an educational program provided for all employees in a long-term care facility, the successes and the lessons learned.

Part V: Applying Quality Improvement in Various Clinical Settings

As patients have been moving across settings of care with increasing rapidity, the locus of post-acute care has shifted earlier and earlier to other settings including rehabilitation, subacute, and long-term care facilities and into the patient's home. Although there is no widespread evidence (only anecdotal reports) that these shifts have adversely affected patients, many observers have voiced concern that such transitions can disrupt continuity of care and result in quality problems. Patients frequently report that the time of discharge from the hospital is fraught with anxiety, faulty communication, and uncertainty about what will happen next.

Thirteen clinical settings (seven new settings and six extensively revised and expanded settings in this second edition) have been provided for readers working in Ambulatory Care; Home Care; Home Medical Equipment: Home Oxygen and Durable Medical Equipment; Hospice; Integrated Health Care Systems; Long-term care; Managed Care: An HMO example; Natural and Alternative Therapies; Psychiatry; Public Health; Rehabilitation; Subacute Care, and Partnerships between Integrated Systems and the Community, describing a shift from an integrated system's needs and expectations for providing quality care to establishing priorities based on a communities' health care needs and expectations.

Creating a new program or assessing an existing one is an easier process when materials can be reviewed in light of what others have experienced and produced; reinventing the wheel is senseless when experts can share their experiences, successes and lessons learned. Chapters 20 through 32 provide descriptions of applicable standards, quality improvement plans,

examples of key indicators, tools and techniques used to measure quality performance, evaluation plans, and consumer satisfaction measurements.

Speaking the same language is critical for TQM/CQI to succeed. Recognizing that an extensive, common lexicon for words and concepts related to quality does not exist, a **glossary** has been included. Readers will find selected **quality-related references** to enhance their understanding of quality and selected **quality-related Internet sites** in the Bibliography.

The United States health care industry faces the greatest need for change in several decades. As the next millennium rapidly approaches, the way we view and achieve health care will determine the survival or demise of the industry. The organization's vision of quality and the transformational leaders championing the changes that must occur in their people, culture, and resources are creating a paradigm shift. This shift is characterized by mutuality and affiliation, collaboration with multifunctional activity, and multidisciplinary teams. Learning organizations foster creativity, innovation, risk-taking, and the empowerment and self-governance of all employees so that services can be integrated along the full continuum of care, an "authentic health care system" that ensures the best outcomes for the patient.

Building a quality improvement program around the delivery of patient care means continually improving methods of assessment to meet and exceed the needs and desires of both internal and external customers. Providing compassionate, high-quality and cost-effective health care that incorporates patients' preferences in shared decision-making processes is key to success. Whether patients have a right *or* a shared right *and* a responsibility to health care is still a matter of public debate; they do, however, have a right to high quality care provided by competent practitioners.

Claire Gavin Meisenheimer

REFERENCES

————. 1997 Health Care Industry Outlook, *Healthcare Trends Report, 11*(1), 15.

Lipman-Blumen, J. (1996). *The connective edge*. San Francisco: Jossey-Bass.

## PART I

Understanding the Foundation for Quality Improvement

## CHAPTER 1

Lessons from the Past: Vision for the Future of Quality Care

Margaret J. Bull

CHAPTER OBJECTIVES

After completing this chapter, the reader will be able to

- describe significant historical events that have contributed to improving quality
- identify major forces influencing quality in the health care system
- detail the quality journey through the emphasis on structure, process, and outcomes indicators
- relate the interrelationship of cost to quality of care

What is quality care? The response depends on who is asking, and on whose perspective is considered: Professionals'? Payers'? Patients'? In a general sense, *quality* refers to the degree of excellence a thing possesses. Various forces influence quality care and quality improvement efforts (Figure 1–1). Although the role of these forces has fluctuated throughout history, professional accountability has played a persistent role as providers continue to care for consumers by continually improving access to, and quality of, services and programs in a cost-effective and efficient manner.

Excellence in health care has been viewed and measured in different ways. Quality has been measured in terms of structure criteria (what goes into care delivery), such as educational preparation of staff and nursing care hours; or as process, or those care-providing activities performed by health care professionals; and outcome criteria, usually changes in the client's health (American Nurses Association [ANA], 1976). However, more recently, outcomes have included the benefits for hospitals and other health care organizations. The shifting emphases on structure, process, and outcome at different points in our history provide lessons on the value of each approach and allow us to use the knowledge gained to create future directions for quality care.

EARLY EFFORTS TO IMPROVE CARE

In Great Britain, from 1854 to 1870, the impetus for systematic evaluation was primarily professional, and the focus included both client outcome and the process of care. During the Crimean War, Florence Nightingale kept statistics on the mortality of British soldiers. Nightingale conducted studies describing the quality of hospital care available to the British army during the war. She used the number of hospital deaths per diagnostic category to describe the unsafe conditions and argued that improvements in sanitation would reduce fatalities and improve outcomes. When Nightingale and her nurses arrived at the Barrack Hospital in 1854, the mortality rate was 32%. Six months after the nurses' arrival, the mortality rate dropped to approximately 2%, clearly demonstrating the effectiveness of nursing care (Nutting & Dock, 1907, p. 142). These accom-

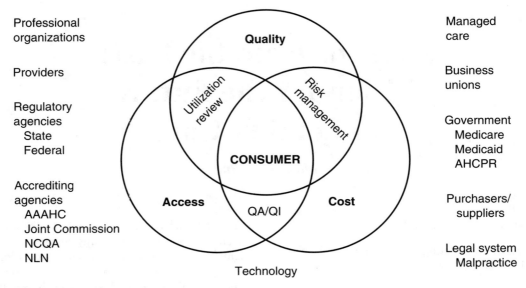

Figure 1–1 Major forces influencing quality in the health care system

plishments aroused public support for the nurses and interest in the care of sick people.

Nightingale also established what might be viewed as early process standards for nursing practice. In *Notes on Nursing* (1860, pp. 12–48), she stated that the first rule of good nursing was to keep the air the patient breathes as pure as the external air, without chilling the patient. In addition, she emphasized the importance of observing signs and symptoms of a change in the patient's condition and indicated that the nurse should always sit down when talking with patients to give them the nurse's complete attention.

In 1863, Nightingale proposed a system to relate the use of hospital beds to indicators of health to promote efficient and effective use of hospital beds. The information collected included the number of patients admitted to the hospital during the year; the number of patients who died in the hospital or who recovered and were discharged; and the number of patients discharged as incurable or unrelieved, or who left the hospital at their own request. From those data, specific medical and surgical treatments were correlated with diagnostic cate-

gories, and mortality rates were calculated (Brook & Avery, 1975, p. 3).

In 1908, Emory W. Groves, a British physician, continued the outcome approach. He surveyed 50 hospitals with more than 200 beds for patient mortality from surgical procedures and found that mortality ranged from 9% for appendectomies to 44% for procedures related to malignant diseases (Groves, 1908). Groves's study raised two points: (1) the need to develop an acceptable standard classification for diseases and operations that would permit comparisons of data from different hospitals and (2) the need to establish a follow-up system for particular categories of diseases, such as malignancies, that would allow assessment of long-term results (i.e., mortality, extent of symptoms, and level of disability).

In the United States, during the early 20th century, the public had a fatalistic view of health care. A poor outcome was not linked to practitioner capabilities or access to care but tended to be accepted as something beyond human control. During this period, health professionals provided the major impetus for quality assurance. The focus on client outcome that began in England continued, and, in addition, an emphasis on structure developed.

Furthermore, the early 20th century was characterized by social reform. Municipal reform usually emphasized efficiency and honest accounting in public administration; structural reforms included independent audits of city accounts. In the medical field, reform-minded physicians recognized the need for changes in medical education as early as 1876. However, the American Medical Association Council knew that instituting the desired educational reform required a new financing structure; a medical school would have to be supported by public or private funds rather than operated on a profit-making basis as in the past. Consequently, the professional association turned to a foundation for assistance. As a result, the Carnegie Foundation undertook a national survey of medical schools and published the results in the Flexnor Report of 1910, which condemned the standards of proprietary colleges, exposed several schools as diploma mills, and indicated that many physicians were poorly educated. As the new standards recommended in the Flexnor Report were instituted, many medical schools closed (Fee, 1982, pp. 286–287).

Also during this time, the first state nurses' associations organized to work for legislation mandating the registration of nurses. Concern for improving the educational base for nursing was linked to licensure efforts. State licensure laws addressed four areas of legal requirements: (1) preliminary education, (2) professional training, (3) licensing tests, and (4) registry. By 1912, 6 states required completion of high school, 4 states required 1 year of high school, 3 states required completion of grammar school, and 19 states had no regulation regarding education. Professional education requirements also varied considerably: 21 states required a 2-year course; 9 states, a 3-year course; and 2 states did not have any requirements. All states required a licensing examination; however, nurses registered in one state could obtain a waiver to practice in another state (Goodrich, 1912).

The focus on structure standards also was reflected in the 1912 criteria for community health nurses developed by the Joint Committee for Consideration of the Standardization of Visiting Nurses. These first standards were that a nurse be a graduate of a recognized general hospital of not fewer than 50 beds and have at least 2 years of training, with a course in obstetrics; and that a nurse applying from a state "where state regulation pertains" must be a graduate of a hospital acceptable to the state board registration (Wald, 1912). The intent of nurses and physicians in establishing structure standards was to protect the public from unsafe practitioners.

In addition to the focus on structure, this era saw the proposal of a patient follow-up system that emphasized outcome-oriented medical audits. Dr. Ernest Codman (1914), a surgeon at Massachusetts General Hospital in Boston, recommended that each patient be examined 1 year after surgery to determine whether the operation had alleviated symptoms. His efforts led to the creation of the American College of Surgeons' Hospital Standardization Program in 1918. This program included the use of standards, hospital visitation and evaluation, and the granting of accreditation for recognized compliance with standards. Later, the patterns from this program were adopted by the Joint Commission for the Accreditation of Hospitals (renamed the Joint Commission on Accreditation of Healthcare Organizations in the 1990s).

A key lesson from early efforts to improve care was that nursing care improved outcomes for the British soldiers. Equally important was the lesson that professional achievements in improving client outcomes generated public support that advanced the work of the nurses.

1920–1940: LULL IN THE QUALITY EMPHASIS

Little substantive work in the area of quality assurance occurred from 1920 to 1940. The reasons are unclear. However, one might speculate that the public was engrossed in recovery from World War I during the 1920s and occupied with the collapse of the economy in the 1930s. In terms of health care, the period was marked by attempts to increase access to health care for all income groups. During the 1930s, several bills proposing national health insurance programs were introduced in Congress. In addition, some states introduced legislation, such as the Biemiller bills in Wisconsin, which advocated compulsory health insurance. However, compulsory health insurance was not enacted; instead, voluntary health insurance programs emerged (Kingsbury, 1939, pp. 151–153).

One evaluation study, conducted during the late 1920s by the Committee on the Grading of Nursing Schools, focused on labor needs in nursing, patient satisfaction with nursing care, and physician satisfaction with nurses and nursing care. The findings of the study indicated a need for more graduate nurses in hospitals and for nurses with preparation in community health (Burgess, 1928, pp. 112–113). The committee found that 90% of the 23,500 physicians in the sample were satisfied with the nurses and the care given their patients (Burgess, 1928, pp. 121–122). The physicians in the sample wanted nurses to meet the following criteria: possess skill in giving general care and making patients comfortable, possess skill in observing and reporting symptoms, exercise care in following medical orders, and have an attractive personality and "good breeding" (Burgess, 1928, pp. 151–152).

The study also found that 86% of the patients were satisfied with their care and would have liked the same nurse again. The patients felt the most difficult problem was to get the "right" nurse and cited the following qualities of good nursing: adaptability, patience, gentleness, and loyalty to the family and the physician. Patient dissatisfaction with nursing care focused on hospital nursing and included some of the following complaints: being awakened at 5 AM or 6 AM for early morning care (patients stated sick people need all the rest they can get); having shortages of nurses to care for their needs; being given dirty bedpans; and having nurses unreceptive to suggestions from the patients regarding their care (Burgess, 1928, pp. 204–229).

Although quality improvement was not stressed during this period, two critical lessons were apparent. First, patients and health care professionals had somewhat different perspectives on what constituted quality care. Second, patients did not perceive the health care delivery system as organized to meet their needs. Although nursing provided leadership in obtaining the data on patients' perspectives, there was little evidence of any action taken to incorporate these perspectives into standards of care or to modify delivery systems to be more responsive to patients' needs for rest.

1940–1960: EMPHASIS ON PROCESS AND STRUCTURE

When interest in assessing the quality of care resumed in the late 1940s and 1950s, the emphasis was on process and structure rather than outcome. This change in focus may have been related to practicality and accessibility of information regarding structure and process. Also, during this period, the public developed greater interest in the organization, planning, and evaluation of health services. The increased level of education of the public and the emphasis on goal-directed planning by business probably contributed to consumer interest in health services and the demands for accessibility to health care. This led to the Hill-Burton Act of 1946, which provided funds for the expansion of hospitals.

A few years later, in 1952, the Joint Commission on Accreditation of Hospitals was formed as an outgrowth of the Clinical Congress of Surgeons (Woody, 1976, p. 23). The criteria developed by the Joint Commission illustrate the emphasis on structure standards. For instance, hospitals were required to post signs in areas where oxygen was used. It was assumed that meeting those standards would automatically result in high-quality care.

Also during the 1950s, three landmark studies involving medical care were published. Each of these studies focused on the process of care; however, each used a different method. Dr. O.L. Peterson studied the quality of care delivered by general practitioners while they were providing care. He scored their practice on the basis of adequacy of the history, physical exam, therapy, and amount of follow-up care. A few years later, Dr. M.A. Morehead studied the quality of ambulatory care provided in the Health Insurance Plan, a prepaid group practice in New York. He relied on physicians' judgments on the process of care, talked with the physicians, and reviewed the medical record. Dr. B.C. Payne studied the care given in a select group of short-term general hospitals in Michigan by comparing the information contained in the medical record against a set of disease-specific criteria established by a group of physicians. All three found major deficiencies in care (Brook & Avery, 1975, p. 6).

Nursing studies during the 1950s described the process of nursing care. Several studies by psychiatric nurses centered on nurse–patient interaction and proposed methods of securing data for the analysis of nurse–patient interaction. For example, Wandelt (1954) studied planned instruction versus incidental instruction of hospitalized patients with tuberculosis and found that patients who received planned instruction had a better understanding of their disease. In addition, nurses proceeded with the development of structure standards. For instance, in 1959, the ANA published its *Functions, Standards and Qualifications for Practice* and the National League for Nursing (NLN) published *What People Can Expect of a Modern Nursing Service.*

Lessons from this period suggested that a variety of approaches might be used to measure the process of care delivery. Although direct observation, record audits, and interviews were three approaches evident in the studies of this period, there was little discussion of the benefits of one approach versus another. Also, Morehead's study provided an early example of triangulating methods (using both interview and medical chart audit) to evaluate the quality of care.

1960s: BEYOND PROCESS

As the 1960s evolved, the public developed greater expectations of health care. The decade was marked by concern for consumer protection, human rights, and the concept of health care as a right. Also, the federal government became involved in financing health care through the enactment of Medicare and Medicaid, and with that involvement came government regulations regarding the cost and quality of services. The Social Security Amendment of 1965, which enacted Medicare and Medicaid, provided funds for medical care of the aged and low-income populations. The legislation flowed from current views of health care as an individual's right, and it brought government regulation, particularly structure standards, to nursing homes and acute-care settings.

Medicare and Medicaid were closely followed by the Comprehensive Health Planning Act of 1966, which attempted to tie spending to better planning and to establish priorities for federal and state funding. The Regional Medical Program Act of 1966 represented an attempt to merge two goals: the promotion of scientific research and the development of improved service in the application of knowledge. This act provided funds for scientific research, and implementation occurred at the state level (Taft & Levine, 1977, pp. 36–41).

Dr. John Hirschboeck, executive director of the Wisconsin Regional Medical Program, called an invitational meeting that included nurses less than 1 month after the formal organization of that program in 1976. Within 1 year, this group formally appointed a nursing committee to define the needs of nursing in Wisconsin (Hinsvark, 1976, pp. 2–4). The nursing committee laid the groundwork for quality assurance activities in the decade that followed. One of the goals of the committee was to improve the delivery of nursing services to patients, families, and the community. The committee did not limit its efforts to Wisconsin but held a national workshop for nurses involved in regional medical programs. From 1969 to 1974, quality assurance studies such as Nurse Utilization, conducted by Janet Kraegel, Patient Health Outcome by Nurse Peer, conducted by Marie Zimmer, and Film Script for Quality Assurance, developed by J. Lund, were among the nursing projects funded by the Wisconsin program (Hinsvark, 1976, p. 14).

In the professional sector, nursing focused primarily on the methods of assessing process. A well-known process audit developed by Maria Phaneuf (1964, 1972) was based on the seven functions of nursing defined by Lesnik and Anderson (1955). Another process audit developed by Eleanor Lambertsen (1965) consisted of six basic standards with substandards. The evidence required for each substandard varied from service to service. This system allowed nurses who provided the care on different services to develop their own measurements.

Although the primary focus of quality improvement during the 1960s was on process, elements of structure persisted in the Joint Commission requirements. A study conducted by Myrtle Aydelotte and Marie Tener (1960, pp. 47–76), *An Investigation of the Relation between Nursing Activity and Patient Welfare*, represented an early attempt to link structure, process, and outcome. The study included the following measures: number of professional nursing care hours; length of hospital stay; number of fever days patients experienced; number of postoperative days; administration pattern for analgesic, narcotic, and sedative use; and scaled measures of patients' physical and mental status. The results indicated that the relationship between nursing activity and patient outcome was not statistically significant. In the medical sector, Avedis Donabedian (1966) described the difference between structure, process, and outcomes and urged the development of criteria for evaluating outcomes. Thus the importance of giving simultaneous attention to structure, process, and outcome criteria was a key lesson from this period, and it set the stage for the focus in the decade that followed.

1970s: PERIOD OF RAPID GROWTH

During the 1970s, a number of forces contributed to the growth of quality improvement. Specifically, the public's increased concern about inflation and rising health care costs led to greater interest in professional accountability. Also, a combination of concerns about cost and legislation prompted consumer involvement in health planning. At the same time, government and other third-party payers' concerns about health care rising costs led to a number of proposals for national health insurance. None of the proposals was enacted; however, they did stimulate discussions of cost and quality.

Continued concern for rising costs resulted in the passage of two bills. First, in 1972, the Bennett Amendment established professional standards review organizations (PSROs; Office of Professional Standards Review, 1974, p. 1). This legislation was strongly physician oriented. Under this law, the medical care delivered to people in federally financed programs was reviewed. The law provided for medical care evaluation, continued stay review, and admissions certification. However, only services rendered in a hospital or nursing home were subject to review. Reactions to PSROs were mixed: A number of established interests felt threatened and many physicians viewed PSROs as a government attempt to control their livelihood; hospital administrators were placed in the position of bystander because they were not guaranteed a seat at the PSRO table even though hospitals were responsible for absorbing the economic impact of PSROs. The Joint Commission viewed PSROs as a competitor—after all, PSROs might eliminate the need for the Joint Commission (Kinzer,

1976, pp. 106–113). Such reactions from special interest groups hindered the implementation of PSROs.

Although nursing was not specifically mentioned in the PSRO legislation, the government in 1974 awarded a contract to the ANA to develop model sets of screening criteria to measure the quality and effectiveness of nursing care and also to formulate guidelines for the involvement of nurses in review processes and in PSROs (Lang, 1976). However, it was not until 1982 that a nurse, Norma Lang, was appointed to the board of the National Professional Standards Review Council ("Norma Lang Named," 1982, p. 32).

The second bill, the National Health Planning and Resource Development Act of 1974 (P.L. 93-641), was an attempt to correct the maldistribution of health care facilities and labor. The intent of the law was to enable decision making about the allocation and development of health resources to be free from provider control. The law created health systems agencies to develop ways to improve the delivery of health care; however, the health system agencies were not granted any power or authority to carry out their mission. Professional forces continued to be active in the 1970s. Early in the decade, the ANA developed standards of practice that emphasized both structure and process. Standards for specialty groups such as maternal–child health, community health, and oncology followed. The ANA (1976, p. 18) also adopted a model to guide quality improvement efforts. The purpose of the model was to assist individual nurses and groups of nurses in the implementation of programs to ensure quality nursing care. The model can be used to evaluate nurse performance, patient care, or an organizational setting. As illustrated in Figure 1–2, the components of the model include

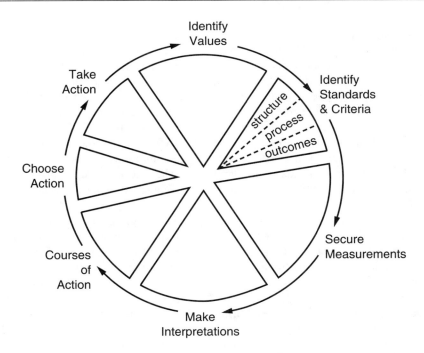

Figure 1–2 Quality Assurance Model. *Source:* Reprinted with permission from *American Nurses Association Quality Care Assurance Workbook*, ©1976, American Nurses Association.

- identifying values, because societal, professional, and scientific values will determine standards
- identifying structure, process, and outcome standards and criteria
- securing measurements needed to determine the degree of attainment of standards and criteria
- making interpretations about the strengths and weaknesses of nursing practice based on the measurement results
- identifying alternative courses of action
- deciding on a course of action
- taking action

One of the strengths of the model is that it allows for the use of structure, process, and outcome methods in assessing and improving the quality of care. The circular path of the arrows denotes that quality improvement is an ongoing process. The model also encourages nurses to focus on patient outcomes and the relationship between structure, process, and outcomes.

The literature on quality improvement increased rapidly during the 1970s. However, there were three times as many discussion articles as studies of quality care (Oliver, 1979, pp. 34–36). Some articles described the development of process tools; others described outcome criteria for specific patient populations based on medical diagnosis or populations at risk. One of the outcome criteria sets developed by Marie Zimmer, Norma Lang, and Doris Miller through the Wisconsin Regional Medical Program included outcomes for patients with essential hypertension, normal first pregnancy, psychogenic depression, chronic obstructive pulmonary disease, cerebral vascular accident in nursing home setting, and immobilization due to low back pain (Zimmer, Lang, & Miller, 1974, pp. 11–12).

Two process tools were developed during this period: the Slater Nursing Competencies Rating Scale, which measured competencies displayed by nurses, and the Quality Patient Care Scale, which measured the quality of

nursing care received by a patient while care is ongoing (Wandelt & Ager, 1974; Wandelt & Stewart, 1975). In addition, the Medicus Systems Corporation outlined an evaluation system focusing on outcomes of care (Jelinek, Haussman, Hegevary, & Newman, 1974, pp. 4–15). In this system, desired patient outcomes are identified. Then nursing processes or strategies are developed to produce the desired outcome. Another method focusing on outcomes was introduced by the Joint Commission in the form of the Peer Evaluation Program Primer (Jacobs & Jacobs, 1974), a methodology that included a retrospective process audit that could be used if the outcome audit identified a particular nursing care problem. Quality of professional services was added to the Joint Commission manual in 1976, and, in 1979, quality assurance was announced as a mandatory Joint Commission standard for 1981.

Also during the 1970s, the American Public Health Association surveyed public health agencies about their quality improvement activities (Januska, Engle, & Wood, 1976). They found that supervisory and record audits were the most common methods of assessing the quality of care. Few agencies reported the use of outcomes. Continued emphasis on structure standards was evident during this time in the development of criteria for clinical practice certification and the NLN criteria for accrediting community health nursing services (1980).

The National Conference Group on Nursing Diagnosis stimulated further developments in quality improvement. The work of the group in identifying, developing, and classifying nursing diagnoses provided an important approach for identifying patient populations for quality improvement studies. From its inception in 1973, the group maintained a liaison with the ANA Congress on Nursing Practice to facilitate information exchange. The Congress on Nursing Practice was interested in quality improvement issues such as the implementation of practice standards, nursing process, and the development of outcomes based on a classification scheme (Gordon, 1982, pp. 2–5). The fruits of this liaison became evident in the quality improvement studies of the 1980s.

Clearly a number of factors related to legislation, professional accountability, consumer demands, and health care reimbursement combined to influence the rapid growth of quality improvement efforts during these years. The lessons from the 1970s produced a number of tools to measure the quality of care. Many of these instruments were used in the decades that followed. The 1970s also was a decade of renewed emphasis on patient outcomes.

1980s: EMPHASIS ON COSTS OF CARE

The advent of the 1980s witnessed a change in values, technology, and the challenges faced by people concerned with the quality of care. Concerns about rising health care costs superseded quality of care issues. Cost-containment efforts dominated health care delivery in the 1980s. The government responded by evaluating the impact of legislation enacted in the previous decade. The PSROs were created to curtail costs as well as monitor quality, yet, a decade later, the escalation of health care costs continued. Therefore, PSROs faced budget cuts and extinction. In a similar manner, the effectiveness of health systems agencies was reviewed. The intent of the legislation that created health systems agencies was to correct the maldistribution of health care facilities and labor. However, the maldistribution persisted, and health system agencies were also faced with budget cuts and the possibility of extinction.

In another attempt to curtail health care costs, Congress enacted the Tax Equity and Fiscal Responsibility Act of 1982 (TEFRA). This act placed a ceiling on Medicare reimbursement for hospital services and set the stage for the competitive approach evident in the 1983 Social Security amendments, which mandated a prospective reimbursement system based on diagnosis-related groups (DRGs) for Medicare recipients. The objectives of the prospective payment legislation were to restructure economic incentives for hospitals, establishing marketlike forces; link payment to diagnosis, basing payment on a system that was believed to more accurately identify the product being purchased for Medicare recipients; establish the federal government as a prudent buyer of services; and restrain the rate of hospital cost increase and therefore moderate the outflow from the Medicare trust funds ("Medicare Program," 1984). Under the prospective payment system, hospitals were paid a predetermined rate for each case within a given DRG, regardless of the length of stay. However, DRGs did not address differences in the need for professional nursing care that can exist among patients with the same medical diagnosis.

In addition to mandating prospective payment, the 1983 Social Security amendments specified rules for implementing professional review organizations (PROs) by October 1984. The intent was to replace PSROs. The new rules required that the 1980 PSRO areas currently in existence be consolidated into designated state and territory areas. PROs differ from the PSROs in several respects. First, PROs oversee either for-profit or nonprofit organizations. Second, PROs either include physicians or have access to them; PSROs were required to include at least 25% of the physicians in the PSRO area in their membership. Third, PROs define their operational objectives; PSROs were not required to do so. Fourth, PROs were required to consult with nurses and other nonphysician health care providers with respect to the responsibilities of the PROs for the review of nurses' (and other health care providers') professional activities ("PRO Regulations," 1984). Furthermore, hospitals were required to contract with PROs, or a PSRO that had a PRO contract, for utilization review. If the PRO found that a hospital had questionable admission patterns, corrective action could be taken. The action might range from a more intensive review of hospital admissions and physician cases to punitive steps, such as monetary fines imposed on the hospital or physician ("Federal Health Insurance," 1983).

Also during the 1980s, the Joint Commission implemented new standards that required the integration and coordination of quality assurance activities into a hospitalwide program that was comprehensive in nature and focused on problems relating to patient care. During the latter part of the decade, the Joint Commission began compiling state and national averages to demonstrate how the health care industry complied with accreditation standards. Preliminary reports indicated that 27.8% of hospitals had difficulty meeting the standard that required a systematic process for monitoring and evaluating patient care; 56% of the hospitals lacked adequate procedures for measuring quality of medical care ("New JCAHO Data," 1990).

Although the 1980s were characterized by cost containment, the latter part of the decade witnessed a resurgence of issues relating to quality of health care. Questions were raised whether the measures of quality selected for acute care were applicable to long-term care, and whether quality of care differs for different cohorts (Kane & Kane, 1988). Also, the belief that cost containment automatically led to decreased quality was dispelled by the diffusion of the business philosophy espoused by Crosby, Deming, and Juran to health care organizations. Each of the three business leaders suggested slightly different ways to achieve quality in an organization, but they agreed that a management systems approach to quality improvement was essential in creating a culture of quality (Crosby, 1984; Deming, 1984; Juran, 1988). Belief in quality as a mechanism for organizational improvement continued into the 1990s.

A key lesson from the 1980s was that survival of hospitals and health organizations became an outcome, one that nearly superseded patient outcomes in importance. This lesson raised two questions: How does a focus on cost issues redefine quality of care? What happens to the patient in this type of environment?

1990s: COST AND QUALITY

Quality became the watchword of the 1990s. As part of its Agenda for Change, the Joint Commission on Accreditation of Hospitals changed its name to the Joint Commission on Accreditation of Healthcare Organizations, introduced the ten-step model for monitoring and evaluating, and emphasized the concept of continuous quality improvement. The Joint Commission's standard focused on total quality management and provided for input from the health care consumer in evaluating care (Joint Commission, 1992). The competitive health care environment of the 1980s provided an impetus for health care organizations to develop new marketing strategies; delivering high-quality services became one mechanism for an organization to distinguish its services from those of its competitors. In addition, the new philosophy proposed by Deming (1984) postulated that gains in quality attract new users and result in gains in efficiency and productivity, which translate into lower costs. Ensuring quality in the process of delivering health care is cost-effective. Deming's and Crosby's (1984) strategies for quality improvement were based on the premise that an organization's quality problems reside predominantly in its systems, not in its people. Consequently, quality improvement necessitated an organizational culture committed to quality. Using these strategies in health care calls for a commitment to an interdisciplinary approach to quality improvement because of the different professionals, paraprofessionals, and vendors involved in the delivery of services.

The focus on outcomes continued in the 1990s with an emphasis on relating costs to outcomes of care (Crosby, 1984; Deming, 1984). This period witnessed renewed interest in identifying and conducting clinical research related to client outcomes (Lang, Kraegel, Rantz, & Krejci, 1990). Attempts were made to classify outcomes to achieve a standard framework for client data (Lang & Marek, 1990). Deming's systems approach and the need for classifying outcomes challenge health professionals to develop a classification system that can be used by all disciplines involved in delivering care, rather than to focus on outcomes for a single discipline.

Nursing studies also reflected the emphasis on outcomes. Martin and colleagues (1986, 1992) worked with the Visiting Nurse Association of Omaha, Nebraska, to develop a patient classification system for community health nursing. As part of the Omaha project, outcomes were classified in categories of knowledge, behavior, or status. Lalonde (1986) also studied outcomes for home health care. The outcomes measured in the project included general symptom distress, the taking of prescribed medications, discharge status, caregiver strain, functional status, physiologic indicators, and knowledge of the health problems. Later, quality indicator groups that incorporated both global and focused measures of outcome were developed for home care (Shaughnessy & Crisler, 1995). The global measures applied to all patients, whereas the focused measures pertained to a specific group of patients (e.g., those with pressure ulcers or chronic obstructive pulmonary disease).

Also during the 1990s, a number of efforts focused on developing instruments to measure the care provided. The Agency for Health Care Policy and Research funded 94 Medical Treatment Effectiveness Program research grants and contracts in fiscal year 1991 (Cummings, 1992). The Department of Health and Human Services (DHHS), Health Care Financing Administration, developed a Uniform Needs Assessment for Posthospital Care, whose intent was to evaluate patient needs for nursing home care, rehabilitation services, or home care following hospitalization (DHHS, 1992). Also during this period, Werley and Lang (1988) developed a nursing minimum data set to establish uniform standards for collecting essential nursing data. The essential nursing care elements in the nursing minimum data set included nursing diagnosis, interventions, outcomes, and intensity of nursing care.

The Agency for Health Care Policy and Research also emphasized the processes of care through its Office of the Forum for Quality and Effectiveness in Health Care. The primary responsibility of the forum was to facilitate the development, periodic review, and update of practice guidelines that assist practitioners in managing clinical conditions (DHHS, 1994). Between 1992 and 1994, a number of practice guidelines addressing such diverse conditions as acute pain, cancer pain, pressure ulcers, sickle cell disease, depression, and unstable angina were published.

Hospitals and home care organizations also emphasized process criteria in developing critical pathways and caremaps (Goodwin, 1992; Graybeal, Gheen, & McKenna, 1993). *Critical pathways* and caremaps define the timing and sequence of health professionals' activities for a specific procedure or diagnosis (Coffey, Othman, & Walters, 1995). The goal is to use resources efficiently. The focus of these efforts was primarily on standardizing practice or plans of care for specific populations. Few hospitals integrated patient outcomes in their plans or developed pathways that followed patients' postdischarge (Woodyard & Sheetz, 1993; Zander, 1992).

The development of practice guidelines might be viewed as one mechanism for defining the work process and ensuring quality care. However, implementation of practice guidelines presents a major challenge. Even with the same geographic area, hospitals and other health care organizations work within the confines of their own organization to develop guidelines. Sharing guidelines with other institutions often is impeded by the organization's need to maintain a competitive edge in the marketplace. Yet applying continuous quality improvement principles to health care generates an awareness that the provision of quality care demands going beyond integration and communication among providers on a particular unit or in a specific setting. Health care providers need to go beyond their institutional or organizational boundaries and work together to provide quality care across settings. Also, the issue of whether measures of quality used for acute-care clients apply to long-term care can be addressed more readily when providers collaborate across institutional boundaries.

A key lesson from the 1990s was that process, or the way in which care is delivered, is critical to quality and cost issues. Resources will continue to be limited, yet the challenge is to improve the efficiency of delivery while maintaining quality.

VISIONS FOR THE FUTURE

The reengineering and restructuring of health care organizations that occurred during the 1990s challenge health care professionals to provide quality care with fewer resources. Although managed care systems (i.e., systems of administration used to coordinate care providers and services) became popular during the 1990s, research about their effectiveness is scarce. Managed care environments with their focus on cost containment and, in some instances, the rationing of care, provide an impetus for a systematic examination of client outcomes. Given the limited resources, collaboration among members of the health care team will become increasingly important. Interdisciplinary approaches to patient care may predominate, particularly in meeting more complex health care needs. Quality improve-

ment efforts might focus on the effectiveness of the team in improving outcomes. Attention to mechanisms that facilitate continuity or seamless care, particularly for populations that require long-term care, will become increasingly important.

The survival of hospitals and health care organizations is an important outcome for health care providers within the institutions, and perhaps for society. However, the focus of professional practice has been the patient, and professional accountability mandates a focus on patient outcomes. As health care professionals enter into the 21st century, they will be called upon to reexamine their values and to justify their existence. In doing so, they can draw on the lessons learned from the past. History teaches us that nurses succeeded in improving patient outcomes, and this achievement resulted in public support for the nurses' work. In the future, health care professionals will need to become adept at marketing their successes and systematically documenting their achievements through clinical research. Partnerships with clients to produce desired outcomes are likely to benefit both patients and professionals. Key questions that health care professionals will need to address in planning actions are: What is the goal of health care for client populations? What can we do to facilitate achievement of the goal? What mechanisms will effectively disseminate our achievements to society?

REFERENCES

American Nurses Association. (1976). *Quality assurance workbook*. Kansas City, MO: American Nurses' Association.

Aydelotte, M., & Tener, M. (1960). *An investigation of the relation between nursing activity and patient welfare*. Ames, IA: State University of Iowa.

Brook, R., & Avery, A. (1975). *Quality assurance mechanisms in the United States: From there to where?* Santa Monica, CA: Rand.

Burgess, M.A. (1928). *Nurses, patients, and pocketbooks*. New York: Committee on the Grading at Nursing Schools.

Codman, E. (1914). The product of a hospital. *Surgical Gynecology and Obstetrics*, *18*, 491–494.

Coffey, R., Othman, J.E., & Walters, J. (1995). Extending the application of critical path methods. *Quality Management in Health Care*, *3*(2), 14–29.

Crosby, P. (1984). *Quality without tears: The art of hassle-free management*. New York: McGraw-Hill.

Cummings, M. (1992). Patient outcomes research—nursing, an important component. *Journal of Professional Nursing*, *8*(6), 318.

Deming, W.E. (1984). *Quality, productivity, and competitive position*. Cambridge, MA: Massachusetts Institute of Technology.

Donabedian, A. (1966). Evaluating the quality of medical care. *Milbank Memorial Fund Quarterly*, *44*, 194–196.

Federal health insurance for the aged and disabled. (1983). *Federal Register* 48, No. 171 (Sept. 1), 39807.

Fee, E. (1982). A historical perspective on quality assurance and cost containment. In J. Williamson & Assoc. (Eds.), *Teaching quality assurance and cost containment in health care* (pp. 286–287). San Francisco: Jossey-Bass.

Goodrich, A. (1912). A general presentation of the statutory requirements of the different states. *American Journal of Nursing, 12,* 1001–1005.

Goodwin, D.R. (1992). Critical pathways in home health care. *Journal of Nursing Administration, 22*(2), 35–40.

Gordon, M. (1982). Historical perspective: The national conference group for classification of nursing diagnoses. In M. Kim & D. Moritz (Eds.), *Classification of nursing diagnoses* (pp. 2–5). New York: McGraw-Hill.

Graybeal, K., Gheen, M., & McKenna, B. (1993). Clinical pathways development: The Overlake model. *Nursing Management, 24*(4), 42–45.

Groves, E. (1908). A plea for uniform registration of operation results. *British Journal of Medicine, 2,* 1008–1009.

Hinsvark, I. (1976). *And the winds of change blew: A report of the Nursing Committee of the Wisconsin Regional Medical Program.* Milwaukee, WI: Wisconsin Regional Medical Program.

Jacobs, N., & Jacobs, C. (1974). *The PEP primer.* Chicago: Joint Commission on Accreditation of Hospitals.

Januska, C., Engle, J., & Wood, J. (1976). *Status of quality assurance in public health nursing.* New York: American Public Health Association.

Jelinek, R., Haussman, R., Hegevary, S., & Newman, J. (1974). *A methodology for monitoring quality of nursing care.* Bethesda, MD: Department of Health, Education, and Welfare.

Joint Commission on Accreditation of Healthcare Organizations. (1992). *Manual for hospitals.* Chicago: The Joint Commission.

Juran, H. (1988). *Juran on planning for quality.* New York: Free Press.

Kane, R.A., & Kane, R.L. (1988). Long-term care: Variations on a quality assurance theme. *Inquiry, 25,* 132–146.

Kingsbury, J. (1939). *Health in handcuffs.* New York: Modern Age Books.

Kinzer, D. (1976). Inpatient quality assurance activities: Coordination of Federal, State, and private roles—the hospital's views. In R. Egdahl & P. Gertman (Eds.), *Quality assurance in health care* (pp. 106–113). Gaithersburg, MD: Aspen.

Lalonde, B. (1986). *Quality Assurance Manual for the Home Care Association of Washington.* Edmonds, WA: The Home Care Association of Washington.

Lambertsen, E. (1965). Evaluating the quality of nursing care. *Hospitals, 39,* 61–66.

Lang, N. (1976). Issues in quality assurance in nursing. In American Nurses' Association (Ed.), *Issues in evaluation research.* Kansas City, MO: American Nurses' Association.

Lang, N., Kraegel, J., Rantz, M., & Krejci, J. (1990). *Quality of health care for older people in America.* Kansas City, MO: American Nurses' Association.

Lang, N., & Marek, K. (1990). The classification of patient outcomes. *Journal of Professional Nursing, 6*(3), 158–163.

Lesnik, M.J., & Anderson, B.E. (1955). *Nursing practice and the law.* Philadelphia: J.B. Lippincott.

Martin, K., Scheet, N., & Crews, C. (1986). *Client management information system for community health nursing agencies: An implementation manual.* Rockville, MD: Division of Nursing, US DHHS, PHS, HRSA. (NTIS no. HRP-0907023).

Martin, K., & Scheet, N. (1992). *The Omaha system.* St. Louis, MO: Mosby.

Medicare program: Changes in the inpatient hospital prospective payment system. (1984). *Federal Register* (49, 27422).

National League for Nursing. (1980). *Criteria and standards manual for NLN/APHA accreditation of home health agencies and community nursing services* (No. 21-1306). New York: Author.

New JCAHO data spotlights quality problems. (1990). *American Journal of Nursing, 90,* 18.

Nightingale, Florence. (1860). *Notes on nursing: What it is and what it is not.* New York: Appleton.

Norma Lang Named to Standards Council, 1st Nurse Appointed. (1982). *American Nurse, 14*(4), 32.

Nutting, M.A., & Dock, L. (1907). *A history of nursing.* New York: G.P. Putnam's Sons.

Office of Professional Standards Review. (1974). *PSRO program manual.* Rockville, MD: Department of Health, Education, and Welfare.

Oliver, N.R. (1979). Diffusion of knowledge in a scientific community: The growth of quality assurance in nursing literature. Master's thesis, University of Wisconsin, Milwaukee.

Phaneuf, M. (1964). A nursing audit method. *Nursing Outlook, 12,* 67.

Phaneuf, M. (1972). *The nursing audit: Profile for excellence.* New York: Appleton-Century-Crofts.

PRO regulations issued by HCFA. (1984). *Capital Update, 2*(3), 7.

Shaughnessy, P., & Crisler, K. (1995). *Outcome-Based quality improvement.* Denver, CO: Colorado Center for Health Policy and Services Research.

Taft, C., & Levine, S. (1976). Problems of federal policies and strategies to influence the quality of health care. In R. Egdahl & P. Gertman (Eds.), *Quality assurance in health care* (pp. 36–41). Gaithersburg, MD: Aspen.

U.S. Department of Health and Human Services, Health Care Financing Administration. (1992). *Report of the Secretary's Advisory Panel on the Development of Uniform Needs Assessment Instrument(s)*. Washington, DC: U.S. Government Printing Office.

U.S. Department of Health and Human Services. (1994). *Unstable angina: Diagnosis and management*. (AHCPR Publication No. 94–0602). Rockville, MD: Author.

Wald, L. (1912). Report of the Joint Committee Appointed for Consideration of the Standardization of Visiting Nurses. *American Journal of Nursing, 12*, 894–897.

Wandelt, M. (1954). Planned versus incidental instruction for patients in tuberculosis therapy. *Nursing Research, 3*, 52–59.

Wandelt, M.A., & Ager, J. (1974). *Quality of patient care scale*. New York: Appleton-Century-Crofts.

Wandelt, M.A., & Stewart, D.S. (1975). *Slater nursing competencies rating scale*. New York: Appleton-Century-Crofts.

Werley, H.H., & Lang, N. (1988). The consensually derived nursing minimum data set: Elements and definitions. In H. Werley & N. Lang (Eds.), *Identification of the nursing minimum data set*. New York: Springer.

Woody, M. (1976). Where is nursing in quality assurance? In National League for Nursing (Ed.), *Quality assurance models for nursing education*. New York: National League for Nursing.

Woodyard, L., & Sheetz, J. (1993). Critical pathway patient outcomes: The missing standard. *Journal of Nursing Care Quality, 8*(1), 51–57.

Zander, K. (1992). Focusing on patient outcome: Case management in the 90s. *Dimensions of Critical Care Nursing, 11*(3), 127–129.

Zimmer, M., Lang, N., & Miller, D. (1974). *Development of sets of patients health outcome criteria by panels of nurse experts*. Milwaukee: Wisconsin Regional Medical Program.

CHAPTER 2

Quality Outcomes Management: Executive Role Imperative

Ellen M. Lewis, Lori C. Marshall, Ann Marie Vonglis, and Nancy E. Donaldson

CHAPTER OBJECTIVES

After completing this chapter, the reader will be able to

- define multiple components of the patient care executive's role in managing quality
- apply the role of leadership in quality outcome using a Plan-Do-Check-Act framework
- specify various patient-focused structure, process, and outcomes indicators

Forecasters predict the current era of health care revolution and reform has only just begun. Clearly, patient care executives (PCEs) who lead successful organizations and institutions into the future will need to acquire new skills to manage the health care risk of enrolled lives, maximize clinical productivity and effectiveness, transform the professional/technical clinical work force with the skills demanded in the new millennium, and delight customers. PCEs, who will have strategic roles in organized delivery systems that will continue to evolve, will be expected to address clinical quality, cost, technology, and information management. PCEs must understand and embrace the knowledge that prediction and management, provider–patient partnerships, and population-based foci are the new principles driving health policy and care delivery. Also, managed health care and capitation are expected to expand exponentially, and purchasers will continue to ratchet premiums and costs downward. As the transformed health care market compresses costs, reducing the value of cost-per-case comparisons, the significance of quality as *the* variable on which comparisons between providers and institutions are based comes strategically into focus. The capacity to respond to increasing payer, purchaser, employer, consumer, and regulatory demands for evidence of continuous quality improvement (CQI) requires access to sophisticated clinical and financial data systems and systematic integration of institutional quality planning, monitoring, and improvement. In today's health care environment, measuring clinical outcomes and costs of quality go hand in hand. A review of the literature demonstrates that processes to achieve cost containment while preserving or improving quality of care can and are being achieved today (Clare, Sargent, Moxley, & Forthman, 1995; Finnigan, Abel, Dobler, Hudon, & Terry, 1993; Gagen & Holsclaw, 1995; Gates, 1995; King, McDonald, & Good, 1995; Lucas, Gunter, Byrnes, Coyle, & Friedman, 1995). Ultimately, effective management of clinical, service, and financial processes and outcomes will determine the health care providers and institutions that will compete and survive in the reforming health care delivery system of the future.

Executive level leadership is crucial to linking organizational strategic priorities with quality improvement efforts, optimizing the impact of quality management on organizational performance as a whole. However, the PCE is key to establishing the philosophical commitment to CQI as a core value of patient care services. Patient care–focused quality management activities must engage all staff, and the PCE must ensure and support staff development related to clinical process improvements.

A fundamental challenge is to capture reliable data as the basis for measuring baseline care and managing clinical variation. Ongoing clinical process measurement is key to tracing the impact of quality improvement interventions on quality outcomes and delivering data-driven feedback to clinical staff. Phase I of the American Nurses Association (ANA, 1995) nursing quality report card project, undertaken in response to demand for nurse-sensitive quality indicators and in consultation with Lewin-VHI, Inc., yielded 11 quality indicators (Exhibit 2–1) for integration into clinical data systems. Phase II of the project produced 7 priority indi-

Exhibit 2–1 Acute-Care Nursing Quality Indicators

PATIENT-FOCUSED OUTCOME INDICATORS

- Mortality Rate
- Length of Stay
- Adverse Incidents
  - Adverse Incident Rate (total)
  - Medication Error Rate
  - Patient Injury Rate*
- Complications
  - Total Complication Rate
  - Decubitus Ulcer Rate
  - Nosocomial Infection Rate (total)*
  - Nosocomial Urinary Tract Infection Rate
  - Nosocomial Pneumonia Rate
  - Nosocomial Surgical Wound Infection Rate

- Patient Family Satisfaction with Nursing Care*
  - Patient Willingness to Recommend Hospital to Other/Use Hospital Again
- Patient Adherence to Discharge Plan
  - Readmission Rates
  - Emergency Room Visits Post-Discharge
  - Unscheduled Physician Visits Post-Discharge
  - Patient Knowledge of Disease/Condition and Care Requirements

PROCESS OF CARE INDICATORS

- Nurse Satisfaction
- Assessment and Implementation of Patient Care Requirements
  - Assessment of Patient Care Requirements*
  - Development of a Nursing Plan
  - Accurate and Timely Execution of Therapeutic Interventions and Procedures
  - Documentation of Nursing Diagnosis
  - Therapeutic Objectives, and Care Given
- Pain Management*
- Maintenance of Skin Integrity*

- Patient Education
- Discharge Planning
- Assurance of Patient Safety
  - Overall Assurance of Patient Safety
  - Appropriate Use of Restraints (all)
  - Appropriate Use of Pharmaceutical Restraints
  - Appropriate Use of Physical Restraints
- Responsiveness to Unplanned Patient Care Needs

continues

Exhibit 2–1 continued

STRUCTURE OF CARE INDICATORS-NURSE STAFFING PATTERNS

- Ratio of Total Nursing Staff to Patients
  - RN/Patient Ratio
  - LPN/Patient Ratio
  - Unlicensed Workers/Patient Ratio
- Ratio of RNs to Total Nursing Staff
  - Mix of RNs, LPNs, and Unlicensed Workers
- RN Staff Qualifications
  - RN Staff Experience
  - RN Staff Education (i.e., MSNs, BSNs)
- Nursing Staff Injury Rate

- Total Nursing Care Hours Provided per Patient* (Case Mix, Acuity Adjusted)
  - RN Hours per Patient
  - LPN Hours per Patient
  - Unlicensed Worker Hours per Patient
- Staff Continuity
  - Use of Agency Nurses
  - Use of Float Nurses
  - Unsafe Assignment Rate
  - Nurse Staff Turnover Rates
- RN Overtime

˙ Phase I quality indicators.
* Phase II priority indicators.

Source: Reprinted with permission from *Nursing Report Card for Acute Care,* p.17, © 1995, American Nurses Association.

---

cators (identified in Exhibit 2–1). The ANA indicators may be critical to patient care leaders in the midst of work redesign and skill mix changes geared to reduce costs and optimize the role performance of patient care professionals and technical workers. Indicator data may be invaluable to identify potential thresholds for staffing and outcome correlations, suggesting a clinical safety net to guide reengineering efforts.

Quality management thrives in flexible organizations with the capacity to plan, design, and refine care processes. Learning organizations, characterized by openness to innovation and efficient internal dissemination of lessons learned in one arena to other applicable units and settings, have the vital capacity to undertake practice and outcomes improvements. The challenge of the PCE is to focus a myriad of quality improvement projects on strategic imperatives and to ensure the interdisciplinary and interdepartmental integrity of project teams.

Furthermore, PCEs must pursue local, regional, and national opportunities to share data, validate conclusions, and identify benchmarks to drive ongoing performance improve-

ment. As the ANA nursing quality report card initiative advances, it is likely that a centralized database will evolve, providing an opportunity for PCEs to measure patient care structure, process, and outcomes using increasingly refined clinical quality indicators and standardized definitions, submit institutional data to regional and national data repositories, and obtain valid comparison data for benchmarking. Ultimately, through the ANA's initiative, "best practices" will emerge. PCEs will then have the opportunity to accelerate performance improvement using this information of best practices between collaborating institutions.

APPLICATION OF THE PCE ROLE

Each organization selects a quality management methodology to guide organizational performance planning, measurement, and improvement. This chapter applies elements of the Plan–Do–Check–Act (PDCA) framework refined and popularized by Deming (1986) to examine and illustrate the PCE and leadership roles in quality outcomes management. Major areas addressed are the vision, culture, commitment, education, structure, process, and outcomes (Table 2–1).

Plan

Developing an organizational quality plan is an essential role of the PCE. To initiate this process, the key PCE function is to link the plan with the organization's vision and mission. The vision must establish strong links between the organizational goals and quality. A vision guides the PCE and leadership to effectively manage resources, provide services matching customer needs, and remain attentive to quality of the service delivery process.

The mission and values of the organization must be used to identify existing quality components and processes, and then assessed for elements that both positively and negatively influence organizational quality culture. For example, do the mission statement and values discuss quality when describing the care delivery process? Does the mission identify other behaviors that may support a quality improvement culture? The PCE should identify behaviors necessary to support the quality culture that are not contained in the mission and values, and then evaluate these behaviors for inclusion or exclusion in the quality plan. It would be appropriate to incorporate the quality culture behaviors into role descriptions and standards for employee performance appraisals.

All organizational leadership, including the PCE's, influences the development of organizational culture. It is important to build on successful practices and the established organizational culture when developing a quality improvement plan. Although organizational cultures vary, there are several quality improvement culture elements that positively predict organizational quality performance. Yearout (1996) identified eight best practices that contribute to an effective quality improvement culture: (1) cascading leadership, (2) strong consistent customer focus, (3) establishment of an alliance between employees and the quality

vision, (4) total commitment to quality improvement, (5) variety of methods to measure improvement, (6) change management, (7) innovative functioning, and (8) adoption of a framework for quality improvement. As a first step to understanding the culture, the PCE must examine the quality management responsibility of each leadership staff and identify how to link his or her own responsibility with the overall organizational quality structure. To evaluate the quality process and team structure, a PCE must ask: Who is involved? How are the teams structured? What are the current leadership roles? What types of teams exist? What are the purposes of the teams? What are the quality improvement outcomes of the teams?

Organizations often start with professional standards over customer expectations. However, a PCE must help the organization to always maintain a strong consistent customer focus when performing quality improvement activities (Yearout, 1996). Quality improvement should not be separate from the improvement of customer service (Reeves, Matney, & Crane, 1995). To support a customer focus, it is paramount to establish an alliance between employees and organizational goals.

Employees must have a clear idea of their role in quality improvement and know the organization's mission and goals. The connection between an employee's contribution to the quality process and outcomes must be specified as it relates to achieving the mission and goals. In addition, a commitment to quality improvement must be cultivated in every employee (Yearout, 1996). The quality process begins with hiring people who share the same level of commitment to quality as established by the organization. Current employees will need mentorship from PCEs and leadership to develop behaviors that foster a commitment to the quality process.

Education and training are essential when implementing any quality program, and the PCE must ensure that educational support remains an organizational priority as well as provide budget support. Cost centers should be

Table 2–1 PCE and Leadership Roles in Quality Outcomes Management

Plan	Do	Check	Act

Vision and mission
• Use vision to
  – Guide management of resources
  – Provide services to match customer needs
  – Increase attentiveness to quality of service
• Determine quality components in mission
  – Identify needed behaviors not contained in mission and values
 	
Culture
• Examine responsibilities of leadership staff
• Link own responsibility with quality structure
• Develop quality plan
  – Build on successful practices
  – Link with established culture
 	
Commitment
• Start with customer expectations
• Establish alliance between employees and organizational goals
 	
Education
• Determine education content
• Draft budget for education
• Determine educational provider
	Motivation
	• Engage staff and physicians
	• Break down barriers for shifts, departments, workgroups, and individuals
	  – Extend quality improvement structure to all shifts
	  – Minimize perception of job loss
	
	Structure
	• Manage change and transition
	  – Regulate excessive and undirected quality activity
	• Prevent parallel activities
	• Provide clear sense of direction
	  – Expectations
	  – Time frame to complete
	  – Quality improvement methods to use
	
	Process
	• Determine complexity of quality issues
	• Determine complexity of quality change
	• Recognize problems with quality teams
	• Provide PCE support from onset of team
		Measurement
		• Ensure measurement of key indicators of organizational performance that are consistent with strategic goals, key functions, dimensions of performance, and so forth
		• Encourage use of aggregated, trended data over time
		• Measure costs, use, and outcomes
		• Use budget and support automation and integration of data to determine links with costs and quality
		Assess performance/outcomes
		• Assist others in determining opportunities for improvement
		• Compare health outcomes to "best practices" in other health care settings
			Actions
			• Review and approve recommendations for improvements to be made
			• Support access to information throughout the organization
			
			Budget
			• Provide a budget and develop a cost center to track expenses related to quality processes
			
			Mentoring
			• Provide mentorship to all participants throughout the quality improvement process
			
			Communication
			• Promote ongoing communication of everyone's efforts in the CQI process

developed to assist in tracking expenses related to quality processes. An organization must plan and budget the dollars associated with all process and system improvement teams. Specifically, an organization must provide

- initial and ongoing training of teams, conferences, and travel
- development of internal data capture, analysis, reporting, and retrieval systems to support quality management measurement and reporting
- access to external databases, including published and unpublished sources
- labor costs for research, team meetings, data retrieval, analysis, and presentation
- support for recommendations from teams to effect improvements related to costs of supplies, equipment, additional staff, new protocols, education, and training
- benchmarking or "best practices" activities, as appropriate

The PCE should evaluate existing organizational resources for ongoing training. If internal educational resources are unavailable, education may need to be provided using an outside consultant well versed in quality, change theory and management, and CQI tools. A program curriculum including an overview of CQI, information management, decision making, outcomes management, quality measurement tools, and evaluation of quality outcomes should be implemented for all organizational staff as well as for the board of directors. (It is important not to assume that the board of directors of a health care organization has a working knowledge of CQI.) Employees learn concepts that are a key to successful implementation of a CQI program. For example, CQI requires employees to focus on roles and not just job tasks. It may take some time to help employees learn to develop this view through guided interactive learning experiences. Another important benefit of education is that employees both learn how to use tools to measure CQI and acquire the decision-making skills to integrate CQI data into care and ser-

vices provided (Caltrinder, Pattison, & Richardson, 1995; Chaudron, 1995). Initial education should address CQI tools such as *process mapping,* which includes the timing of events in the process; *flow charting*, the sequence of events for a process; and *fishbone diagrams*, which establish cause-and-effect relationships.

Do

Do is the implementation of a quality plan. Successful implementation of an organization-wide quality improvement plan requires the PCE to engage staff and physicians in the improvement process. Engaging large groups of people is often difficult; one method to engage teams is to break down barriers between shifts, departments, work groups, and individuals. Shift work greatly influences CQI activities (Penkala, 1995). To engage late and weekend shifts, it is critical that the PCE conveys management's commitment and increased visibility, and ensures support. Limited involvement of late and weekend shift workers is further perpetuated by virtue of scheduling the quality activities such as team meetings and task forces. A quality improvement structure allowing for extended shifts increases the likelihood of a successful quality plan implementation. Thus, linking performance rewards or incentives with quality outcomes, creating involvement opportunities for employees, providing ongoing education and training, and supporting a collaborative program structure spanning all shifts will contribute to increased employee participation.

It is important to recognize that decreased staff participation may be due to the perceived threat of job loss or role function changes evolving from the redesign of organizational processes (Feinberg, 1995). To help minimize this phenomenon and provide an environment where employees will be motivated to participate, the PCE will need to help employees focus on viewing their work as a *role* in the organization and not simply a *job*. Moreover, excessive change and unplanned rapid improvement for the sake of quality may become a barrier to successful implementation of quality activities by increasing employees' and managers' frustration levels. In some instances, misdirected frustration may lead to poor-quality performance. The PCE must help manage transition and change by carefully regulating excessive and undirected quality activities. Although innovation drives important quality changes, the PCE must help manage change while keeping improvements flowing.

To produce desired outcomes, the PCE must ensure that the quality teams are effectively structured. A goal is to have CQI teams remain connected with the mainstream organization and to avoid parallel team functioning. For example, a CQI team may produce worthwhile activities; however, in the aggregate, the quality team's activities may be meaningless (Scholtes, 1995). To help keep teams working synergystically, the PCE must provide the team with a clear sense of direction and scope including how the team's activity integrates with the other CQI teams. When organizing a team, the PCE should assess if the team will be active for an extended period and consider having enough team members to allow for team member turnover (Scholtes, 1995). Depending on the focus of the team, the time frame for project completion may be 3 months to 1 year. Executive-level strategic coordination of teams ensures alignment of CQI teamwork with evolving organizational priorities.

A quality team structure is enhanced when the PCE and leadership maintain the integrity of the team process. The complexity of the CQI issue and the complexity of implementing the CQI change(s) drives the team process. If an issue is complex, the team process may involve a divide-and-conquer strategy. For example, a quality team as a whole may address an issue such as patient injury. Parts of this quality improvement activity, however, may be subdivided among team members to evaluate this issue across the continuum of care. A team that spans more than one department or discipline may involve more than one type of staff role that becomes cross-functional in focus. A team member from each role or area influenced by the issue or problem being addressed will be critical to achieving quality improvement. The team process is enhanced when team composition includes individuals with a variety of perspectives (Scholtes, 1995). For instance, a team may need to assign a "devil's advocate" to help examine all aspects of a particular issue or problem. In addition, successful implementation of CQI change may be increased when leaders and employees who have the potential of becoming barriers to the change process are added to the QI team (Scholtes, 1995).

The PCE must recognize the problems with CQI teams and help maximize team involvement and effectiveness (Chaudron, 1995). If a team is no longer effective or useful, the PCE must decide whether to continue or disband the team. A common mistake made by a PCE or leader is to remain on the periphery of team activity. A lack of management support is one reason quality improvement teams fail. It is important for the PCE to become part of the team process from the beginning and not wait until the team is in trouble to provide support and direction. It is critical that the PCE and leadership provide the quality teams with clear guidelines regarding the time they have to complete a process, the expected results, and the quality improvement methods to be used by the team (Caltrinder et al., 1995; Chaudron, 1995; Margerison & McCann, 1995). Additional PCE support may include assisting the team to remove barriers and obstacles and helping the team to relinquish old ways of providing care and services.

Check

Check, the next component of the model, includes measurement of key indicators and assessment of performance. The PCE's role in ensuring access to organizational measures of performance is essential to the success of the CQI process. The measurement of aggregate, trended data over time reveals the extent to which clinical processes vary within or between units and suggests whether the observed variation exceeds expected levels. Typically, the following indicators measure the organization's performance:

- customer satisfaction—patients, employees, physicians, and third-party payers
- medication errors
- adverse drug reactions
- patient injuries
- workers' compensation claims
- employee turnover
- security incidents
- patient falls
- staff completion of new employee orientation
- staff completion of health and safety programs
- antibiotic appropriateness
- nosocomial infections
- readmissions
- pain management
- patient education effectiveness
- functional health status
- quality of life

The business community now demands evidence that an organization has controlled the growing costs of purchasing health care for its membership. Hospitals must "give in" to the demands of third-party payers and other agencies. As the health care market becomes more competitive, major advances will be made in information processing, which has made formerly proprietary information more accessible to the public. Data on use, costs, and outcomes have enabled government and regulatory agencies, insurers, and customers to conduct their own analyses of hospital costs (Lucas et al., 1995). Interest in health care information has moved from the professional to the public domain as various groups have gained access to these data. They now measure the value received for their money, evaluate the relative effectiveness of various treatments, and compare health outcomes in different hospitals.

The process the leadership team uses in determining the measures of organizational performance may vary, but usually will include data already collected in the organization. The selection process also may include the use of a priority or decision-making tool (Exhibit 2–2) comprising areas such as:

- consistency with organizational goals or key strategy foci
- key functions as described by the Joint Commission on Accreditation of Healthcare Organizations, such as patient assessment, patient care and treatment, patient rights, care environment, patient and family education, and human resources management
- dimensions of performance as described by the Joint Commission, such as timeliness, efficiency, efficacy, effectiveness, appropriateness, respect, and caring
- high-volume, high-risk, problem-prone areas (Joint Commission, 1996)

Once the organizational measures are collected, a reporting tool (Exhibit 2–3) is used that lists the indicators with their corresponding results for each month. Typically, this report is presented on at least a quarterly basis to the leadership team for review and discussion, with subsequent reporting to the governing board. Periodically, additional indicators may be selected for review and others, once reviewed over time, may be removed from the report.

CQI project teams design, implement, and monitor such processes as clinical pathways and then benchmark with other organizations to develop best practices guidelines. "Hospitals must forge a partnership between the administration and medical staff" (Clare et al., 1995, p. 58). With the assessment of a pathway or clinical condition such as pneumonia, total knee replacement, total hip replacement, CABG, head and neck surgery, and so forth, the participation of the medical staff in the entire process is crucial to achieving improved clinical and financial outcomes. To gain their

Exhibit 2–2 Sample Decision-Making Tool

WESTERN MEDICAL CENTER
1996 PERFORMANCE IMPROVEMENT ACTIVITIES

Chartered CQI Teams or Key Function Teams:
Key Function Teams:
Anesthesia Care: GI Lab, PICU/PEDS, PACU, L&D, ICU
Assessment/Continuum of Care: ER, Education 4th Flr, Case Mgmt
Medication/Nutrition: 7th Flr, ICU, Education
Blood Administration: OR, ER/Trauma, 7th Flr

NURSING STAFF PARTICIPATION IN THE FOLLOWING CQI TEAMS:
Tests & Treatments: PICU, 4th Flr, ER, Education, Outpatient Surgery
Service Location: L&D
Late Charges: ER, L&D, 6th Flr
C-Section: L&D, Prenatal, ICU, Case Mgmt, OR
Antibiotic Utilization: PEDS, Education, ER, 7th Flr, 4th Flr

OUTPATIENT PLANNING
OR, Outpatient, PEDS, 4th Flr, Case Mgmt

MULTIDISCIPLINARY OR DEPARTMENTAL TEAMS/PROJECT INDICATORS

ACTIVITY	DISCIPLINES	START DATE	M&CQ OUTCOMES	IMP CUST SATIS	REDUCE COSTS	I&D AREAS EXCEL	PATIENT RIGHTS	ASSESSMENT	CARE OF PATIENTS	PATIENT EDUCATION	CONTINUUM	ENVIRONMENT OF CARE	HUMAN RESOURCES	MAN OF INFORMATION	INFECTION CONTROL	EFFICACY	APPROPRIATE	AVAILABILITY	TIMELINESS	EFFECTIVENESS	CONTINUITY	SAFETY	EFFICIENCY	RESPECT/CARING	MEDICATION USE	BLOOD USE	SCR/OP/IP	HIGH VOLUME	HIGH RISK	PROBLEM PRONE
Restraints (Indicators)	Medical Staff/Nursing	Ongoing	X				X		X	X							X	X	X	X	X	X		X					X	X
Conscious Sedation (Indicators)	Medical Staff/Nursing	Ongoing	X					X	X	X							X	X	X	X		X	X						X	
Patient Falls (Events)	Nursing	Ongoing	X					X	X								X	X	X	X		X	X						X	
Medication Errors (Events)	Pharmacy/Nursing	Ongoing	X						X			X					X	X	X	X		X							X	
Skin Integrity (Indicators, Events)	Medical Staff/Nursing	Ongoing	X	X				X								X	X	X	X	X	X	X		X				X		
Patient Satisfaction (Survey Indicators)	Nursing	Ongoing	X	X					X								X	X	X	X	X			X						
Nutritional Care (Indicators)	Nutrition Service/Nursing	Jan-96	X																X											
Food/Drug Interaction Instruction	Nutrition Service/Nursing	Ongoing	X							X							X		X			X						X		X
Medical Record Documentation (Indicators)	Multidisciplinary	Jan-96	X	X					X	X	X			X		X	X	X	X	X	X	X		X	X	X	X	X	X	X

Column groups: GOAL (M&CQ OUTCOMES, IMP CUST SATIS, REDUCE COSTS, I&D AREAS EXCEL); FUNCTIONS (PATIENT RIGHTS, ASSESSMENT, CARE OF PATIENTS, PATIENT EDUCATION, CONTINUUM, ENVIRONMENT OF CARE, HUMAN RESOURCES, MAN OF INFORMATION, INFECTION CONTROL); DIMENSIONS (EFFICACY, APPROPRIATE, AVAILABILITY, TIMELINESS, EFFECTIVENESS, CONTINUITY, SAFETY, EFFICIENCY, RESPECT/CARING); MONITOR (MEDICATION USE, BLOOD USE, SCR/OP/IP); TYPE (HIGH VOLUME, HIGH RISK, PROBLEM PRONE). STOP DATE column not marked.

Legend for Abbreviations:
M&CQ Outcomes—Measure and Communicate Quality Outcomes
Imp Cust Satis—Improved Customer Satisfaction
I&D Areas Excel—Investigate & Develop Areas of Excellence
Man of Information—Management of Information
SCR/OP/IP—Surgical Case Review, Operative Procedures, Invasive Procedures

Authors wish to acknowledge Janet Callahan, RN, MS, CPHQ, Director, Quality Resources.
Courtesy of Western Medical Center, Santa Ana, California.

Exhibit 2–3 Sample Reporting Tool

Project/Activity	Jan.	Feb.	Mar.	April	May	June	July	Aug.	Sept.	Oct.	Nov.	Dec.
Customer satisfaction of patients, employees, physicians, payers												
Medication errors												
Adverse drug reactions												
Patient injuries												
Workers' compensation claims												
Employee turnover												
Security incidents												
Patient falls												
Staff completion of new employee orientation												
Staff completion of health and safety programs												
Antibiotic appropriateness												
Nosocomial infections												

support, the PCE and leadership team must invite key members to participate in the CQI process. This participation may result in a potential loss of income for some physicians who may give the considerable time required for CQI meetings and outside research. Therefore, the PCE and leadership team might consider recognizing key members and providing incentives to them; however, the benefits will only be realized with this partnership.

As clinical pathways are developed and implemented, internal best practices will emerge. In addition, external benchmarks or best practices may also be used as comparisons. CQI teams measure and compare the following:

- length of stays per episode
- customer satisfaction
- use of laboratory, radiology, and other diagnostic services
- timeliness of services, turnaround time
- costs and quality of clinical care
- inappropriate variation in provider practice patterns
- use of CQI tools and techniques to improve system performance

The creation and implementation of information technologies allow the PCE to integrate data to identify direct links between costs and quality. However, organizations still face obstacles in accessing those resources. Florence Nightingale in 1863 stated the following:

> In attempting to arrive at the truth, I have applied everywhere for information, but in scarcely an instance have I been able to obtain hospital records fit for any purpose of comparison. If they could be obtained they would enable us to decide many other questions besides the one alluded to. They would show the subscribers how their money was being spent, what good was really being done with it, or whether the money was not doing mischief rather than good.

In more recent times, Gagen and Holsclaw (1995) stated that "the problem in outcomes research is not the availability of raw data; hospitals are swamped in a sea of data. The real need is to provide cost-effective and usable access to just the right information to develop the appropriate conclusions" (p. 26). Access to data is still an issue, and thus the PCE is accountable for ensuring that the technological tools are in place that facilitate those processes for effective decision making.

It is essential to have an infrastructure that allows computerized programs to interface several health care feeder systems and combine them into a single database. One type of tool is a decision support system that integrates all clinical and financial patient case data. Such a system is able to process information to reflect complex relationships among patient, procedural, financial, and quality data. Components of this system include costing information, case mix, flexible budgeting, and clinical and financial forecasting. Furthermore, the decision support system can help answer the following questions:

- What is the most effective and efficient clinical practice center for any one procedure?
- What resources have been used, and what is the standard for a given condition?
- What are the various complication rates?
- What are the key clinical variables affecting resource use and outcomes?
- Which resources are critical to the most efficient treatment process? At what point should they be delivered, and what, if any, resources can be eliminated?

Reaching the optimal quality–cost level at which excellent quality is achieved at a reasonable cost is the objective of health care providers and administrators alike. A decision support system assists in the achievement of both objectives, whereby programming of system rules can then scan the database to identify when certain events occur. The system can detect potentially inappropriate patient case management in terms of quality or cost, and, thus, appropriate follow-up can occur.

The automation of quality improvement activities provides for automatically quantifying clinical indicators and screening for complications for all patient cases. This tool provides a mechanism for continuous improvement in utilization review, risk management, infection control, and the quality improvement program. A decision support system can facilitate change in the organization's management culture and can aid in the redesigning of the treatment process. Information about quality and resource use is more meaningful to physicians and administrators when it is linked with the clinical process (Raco, Shapleigh, & Cook, 1989).

Act

The last component of the PDCA cycle is *Act*. Once data are measured and transformed into usable and meaningful information, an assessment is made whether any opportunities need improvement. Actions are decisions made and guide the ongoing cycle back to the Plan step. The leadership team plays a key role in supporting this phase of the process, as well as the clinical teams.

The Act phase includes improvement actions based on measurement and assessment. For example, if measurement and assessment determine that inadequate staffing patterns resulted in treatment delays for patients, then an improvement action would be to change those staffing patterns. Other examples of actions would include

- redesigning patient education information so that home care patients are knowledgeable regarding their care and access to health care
- implementing a skin integrity risk assessment tool to better identify patients at risk for developing pressure ulcers
- developing critical pathways to better coordinate patient care across the continuum

- changing staffing levels according to patient activity (Joint Commission, 1995)

The PCE and leadership team should actively play a role in reviewing a CQI team's recommendations for all improvements, and not only when there is a financial component included. A cost analysis and justification are presented to the leadership team with subsequent decisions made that may or may not support the costs of improvement. If financial support is approved, the CQI team may continue on its journey to obtain the desired products, services, or resources. If not approved, the leadership team will provide a rationale and other possible actions or directions for the CQI team.

For clinical teams to develop effective action plans that can result in clinical or system improvements, the PCE and administration should provide the support to access information across the organization. Systems must be in place to facilitate clinical and administrative decision making.

During a health care organization's accreditation survey, interview questions are posed to the organization's leadership, including the PCE, to determine the organization's commitment and support of the CQI processes throughout the organization. Questions may include the following:

- How does the organization budget for quality efforts?
- What does quality mean to you?
- How do you measure success for the organization?
- What is cost containment for this organization?

The responses to these questions demonstrate not only the organization's support of CQI efforts, but also give a measure of the organization's culture as well as indicate the preparedness of the leadership team to face the current challenges in such a dynamic environment.

Another key role leadership plays in supporting quality improvement in the health care setting is the ongoing communication of every-one's efforts along the quality journey. Communication is demonstrated by

- obtaining input from employees, physicians, and customers for potential quality projects (e.g., CQI hotline, employee–physician newsletter, or CQI suggestion boxes)
- publishing a team's charter (i.e., the mission, goals, scope, members, and so forth) in the employee–physician newsletter and providing such information on posters
- presenting a team's progress to key committees and forums
- describing a team's journey and accomplishments by means of posters or storyboards located in key areas throughout the health care setting

The PCE's role in the Act phase cannot be understated. It is one that requires great visibility and active participation throughout the entire process.

CONCLUSION

The PCE's key role now and in the future will be to minimize costs and maximize rev-enues while providing excellence in patient care. Economic pressures, consumer expectations, care rationing, and access to care affect future managerial decisions. Appropriate allocation and resource use with the ability to adjust resource components will help ensure cost-effective delivery of services. CQI activities should be quantifiable in terms of labor and other resources. Good management techniques will enhance the PCE's ability to scrutinize CQI programs for cost-effectiveness and efficiency. Furthermore, a successful organization is one in which every department is able to not only articulate and demonstrate what quality is, but respond quickly to changes in strategic direction. The PCE and the leadership team play a pivotal role in ensuring that the organization is equipped to respond to changing forces in the health care arena. Equally important is the role that each member plays in mentoring staff throughout the CQI process. Only with this commitment and visible support will there be the outcomes organizations need to not only gain a competitive market advantage, but truly achieve the quality services and quality of care for patients and families.

REFERENCES

American Nurses Association. (1995). *Nursing's report card for acute care settings: Executive summary.* Washington, DC: Author.

Caltrinder, J., Pattison, D., & Richardson, P. (1995). Can cost control and quality care coexist? *Management Accounting, 77*(2), 38–42.

Chaudron, D. (1995). An effective quality team. Not! *Human Resources Focus, 72*(8), 6–7.

Clare, M., Sargent, D., Moxley, R., & Forthman, T. (1995). Reducing health care delivery costs using clinical paths: A case study on improving hospital profitability. *Journal of Health Care Finance, 21*(3), 48–58.

Deming, W.E. (1986). *Out of control.* Cambridge, MA: Massachusetts Institute of Technology.

Feinberg, S. (1995). Overcoming the real issues of implementation. *Quality Progress, 28*(7), 79–81.

Finnigan, S., Abel, M., Dobler, T., Hudon, L., & Terry, B. (1993). Automated patient acuity: Linking nursing sys-tems and quality measurement with patient outcomes. *Journal of Nursing Administration, 23*(5), 62–71.

Gagen, T., & Holsclaw, R. (1995, June). Tying outcomes to cost and quality. *Health Management Technology,* 26–28.

Gates, P. (1995). Think globally, act locally: An approach to implementation of clinical practice guidelines. *Journal on Quality Improvement, 21*(2), 71–85.

Joint Commission on Accreditation of Healthcare Organizations. (1995). *Cycling for performance: A pocket guide.* Oakbrook Terrace, IL: Author.

Joint Commission on Accreditation of Healthcare Organizations. (1996). *Accreditation manual for hospi-tals.* Oakbrook Terrace, IL: Author.

King, M., McDonald, B., & Good, D. (1995). Redesigning care using total quality management and outcome/vari-ance analysis. *Aspen's Advisor for Nurse Executives, 10*(5), 3–5.

Lucas, J., Gunter, M., Byrnes, J., Coyle, M., & Friedman, N. (1995). Integrating outcomes measurement into clinical practice improvement across the continuum of care: A disease-specific episode of care model. *Managed Care Quarterly*, *3*(2), 14–22.

Margerison, C., & McCann, D. (1995). Quality in teamwork. *Journal for Quality and Participation*, *8*(2), 32–35.

Nightingale, F. (1863). *Notes on hospitals*. London: Longman, Green, Longman, Roberts & Green.

Penkala, D. (1995). It's 10 p.m.: Do you know where your quality program is? *Quality Progress*, *28*(2), 91–93.

Raco, R., Shapleigh, C., & Cook, D. (1989). Decision support in the 1990's: The future is now. *Computers in Healthcare*, *2*(12), 24–26.

Reeves, S., Matney, K., & Crane, V. (1995). Continuous quality improvement as an ideal in hospital practice. *Health Care Supervisor*, *13*(4), 1–12.

Scholtes, P. (1995). Teams in the age of systems. *Quality Progress*, *28*(12), 51–59.

Yearout, S. (1996). The secrets of improvement-driven organizations. *Quality Progress*, *29*(1), 51–56.

## PART II

Quality Improvement Process: Components of a Program

## Chapter 3

Standards: The Basis of a Quality Improvement Program

Shirley Ann Larson

CHAPTER OBJECTIVES

After completing this chapter, the reader will be able to

- define the concept of "standard"
- differentiate between structure, process, and outcome standards
- compare various standards developed by professionals and accrediting bodies

The provision of quality care is a key expectation for health care organizations. The health care providers who work within the organization commit themselves to providing care to their customers (i.e., patients, clients, and residents) that will meet standards of quality, which are defined in a variety of ways. The patients, clients, or residents anticipate that they will receive quality services. The payers of health care bills expect to pay for care that has met quality of care standards. In a global view, the public and health care providers seek organizations that can be accessed by the public, demonstrate fiscal responsibility, and are recognized for quality care. The thread that would seem to tie these expectations together is that all are seeking standards that translate into an ongoing improvement in the quality of care. To define those standards is indeed a challenge.

In today's health care arena, the Joint Commission on Accreditation of Healthcare Organizations (Joint Commission) has a repu-

tation and a high profile for using a survey process that is based on standards and for challenging the organizations it surveys to demonstrate quality improvement programs. Professional organizations and governmental and private agencies have intensified the development and dissemination of standards that serve as the basis for quality improvement initiatives. The Agency for Health Care Policy and Research (AHCPR), created by the U.S. Department of Health and Social Services in 1989, has become one of the most visible agencies for the development of patient care guidelines. The Malcolm Baldrige National Quality Award, created by P.L. 100–107 in 1987, is managed by the U.S. Department of Commerce and is predicated on multiple standards organized into seven areas. Organizations and others who are seeking the award use these quality criteria as the guiding direction for their quality improvement programs.

ROLE OF STANDARDS IN A QUALITY IMPROVEMENT PROGRAM

A *standard* refers not necessarily to an optimum level of achievement but more accurately to an acceptable level of achievement, based on the realistic availability of resources and on the practice environment. Because standards are based on values and expectations that are tempered by reality, there is often a significant discrepancy between optimum and acceptable levels of achievement. An organization or profession needs to strive to identify optimum and acceptable standards that are not at the extremes of the continuum. Ultimately, the organization or profession will use the standards to identify opportunities to improve patient care, thus making standards dynamic. Standards are not static or permanent; rather, they are in a constant state of transition. They are continually modified by changes in values, advances in science and technology, and alterations in the policies and regulations of governmental, institutional, and regulatory agencies. Perhaps the ultimate function of standards is to reflect progressively higher levels of acceptable achievement, thus ensuring continual refinement of the concept of quality patient care.

In the current health care environment, process and outcome standards are the basis for continuous quality improvement (CQI) programs. *Process standards* flow from those functions carried out by health care providers in the delivery of patient care. Those functions include the assessment and evaluation of patient needs and those of the patient's significant others, individualized treatment planning, the technical aspects of performing treatments and providing direct patient care, and the management of critical events and complications. For nurses, these functions can be translated into the use of the nursing process. One of the key concepts of a quality improvement program is to prioritize, evaluate, and improve processes. In 1996, the Joint Commission organized its standards into 11 functions, defined as patient care functions and organizational functions (Exhibit 3–1).

Outcome standards are patient focused and are currently receiving the highest level of attention in the quality improvement literature and in the organizations that are influential in establishing the direction for standards that will become the basis of quality improvement activities. Outcome standards reflect the anticipated change for a patient and his or her significant others as a result of the care provided by the health caregivers of the organization that

the patient has entrusted to meet his or her health and illness needs. Outcomes include complications, adverse events, short-term results of specific procedures and treatments, and the patient's longer term health and functioning status. Overall, successful quality improvement programs are designed to incorporate process and outcome standards in a balance that meets the optimal improvement in the patient care provided by a given organization.

THE JOINT COMMISSION ON ACCREDITATION OF HEALTHCARE ORGANIZATIONS

The Joint Commission, established in 1951 by the American College of Surgeons, American College of Physicians, American Hospital Association, American Medical Association, and Canadian Medical Association, is a voluntary organization designed to establish and evaluate standards for the optimum functioning of health care organizations. The Canadian Medical Association withdrew in 1959; the American Dental Association became the fifth corporate member in 1979. In 1965, Medicare legislation recognized the Joint Commission standards as the norm in determining quality levels of patient care.

The Joint Commission uses research and input from many health care professionals to develop the standards for evaluating organizations. It responds to voluntary requests from organizations for accreditation by sending an on-site team of professional surveyors to evaluate each organization via the standards and to serve in an educational and consultative role.

In 1951, the Joint Commission standards included quality assurance requirements to enhance the quality of care in the hospitals and other organizations that receive accreditation. The emphasis of the quality standards has shifted from peer review to criteria-based audit, to ongoing monitoring and evaluation, and then to assessment and improvement. Each of these phases has reflected increased knowledge in how to effectively assess and improve care. The

Exhibit 3–1 The 11 Joint Commission on Accreditation of Healthcare Organizations Functions

Patient-Focused Functions

1. Patient Rights and Organization Ethics
2. Assessment of Patients
3. Care of Patients (planning and providing care; anesthesia care; medication use; nutrition care; operative and other procedures; rehabilitation care; and special procedures such as physical restraint use)
4. Education (Patient and Family)
5. Continuum of Care

Organization Functions

6. Improving Organization Performance
7. Leadership
8. Management of Environment (physical and social environments)
9. Management of Human Resources (competencies; staff education)
10. Management of Information
11. Surveillance, Prevention, and Control of Infection

Structures with Functions

Governance
Management
Medical Staff
Nursing

Source: Data from *1997 Comprehensive Accreditation Manual for Hospitals,* Joint Commission on Accreditation of Healthcare Organizations.

Joint Commission presently uses the term *improvement of performance.* Now, with quality improvement in the computer era and greater emphasis being placed on accurate data collection and analysis, outcome information, and organizational performance, the Joint Commission continues to lead with initiatives for change. The 1996 Joint Commission standards are organized by functions and emphasize organizational quality improvement. The improvement of performance (quality improvement) standards focus on design, measurement, assessment, and improvement. A quality improvement program needs to be organization-wide, interdisciplinary, and designed to evaluate and improve processes and outcomes in clinical, support, management, and governance functions. The Joint Commission (1997) developed a flowchart to illustrate the cycle for improving performance and outcomes (Figure 3–1).

The Joint Commission cycle for improving performance and outcome is ongoing and is designed to consider the external and internal environments of a health care organization. A health care organization can use the cycle in multiple improvement efforts, for example, designing a new program or service, creating a flowchart of a clinical process, measuring patient outcomes, comparing its performance to other organizations, establishing quality improvement priorities, or piloting innovations. The cycle can be entered at any stage but is described in this chapter as being initiated in the design stage.

Design Stage

In the design stage, the staff have clearly identified the process or outcome they wish to improve. They address the relationship of the

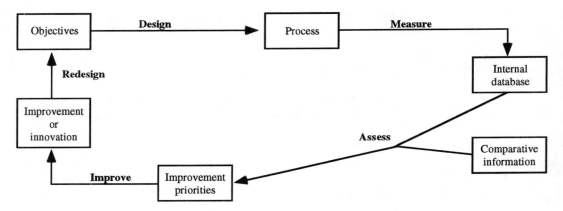

Figure 3–1 Improving organization performance function. *Source: 1997 Comprehensive Accreditation Manual for Hospitals,* Joint Commission on Accreditation of Healthcare Organizations, ©1997.

process to the organization's mission, vision, values, and priorities. The needs and expectations of the customers or patients affected by the process must be determined and influence the design phase. The staff need to develop clear objectives to guide the process improvement. State-of-the-art knowledge about the process must be researched and considered in the proposed design. Baseline performance expectations are established to guide the next two stages: measurement and assessment.

Measurement Stage

Measurement is the foundation for all improvement activities. The leaders for the improvement of performance should delineate the measures that will be necessary to assess the process initially, support the changes, and evaluate the improved process and outcomes. Potential measurements include outcomes, process parameters, customer or patient satisfaction, and costs associated with the process improvement and outcomes. The leaders and staff of an organization must determine the scope, focus, and priorities for measurement activities. Then the organization must organize the measurement activities into a systematic approach, determine the frequency and inten-

sity of each measure, and incorporate the measurements into daily work processes. This data collection may be periodic and ongoing or more intensive. A balanced approach to measurement includes both outcomes and process measures. Outcomes are measured to understand results and processes, to understand the causes of results.

Assessment Stage

The assessment stage may now be initiated and should be systematic and interdisciplinary. Assessment is supported by a variety of methodologies, including the use of statistical analysis tools, graphic tools, cause-and-effect diagrams, peer review, and comparative information. Cause-and-effect (fishbone) diagrams and flowcharts are often used early in the assessment phase. Comparative information includes assessing the organization's own performance and comparing it with others. A control chart is an example of internal performance, and *benchmarking* is a method of comparing with others (discussed later in this chapter). A health care organization may use a variety of assessment frameworks, for example, internal comparisons over time, comparison with practice guidelines or parameters, comparison with reference databases, or benchmarking.

Improvement and Design/Redesign Stages

In the improvement stage, an improvement process model should be used. An organization can improve its processes and outcomes by designing new processes or redesigning current processes. The leaders and staff identify the potential improvement, test or pilot an improvement strategy or innovation, assess data to determine if the improvement produced the desired results, and implement the improvement systemwide if the improvement is effective. Ongoing measurement and assessment are needed to verify that the improvement is maintained.

The staff who have implemented an improvement may determine, through ongoing measurement and assessment, that the design/redesign stage may be indicated again. The Joint Commission cycle for improvement supports a philosophy of continuous improvement.

STANDARDS OF CLINICAL NURSING PRACTICE, CARE, AND PROFESSIONAL PERFORMANCE

Standards of Clinical Nursing Practice

Florence Nightingale defined and wrote standards for nurses in the 1800s. Since that time, multiple definitions have been used to describe standards. In 1991, the American Nurses Association (ANA) published *Standards of Clinical Nursing Practice*. Standards of clinical nursing practice are authoritative statements that describe a level of care or performance common to the profession of nursing (Dean-Baer, 1993). These standards, which can be used to assess the quality of nursing practice, are further described as standards of care and standards of professional performance. The standards of clinical nursing practice include criteria that are relevant and measur-

able and broad enough to encompass all nurses in all practice settings, regardless of patient population. The best possible level of care for patients is defined by the setting in which nursing care is delivered and the length and intensity of the nurse–patient relationship. For standards to be useful and relevant, these realities must be reflected.

Standards of Care

The standards of care, as defined by the ANA, reflect the nursing process. These standards include assessment, diagnosis, outcome identification, planning, implementation, and evaluation. Throughout the standards of care is an emphasis on nursing practice that establishes priorities, is realistic, and is relevant to the patient's immediate condition or needs (Dean-Baer, 1993). Criteria also require each component to be documented in a retrievable record. Another common thread is the inclusion of the patient, family, and significant others and other health care disciplines. The outcome identification standard is especially powerful and requires the nurse to identify outcomes that are individualized for each patient.

Standards of Professional Performance

The standards of professional performance include activities that may not be directly evident in the provision of care but are integral to the professional nursing role and are indirectly reflected in the provision of direct patient care (Dean-Baer, 1993). These standards include quality of care, performance appraisal, education, collegiality, ethics, collaboration, research, and resource use. The degree or level of involvement in these activities may depend on the individual nurse's education, position, and practice environment.

The quality of care standard focuses on participation in quality activities and the use of results to initiate changes in nursing and throughout the health care system. The collaboration and resource use standards most clearly reflect the changes in the practice environment for the 1990s. The collaboration standard focuses on the increasing need for interdisciplinary provision of patient care and the attainment of patient outcomes. The resource use standard defines the nurse's role in considering patient care factors related to safety, effectiveness, and cost. This standard provides guidance as nurses make choices in the planning and delivery of care and in identifying and securing appropriate services for health-related patient needs.

Standards of care and practice, developed by nurses as the basis for nursing care, remain necessary and are valued. The standards have multiple new dimensions in the quality improvement programs now and will have them in the future. Quality programs are designed to be interdisciplinary and organization-wide. Processes are evaluated and improved for the clinical, support, management, and governance components of the organization. Patient outcome measures are designed for patient populations to ensure the same level of care for patients across all care settings. The continuum of care for patients is also a focus. Overall, these standards, as defined by ANA, have significant implications for nurses. They may serve as the foundation for quality improvement activities and related database systems.

Establishment of Standards by Professional Nursing Organizations

Nursing leaders continue to recognize the role and responsibility that professional nursing organizations have in establishing standards of care and practice. Dissemination and education are components inherent in this responsibility. Multiple organizations have accepted that quality improvement in health care is rooted in the professional practice of the disciplines responsible for the delivery of health care. Many professional nursing organizations have provided substantial support in channeling professional energies and resources into the provision of safe, cost-effective, and quality patient care. Such organizations have developed research-based outcome criteria, standardized care plans, core curricula, and guidelines for care and practice. These professional groups have established standards of care that not only set forth a legitimate scope of practice, but also provide a basis for organizing practice philosophies and the nursing process (Patton, 1993).

The ANA (1991) *Standards of Clinical Nursing Practice* apply to the care that is provided to all clients. These standards are generic in nature and are intended to apply to all registered nurses engaged in clinical nursing practice, regardless of their educational preparation, setting for practice, or clinical specialty (i.e., patient population receiving nursing care).

ANA has more recently reported its Nursing's Quality Report Card Outcomes Project (ANA, 1996). ANA has defined clinical quality indicators to assess the impact of nursing actions, structures, and processes on patient outcomes. The project is based on the concept that all nurses must become more knowledgeable about the measurement, benchmarking, and improvement of clinical costs and quality outcomes specific to nursing. The seven nursing quality indicators, identified by the project, are: (1) nosocomial infection rate; (2) patient injury rate; (3) patient satisfaction related to nursing care, pain management, and patient education; (4) maintenance of skin integrity; (5) nursing staff satisfaction; (6) staff mix; and (7) nursing care hours per patient day (Warzynski, 1996). The goal of the project is to promote the participation of nurses in the quality improvement activities in their respective health care organizations.

Over the past 20 years, multiple specialty nursing organizations have developed standards for the specialty area in which their members practice (Exhibit 3–2). Many of these organizations have collaborated with ANA. These standards serve as a framework for guiding and evaluating nursing practice.

Disch (1991) has defined eight primary responsibilities of specialty nursing organiza-

Exhibit 3–2 Nursing Professional Organizations That Have Developed Standards

American Nurses Association (ANA)
American Association of Critical Care Nurses (AACN)
American Society of Post Anesthesia Nurses (ASPAN)
Association of Operating Room Nurses (AORN)
Association of Rehabilitation Nurses (ARN)
Association of Women's Health, Obstetric, and Neonatal Nurses (AWHONN)
Dermatology Nurses' Association (DNA)
Hospice Nurses Association (HNA)
National Association of Orthopaedic Nurses (NAON)
National Consortium of Chemical Dependency Nurses (NCCDN)
National League for Nursing (NLN)
Oncology Nursing Society (ONS)
Society for Vascular Nursing (SVN)

Note: This list is not all-inclusive.
Source: Reprinted with permission from *1995 Encyclopedia of Associations*, Vol. 1, 29th Edition, ©1995, Gale Research, Inc.

tions in defining standards. One of these primary responsibilities is to define the specialty practice and the scope and standards of practice. A second major responsibility is to establish the standards that define the specialty practice base and become the cornerstone of the specialty. Development of appropriate practice guidelines is the third. Practice guidelines are patient focused and must be supported by the standards. Fourth, specialty organizations are responsible for educating their practitioners and other constituencies about the existence, role, and benefits of standards. A fifth responsibility is to develop the measures for judging the competencies of nurse practitioners in the specialty practice area. The sixth responsibility requires these organizations to conduct and fund research and clinical trials. A seventh responsibility is to generate rich databases that will contribute to an enhanced understanding of nursing practice, patient care outcomes, and health care issues. The eighth responsibility is that specialty nursing organizations should collaborate with each other and the ANA to develop standards and practice guidelines to create a framework that accurately represents the entire spectrum of nursing practice.

Nurses who accept the responsibility to define or refine the nursing standards in their organization should explore the potential of using standards from their professional organizations. For example, the Oncology Nursing Society (ONS) played a principle role in establishing standards of care for nurses practicing oncologic nursing. One of the primary objectives for ONS was the perceived need to standardize care delivered by professional nurses to patients with a diagnosis of cancer. ONS has developed 11 outcome criteria, each supported by detail describing patient outcome behaviors: (1) nutrition, (2) mobility, (3) protective mechanisms, (4) information, (5) sexuality, (6) ventilation, (7) detection and prevention, (8) coping, (9) circulation, (10) elimination, and (11) comfort (Patton, 1993). Furthermore, nurses who define standards should consider research-based standards, evaluate patient care for their area of practice by way of peer review, and be committed to peer education and feedback. The standards then become the keystone for the quality improvement program and the development of interdisciplinary plans of care and clinical guidelines and pathways.

Each health care organization continues to have the option of developing its own standards, but many professional organizations are defining and disseminating standards. Agencies such as AHCPR have been established for the purpose of establishing standards and guidelines. Standards are the cornerstones of clinical practice guidelines, practice parameters, clinical pathways, caremaps, and outcomes management programs. The establishment of national standards serves as the basis for participation in national programs that recognize quality improvement initiatives and enable benchmarking with the "best practice" organizations.

Clinical Pathways

Clinical pathways have become one of the most frequently used methodologies for defining an interdisciplinary plan of care. A clinical pathway is grounded in standards; therefore, nursing process and outcome standards are vital for nursing input into the development of a clinical pathway. Clinical pathways provide guidance for the hourly or daily care of patients in the population defined in the pathway. The pathways are used to establish process and outcome measures for quality improvement programs. The premise is to identify and evaluate variances from the pathway.

A clinical pathway program needs to be well defined and needs the demonstrated commitment of the organization's leadership. A clinical pathway program can reduce practice variation among individual providers, improve clinical outcomes, increase satisfaction of external and internal customers, and reduce cost and length of stay for inpatients. Malpractice risks may be reduced and compliance with the Joint Commission's standards for improving organizational performance may be enhanced (Cook, 1994).

Each health care organization needs to determine if clinical pathways will be used. Pathways are designed for a specific patient population and are often defined by diagnosis, although other definitions may be used. Initially, pathways were primarily used for

acute-care hospital inpatients and were developed along the parameters of days of care. The value of pathways has been recognized, and they have been adapted for patient care in ambulatory, home care, and long-term care settings. A pathway can be described for all patients receiving a primary care visit and a specified type of anesthesia, procedure, or treatment. Nurses have been and continue to be in the forefront of pathway development.

Clinical pathways are based on the standards of care for nursing and other disciplines for a specified patient population. Pathways are interdisciplinary and have predetermined criteria that include resource needs, time frames, and expected patient outcomes. The use of pathways should be built into quality improvement programs. For the highest level of effectiveness, path-based patient care must incorporate the component of concurrent review and intervention along with a retrospective analysis of variance measurement data. Improvement of performance opportunities is identified and actions prioritized by using the findings from the evaluation of pathways. Clinical pathways can help patient care providers "do the right thing the first time" for the patients (Spath, 1995, p. 26).

AHCPR

Clinical guidelines are patient focused and may be based on diagnosis, a procedure, a clinical condition such as pain or incontinence, or a health care need such as lifestyle modification to prevent some form of illness or condition (Urban, Greenlee, Krumberger, & Winkelman, 1995). In recent years, clinical guidelines have become well known and better understood through the work of AHCPR, an agency created in December 1989 under P.L. 101–239 to enhance the quality, appropriateness, and effectiveness of health care services and access to these services. AHCPR conducts and supports general health services research, including medical effectiveness research; facilitates the development of clinical practice guidelines; and disseminates the research findings and guidelines to health care providers, policy makers, and the public. Expert panels of interdisciplinary practitioners research, develop, and write the clinical practice guidelines. The guidelines are designed to assist practitioners in the prevention, diagnosis, treatment, and management of clinical conditions. The agency has published 19 guidelines, as of September 1996 (Exhibit 3–3). AHCPR selects clinical conditions based on three criteria: (1) high volume, (2) high cost, or (3) high degree of practice variation (Clinton, 1993). The guidelines are based in outcomes-based research whenever possible. They include a description of the condition, the specific expected outcome criteria, and interventions based on assessment. Algorithms are used in some guidelines to support the assessment to intervention approach. The guidelines do pro-

vide for individual patient variance. They are intended to promote the concept of including the patient in the decision-making process. Each clinical practice publication includes the guideline, a quick reference guide for clinicians, and a patient brochure that describes what the patient can expect in terms of care for the clinical condition described.

Health care organizations throughout the country have adopted the AHCPR clinical guidelines. The guidelines have become the cornerstone for practice decisions, clinician and patient education, and measurements for quality improvement programs.

NATIONAL COMMITTEE FOR QUALITY ASSURANCE (NCQA)

NCQA is an independent, private, not-for-profit organization dedicated to assessing and

---

Exhibit 3–3 AHCPR Guidelines

1. Acute Pain Management
2. Urinary Incontinence (1996)
3. Pressure Ulcers in Adults
4. Cataract in Adults
5. Depression in Primary Care: Volume 1. Detection and Diagnosis; Depression in Primary Care: Volume 2. Treatment of Major Depression
6. Sickle Cell Disease
7. Evaluation and Management of Early HIV Infection
8. Benign Prostatic Hyperplasia
9. Management of Cancer Pain
10. Unstable Angina
11. Heart Failure
12. Otitis Media with Effusion in Young Children
13. Quality Determinants of Mammography
14. Acute Low Back Problems in Adults
15. Treatment of Pressure Ulcers
16. Post-Stroke Rehabilitation
17. Cardiac Rehabilitation
18. Smoking Cessation
19. Alzheimer's Disease

Source: Reprinted from the Agency for Health Care Policy and Research, 1996.

reporting on the quality of managed care plans. Initiated in 1991, the NCQA's mission is to provide information to enable purchasers and consumers of managed health care to, based on quality, distinguish among plans, thereby promoting more informed decisions. NCQA has two major activities: (1) accreditation of managed health care plans and (2) establishment of standards and performance measures.

The accreditation process evaluates how well a health care plan manages all parts of its delivery systems—both providers (e.g., physicians and hospitals) and administrative services—to continuously improve health care for its members. The accreditation standards represent excellent business practice in six areas:

1. quality improvement: a focus on program structure and coordination, member access to care, and ability to demonstrate CQI
2. credentialing: physician credentials and performance; review of health care delivery organizations
3. members' rights and responsibilities: communications to members regarding access, physician selection, and complaint process; responsiveness to members; satisfaction surveys
4. preventive health services: encouragement and delivery of preventive care by physicians; the monitoring and improvement of preventive care as indicated
5. utilization management: reasonable and consistent process for determining appropriateness of individual health services; protection against underuse
6. medical records: consistent with NCQA standards for documentation (e.g., follow-up for abnormal lab results)

NCQA accreditation reviews are rigorous on-site and off-site evaluations. As of early 1996, NCQA had reviewed almost half of the nation's 574 health maintenance organizations.

Performance measures provide information that complements the accreditation. In August 1996, NCQA announced the establishment of *Quality Compass*, a database that includes comparative information for more than 200 managed care plans that cover approximately 18 million lives. The system includes accreditation status and lists scores for the indicators in the Health Plan Employer Data and Information Set (HEDIS). Performance measures, which meet purchaser and consumer needs for objective information, are focused on four key areas: (1) standard performance measurement set; (2) audit process for HEDIS data; (3) national database (*Quality Compass*); and (4) consumer research. The standard performance measures report on quality access and patient satisfaction, membership and use, and finance (NCQA, 1996; Ruth & Detmer, 1995). The NCQA leadership believes that the *Quality Compass* system will establish standards and be a catalyst for plans to be accountable to the purchasers and the public.

Moreover, the new system should benefit several groups. Consumers will be able to select a plan by reviewing comparative information from a single source. In addition, health plans will be aided in their quality improvement efforts by being able to compare their scores with regional and national averages. Benchmarks will provide data to approximate best practices. Employers will benefit from a single source authority. Employers require the managed care data for use in negotiating agreements. This national effort to establish standards for a large group of organizations is a new initiative in health care and has potential impact for the multiple professionals who work in the managed care environment.

PATIENTS AS PARTNERS IN QUALITY IMPROVEMENT PROGRAMS

Reflecting on the earlier definition that a standard of care is what the patient and his or her family or significant other can expect from the care provider, patients should be viewed as partners in the professionals' standards and the quality improvement program. "The concept of partnering of the patient and the provider in healthcare is one that is taking on new meaning" (Cramer & Tucker, 1995, p. 54). The role of the patient as a health care recipient has evolved into a partnership in which patients and providers share responsibility for the development of desired outcomes and the implementation of interventions. This dimension of the use of patient care standards depends on the care providers' commitment to include patients in the development of the standards that were previously the domain of professionals.

Clinical pathways can be an excellent vehicle for communicating the collaboration of patients and providers. Feedback from patients should be sought as pathways are developed. Communication and educational tools for the patient should be created from the patient's perspective. For example, at the Zablocki Veterans Affairs Medical Center in Milwaukee, Wisconsin, a clinical pathway for patients undergoing a total hip replacement was the initial pathway developed. The quality improvement team that developed the pathway included feedback from the veteran patients. The outcome of this feedback included an extensive revision of the preoperative and postoperative patient education program. A patient booklet was developed that paralleled the clinical pathway preadmission, during hospitalization, and postdischarge. The booklet was written in the language of what the patient should expect from nursing, occupational therapy, physical therapy, medical staff, and what the patient needed to do to participate to attain optimal outcome. The booklet has ample illustrations and instructions, such as for exercises. The patient receives the booklet and verbal education in the outpatient setting as soon as the decision for surgery is made. The quality improvement program included patient outcome measures.

BENCHMARKING

The quality improvement and management tool of benchmarking was initiated in industry in the late 1970s and is now being deployed in health care organizations. Camp (1989) has defined *benchmarking* as "the continuous process of measuring products, services, and practices against the toughest competitors or those companies recognized as industry leaders"(10). Benchmarking became increasingly recognized as a premier quality tool when it was included in the criteria for the Malcolm Baldrige National Quality Award. Health care organizations have often compared themselves with each other, but the recognition and use of benchmarking have added a significant dimension to the improvement of performance. When health care organizations use the tool of benchmarking, they measure, assess, and compare its practices, processes, and outcomes with other organizations that are considered comparable with them in scope of service or have been best recognized for best practices.

Benchmarking can be comparative or process (Patrick & Alba, 1994). In *comparative benchmarking*, an organization compares its performance with the performance of others by using performance measures and indicators. Benchmark studies are valuable for examining major care systems, product lines, products, and functions. Findings from benchmarking studies often serve as the catalyst for chartering a CQI team or some other mechanism to improve performance. *Process benchmarking* may start as a comparison of data but evolves into the evaluation of a process or processes. The evaluation of processes is necessary to recognize and identify the best practices. Health care organizations usually benchmark critical processes such as flow through an operating room or an outpatient diagnostic testing center. The success of benchmarking and improvement actions depends on leadership support, interdisciplinary collaboration, and a commitment to improve patient outcome, organizational processes, and practitioners' practice.

MALCOLM BALDRIGE NATIONAL QUALITY AWARD

During the 1980s, leaders in the United States believed that strategic planning for quality and quality improvement programs, through a commitment to excellence, was becoming increasingly essential to the well-being of the U.S. economy and our ability to compete effectively in the global marketplace. Initially, the criteria of the Malcolm Baldrige National Quality Award, signed into law in 1987, were written for and applied in industry. They were used to recognize achievements for a small number of industries. However, in 1995, it was recognized that the criteria should be adapted for health care and education. The award established guidelines and criteria for self- and external evaluation of an organization's quality improvement efforts. The criteria, grouped into seven categories (Exhibit 3–4), are now used to establish the framework for quality improvement within an organization.

CONCLUSION

Standards are the foundation for all monitoring and evaluation processes; they provide the basis on which the quality of patient care is judged and subsequently improved. Standards of practice, care, and performance must

- be consistent with national norms established for the profession
- be consistent with the indicators of quality and appropriate care
- be integrated with the findings of quality assessment
- be complementary to the expectations of regulatory and accreditation bodies
- be consistent with legal definitions of practice (e.g., professional practice acts such as the state nurse practice act)

Exhibit 3–4 Malcolm Baldrige National Quality Award

Core Values and Concepts
Customer-Driven Quality
Leadership
Continuous Improvement and Learning
Employee Participation and Development
Fast Response
Design Quality and Prevention
Long-Range View of the Future
Management by Fact
Partnership Development
Corporate Responsibility and Citizenship
Results Orientation

Criteria Categories
Leadership
Information and Analysis
Strategic Planning
Human Resource Development and Management
Process Management
Organizational Performance Results
Focus on and Satisfaction of Patients and Other Stakeholders

Source: Reprinted from Malcolm Baldrige National Quality Award Health Care Pilot Criteria, 1995, U.S. Department of Commerce.

- reflect the mission and philosophy of the organization, service, or program
- be achievable
- be measurable using well-defined criteria and indicators
- provide benchmarks for comparing data
- be understood, valued, and effectively integrated into daily patient care

Health care professionals have always been committed to evaluating the impact of the care provided on patient outcomes and to implementing change in care or performance when improvement warrants. Standards provide caregivers and professionals, patients and their families, health care organizations, payers of health care costs, and regulatory and accreditation agencies with information on which to formulate expectations regarding the quality of the health care services available to those who access the system.

REFERENCES

Agency for Health Care Policy and Research. (1996). *Clinical practice guidelines.* Rockville, MD: U.S. Department of Health and Human Services.

American Nurses Association. (1991). *Standards of clinical nursing practice.* Kansas City, MO: Author.

American Nurses Association. (1996). *Nursing's quality report card outcomes project.* Washington, DC: Author.

Camp, R.C. (1989). *Benchmarking: The search for industry best practices that lead to superior performance.* Milwaukee, WI: Quality Press.

Clinton, J.J. (1993). Agency for health care policy and research: Improving healthcare through guidelines and outcomes research. *Hospital Formulary,* (28), 933–934.

Cook, J. (1994). Clinical pathways improve organizational performance. *QRC Advisor, 10*(11), 1, 5–8.

Cramer, D., & Tucker, S.M. (1995). The consumer's role in quality: Partnering for quality outcomes. *Journal of Nursing Care Quality, 9*(2), 54–66.

Dean-Baer, S.L. (1993). Application of the new ANA framework for nursing practice standards and guidelines. *Journal of Nursing Care Quality, 8*(1), 33–44.

Disch, J.M. (1991). The role of professional organizations in establishing standards of practice and guidelines. In I.E. Goertzen (Ed.), *Differentiating nursing practice into the twenty-first century.* Kansas City: American Nurses Association Publications, American Academy of Nursing.

Joint Commission on Accreditation of Healthcare Organizations. (1997). *Accreditation manual for hospitals.* Oakbrook Terrace, IL: Author.

National Committee for Quality Assurance. (1996). *1996 Standards for Accreditation of Managed Care Organizations.* Washington, DC: Author.

Patrick, M., & Alba, T. (1994). Health care benchmarking: A team approach. *Quality Management in Health Care, 2*(2), 38–47.

Patton, M.D. (1993). Action research and the process of continual quality improvement in a cancer center. *Oncology Nursing Forum, 20*(5), 751–755.

Ruth, L.C., & Detmer, E.J. (1995, April–June). Assessing health plan quality. *Benefits Quarterly,* 32–36.

Spath, P.L. (1995). Path-based patient care should build quality into the process. *Journal of Healthcare Quality, 17*(6), 26–29.

Urban, N., Greenlee, K.K., Krumberger, J., & Winkelman, C. (1995). *Guidelines for critical care nursing.* St. Louis, MO: C.V. Mosby.

Warzynski, D. (1996, July). Nursing's quality report card outcomes project. *STAT Bulletin.*

## Chapter 4

Building a Quality Improvement Program around Patient Care

Claire G. Meisenheimer

CHAPTER OBJECTIVES

After completing this chapter, the reader will be able to

- describe the characteristics of a learning organization
- assess an organization's readiness for change
- compare quality assurance and quality improvement and draw the linkages between the two processes
- develop a QI plan around patient care

Changes occurring in the health care industry are substantive and constitute a paradigm shift in thinking and behaving. Moving from vertically organized hospitals and concern for *a* department or unit to horizontally organized, integrated health care systems with accountability for cost-effective, patient care outcomes across the continuum of health care requires commitment, flexibility, speed, and a thorough understanding of the momentum that is driving the health care industry. This new way of thinking and behaving requires a "learning organization," that is, leaders with a vision of the continual development of the organization, its people, its capabilities, and its capacity to enhance or to create its own future.

LEARNING ORGANIZATIONS

A learning organization is on a continual mission with

- a strong sense of shared vision ("co-authored" by people at the top and on the front lines who are able to articulate their actual work contribution toward the same goal)
- people who are open to new ideas and perspectives and valued for their opinions (legitimate disagreements can be shared)
- a genuine sense of curiosity that is congruent and diffused throughout the organization
- an ability to produce extraordinary results (a natural byproduct of learning)

Learning organizations delve into the hard work of surfacing the deep-rooted assumptions about how they organize and how the work gets done, hence challenging the existing culture (Flower, 1996).

Two complementary methods of advancing learning in an organization are total quality management (TQM) and systems thinking. The value of TQM, a philosophical approach to participatory management, is in operational learning—the methods, tools, and processes that can be used to examine the complexity of a problem or issue needing improvement. Systems thinking promotes a larger, whole system perspective of the interconnectedness of an issue with other parts of a system. These two methods are required if an organization intends to make the transformation from the traditional quality assurance (QA) driven by accreditation and regulatory requirements to reorganizing quality management around patient care, resulting in cross-functional, clinical, and operational processes that are integrated and work seamlessly across the system.

A successful quality improvement (QI) program is flexible, effective, and efficient in monitoring and improving patient care and professional practice. The design of such a program demands fundamental and sweeping changes in existing philosophies and work processes. It requires a well conceived *vision* of an organization's expected future before the organization systematically plans well-defined goals and objectives, assesses existing activities, and develops an integrated quality process that will successfully improve operations and performance consistent with the needs and expectations of consumers, professionals, and regulatory, accrediting, and reimbursement bodies. The QI program recognizes that quality, cost, and access are interrelated and are included in the strategic planning process.

STRATEGIC PLANNING: BUILDING A QI PROGRAM AROUND PATIENT CARE

Although strategic planning and a QI program are not synonymous, they are intimately linked. Leaders in an organization who are developing the strategic plan must also be involved with the Quality Improvement Council. These leaders are responsible for changing an organization's strategic and operational systems to match the new QI structure. Quality must be incorporated into the organization's overall vision and mission statements; a separate statement regarding quality is perceived as an add-on program and not part of daily work.

Planning a QI program requires knowledge of what constitutes quality and time to process the implications so that organizational and professional prerogatives can be balanced. As consumers both internal and external to the organization place added value and emphasis on quality issues, an effective strategic vision must go beyond just understanding quality

concepts to believing in the absolute necessity for continually improving. Dual directionality must be evident in a QI program; governing boards and top management must "live" the philosophy of TQM from the top down; every other member of the organization must believe and participate from the bottom up. TQM focuses on internal and external consumers and requires a continuous quality improvement (CQI) "mentality" in the total process of providing patient care.

In building the concept of quality into every aspect of an organization's business, day-to-day work meshes with strategic planning; strategic quality planning takes traditional QA and the need for measurement and integrates QA with CQI. Although QA and QI are not synonymous, the relationship is symbiotic. The measurement of quality is one step in the QI process; monitoring quality of care and performance indicators that suggest potential problems may exist should result in recommendations for improving care and performance. QA programs should be incorporated into the structure of the organization's QI program. QI supports and enhances the measurement of key clinical processes and outcomes (QA); it also includes financial and other operational data and works in concert with strategic planning and other sources to improve the overall quality of patient care (Day, Gardner, & Herba, 1995). Exhibit 4–1 compares and contrasts some of the similarities and differences between QA and QI.

ASSESSING AN EXISTING QUALITY PROGRAM: READINESS FOR CHANGE

To survive the global rapid changes, organizations must constantly rethink their assumptions about society, the community of customers, their values and mission, their core competencies, their competitors, their markets, technology, and their strengths and weaknesses. Their theory of business must mirror current

Exhibit 4–1 Comparing QA and QI

QUALITY ASSURANCE	QUALITY IMPROVEMENT
Is coordinator/committee driven	Has prepared leaders; is management/"team" driven; has QI Council support; everyone is accountable
Is problem and people focused	Is processes and systems focused
Is reactive; inspects for quality; quality costs not emphasized	Is proactive; builds in quality up front; quality costs are emphasized
Has limited customer input; has regulatory compliance	Is customer driven: internal, external
Is monitoring and measurement driven; has unit-based and multidisciplinary QA committees	Has involved/knowledgeable "teams"; has cross-functional teams
Identifies scope and aspects of care	Has defined QI initiative (precedes organizing a "team")
Establishes indicators and thresholds	Establishes indicators; clarifies current knowledge of QI initiative and process
Focuses on "outliers," special causes, provider or practitioner	Theorizes reasons for defects in the system; strives for improvement by reducing common causes
Monitors care by collecting and organizing data for each indicator; rudimentarily uses statistical methods	Goes beyond collecting data for each indicator; uncovers root causes of variation; considers/implements solutions; collects data; uses analytical and statistical process control tools (SPC)
Evaluates care against thresholds; identifies areas to improve	Compares data with theory; benchmarks/ identifies "best practices"; addresses resistance to change
Takes action to improve care	Implements solutions to improve care/ systems
Assesses effectiveness of actions; documents improvement	Assesses effectiveness of system; checks performance and lessons learned
Communicates results	Communicates results; monitors control system (acts to hold gain); continues to improve system

reality. Acknowledging the many approaches to CQI, O'Brien et al. (1995) stated that all organizations share the premise that producing high quality requires leaders who are committed to and involved in improvement efforts, frontline employees who are empowered to identify and solve quality problems, and caregivers who are trained in CQI methods.

The challenges of CQI activities arise from the interplay of dynamic processes that can be framed in relation to four dimensions: technical, cultural, strategic, and structural. The *technical dimensions* include training in CQI techniques and tools, data collection and analysis, decision making, and a comprehensive understanding of how daily work is produced and delivered. The *cultural dimension* involves the beliefs, values, norms, and behaviors exhibited in everyday work, which demonstrate a commitment to a shared purpose—patient care, teamwork, and cooperation in formal and informal social interactions and in the systems used to reward performance. The *strategic dimension* links the organization's key strategic priorities—core clinical and administrative processes, competencies, and capabilities—and its CQI efforts. The *structural dimension* encompasses the specific organizational structures and systems, such as committee structures, information systems for data gathering and analysis, and mechanisms for promoting continuous learning (O'Brien et al., 1995).

Quality activities exist in every organization, department, or service. However, the comprehensiveness of a program, its effectiveness, and its efficiency need to be periodically reviewed and evaluated. The availability, acceptability, and appropriateness of staff, facilities, and support need analysis. The concept of quality assessment/assurance (QAA), that is, the measurement of the level of care provided and the mechanisms to improve it, must be clearly and personally defined, implemented, and evaluated. Drucker (1995) noted that assessing the QI program will help prevent organizations from becoming complacent with the status quo, from not fostering opportunities for innovation and misappropriating human resources.

Although the assessment analysis of a program may take many forms, several questions must be answered when examining the program's purpose, scope, and effectiveness in fostering the approach to continually improving quality.

- Are the leaders in the organization intimately involved in the quality program (i.e., are leaders members of the QI Council or cross-functional teams)?
- Is there a clearly written QI plan beginning with a succinctly articulated vision statement?
- Based on the vision statement, does the stated philosophy or mission drive comprehensive, realistic, measurable, and achievable goals and objectives within available resources?
- Do the philosophy and mission statements meet all of the requirements of various internal and external review bodies (i.e., consumers, professional organizations, accrediting agencies, and state and national governments)?
- Does the program articulate systems thinking, a complete cycle that begins with problem identification and promotes sustained problem resolution with continuous improvement?
- Are all resources and support systems appropriately coordinated and used?
- Are roles and responsibilities defined in terms of integrated strategies and quality related goals (i.e., are authority, accountability, and confidentiality clearly designated)?
- Does the patient care or support system of concern need to be reengineered from scratch, or can it be redesigned and improved through incremental change (CQI)?
- What program strengths can be enhanced?
- What program weaknesses require improvements?

Human attitudes and perceptions make or break an organization's efforts to improve quality. Although a program may include all the technical elements, its effectiveness and efficiency can be limited by misunderstanding and lack of true involvement and commitment. When conducted anonymously, an assessment tool such as that shown in Exhibit 4–2 may more honestly reveal hidden rejection or minimal or full support regarding CQI. A tool, designed to elicit a yes/no response with an expectation for comments, should be distributed to all people in the organization and to critical and involved external consumers for education regarding the intent of the QI program as well as for assessment purposes.

Everyone owns the organization's QI program. By challenging the current processes, everyone becomes involved, not just as part of the problem, but as part of the solution. Understanding the intent of the QI program is essential to setting priorities consistent with the strategic plan and the organization's core functions and processes.

The aggregate data will identify perceptions of purpose and scope of program, activities that are performed effectively, and those requiring strengthening. Perceptions of overlap in authority and responsibility, duplication in efforts, and approaches for enhancing integration and coordination of activities can provide valuable opportunities for clarification and education. An assessment of "what exists" will provide the basis for designing a well-defined, comprehensively organized QI plan to objectively measure and improve patient care and professional practice.

DESIGNING A QI PROGRAM

When key leaders in an organization are educated in the principles of TQM and CQI, and managers and all employees become comfortable with the team approach to studying opportunities for improvement, quality becomes an integrated way of managing. The acceptance that the goal of quality programs is to continually improve processes, products, and services is critical; avoid finger-pointing and the "bad apple" syndrome. Avoid useless and meaningless jargon! The language used to reflect that commitment is important only to the degree that it has meaning for everyone involved. Whether TQM, CQI, QI, QA, QAA, quality resource management (QRM), or some other term or acronym is used to reflect an organization's commitment to its internal customers (i.e., all employees) and external customers (e.g., patients, physicians, members of the business community, accrediting and other review bodies, third-party payers) to continually examine processes for the purpose of improving is of less importance than achieving consensus so that all individuals are committed and willing to expend the time, energy, and resources necessary to provide a system of accountability. For purposes of this chapter, the term *quality improvement* (QI), with occasional variation, will be used. Readers should take the opportunity to insert terms that may have greater meaning for them and their colleagues.

Assuming that every process can be improved, there is a shared responsibility by all employees to build quality into every service; no one person, department, or discipline alone is responsible. Although traditional quality activities have been perceived primarily as an oversight concept designed to enhance public accountability, a comprehensive, integrated QI program will always require *professional clinical judgment* as well as the *consumer's perception* of care or a service to successfully improve operations and performance by removing waste and unpredictability, and to comply with regulatory, accrediting, and payer entities.

Adopting CQI methods as the foundation of a solid, ongoing quality program requires a long-term commitment; the process is evolutionary, time-consuming, and requires significant resources. A passion for improving quality and a change in culture may not really occur for 1, 3, 5, or even 10 years. Information alone, knowing the jargon, and a desire to "do good"

Exhibit 4–2 QI Program Assessment

Dear Members of the _____ Organization/Agency:

Your input is critical in assessing our *current* quality improvement plan. As you know, quality improvement—the ongoing measurement of key processes and outcomes, in conjunction with strategic planning and other sources to improve clinical and administrative performance—is only as effective as we make it.

Please place an X in the Yes/No columns *with* explanations or suggestions of **who, what, where, how, and/or when** in the Comments column.

	Yes	No	Comments
A. Does our organization's culture: 　1. demonstrate commitment from leaders and foster our vision?			
2. exhibit transformational leadership by using systems thinking and processes and shared governance behaviors throughout the organization?			
3. promote total quality management (TQM) in our "customer-driven" strategic planning?			
4. emphasize continuous quality improvement (CQI) as a key value in our philosophy/mission, goals, and objectives?			
5. create a constancy of purpose in aligning our philosophy/mission statement, goals, and objectives with services and programs?			
6. link all quality initiatives with the strategic plan, budget, policies, and procedures? (Are quality efforts integral or parallel to the daily workings of the organization?)			
7. value the uniqueness and contributions of all individuals in the organization; all are treated equally?			
8. support an integrated network with a cross-functional team approach; go beyond the traditional boundaries in learning to build patient-centered integrated models of care vs. professional-centered models of care?			

continues

Exhibit 4–2 continued

	Yes	No	Comments
9. provide a human resources program that supports interdependent team-work and a customer focus on the basis of the performance evaluation and compensation system?			
10. value learning and risk-taking with adequate resources?			
11. provide adequate human and technical resources to define, capture, statistically analyze, and report useful, understandable data?			
12. communicate how best practice strategies and benchmarking significantly impact our competitive strategies?			
13. encourage replicating internal and external successful practices across the organization to accelerate the rate of improvement?			
14. understand the culture of our competitors; suppliers?			
B. Does our quality improvement (QI) plan:			
15. use an understandable framework (i.e., Juran's Trilogy, Deming, Systems, Donabedian)?			
16. state our quality vision?			
17. clearly define our goals that stretch us, with achievable objectives?			
18. outline our program's scope of care and services?			
19. identify person(s) or position(s) responsible for coordinating/facilitating the program?			
20. describe our QI Council: purpose, functions, membership, roles?			
21. address the issue of responsibility and authority?			
22. delineate lines of communication including reporting mechanisms?			
23. address confidentiality?			

continues

Exhibit 4–2 continued

	Yes	No	Comments
24. delineate the approach to measuring dimensions of performance related to functions, processes, and outcomes?			
25. include a plan for periodic evaluation?			
C. As a result of *our* QI efforts, do *you* think:			
26. *all* employees support and can articulate our organization's core values and culture?			
27. *all* employees can describe the CQI process and how it is working?			
28. we use QI language appropriately (no meaningless jargon/buzzwords)?			
29. we appropriately use standards established by:			
a. professional organizations?			
b. Joint Commission on Accreditation of Healthcare Organizations, National Committee for Quality Assurance, National League for Nursing Community Health Accreditation Program, and other voluntary accrediting bodies?			
c. state and/or federal government (i.e., Medicare, Medicaid, Agency for Health Care Policy and Research, etc.)			
30. care plans, clinical guidelines, and caremaps are written and used well across the continuum of services?			
31. "critical processes" are known and continuously improved?			
32. *you* have assumed greater ownership of the work structures and the CQI processes (more self-motivated, self-managed, patient focused vs. professionally self-focused); (feeling empowered)?			
33. *your* practice has improved, including patient outcomes?			

continues

Exhibit 4–2 continued

	Yes	No	Comments
34. ways to document patient care, including patient/family involvement, have improved?			
35. we have eliminated professional and service organizational barriers/ boundaries to achieve the necessary integrated work processes?			
36. staff performance appraisals are linked to job descriptions, expected competencies, and realistic performance outcomes?			
37. we competently ensure patient and staff safety including reducing the risk of infection?			
38. patient and family education has been enhanced, fostering relevant and improved outcomes?			
39. internal and external customer satisfaction has increased; needs and expectations are met?			
40. we use our QI program to improve clinical and administrative performance and to minimize costs and other resource consumption?			
41. risks of litigation for our organization have decreased?			
42. we value learning and self-development: orientation, continuing education, and competency systems work well?			
43. we use our QI data as a marketing strategy?			
44. your involvement with state, federal, and voluntary surveyors/accreditors has been helpful to our QI efforts?			
45. we evaluate our performance improvement requirements, successes, and "lessons learned" (at least) on an annual basis?			

D. Additional Comments:

_____

Name and Service (Optional)

will not automatically bring about immediate change. A learning culture in which risk and pilot projects are expected and supported takes time to evolve. A cultural change within the organization requires a philosophy and policy change that communicates commitment and direction to employees and external customers.

Vision

The Joint Commission on Accreditation of Healthcare Organizations (Joint Commission) (1996) has emphasized that the role of leader involves clinical leaders and staff managers as well as the governing body, chief executive officer, and other senior managers. Together, this body must develop a vision that

- is based on an organization's core business—why we exist
- is brief, succinct, tied to individual motivation, stretching but achievable, and is explicit in the mission statement
- drives the organization's mission and goals—where are we, where do we want to go
- addresses internal and external consumer's needs and expectations
- respects everyone's knowledge and contribution to the CQI process
- eliminates barriers between services and disciplines to enhance team building and promote communication and uses a scientific approach to problem solving
- requires ongoing education and training
- expects performance measures consistent with organizational and professional goals
- requires quality to be built into the process, which reduces process variation and emphasizes prevention rather than inspection

The organization's culture as reflected in its mission statement encourages employees to be proactive and outcome oriented, identifying the outcome and working backward through structure and processes that increase efficiency, productivity, and profitability. As described by Day et al. (1995, p. 22), the mission statement of a fully integrated system guides the organization's activities relating to

- people: the creation of an environment that attracts, retains, and supports the development of people who share the organization's values and culture
- customers: clear evidence that service is of demonstrated value for patients, families, physicians, payers, and purchasers
- community: improvement of the health status of the communities the organization serves
- system integration: positioning the organization to be successful in the changing health care industry
- finances: increasing the organization's financial strength

Goals/Objectives

All quality activities support the accomplishment of goals, which are stated in relatively broad but measurable terms, address rights of patients to maximum health care, reduce liability, and expect proper use of resources by competent practitioners. The statement of purpose in the QI plan may incorporate these goals.

Objectives, derived from the program's goals and written in specific, measurable terms, are related to the eventual achievement of the goals. Objectives may address the achievement of an optimum level of care in a cost-effective and safe manner, compliance with specific standards governing practice, methodologies used, and integration with other processes and programs. Goals and objectives may periodically change. New ones are set as old ones are achieved or become inappropriate as the organization assumes new directions.

Once goals and objectives are established for the organization's QI program, each discipline, service, or product can determine its unique methods and approaches to achieving the overall goals and objectives, recognizing the needed interrelatedness with others to serve and improve the outcomes for their populations. Program goals and objectives provide the concrete basis for evaluating the status of all existing quality activities as well as providing a foundation for future quality initiatives. Such initiatives will be implemented through strategic quality planning, quality assurance/quality control, and other QI improvements, using a consistent methodology such as Shewhart-Deming's Plan–Do–Check–Act (PDCA); the Hospital Corporation of America FOCUS-PDCA, which added to the Shewhart-Deming cycle; Juran's Triology: quality planning, quality control/quality assurance, and QI (Juran, 1988); Donabedian's (1980) structure, process, outcome model; or another methodology that provides a useful QI framework. Exhibit 4–3 provides a modified synopsis of various quality gurus' principles.

Standards

Because each health care organization is different in purpose, size, and resources, its QI program should reflect its uniqueness. It should use the data gathered from an extensive assessment, as well as the appropriate standards and suggested formats established by various review bodies, including the Joint Commission; the National Committee for Quality Assurance (NCQA); professional organizations such as the National League for Nursing Community Health Accreditation Program and "Benchmarks for Excellence in Home Care"; and governmental groups such as Medicare (OASIS) and Medicaid (the NCQA Health Plan Employer Data and Information Set [HEDIS 3.0]), or other applicable standards. The National Library of Healthcare Indicators (NLHI) has been developed by the Joint Commission to complement the measures developed by the Agency for Health Care Policy and Research (AHCPR) and its recently established indicator typology initiative known as CONQUEST (a computerized needs-oriented quality measurement evaluation system); NLHI

is focused on supporting QI activities in relation to the accreditation process (Loeb, 1996).

In addition to the preceding standards, the Malcolm Baldrige National Quality Award is given to organizations that best exemplify QI that has had a sustained impact. The International Standards Organization (ISO) has produced the ISO 9000 and ISO 14001 series of quality management and quality assurance standards. These standards apply to any organization doing business in the international market. Business and industry are examining organization performance in the areas of customer satisfaction, market share and profitability, quality and cost, and employee relations. Thus, these organizations are expecting the same scrutiny of health care organizations.

The QI Plan

As multiple organizations integrate, a quality (performance) improvement plan such as shown in Exhibit 4–4 and a communication flowchart (Figure 4–1) should evolve with the following components supporting a collaborative program to promote high-quality and efficient care for the welfare of its patients and the community:

- vision statement, purpose
- plan goals and objectives
- organizational structure
- dimensions of performance
- roles and responsibilities
- approaches and methodologies
- communication patterns
- confidentiality
- transition of medical staff, other members of the organization
- evaluation

Other tools that may be useful to facilitate members of the organization to provide and receive information in an organized and consistent manner include the following:

Exhibit 4–5: Proposed Quality Improvement Activity

Exhibit 4–3 Overview of Quality Gurus

Deming's 14 Points

1. Create consistency of purpose.
2. Adopt the new philosophy.
3. Cease dependence on inspection.
4. End the practice of awarding business on the basis of price alone.
5. Improve constantly.
6. Institute training/retraining on the job.
7. Institute leadership for system improvement.
8. Drive out fear.
9. Break down barriers between departments/programs.
10. Eliminate arbitrary quotas, slogans without providing resources.
11. Eliminate work standards (quotas) for management.
12. Remove barriers to pride of workmanship.
13. Institute education and self-improvement for everyone.
14. Transform everyone's job, the organization.

Crosby's 14 Steps

1. Management commitment
2. QI team
3. Quality measurement
4. Cost of quality evaluation
5. Quality awareness
6. Correction action
7. Ad hoc committee for zero defect planning
8. Supervisory training
9. Zero defects day
10. Goal-setting
11. Error/cause removal
12. Recognition
13. Quality councils
14. Do it over again

Donabedian's Model

• Structure
• Process
• Outcome

Juran Trilogy

I. Quality Planning
   1. Determine current/future customers.
   2. Determine customers' needs.
   3. Enable team.
   4. Develop service to meet needs.
   5. Develop processes to deliver service.
   6. Transfer new process to operation.
II. Quality Control/Quality Assurance
   1. Measure performance.
   2. Compare actual performance to goals/benchmarks.
   3. Reduce undesired variation.
III. Quality Improvement
   1. Identify needed improvement projects.
   2. Establish project teams.
   3. Provide teams with
      • resources
      • motivation
      • training
      to determine causes, stimulate solutions, establish standards, and hold gains.
   4. Identify opportunities to replicate the remedy.

Source: Adapted from *Out of the Crisis* by W. Edwards Deming by permission of MIT and The W. Edwards Deming Institute. Published by MIT, Center for Advanced Educational Services, Cambridge, MA 02139. Copyright 1986 by W. Edwards Deming; Adapted with the permission of The Free Press, a division of Simon & Schuster from JURAN ON PLANNING FOR QUALITY by J.M. Juran. Copyright 1988 by Juran Institute, Inc.; Adapted from Crosby, 1979.

Exhibit 4–4 Community Hospitals of Central California (CHCC) Performance Improvement Plan

CHCC Hospitals of Central California
Performance Improvement Plan
1995

Executive Summary

Community Hospitals of Central California (CHCC) is a not-for-profit institution dedicated to improving the health status of the CHCC we serve.

CHCC has implemented a Shared Governance organizational structure which is committed to **continuous quality improvement** (CPI). It is our belief that continuous improvement is achieved in a culture driven by a commitment to consistently meet or exceed our customers' expectations **while documenting better outcomes**. We have begun the transition from Quality Assurance (monitoring competency and consistency) to Continuous Quality Improvement, which is process oriented. Our goal is to achieve Performance Improvement, which is a systems oriented model that creates "best practice" by improving outcomes. (Diagram 1)

The following goals have been established to integrate the **Continuous Improvement Plan** through our health system:

- Educate leadership and staff at point of service on performance improvement process.
- Utilize Shared Governance Model to identify multidisciplinary stakeholders in performance improvement activities.
- Implement the Performance Improvement Process: Six Step Model.
- Develop and implement Patient Care Protocols to improve clinical outcomes.
- Utilize aggregated data to assess, follow up, and improve system or quality performance.

Plan for Quality

CHCC commitment to quality is evidenced in our Mission House:

Diagram 1

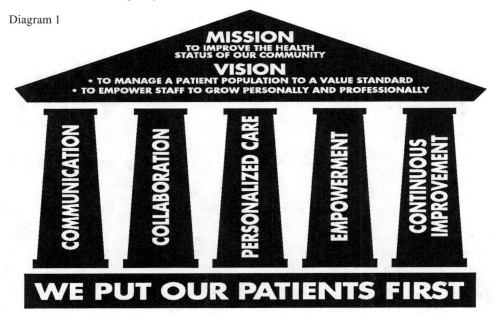

continues

Exhibit 4–4 continued

To achieve our corporate mission and vision, **CHCC** identifies the pillars to support the foundation of all activity. . . . **"We put our patients first."** Exceptional customer service is the core value. To communicate this to all members of the team, there is a basic philosophy, which states, "We are caring professionals serving every person we meet with compassion and respect."

This is accomplished through:

- **Communication**: Information is truly a shared resource for all members of the organization.
- **Collaboration**: CHCC is part of a larger network of systems, services, and facilities that collaboratively supports the mission of improving the health status of our community.
- **Personalized Care**: Personalized patient care services at CHCC are provided in a caring environment by multidisciplinary, self-directed teams.
- **Empowerment**: To create an environment that encourages individuals to acquire the tools, skills sets, and emotional freedom and results in a sense of satisfaction at the point of service so that the highest quality of service will be achieved.
- **Continuous Improvement**: Continuous improvement of outcomes begins with individual accountability. The people of **CHCC** are internally motivated to pursue lifelong learning and the leadership fosters an environment for achieving personal growth and accountability, allowing employees to tap into higher purpose.

CHCC Cascade
MISSION: To Improve the Health Status of Our Community

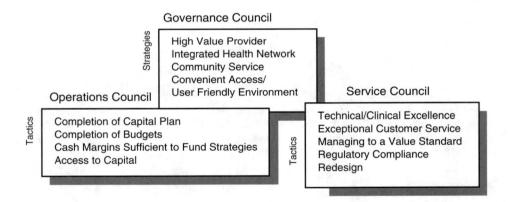

In an effort to meet **CHCC's** mission, the organization has developed an Outcome Matrix Model referred to as the **"Cascade."** This is the method for showing the connection of all work done in the system to the originating tactics, strategies, and ultimately back to the mission and vision. The Governance Council translates the vision and strategies as approved by the Board of Directors and communicates them back to the other councils as strategic outcomes and indicators. Operations and Service Council then develop tactics based on strategic needs and ideal care delivery. Pathways then develops process/function outcomes, statements, indicators, and implementation plans. The cascade in reverse is the reporting mechanism and the way progress is tracked by Councils (Diagram 2, detail Cascade).

continues

Exhibit 4–4 continued

Diagram 2—CHCC Cascade: Translating the Mission and Vision to the Point of Service

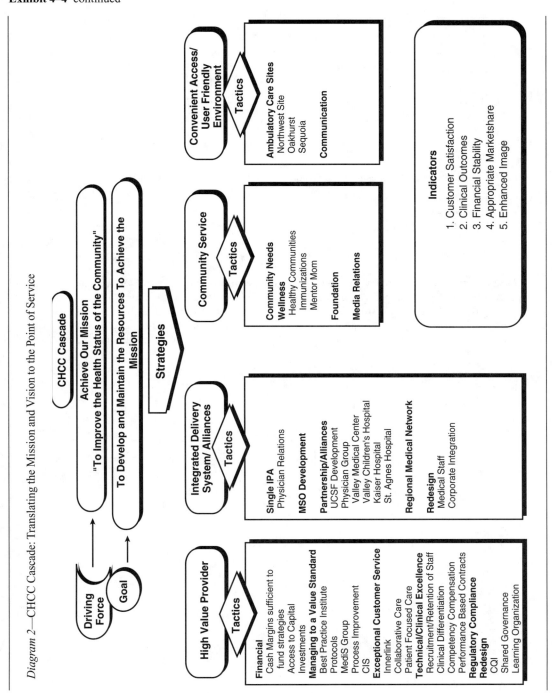

CHCC Cascade

Driving Force

Goal

Achieve Our Mission
"To Improve the Health Status of the Community"

To Develop and Maintain the Resources To Achieve the Mission

Strategies

Convenient Access/User Friendly Environment

Tactics

Ambulatory Care Sites
Northwest Site
Oakhurst
Sequoia

Communication

Community Service

Tactics

Community Needs
Wellness
Healthy Communities
Immunizations
Mentor Mom

Foundation

Media Relations

Integrated Delivery System/ Alliances

Tactics

Single IPA
Physician Relations

MSO Development

Partnership/Alliances
UCSF Development
Physician Group
Valley Medical Center
Valley Children's Hospital
Kaiser Hospital
St. Agnes Hospital

Regional Medical Network

Redesign
Medical Staff
Corporate Integration

High Value Provider

Tactics

Financial
Cash Margins sufficient to fund strategies
Access to Capital
Investments
Managing to a Value Standard
Best Practice Institute
Protocols
MediS Group
Process Improvement
CIS
Exceptional Customer Service
Innerlink
Collaborative Care
Patient Focused Care
Technical/Clinical Excellence
Recruitment/Retention of Staff
Clinical Differentiation
Competency Compensation
Performance Based Contracts
Regulatory Compliance
Redesign
CQI
Shared Governance
Learning Organization

Indicators
1. Customer Satisfaction
2. Clinical Outcomes
3. Financial Stability
4. Appropriate Marketshare
5. Enhanced Image

continues

Exhibit 4–4 continued

Governance has established five indicators and prioritized them to provide context for decision making and CPI activities. The indicators are:

- **Customer Service**
- **Clinical Outcomes**
- **Financial Stability**
- **Appropriate Market Share**
- **Enhanced Image**

A. Organization Structure:

In May 1994, a corporate redesign plan was outlined with the following conceptual cornerstones:

- **Shared Governance**
- **Collaborative Care**
- **Individualized/Patient Focused Care**

1. Shared Governance

The goal was to radically redesign to gain major improvements in quality and service while creating a product that was cost competitive for the current marketplace and into the future. The patient is the center focus for all activities. (Structure and Design: Organization Charts)

Shared Governance is an organizational model that encourages the majority of decisions to be made at the point of service and builds a structure that supports accountability in the decision maker. There are three corporate councils:

- **a. Governance**
- **b. Service**
- **c. Operations**

continues

Exhibit 4–4 continued

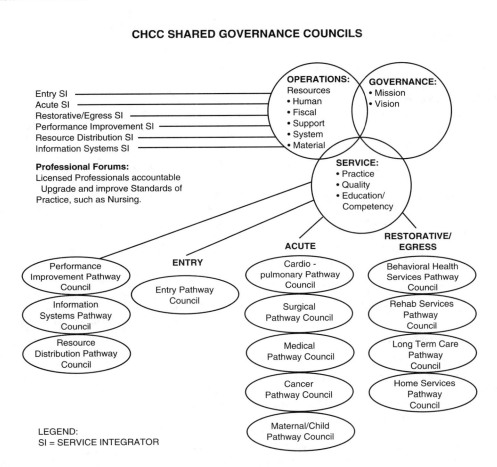

CHCC SHARED GOVERNANCE COUNCILS

Entry SI
Acute SI
Restorative/Egress SI
Performance Improvement SI
Resource Distribution SI
Information Systems SI

OPERATIONS:
Resources
• Human
• Fiscal
• Support
• System
• Material

GOVERNANCE:
• Mission
• Vision

Professional Forums:
Licensed Professionals accountable
Upgrade and improve Standards of
Practice, such as Nursing.

SERVICE:
• Practice
• Quality
• Education/
 Competency

**RESTORATIVE/
EGRESS**

ACUTE

ENTRY

Performance
Improvement Pathway
Council

Entry Pathway
Council

Cardio -
pulmonary Pathway
Council

Behavioral Health
Services Pathway
Council

Information
Systems Pathway
Council

Surgical
Pathway Council

Rehab Services
Pathway
Council

Resource
Distribution Pathway
Council

Medical
Pathway Council

Long Term Care
Pathway
Council

Cancer
Pathway Council

Home Services
Pathway
Council

Maternal/Child
Pathway Council

LEGEND:
SI = SERVICE INTEGRATOR

a. Governance Council

The Governance Council defines the Mission and Vision and translates that into strategic directives for the corporation.

> **Mission: To Improve the Health Status of our CHCC.**
>
> **Vision: To manage a patient population to a value standard.**
> **To empower staff to grow personally and professionally.**

Definition of Quality

The Governance Council has defined the term **"Value Standard"** in the **CHCC** Model of Care to mean a series of cost, quality service, and time standards that are organized by patient care protocols and ambulatory care practice parameters into a value standard system.

continues

Exhibit 4–4 continued

$$\text{Value} = \frac{\text{Quality}}{\text{Cost}} \times \frac{\text{Service}}{\text{Time}}$$

b. Service Council
Accountability for Quality

I. Patient Care Services

  a. There is a definition of the scope of patient care services.

  b. The professional goals and objectives of patient care/services are defined within the resources available.

  c. There is a conceptual framework for professional practice in **CHCC** that is the Innerlink model, which is based upon a multidisciplinary approach to patient focused care, whole system shared governance, CPI, and collaborative care.

  d. There is a defined delivery care model within the context of resources available.

  e. There are established Standards of Practice, Standards of Care, and Patient Care Protocols, which provide a foundation for quality of care.

  f. There is a mechanism to define and evaluate staff accountabilities to reflect changing roles, responsibilities, values, resources, and expectations.

  g. There is an effective clinical information system for recording and evaluation of patient care.

  h. There is a mechanism that promotes and ensures multidisciplinary relationships in patient care.

II. Quality/Performance Improvement

  A. There is a planned, systematic, organization-wide mechanism that designs, measures, assesses, and improves the quality of patient care and organizational functions.

    1. **Design**

      a. will integrate all systems Performance Improvement Plans

      b. will be based on:

        (1) Organization's Mission, Vision, and Plans

        (2) needs and expectations of patients, staff, and others;

        (3) up-to-date sources of information about designing processes; and

        (4) the performance of the processes and their outcomes in other organizations

    2. **Measurement**

      a. will include collection of data needed to assess functions, processes, performance, and outcomes.

      b. will determine whether implemented changes improve the process

    3. **Assessment**

      a. will determine the level of performance and the priorities for improvement throughout the system and,

      b. will determine actions to improve performance and whether changes implemented resulted in improvement.

    4. **Improvement**

      a. The mechanism ensures systematic improvement in the performance of existing processes and outcomes.

continues

Exhibit 4–4 continued

B. There is a mechanism to measure and maintain competency by:
1. monitoring staff through credentialing, privileging, use of performance standards and performance-based/outcome-based evaluations. (Benner Model)
2. a mechanism that reflects multidisciplinary clinical practice guidelines (patient care protocols) that evaluate the relationship between the team processes and its outcome.
3. competency based compensation

III. Education/Research

A. There is a commitment to be a Learning Organization.
1. It will promote continuing staff education.
2. It will identify and prioritize learning needs.
3. It will integrate and coordinate services based education programs with goals and objectives to promote role competency.
4. It will evaluate the plan and the effectiveness of the programs.
5. It will identify available resources.
B. There will be effective communication through the pathways.
C. There is a system that defines the relationship between the service pathway and academic institutions.
D. There is a system that supports research.

c. Operations Council

It is the accountability of our operations council to provide the linkage between Service & Governance as it relates to **Fiscal Resources** by:

1. Development of annual operating budget to ensure access to capital to fund strategies.
2. Review performance against budget.
3. Review resources available to provide care and meet patient needs.

Operations Council has accountabilities in functional issues of Service integration such as:

Material Resources
Human Resources
Support to Staff
System Management

2. Collaborative Care

This is a patient empowerment model whose focused goal is to demystify, humanize, personalize, and deinstitutionalize the hospital experience. This is accomplished through:

- Supportive environment that fosters compassion and comfort
- Home-like surroundings that nurture and heal
- Choice and personal control
- Access to information
- Entertainment and the healing arts

continues

Exhibit 4–4 continued

3. Individualized/Patient Focused Care

The basic principles of Patient Focused Care is that the system, roles, functions, and processes are designed around the needs of the patient. **CHCC** has implemented unique systems to achieve this mission.

- Partner Model
- Multidisciplinary practices
- Unit based disciplines
- Environmental/architectural design

B. Critical Organization-Wide Functions

1. **Corporate Quality Initiatives: CHCC** has identified two major organization-wide initiatives, **Patient & Family Education** and **Pain Management**. These are critical issues addressed at the point of service to attend to the needs of all our patients.
2. **CHCC** has identified the following organization-wide functions as most important to the delivery of patient care services and to patient outcomes.
Patient Focused Functions

   * Patient Rights and Organizations Ethics
   * Assessment of Patients
   * Care of Patients
   * Education
   * Continuum of Care

Organizational Functions

   * Improving Organizational Performance
   * Leadership
   * Management of the Environment of Care
   * Management of Human Resources
   * Management of Information
   * Surveillance, Prevention, and Control of Infection

3. Dimensions of Performance

The organization-wide functions shall be measured and assessed in terms of the appropriate dimensions of performance. Processes involved in the continuous improvement of these functions may include those related to governance, leadership, clinical and/or support activities.

- **Efficacy**—the degree in which care of the patient has shown to accomplish desired or expected outcomes.
- **Appropriateness**—relevant care for the clinical needs of the patient.
- **Availability**—appropriate care is available and given to meet the specific needs of the patient.
- **Timeliness**—the degree to which care is provided to the patient at the most beneficial or necessary time.
- **Effectiveness**—the degree to which care is provided in the most appropriate manner, given the current state of knowledge, to achieve the desires or expected outcomes.
- **Continuity of service/practitioners and providers**—the degree to which care is coordinated and consistent through the organization following patient care protocols.
- **Safety**—the degree to which intervention and environmental risks are minimized for patients, partners, physicians, and others.

continues

Exhibit 4–4 continued

- **Efficiency**—relationship between outcomes and resources to deliver quality patient care. Achieving the Value Standard established.
- **Respect and Caring**—the degree to which the patient is involved and empowered with his or her own care (Collaborative Care Model). Care providers are sensitive to the individualized needs of each patient and service is provided with respect, caring, and dignity.

4. Pathways

At the point of service, there is a process for analyzing and assessing the effectiveness of performance improvement. Additionally, there is a mechanism for the deliberation of conflicts between systems, services, cost, or providers affecting the achievement of the mission. **CHCC** has identified critical success factors through the pathways. The success factors and examples of measurements are:

Work Environment
Cost Efficiency
Quality/Clinical Outcomes
Service Efficiency

5. Staff Participation in Performance Improvement

Employee will participate in CPI activities through redesign, task forces, provider teams, service teams, and at the point of service in direct patient care. At **CHCC**, Performance Improvement is a continuous process owned by each pathway. We are currently in transition and in the process of training all staff on the CPI process.

6. Performance Improvement Knowledge and Skill Training

The Performance Improvement knowledge and skill training needs of the Governing Board, Governance Councils, Medical Staff Leadership, and pathway partners shall be continually assessed and training provided.

Council leaders have been trained on principles and tools of CPI, including practical application. Performance Improvement (PI) Pathway partners receive additional training in facilitation and mentoring CPI activities.

Performance Improvement Representatives—Each pathway has an identified PI representative to assist with design, measuring, and translating the data into an operational plan.

Learning Coach—Their role is to support staff in their identified pathway to implement the Shared Governance Model and mentor partners in their new roles. Additionally, the learning coaches will identify and meet the educational needs of the staff via training, support, and guidance.

Employees will be introduced to the CPI concepts and objectives during new employee orientation, pathway council meetings, Share Points, electronic communications, and working sessions as **CHCC** transitions into this organization-wide program.

continues

Exhibit 4–4 continued

7. Established Priorities for Performance Improvement

CHCC has established priorities for Continuous Performance Improvement in collaboration with Corporate Councils, Medical Staff Leadership, and point of service partners. The criteria utilized are:
- **CHCC's** mission, vision, Strategic Plan
- CHCC needs assessment
- Needs and expectations of patients and families
- Input from medical staff and partners
- High volume diagnoses/procedures/processes
- High risk diagnoses/procedures/processes
- High cost diagnoses/procedures/processes
- Problem prone procedures and processes
- Input from external sources (regulatory agencies, etc.)
- Clinical competencies
- Educational needs
- Resources necessary to implement improvement

C. Structure and Design

CHCC ORGANIZATION

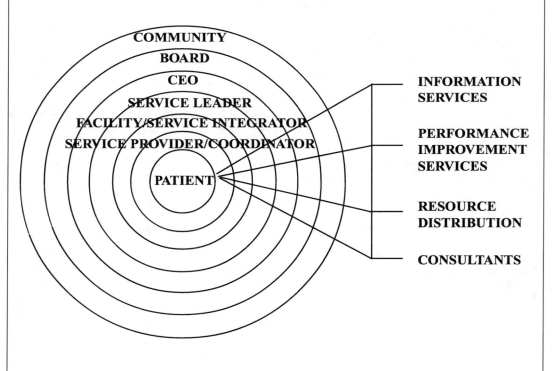

COMMUNITY
BOARD
CEO
SERVICE LEADER
FACILITY/SERVICE INTEGRATOR
SERVICE PROVIDER/COORDINATOR
PATIENT

INFORMATION SERVICES

PERFORMANCE IMPROVEMENT SERVICES

RESOURCE DISTRIBUTION

CONSULTANTS

continues

Exhibit 4–4 continued

D. Roles & Responsibilities

The role and accountabilities of the Shared Governance Model are:

Key positions	Accountabilities
Governance Council	• Translates the Mission, Vision of the CHCC into strategies. • Provides the framework for accomplishing the mission. • Ensures that there is seamless and effective integration of policy, operations, and service. • Ensures effective leadership is demonstrated throughout the organization. • Provides a mechanism for the deliberation and resolution of conflict between systems, services, cost, or providers affecting the achievement of **CHCC's** mission.

Service Council	• Patient Care Services
	• Quality and Continuous Performance Improvement: a planned, systematic organization-wide mechanism that designs, measures, assesses, and improves the quality of patient care and organizational functions.
	
	    Clinical protocols
	    Standards development/Competency
	    Education/Research
	    Sets Key Quality Initiatives
	
	• Receives reports on CPI activities
	• Oversees Performance Improvement activities that cross pathways to improve:
	    Delivery System/Models
	    Interdisciplinary Relationships
	• Communicates results through Share Points and through council system.

Operations Council	• Resource Allocation to Support CPI process: human, material, and support services • Ensuring work area systems are in alignment with the corporate mission and goals implementing a whole system framework • Implementation of clinical information system to meet the needs of patient focused care
Pathway Councils Provider Teams	• Design, Measure, Assess, and Improve Systems, functions, and process that achieve managing the member population to a value standard • Sanction Policy specific to service area • Identify teams to perform CPI projects • Review Feedback from Customer Satisfaction, CPI Task Forces, Risk Safety, Infection Control, Utilization reports

continues

Exhibit 4–4 continued

Key positions	Accountabilities
	• Collaborate with other stakeholders to improve process that crosses pathways • Work with PI Pathway Representatives and Learning Coaches to identify education or performance improvement needs • Communicate via Council's CPI results
Medical Executive Committee, Quality Management Committee Medical Staff Departments Professional Affairs: Linkage to Governing Body	• The Medical Executive Committee shall be responsible for the ongoing quality of medical care and professional services provided by all individuals with clinical privileges, and 1) participate in organization-wide measurement and CPI activities, 2) have representation on Service and Governance Council, 3) involve Medical Staff members in departmental Performance Improvement activities, development of patient care protocols, and peer review. • In conjunction with Service Council and the Performance Improvement Pathway, the Medical Executive Committee shall have oversight responsibilities for Medical Staff related improvement activities and QMC. • The Medical Executive Committee shall review QMC, infection control, medical records, surgical and other invasive procedures, credentialing, clinical risk management, and safety activities impacting services. Confidentiality is maintained. • Each Medical Staff Committee shall determine: 1) important aspects of care and PI priorities, 2) critical indicators/performance measures, and 3) comparison levels or triggers for action when patterns and trends are identified. QMC shall also monitor the findings and recommendations of the Pharmacy and Therapeutics Committee and Infection Control.

E. Approach & Methodology

CHCC has implemented the Continuous Improvement Process. This is a six-step process designed to provide the structure for all improvement activity that strives to meet or exceed our customers' expectation and achieving better clinical outcomes. The six steps are:

- Define Problem and Outcome Statements
- Describe the "AS IS"
- Brainstorm the "Ideal"
- Design and Select options
- Implement the Change
- Follow up and Improve

continues

Exhibit 4–4 continued

CHCC also has implemented in the training of the "OZ Principle*." This is a technique that supports accountability at the point of service. The below the line behaviors are the victim cycle and above the line behaviors are **See it, Own It, Solve It, and Do it!** (Diagram 3)

Diagram 3

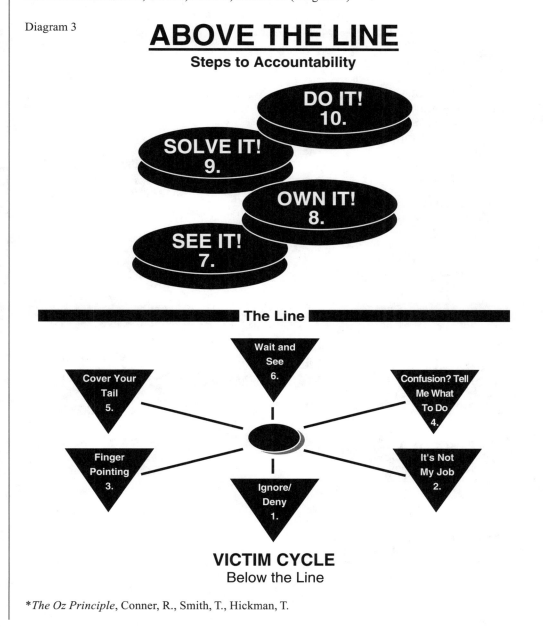

ABOVE THE LINE
Steps to Accountability

DO IT!
10.

SOLVE IT!
9.

OWN IT!
8.

SEE IT!
7.

◼ The Line ◼

Wait and
See
6.

Cover Your
Tail
5.

Confusion? Tell
Me What
To Do
4.

Finger
Pointing
3.

It's Not
My Job
2.

Ignore/
Deny
1.

VICTIM CYCLE
Below the Line

*The Oz Principle, Conner, R., Smith, T., Hickman, T.

continues

Exhibit 4–4 continued

F. Communication of Results of Quality

The review of the CPI process is the accountability of the Service Council. The mechanism is the reverse of the cascade. The CPI activities are identified at the point of service, follow the six-step model, and report outcomes through the system via the Service Council. These outcome data are then shared with others in the organization through

- Presentation at Service Council
- Council representatives report to Governance/Operations
- Corporate Council Minutes, Sharepoints
- Pathway/Provider Team meetings
- Quality Management Committee
- Storyboards at Point of Service
- Publication of Research Articles (Diagram 4)

Diagram 4

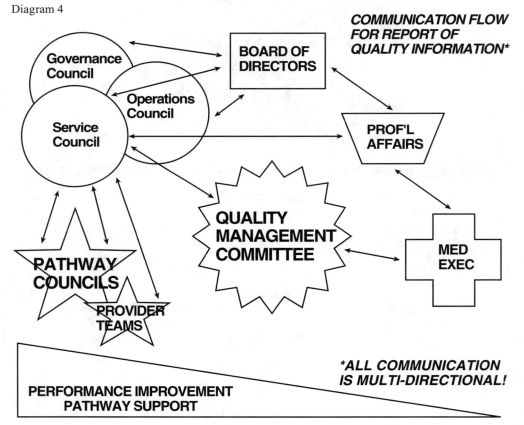

continues

Exhibit 4–4 continued

Confidentiality of Information

Appropriate safeguards have been established to restrict access to highly sensitive and confidential Performance Improvement information, which is protected against disclosure and discoverability through California Evidence Codes 1156 and 1157.

G. Transition of Medical Staff Quality to Continuous Performance Improvement

It is always important to assess the competence and performance of individual providers, but broader improvement is attainable by improving processes. The following goals have been identified to assist in the transition of our Medical Staff Quality Program:

1. Medical Staff Committees will be used as Performance Improvement teams, and membership will be expanded to include representatives from all appropriate clinical disciplines.
2. An environment will be created that allows for exploring opportunities for improvement rather than placing blame.
3. Actions will be based on statistically valid data.
4. Just-in-time training will be provided to committee members.

Performance Improvement results attributable to an individual in licensed dependent practitioners shall be used in determining clinical privileges, periodic performance evaluations, peer reviews, and re-appointment to the medical staff of **CHCC** as per the terms and conditions of the Medical Staff Bylaws. The designated medical Staff Committee shall review all pertinent information available and make recommendations to the Medical Executive Committee.

The Best Practice Institute (BPI) has been approved through the council structure. This is an entity within the system that focuses entirely on continuous research and development, and improvement in care delivery and process standards.

H. Goals: Present and Future

Current Achievements	Future Goals
1. Pathways identify their specific customers and stakeholders and determine their needs and expectations.	1. All Pathways will have a process in place to assess, manage, and improve their customers' satisfaction.
2. The formal process for submitting, approving and coordinating, tracking and supporting cross pathway functions CPI projects is overseen by Service Council.	2. Internal and External benchmarks will be identified and assessed and utilized in all pathways.
3. Pathway and provider teams develop and initiate CPI based upon patient needs and coordinate to the mission and vision.	3. Service Council will take an active leadership role in communicating, educating, and implementing the quality process.
4. Council's visibility and leadership in the CPI process will be evident to all partners and physicians.	4. Medical Staff leadership will be actively involved in the CPI process.
5. An education and training curriculum is designed.	5. Performance Improvement data will be available electronically at the point of service in a timely and reliable manner.
6. Patient Care Protocols are identified as a primary tool to achieve management of a patient to a value standard.	6. Patient Care Protocols will guide the majority of patient care and strategies.

continues

Exhibit 4–4 continued

Current Achievements	Future Goals
7. Multidisciplinary patient and family education and pain management identification has been implemented, documented, and is being measured.	7. Patient Focused Care and Collaborative Care Models will be in place throughout the organization to improve patient outcomes, quality of service, and efficiency of the system. 8. Organization-wide communication of the cascade, which translates the mission and vision into CPI activities at the point of service. 9. There will be a mechanism for decision making utilizing the indicators established by the Governance Council.

I. Evaluation

The purpose, structure, functions, and implementation plan of the CPI process is reviewed on an ongoing basis. Quality Reports and CPI activities are reported on a regularly scheduled basis using the Shared Governance and Medical Staff structures. The Service Council ensures that the projects are achieving the objectives and that they are consistent with the Mission and Vision and other internal and external needs and expectations.

Courtesy of Community Hospitals of Central California, Fresno, California.

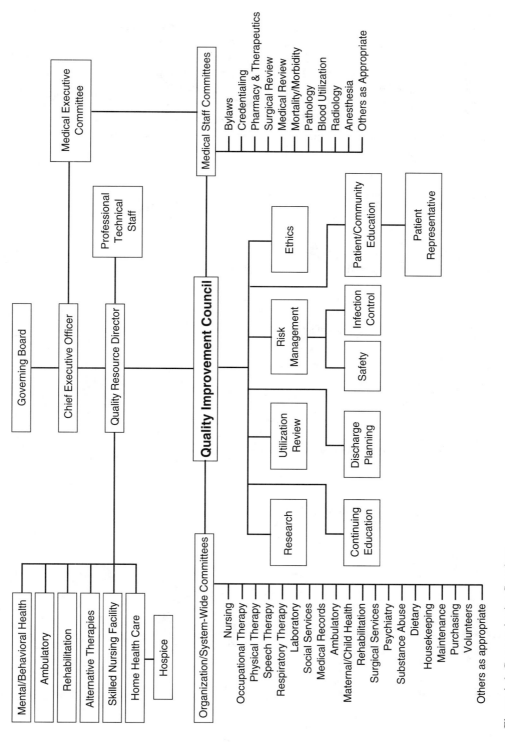

Figure 4-1 Communication flowchart

CONCLUSION

CQI has captured the enterprise of growing numbers of health care organizations and practitioners. Building a CQI program around patient care focuses the daily work of improving how organizations are managed and how services are provided. Although CQI has demonstrated an unprecedented ability to attract the support and involvement of both practitioners and administrators, significant challenges still lie ahead.

As organizations continue to merge and develop new relationships, leaders must be consistent in their modeling behavior to create a cultural transformation; all employees must be consistent in applying CQI tools to reach new benchmarks and hold the gains. Although many organizations are successfully devoting efforts to improving clinical care, most of the activity

Exhibit 4–5 Proposed Quality Improvement Activity

Date:

To: **Quality Resource Director**
         Quality Resource Council

From: _____
         (Department/Service/Individuals composing the team)

1.   Identify quality performance issue/opportunity.

2.   Describe rationale for selection.

3.   List individuals/program/services involved in issue:

4.   Identify type of assistance needed:

Recommendations of Quality Resource Director/Council:

Returned to: _____   **Date:** _____

Recommendations:

Exhibit 4–6 Quality Improvement Opportunity

Objective: To facilitate systematic process by which the _____
team/department/program/service(s) will monitor and evaluate the quality and appropriateness of patient care processes and professional practices.

Date:

Clinical/Nonclinical Area:

Scope of Care/Practice:
(patient/services provided; internal/external consumers)

Aspects of Care/Practice:
(components of program: high-volume, high-risk, high-benefits care; new procedures; new equipment;
appropriate care/service)

Thresholds/Benchmarks:
(current/projected)

Action(s) to be taken:
(relevant individuals/departments/services, etc.; time frames)

QA Coordinator:

Submitted to: Quality Resource Director   **Date:**
Quality Improvement Council   **Date:**

Recommendations:

Exhibit 4–7 Quality Improvement Assessment/Improvement Activity

Clinical/Nonclinical Area Involved: **Suspected Quality Issue/Opportunity for Improvement:**

Team Collecting Data: **Rationale for Selection:**

Time Frame: _____ **to** _____

Assessment (Data Source/Current Knowledge of Problem/Process)	Problem/Issue Causes of Variation (Systems; Knowledge; Performance)	Corrective Action To Improve System/Reduce Variation

Evaluation: Date(s), effectiveness of actions, documentation of improvement, change in thresholds/benchmarks, methodology for continuous improvement, responsible person(s)

Submitted to Quality Resource Director/Council   **Date:** _____

Recommendations:

Exhibit 4–8 Team/Committee Agenda/Minutes

TEAM/COMMITTEE: **AGENDA** FOR MEETING ON:		TIME: PLACE:	
TOPIC		**SPEAKER**	**TIME**
1. 2. 3. 4.			
MINUTES DATE: ____ TIME: _____ TO: ____ LEADER/FACILITATOR: _____ RECORDER: _____ SUBMITTED TO: _____ QRC Council, Other		**MEMBERS PRESENT:** (Sign-in sheet attached) **EXCUSED:** GUESTS:	

TOPIC	SPEAKER	TIME	DISCUSSION	ACTION/TIME FRAME

Exhibit 4–9 Reports: Documentation of Quality Improvement Activities (Trends and Patterns)

Date	Team Involved	Suspected Quality Issue	Selection Rationale	Date Study Initiated

Responsible Person(s)	Monitors/ Indicators	Assessment/ Data Sources	Problem Cause(s) Study Results

continues

Exhibit 4–9 continued

Corrective Action(s), Date(s), Responsible Person(s)	Date Submitted to Quality Resources Director	Date Submitted to Quality Improvement Committee	Recommendations/ Time Frame

Assessment of Improvement Process	Responsible Person(s), Date	Effect of Improvements on Patient Care, Professional/Organization Performance

Exhibit 4–10 Annual Continuous Quality Improvement Review

Date:

To: Quality Resource Director
Quality Resource Council

From: _____
   (Team/Program/Department/Service)

1. List successfully conducted studies/activities/processes examined within the past year; note cost-effectiveness and efficiency.

2. Identify staff involvement in quality improvement activities during the year (i.e., committees, studies, peer review, research).

3. Identify quality issue/process (include previously cited unresolved issues; enumerate difficulties encountered).

4. List studies based on goals to be
   conducted during coming year.   *Time Frame*   *Responsible Person(s)*

5. Identify type of assistance needed in the coming year (i.e., education, study designs, statistical techniques, "team" building, etc.).

Reviewed by: _____   **Date:** _____
         Quality Resource Director

Recommendations:

---

still revolves around administratively oriented projects. A major challenge relates to applying CQI to the care of patients across an episode of illness. Coordination across multiple sites and providers to enhance continuity of care and achieve appropriate, cost-effective patient outcomes is a critical role CQI can help manage.

CQI can also be used to facilitate the development of a systems framework for managing population-based care and disease state management. By integrating effectiveness and outcomes research findings, clinical protocols and critical pathways, QI processes, clinical reengineering, and case management approaches, health care organizations can clarify and improve their performance in relation to functions that are central to their evolving missions (O'Brien et al., 1995). If we are really optimizing the use of available resources, providing good service, and fulfilling the mission, however good we are today, we will be better tomorrow. A learning organization has the capacity to treat its people as assets and recreate itself as something different tomorrow.

REFERENCES

Crosby, P. (1979). *Quality is free: The art of making quality certain*. New York: McGraw-Hill.

Day, G., Gardner, S., & Herba, C. (1995). An integrated approach to hospital strategic planning, quality assurance, and continuous quality improvement. *Journal for Healthcare Quality, 17*(5), 21–25.

Deming, W. (1988). *Out of crises*. Cambridge, MA: MIT Center for Advanced Engineering Study.

Donabedian, A. (1980). *The definition of quality and approaches to its assessment. Volume 1. In exploration in quality assessment and monitoring*. Ann Arbor, MI: Health Administration Press.

Drucker, P. (1995). *Managing in a time of great change*. New York: Truman Talley Books/Dalton.

Flower, J. (1996). How we learn. *Healthcare Forum Journal, 39*(4), 40.

Joint Commission on Accreditation of Healthcare Organizations. (1996). *1997 accreditation manual for hospitals*. Oakbrook Terrace, IL: Author.

Juran, J.M. (1988). *Juran on planning for quality*. New York: Free Press.

Loeb, J. (1996). Putting it (performance measures) together: An interview with Jerod Loeb. *The Joint Commission Journal on Quality Improvement, 22*(7), 518–526.

O'Brien J., Shortell, S., Hughes, E., Forster, R., Carman, J., Boerstler, H., & O'Connor, E. (1995). An integrative model for organization-wide quality improvement: Lessons from the field. *Quality Management in Health Care, 3*(4), 19–30.

CHAPTER 5

Selecting Quality Initiatives and Methodologies

Joann Genovich-Richards

CHAPTER OBJECTIVES

After completing this chapter, the reader will be able to

- describe the two com5ponents of quality measurement
- choose quality initiatives
- develop relevant and useful indicators for measuring quality
- select appropriate data collections methodologies

Options for health services quality programs have expanded to the point of presenting a large palette of choices. From a few specific approaches to quality assurance from the 1960s and 1970s—by analogy the field's primary colors—elements from the original programs have been "mixed" and new elements added, presenting many "colors" from which to choose in designing programs. The challenge for health professionals is to select and blend the options to produce a quality management program that is internally useful, meets the demands of various external entities, and can flexibly adapt to new options and demands.

In these jargon-filled times, commonly agreed on definitions often do not exist. With respect to quality, the language has become fragmented—even to the degree that there are debates about whether *quality* is an adjective or a noun! Nevertheless, the Institute of Medicine's quality definition is highly cited by practitioners and researchers: "Quality of care is the degree to which health services for individuals and populations increase the likelihood of desired health outcomes and are consistent with current professional knowledge" (Lohr, 1990).

In this discussion, *quality management* is an umbrella term for all the activities that occur within an organization to assess and improve the quality of care, reengineer the processes of care, and report information to internal and external customers. Figure 5–1 depicts the general relationship between these components. Conceptually, quality measurement has two components that may be thought of as two sides of the same coin. The first component is the quality of care (sometimes referred to as "technical quality" or "clinical quality"). In general, this is the area of professional peer review about the structures, processes, and outcomes of care. Consumer perceptions are an increasingly important component of quality measurement. Beyond traditional satisfaction surveys, consumer reports about the process of care can be used to verify technical sources of information (e.g., Was your blood pressure taken on your last office visit?). Health status surveys, various quality of well-being tools, and inventories of health behavior risk factors are increasingly being used to profile the health of enrolled populations, plan the care for specific clinical groups, risk adjust and stratify quality measures, and predict trajectories about individuals' course of care.

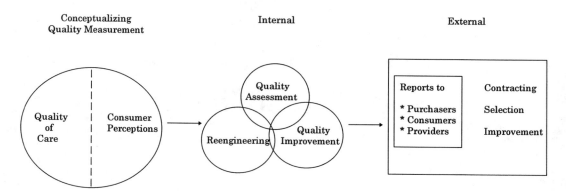

Figure 5–1 Quality management in an age of accountability

Consumer perceptions will be an increasingly important area for research and practice applications over the next decade.

The next section of Figure 5–1 addresses internal quality management. Quality assessment, the traditional core of monitoring and evaluation with its roots in the paradigm of structure, process, and outcome measures (Donabedian, 1966), remains a common building block for quality management programs across health care settings and disciplines. Quality improvement contains a wide range of philosophical and measurement techniques (Crosby, 1979; Deming, 1986; Juran, 1988), which have come into health care since the 1980s (e.g., Berwick, 1989; James, 1989; Laffel & Blumenthal, 1989; McLaughlin & Kaluzny, 1990). *Reengineering*, which addresses the redesign of basic processes rather than improving them (Hammer, 1990), migrated to health care in the 1990s (e.g., Griffith, 1994; Kennedy, 1994).

As shown in Figure 5–1, reports are increasingly demanded by external and internal customers as part of demonstrating accountability for care. If one is in a health plan setting, systematic demands *have* increasingly been made for accreditation and performance measurement data from employers (often referred to as *purchasers*). If one is in a hospital or home care setting, for example, performance information *will be* increasingly demanded by the

health plans—an example of "trickle-down" accountability. Regardless of setting, health care accreditors and regulators require various reports. Consumers are more directly receiving performance information for use in selecting providers, hospitals, and health plans. Accountability is increasingly being demonstrated in report card formats for various audiences (Alsever, Ritchey, & Lima, 1995; Montague, 1996; National Committee for Quality Assurance [NCQA], 1995; see Chapter 8 for additional discussions of accountability to external customers).

QUALITY MANAGEMENT: THE INTERNAL ROAD MAP

Within health care organizations, how can quality management be organized? Figure 5–2 provides a conceptual framework for considering the elements of reengineering, quality improvement methods, and basic quality assessment. This framework is an elaboration of the Shewhart cycle, called the Deming Cycle in Japan—because Deming introduced it there—as well as the Plan–Do–Check–Act cycle, or PDCA (Walton, 1986).

Several premises underlying Figure 5–2 need to be made explicit. First, the organization's leadership is visibly committed to quality. Affective and behavioral development initiatives related to the quality culture, measures,

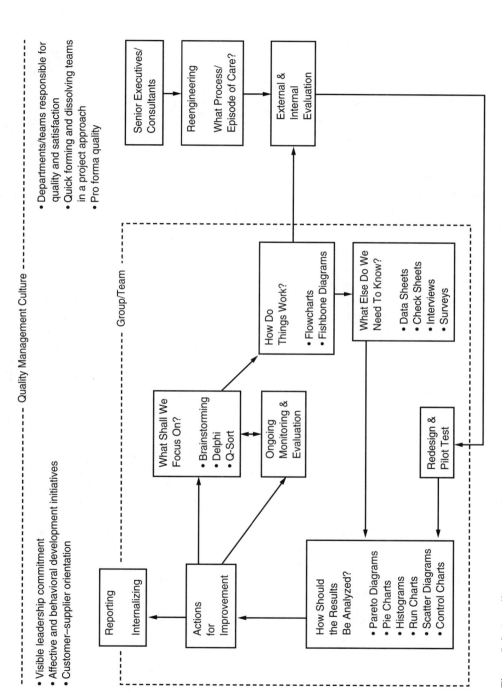

Figure 5–2 A quality management road map

and actions, beginning with the board and executive leadership, have permeated the entire institution, although development is ongoing. As a result, all of the areas have been inculcated in a customer orientation. Strategic planning, financial activities, human resources activities, and information systems throughout the organization are oriented toward quality management. *Pro forma quality*, the process of prospectively planning for the quality evaluation of new or deleted services (Genovich-Richards, 1992), is routinely practiced and reported to the board along with pro forma financial information. Departments are responsible for the quality of their products and the satisfaction of their customers. Each has developed ongoing measures of quality and satisfaction that are routinely reported in the management reporting system. In addition, there are many initiatives underway to improve functions and services involving teams (departmental or interdepartmental) with members from various parts of the organization. Some of these initiatives have resulted in a set of measures that are routinely reported among departments that are in customer–supplier relationships.

What Shall We Focus On?

In a complex enterprise such as health care delivery, teams are likely to have many ideas of areas requiring ongoing measurement or improvement. Therefore, the first task is selection of one area, or at most a few, for inquiry. The most common methods for consensus and prioritization are brainstorming, the Delphi technique, and the Q-sort method. Of course, the group members need to be trained in these techniques before using them. Selection among these methods should be made on the basis of time, resources, and the need for participation from individuals other than team members. This last point is particularly critical if the area of inquiry, subsequent data collection, and later interventions are likely to involve additional individuals. The time involved in

obtaining greater participation in selection of the area for inquiry may prove to be a good investment.

In *brainstorming* (Udinsky, Osterlind, & Lynch, 1981), ideas are put forth without further discussion or judgment in a lively round-robin session. Then, in a subsequent discussion, the items are reviewed, discussed, and clarified. Rankings by the individuals determine the relative priority of each item. Brainstorming can be completed in one or two sessions.

In the *Delphi technique*, input is obtained through several rounds of questionnaires and is continued until opinions converge (Fink, Kosecoff, Chassin, & Brook, 1984). It ensures anonymity in the decision-making process but is usually more time consuming and resource intensive than brainstorming. The technique may be particularly useful when it is desirable to have input from more individuals than those on the team in selecting the area for inquiry. Of particular importance in hospitals is the involvement of staff on the afternoon and evening shifts.

The *Q-sort method* requires the team to meet once to brainstorm the items. The items are subsequently placed on separate cards, and people individually sort them into a predetermined number of piles indicating relative priority. Homogeneity in the rankings is used for selecting the area(s) of inquiry (Udinsky et al., 1981). The technique is moderately time and resource intensive, in between the brainstorming and Delphi approaches. It does provide the opportunity for more people than those on the team to participate without the time and expense of the multiple questionnaires used in the Delphi method.

Monitoring and Evaluation

If the task at hand is to develop an ongoing monitoring and evaluation plan within an organization or a specific department, part of the "What shall we focus on?" discussion needs to consider activities that:

- occur frequently
- affect large number of patients
- place patients at risk by
  - not providing care correctly
  - not providing care when indicated
  - providing care that is not indicated
- produce problems for patients or staff

This list is frequently summarized as the high-volume, high-risk, or problem prone approach.

Next, indicators would be developed for monitoring and evaluation. An indicator is a good "pointer" (Kazandjian, 1996) if it:

- is objective
- is measurable
- is based on current knowledge and clinical experience
- reflects
  - structures of care
  - processes of care
  - outcomes of care

Structure, process, and outcome measures have been a historic cornerstone of quality assessment. Definitions and examples of each type of measure are given in Table 5–1. Outcome measures have received the most emphasis in recent years. They will become increasingly important as the emphasis shifts to the longitudinal review of the continuum of

care. However, the ancient Greek philosophy of "everything in moderation" is appropriate, and a variety of each type of measure should be used.

What makes an indicator objective and measurable? It is essentially a matter of clarity and reproducibility. Indicators that attempt to cover more than one action by linking them with conjunctions or using more than one sentence can be difficult to use in a consistent manner. For example, consider that an indicator statement asks for the signature, date, and legibility of a medical record entry. Technically, if one element is missing, the entire indicator is considered as "not met." This bundled information does not provide useful information for improvement. A better approach is to further specify an indicator with specific substatements or elements (often called *criteria*). In this example, the indicator would address documentation and the subcomponents would address signature, date, and legibility. The reports on this indicator would display the individual items so that efforts toward improvement could be more finely focused on the specific area(s) of concern.

Quality assessment increasingly uses numerical reference points for interpreting the results. These points often are referred to as *goals* if there is a national or research-based reference number, such as the *Healthy People*

Table 5–1 Measures

	Structure	*Process*	*Outcome*
Definition	The inputs or elements that facilitate care	Functions of the care providers	Results of care
Examples	Resources Equipment Numbers of staff Qualifications of staff	Assessment Planning Treatment Timeliness	Short-term results Complications Adverse events Satisfaction Long-term results Changes in health status

Note: This table is illustrative and not comprehensive.

2000 goals (U.S. Public Health Service, 1990), or *benchmarks* if there is an industry source for comparison. External databases are increasingly available for use in developing comparative rates. For example, the Health Care Financing Administration Medicare files are now available on-line.[1] Historically, some parts of the health care industry have also used internal "thresholds" as a quantitative point for triggering further review.

For each indicator used in monitoring and evaluation, a decision has to be made about the data collection frequency and sampling. Each serious complication or death (known variously as adverse events, sentinel events, generic screens, or occurrence screens) is reviewed by the appropriate professional group on an immediate and ongoing basis. As such, sampling is inappropriate for these serious events. Other indicators can be collected on an ongoing or periodic basis, and calendars that display the plan for the data collection activity at the organizational and departmental/unit levels are helpful for describing the quality management program to internal and external audiences.

In recent years, there has been a shift from trying to do a large number of indicator reviews on a continuous basis to doing shorter, staggered data collection activities, as well as a shift from retrospective medical record reviews to concurrent data collection. These shifts have increased the importance of sampling strategies. However, beliefs about appropriate sample sizes vary from one section of the health care industry to another, and may also reflect the available technologies. For example, managed care plans follow the instructions of HEDIS 3.0 (Health Plan Employer Data and Information Set; NCQA, 1996) for randomly

selecting 384 medical records for the quality performance measures but may report on the total population of available cases if administrative databases are available. Periodic data collection in hospitals may be as small as 30 cases. Statistical consultation should be sought in planning the data collection and reporting strategies so that the number of cases obtained and the appropriate statistical treatments or displays can be developed in tandem. Data can be collected from a wide variety of sources. Exhibit 5–1 contains many of the most common ones. Data tool construction is an art. Exhibit 5–2 provides a summary of helpful, time-tested hints to consider.

A review of the literature is one way to demonstrate use of current knowledge in the development of indicators, formulation of data collection strategies, and the setting of performance goals. The citation for the indicator reference may be included in the quality management plan for the area or incorporated into a data collection tool. The Agency for Health Care Policy and Research (AHCPR) is a federal

---

Exhibit 5–1 Internal Sources of Data

- Medical records
- Incident reports
- Infection control reports
- Blood utilization reports
- Pharmacy reports
- Laboratory reports
- Committee/department reports
- Generic screening indicators
- Patient bills
- Staff research and evaluation reports
- Staff surveys
- Patient surveys
- Credentialing reports
- Liability claims data
- Financial data
- Marketing/planning databases

Note: This list is illustrative and not comprehensive.

---

[1] Health Care Financing and Administration Medicare data files are available on the World Wide Web site address <http://www.ssa.gov.hcfa/hcfahp2.html>.

Exhibit 5–2 Tool Construction Hints

1. Routine header information for data collection tool

   - Name of indicator/performance measure
   - Whether data to be collected relates to a high-volume, high-risk, or problem prone area
   - If relevant, the standard of care or practice that is being addressed
   - Appropriate instructions, definitions, glossaries, and legends

2. Patient/client information

   - Identifying number
   - Sex (may not be necessary if there are sufficient data links)
   - Age (may not be necessary if there are sufficient data links)
   - Depending on measure: diagnosis, discharge status, and insurer
   - Unit location and shift
   - Identifier for primary nurse, physician, or therapist

3. Collection information

   - Data source
   - Date data obtained
   - Identifier for collector of information (number or initials)

4. Computer-ready format of data entry Examples:

   - Indicator met or not met recorded as 1 or 0
   - Age recorded by date of birth
   - Time in military time
   - Coding for days of the week and shifts

5. Pilot test any tool before widespread implementation

Exhibit 5–3 Guidelines Available from AHCPR

1. Acute Pain Management: Operative or Medical Procedures and Trauma
2. Urinary Incontinence in Adults
3. Pressure Ulcers in Adults: Prediction and Prevention
4. Cataract in Adults: Management of Functional Impairment
5. Depression in Primary Care: Detection, Diagnosis, and Treatment
6. Sickle Cell Disease: Screening, Diagnosis, Management, and Counseling in Newborns and Infants
7. Early HIV Infection: Evaluation and Management
8. Benign Prostatic Hyperplasia: Diagnosis and Management
9. Management of Cancer Pain
10. Unstable Angina: Diagnosis and Management
11. Heart Failure: Evaluation and Care of Patients with Left Ventricular Systolic Dysfunction
12. Otitis Media with Effusion in Children
13. Quality Determinants of Mammography
14. Acute Low Back Problems in Adults
15. Treatment of Pressure Ulcers
16. Post-Stroke Rehabilitation
17. Cardiac Rehabilitation
18. Urinary Incontinence Update
19. Alzheimer's Disease

source of information that can inform the indicator development process. First, AHCPR has been developing a wide set of clinical practice guidelines. A summary of the available guidelines as of this writing is contained in Exhibit 5–3.[2] In addition to a detailed document for each guideline, a short clinical summary and a related patient brochure are available (some in additional languages). AHCPR has also funded a project to develop a common typology for quality measures (Center for Health Policy Studies/Center for Quality of Care Research and

[2]Information concerning the most recent materials available from AHCPR can be obtained from their World Wide Web site address <http://www.ahcpr.gov>.

Education, 1995). In 1996, AHCPR publicly released a database containing multiple measurement sets based on the typology, known as CONQUEST—Computerized Needs-Oriented Quality Measurement Evaluation System.[3] CONQUEST can be used to

- identify existing clinical performance measures
- compare and select clinical performance measures most appropriate to an organization or department's needs
- examine information about the clinical rationale behind a given performance measure
- identify the methodological assumptions, data source requirements, sampling requirements, clinical setting for which the measure was designed, and methods for "scoring" or analyzing a given measure
- locate the organizations offering the measures

How Do Things Work?

Returning to the main square in Figure 5–2, once the area of inquiry is selected, the question "How do things work?" seeks to outline all the steps and actions that contribute to the area being considered. The two most common approaches are flowcharts and cause-and-effect, or fishbone, diagrams. The flowchart provides a graphic representation of the sequence of a process. It is the technique of choice when trying to streamline processes through elimination of redundancies and misunderstandings. The fishbone or Ishikawa diagram (Ishikawa, 1987) displays potential

---

[3]For additional information on CONQUEST, contact:
Margaret Keyes
Agency for Health Care Policy and Research
2101 E. Jefferson St.
Rockville, MD 20852
Telephone: 301-594-1349
Fax: 301-594-2155
E-mail address: mkeyes@po3.ahcpr.gov

causes of a problem. For example, if postoperative infection is the area of concern, various factors can be identified as causes under the major headings of the patient, surgical care, preoperative preparation, and postoperative care. In examining delays in initiating therapy in septic patients, causes from the physician office systems, transportation, admitting office, pharmacy, and nursing could all be identified (Batalden & Buchanan, 1989). The fishbone diagram allows for easy visualization of potential causes. However, to create one during a group session requires great skill on the recorder's part. It may be easier to brainstorm the causes and have one person prepare the fishbone diagram for the next meeting. During discussion of a fishbone diagram, it is sometimes possible to determine which causes will be most amenable to change.

After the team has developed the flowchart or cause-and-effect diagram, there may be value in circulating it to other staff members. Frequently, the processes in place on the day shift differ from those of the other shifts, and there may be additional changes in processes on weekends. Also, despite the best efforts of any team member, additional insights might be provided by departmental colleagues. Again, the time spent in broader review will probably prove a wise investment, allowing processes to be changed at a later time if needed.

What Else Do We Need to Know?

In most cases, the team realizes it needs additional information and seeks to obtain it in a timely manner over the next several weeks. Knowledge and experience about the data collection tools of traditional monitoring and evaluation methods will be useful in this activity. Data sheets, check sheets, surveys, and interviews all have their uses at this stage. As an example, suppose a team selects the admission process for the area of inquiry. A flowchart graphically portrays the process of patient flow. Through a fishbone diagram, the group identifies delays in patients' departures from the admitting area as a possible cause of delays in the admission process. To proceed with their analysis, the team requires additional information on the delay time attributable to several steps of the process. For 1 week, staff in different parts of the organization record the time required by their step in the process for each patient. The greatest time delays are found to be related to transporter availability. The solution, achieved following some additional analysis by a team of transporters, is initiation of a silent beeper system for the transporters.

How Should the Results Be Analyzed?

Depending on the type of data obtained, a variety of visual display techniques, which supplement those previously described, may be used to analyze and present data. They may be loosely classified into frequency or proportion techniques (Pareto diagrams, pie charts, histograms, run charts, and scatter diagrams) and statistical techniques (control charts, charts with standard deviations, and charts with control limits).

Pareto diagrams provide a visual ranking of the importance of various factors, identifying areas for further inquiry or intervention. The horizontal axis always contains the factors, and the vertical axis, the frequency. A *pie chart* can convey the same information through different sizes and colors of the pie, usually reflected as percentages.

Histograms provide information on the frequency of variation of a specific area. A histogram can be thought of as a vertical stem-and-leaf diagram. The horizontal axis always contains the discrete values that can occur for the topic under study, ordered from lowest to highest. The vertical axis contains the frequency. At a glance, information is provided about outliers and, intuitively, the median value.

Run charts give information about a process over time and can be useful in identifying trends and cycles. The horizontal axis is always in units of time (days, weeks, shifts, and so forth), and the vertical axis provides a frequency count. Over time, the chart can be useful in displaying whether a process change has had an impact (Batalden & Buchanan, 1989).

The *scatter diagram* is a simple depiction of the relationship between the quantities of two items. The two items need not be on the same scale. For example, Walton (1986) has provided an example of active ingredient stability. The horizontal axis displays shelf life in months, and the vertical axis displays the quantity of active ingredient per sample. At a glance, the optimum situation can be roughly determined.

Control charts, of which there are several varieties, provide information about a process or attribute over time, with upper and lower limits based on historical variability. The pure *statistical process control chart* is the most complicated of the techniques discussed in the quality improvement literature. Most articles only give it superficial treatment and do not explain the actual calculations required. Ishikawa (1987) has provided complete details for the calculations. Efforts are being made to use the method. Spoeri (1990) has provided examples for length of stay and mortality data. A large variety of statistical packages with display options are available to make the transition to using these techniques.

Data can be displayed with standard deviations and confidence limits, which serve to visually bound the data similar to a statistical process control chart. Some knowledge of inferential statistics is required to apply confidence limits. However, standard deviations are understood by most people with graduate-level preparation and are easily obtained from the most basic of statistical packages and some handheld calculators. As with other display techniques, various forms of control charts must be "played with" to assess their utility.

Actions for Improvement

The actions possible for improvement usually relate to systems, procedures, policies, resources, and people. Of course, the actions usually reflect an organization's culture (Genovich-Richards, 1995). For organizations that are only superficially committed to quality, one or more classic caricatures of problem solving may exist, impeding substantive improvements:

1. "the ostrich syndrome" of avoiding change by playing "paper chase" through memos
2. "passing the hot potato" by referring the matter to another department or committee
3. "Don't bother me with the details," in which the only interest is in the "bottom line"
4. "cowboys" who operate on "instinct" and the "gut level"
5. "Just the facts," in which professional groups want the data and assume that their members will "do the right thing" if they "have all the facts"

Reporting/Internalizing the Changes

Important linkages between the quality improvement efforts and traditional monitoring and evaluation occur in these later stages. In one direction, a successful team's effort could easily translate into a permanent part of the monitoring and evaluation process based on a few measures. In the opposite direction, when a long-standing indicator begins to demonstrate a negative trend through the ongoing monitoring and evaluation process, there should be a mechanism to mobilize action of an appropriate team to investigate what has changed. As a result, quality improvement work by teams and traditional monitoring and evaluation become mutually reinforcing activities.

There is no inherent requirement for reporting on team activities in the quality improvement literature. However, any state-of-the-art management reporting system, of which the quality reports are one component, should be capturing things to cheer about. Therefore,

mechanisms should be developed to celebrate the successes and to ponder where there are lacks in improvement. The storyboard approach (Elgass, 1990) is one effective way to display progress. Development of nontraditional reports—for example, the use of faces (Chernoff, 1973)—is another area for creative play.

Reengineering

By definition,

> reengineering strives to break away from the old rules about how we organize and conduct business. It involves recognizing and rejecting some of them and then finding imaginative new ways to accomplish work. From our redesigned processes, new rules will emerge that fit the times. Only then can we hope to achieve quantum leaps in performance. (Hammer, 1990, pp. 103–104)

Within health care, reengineering efforts are increasingly focused on the entire episode of care so that "carefully designed, systematized processes that emphasize teamwork and integration along horizontal, patient-focused paths" (Sharp, 1994, p. 32) are the end product. At facilities in the Lovelace Health Systems, Albuquerque, NM, episode of care processes are specifically geared to avoiding breaks in services and evaluating outcomes across the continuum of care (American Health Consultants, 1995). As a major component of redesigning processes, reengineering often focuses on improved information acquisition and transfer. Examples include "smart systems" that suggest best practices based on guidelines, and automatic triggers that activate the critical pathway to be followed by a multidisciplinary team (Kralovec, 1994).

Following the far right-hand boxes of Figure 5–2, the first step is to decide what processes need to be reengineered. Although staff can make contributions to this decision, the targets are often selected by senior executives with the help of consultants (Coffey & Berglund, 1994). Ideally, there is broad participation in the redesign process.

As the process is redesigned, many of the steps previously discussed can be taken. There may be value in gaining some information about current processes so that valuable current steps are identified and retained, whereas problematic ones are slated for redesign. Once the new process is implemented as a pilot test, it will be necessary to gather data about how well the new process is working, analyze those data, report, and improve the new process. As the new process is institutionalized, several measures for ongoing monitoring and evaluation would be incorporated into the quality management plan.

EMERGING ISSUES

There are many interesting emerging trends in quality management. Three will probably have a direct effect on providers in the near future: (1) the need to quantify value, (2) ethical decision making, and (3) community-level quality assessment and improvement.

The evaluation of quality has often been a purely clinical exercise, separated from the economics of health care delivery. Quantifying the value of improved and reengineered processes will become increasingly important. This activity will also be more rigorously tied to guidelines and quantified assessments of patients' needs. For example, in the Kaiser Foundation Health Plan of Southern California, guidelines were developed for the appropriate use of two different types of radiology contrast agents. The more expensive agent would be used with certain high-risk patients. The savings of $3.5 million was redirected to offering colon and breast cancer screening benefits (Eddy, 1992; Sharp, 1995). Other examples include the quantification of savings from more appropriate levels of sedation for intensive care patients, treatment with antibiotics, and the redesign of orthopedic procedures (Berwick, 1995).

Ethics and ethical decision making is an increasingly important component of quality discussions (Buban, 1995; Steeples, 1994). Within health care, debates about ethics and quality will need to be engaged as part of the decisions with purchasers and consumers about the structures of benefits (Friedman, 1993) and shared decision making at the time of care.

The focus of health care is rapidly shifting beyond the walls of health care facilities. As a result, community-level quality assessment and improvement activities will become more common in the next millennium. Quality assessment will shift from the population of a hospital or plan to the health of the population living in the community. The information will be obtained by aggregation of the statistics of health plans, as managed care becomes the dominant insurance mechanism, or through community information systems (Duncan, 1995; McCutcheon & Schumacher, 1994). Improvements will increasingly be geared to the underlying social issues rather than the medicalized version of the problems (Hurowitz, 1993). The community-level emphasis will probably be the vehicle for redeploying the health care work force from the health care facilities to the neighborhoods.

CONCLUSION

Quality management methods have a rich heritage from the history of traditional quality assurance and assessment. They have been enhanced and expanded by quality improvement and reengineering initiatives. As quality management evolves, there will be continuing challenges to develop performance measurement and reporting systems that meet the external demands for accountability in addition to the internal demands. All the evolutions and changes in emphases need to be kept in perspective. It is helpful to remember that only in hindsight does a period of history appear placid: at any given point in time, people consider their current environment as turbulent.

With regard to methods, there is an opportunity to play with the many old and new colors, creating a unique work that is meaningful, complete, and flexible.

REFERENCES

Alsever, R.N., Ritchey, T., & Lima, N.P. (1995). Developing a hospital report card to demonstrate value in healthcare. *Journal of Health Care Quality, 17*(1), 19–28.

American Health Consultants. (1995). Look at outcomes across the continuum of care. *Patient Satisfaction & Outcomes Management in Physician Practices, 1*(6), 65.

Batalden, P.B., & Buchanan, E.D. (1989). Industrial models of quality improvement. In N. Goldfield & D. Nash (Eds.), *Providing quality care: The challenge to clinicians.* Philadelphia: American College of Physicians.

Berwick, D.M. (1989). Continuous improvement as an ideal in health care. *New England Journal of Medicine, 320*(1), 53–56.

Berwick, D.M. (1995). Quality comes home. *Quality Connection, 4*(1), 1–4.

Buban, M. (1995). Factoring ethics into the TQM equation. *Quality Progress, 28*(10), 97–99.

Center for Health Policy Studies/Center for Quality of Care Research and Education. (1995). *Understanding and choosing clinical performance measures for quality improvement: Development of a typology (final report).* Contract No. 282-92-0038, Delivery Order #3. Rockville, MD: Agency for Health Care Policy and Research.

Chernoff, H. (1973). The use of faces to represent points in k-dimensional space graphically. *Journal of the American Statistical Association, 68,* 361–368.

Coffey, R.J., & Berglund, R.G. (1994). Relationships among quality assurance, quality improvement, and reengineering. *The Journal of Healthcare Information and Management Systems Society, 8*(4), 5–10.

Crosby, P.B. (1979). *Quality is free.* New York: New American Library.

Deming, W.E. (1986). *Out of the crisis.* Cambridge, MA: MIT Press.

Donabedian, A. (1966). Evaluating the quality of medical care. *Milbank Memorial Fund Quarterly, 44*(3, Part 2), 166–206.

Duncan, K.A. (1995). Evolving community health information networks. *Frontiers of Health Services Management, 12*(1), 5–41.

Eddy, D. (1992). Applying cost-effective analysis. *Journal of the American Medical Association, 268*(20), 2575–2582.

Elgass, J.R. (1990, July 2). Hospitals' quality quest focuses on customers' needs. *The University Record* (University of Michigan).

Fink, A., Kosecoff, J., Chassin, M., & Brook R.H. (1984). Consensus methods: Characteristics and guidelines for use. *American Journal of Public Health, 74,* 979–983.

Friedman, E. (1993, July/August). Managed care and managing ethics. *Healthcare Forum Journal, 9,* 11, 13–15.

Genovich-Richards, J. (1992). Selecting topics and methodologies. In C.G. Meisenheimer (Ed.), *Improving quality: A guide to effective programs* (pp. 87–118). Gaithersburg, MD: Aspen.

Genovich-Richards, J. (1995). Designing quality management programs for today and tomorrow. In V.A. Kazandjian (Ed.), *The epidemiology of quality* (pp. 55–83). Gaithersburg, MD: Aspen.

Griffith, J.R. (1994). Reengineering health care: Management systems for survivors. *Hospital & Health Services Administration, 39*(4), 451–470.

Hammer, M. (1990, July–August). Reengineering work: Don't automate, obliterate. *Harvard Business Review,* 104–112.

Hurowitz, J.C. (1993). Toward a social policy for health. *New England Journal of Medicine, 329*(2), 130–133.

Ishikawa, K. (1987). *Guide to quality control.* (Asian Productivity Organization, Trans.). White Plains, NY: Kraus International Publications.

James, B.C. (1989). *Quality management for health care delivery.* Chicago: Hospital Research and Educational Trust.

Juran, J.M. (1988). *Juran on planning for quality.* New York: Free Press.

Kazandjian, V.A. (1996). Indicators of performance or the search for the best pointer dog. In V.A. Kazandjian (Ed.), *The epidemiology of quality* (pp. 25–37). Gaithersburg, MD: Aspen.

Kennedy, M. (1994). Reengineering in healthcare. *The Quality Letter for Healthcare Leaders, 6*(7), 2–10.

Kralovec, O.J. (1994). The critical role information systems play in reengineering efforts. *The Quality Letter for Healthcare Leaders, 6*(7), 11–13.

Laffel, G., & Blumenthal, D. (1989). The case for using industrial quality management science in health care organizations. *Journal of the American Medical Association, 262,* 2869–2873.

Lohr, K. (1990). *Medicare: A Strategy for Quality Assurance.* Washington, DC: Institute of Medicine, National Academy Press.

McCutcheon, J., & Schumacher, D.N. (1994). Healthcare transformation and the case for a community-wide health information management environment. *Quality Management in Health Care, 2*(4), 1–17.

McLaughlin, C.P., & Kaluzny, A.D. (1990). Total quality management in health: Making it work. *Health Care Management Review, 15*(3), 7–14.

Montague, J. (1996). Report card daze. *Hospitals & Health Networks, 70*(1), 33–36.

National Committee for Quality Assurance. (1995). *Technical Report: 1994 Report Card Pilot Project.* Washington, DC: Author.

National Committee for Quality Assurance. (1996). *Health Plan Employer Data and Information Set 3.0.* Washington, DC: Author.

Sharp, J. (1994). The new production theory for health care through clinical reengineering: A study of clinical guidelines—Part I. *Physician Executive, 20*(12), 30–34.

Sharp, J. (1995). The new production theory for health care through clinical reengineering: A study of clinical guidelines—Part II. *Physician Executive, 21*(1), 36–38.

Spoeri, R.K. (1990). The inspection of data. In D.R. Longo & D. Bohr (Eds.), *Quantitative methods in quality assessment: A guide for practitioners* (pp. 36–38). Chicago: American Hospital Publishing.

Steeples, M.M. (1994). The quality–ethics connection. *Quality Progress, 27*(6), 73–75.

Udinsky, B.F., Osterlind, S.J., & Lynch, S.W. (1981). *Evaluation resource handbook: Gathering, analyzing, reporting data.* San Diego, CA: EDITS.

U.S. Public Health Service. (1990). *Healthy people 2000: National health promotion and disease prevention objectives* (DHHS 91-50213). Washington, DC: U.S. Government Printing Office.

Walton, M. (1986). *The Deming Management Method.* New York: Dodd, Mead.

## CHAPTER 6

Communicating Quality Outcomes

Karen Ann Lentz

CHAPTER OBJECTIVES

After completing this chapter, the reader will be able to

- describe the conversion of data to information
- explain data characteristics
- summarize the three components involved in communicating 110 activities
- prepare a clear, precise, 110 report
- discuss creative visual methods for presenting data and information
- explain the legal implications of disclosing quality data

An aspect of quality improvement that is essential in the evaluation process is the generation of a report and the communication of information to appropriate individuals. A quality improvement report provides factual information about an organization's practice, professional performance, or issues of significance to patient care. The purpose of such a report is to give direction to those individuals involved in evaluating and enhancing systems of patient care and maintaining practice standards.

Inherent in the reporting of quality improvement activities is the concept of accountability. Quality improvement reports provide the necessary documentation to assure the public and regulatory agencies that performance within an institution is consistent with community and national standards. In addition, documentation of quality improvement activities provides an organization with the information needed to make determinations regarding cost, resources use, quality and appropriateness of care, as well as the reappointment of medical staff members. Thus, quality improvement documentation assists the organization in fulfilling its responsibilities to the public as well as enabling the organization to better monitor and improve the care it provides.

CONVERSION OF DATA TO INFORMATION

Health care organizations need information about process and outcome performance, such as financial performance, resource consumption, medical outcomes, customer satisfaction, and market share, to draw organizationally relevant conclusions about performance. Traditional measures are organized around departments or divisions, but they can be built around diagnostic groupings, service lines, patient groupings, or any other division that makes the data meaningful for the organization (Carter & Meridy, 1996). How do health care providers know whether particular processes are producing optimal results? Processes are evaluated by collecting and analyzing data. Data are the foundation of information used in a quality improvement report.

Raw data are meaningless unless the data are translated into performance information, which is digested in a format that is useful to the decision maker. The process of translating the data into performance information is accomplished by personnel familiar with the quality performance issues related to the process to be evaluated. Because the usefulness of the performance report depends on the data from which it is derived, it is essential that the data collection system be carefully designed to gather the discrete facts that are relevant to the quality performance issue to be evaluated.

Data must have acceptable degrees of relevance, range, reliability, validity, variation, and control to avoid the potential of providing irrelevant information or misinformation that can lead to poor decisions (Joint Commission, 1996b). Data interpreters must evaluate the strength of the clinical performance data using the following six attributes of strong clinical performance data:

1. *Relevance* is the degree to which clinical performance data relate to what organizations do—the functions or processes and the relative importance of these functions or processes. Irrelevant data waste resources (Joint Commission, 1996b).

2. *Range* of health care process and outcomes will give data users a complete portrait to accurately judge an organization's performance. This range will allow data users to invest improvement resources where they will do the most good and avoid causing (or failing to prevent) harm elsewhere in the organization (Joint Commission, 1996b).

3. *Data reliability* is the extent to which data results are consistent across repeated measurements of the same phenomenon by different measurers or at different times by the same measurers. The phenomenon must not have changed in the interval between measurements. All data have a degree of unreliability. Nevertheless, an acceptable level of reli-

ability should be present if data are to provide an accurate representation of the process or outcome undergoing measurement (Joint Commission, 1996b).

4. *Data validity* is the extent to which an indicator and its data measure only what they were intended to measure. The usefulness of data is directly related to the degree that they are valid in the eyes of the users. Data reliability and validity are distinct, but interlinked, attributes that come in degree. Unreliable data will almost always be invalid data. Reliable data, however, may not necessarily be valid data (Joint Commission, 1996b).

5. *Degree of variation* influences improvement opportunities. Wider variation in data usually signals more improvement opportunities, whereas narrower variation means fewer improvement opportunities. A large discrepancy between the average value of a data set and what is generally the established and well-accepted (desired) average signals more improvement opportunities; a small discrepancy means fewer opportunities. Probably the greatest opportunity for improvement comes with data that show both wide variation with respect to their average and have an average that is displaced from the established average. The least opportunity for improvement comes with data that show narrow variation with respect to their average, which is not displaced from the established average (Joint Commission, 1996b).

6. *Control* is the degree to which organizations and clinicians have the authority to determine the methods, timing, and other factors that affect the process to be measured. Without control over the processes and outcomes undergoing measurement, improvement efforts can be both costly and futile (Joint Commission, 1996b).

Strong clinical performance data can easily be transformed into accurate, useful information. This information can assist health care providers in decision making and guide actions for improvement.

REPORT PREPARATION

Quality improvement reports may consist of highly structured forms such as incident reports or freely arranged documents that require the author to systematically organize information in a narrative style. Regardless of the type of format used, consideration should be given to the basic principles of written communication in completing a report. A report should consist of a clear and precise accounting of relevant data and information. Perhaps the most important steps in achieving this goal are to specifically define the subject of the report and develop a corresponding outline. The outline provides a framework for the report and guarantees inclusion of essential material.

A quality improvement report usually includes the following elements:

- a statement of the topic, or problems and study objectives
- an explicit description of relevant data
- a delineation of the conclusions and recommendations
- an assessment of the effectiveness of the actions previously taken
- the identification of corrective action, people responsible for each action, and the date when each action is to be complete

The effectiveness of a report depends on its completeness; therefore, a full account of pertinent details is necessary to enable the reader to gain an understanding of the topic.

Although a report must be readable and understandable, it is not a literary narrative and, therefore, should not be embellished with decorative language. Information in a report is conveyed in a straightforward, concise, and coherent style. However, a report does not have to be dull. Incorporation of variety into the report enhances its interest and readability.

Variations in sentence structure and length enliven the facts. In addition, the correct use of punctuation and grammar facilitates the reader's comprehension of the written word. The author of a report is usually reporting on an event that has already occurred; consequently, the report is written in the past tense. It is recommended that a colleague critique the author's preliminary draft of the report for clarity and readability.

Information in a report is presented in a neat and legible manner to enhance its comprehension. Typing of a report, although not always essential, is recommended to give the report an attractive and professional appearance. Whether the report is handwritten or typed, the information should be clearly labeled and adequately spaced on the paper. In addition, the use of visual aids in a report facilitates the objective presentation of information, provides variety, and captures the reader's attention. Visual aids may include histograms, bar graphs, line graphs, statistical tables, diagrams, or other performance-comparison measurements. A graphic or tabular display is used to supplement the narrative report and to clarify the significance of the information. The creative use of accurate and clear visual aids is encouraged; however, the use of crowded and confusing graphic displays may detract from the purpose of the report. Effective use of graphic displays necessitates that they be clearly labeled and self-explanatory.

The current capability to collect and statistically analyze large amounts of data by computer and then to convert the results into easily readable graphic representations has generated an array of performance-comparison measurements. Foremost among these measurements is the benchmarking technique. *Benchmarking* refers to the concept of setting goals based on ascertaining what has been achieved by others. The concept includes setting goals based on the market—what has been achieved by external competitors. It also considers what has been achieved by internal competitors: subsidiaries, other divisions, or other departments.

Display of benchmarked data helps an organization change its behavior and measure the beneficial consequences of the action taken (Rowland & Rowland, 1996).

A report completed by the Clinical Assessment and Risk Evaluation (CARE) staff at the Zablocki Department of Veterans Affairs Medical Center in Milwaukee, WI, provides an example of the effective use of a visual aid using the benchmarking technique. As indicated in Figure 6–1, the use of a line graph provides a clear and understandable distillation of the essential data needed to review and evaluate the average wait time for the next new patient appointment in the cardiology clinic, compared with the wait time for other comparable hospitals within its network.

It is important to keep in mind that the ultimate objective of quality improvement is to improve patient care. The identification, analysis, and reporting of problems are of little value if the process does not lead to corrective action. Correctly identifying deficiencies but failing to resolve them amounts to an idle gesture. This pitfall is best avoided by specifying corrective action with a high degree of particularity. Therefore, the section of the report containing the recommendations is an essential part of quality improvement documentation because of its potential impact on quality of care. Recommendations are developed from an analysis of the findings and are based on the conclusions. The following items should be included:

- delineation of a specific solution or action to alleviate or eliminate an identified problem or improve a process
- identification of a person(s) responsible for implementation of each of the recommendations

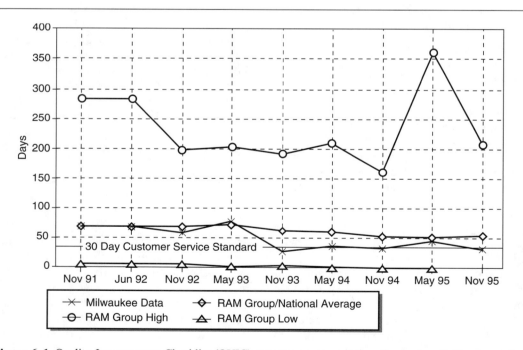

Figure 6–1 Quality Improvement Checklist (QUIC) report average wait time for next available new patient appointment, cardiology clinic. RAM: Resource Allocation Methodology. Courtesy of the Clement J. Zablocki VA Medical Center, 1996, Milwaukee, Wisconsin

- identification of a time frame for implementation of each recommendation
- identification of a time frame for overall or focused evaluation of the problem or process
- prioritization of recommendations

Recommendations that are succinct and clearly stated have the greatest potential for effecting change.

COMMUNICATION SYSTEMS

The communication of an organization's quality improvement activities involves three components:

1. organizational structure
2. reporting systems
3. presentation

The organizational structure reflects lines of communication and authority for the total quality improvement program. Reporting systems consist of the systematic communication of information and feedback related to maintenance of quality standards, the resolution of specific problems, and the improvement in processes. Presentation is the use of visual media and the latest technologies to communicate information.

Organizational Structure

The structure of an organization's quality improvement program should be designed to facilitate the collection, analysis, and reporting of quality improvement data and the implementation of quality improvement activities. Emphasis is on the development and maintenance of effective mechanisms to monitor and evaluate performance standards and processes. The quality improvement structure is organized to encompass all areas for which standards have been established. The Joint Commission on Accreditation of Healthcare Organizations (Joint Commission, 1996) has categorized standards according to the functional classifications as shown in Table 6–1. The organizational structure of a well-designed quality improvement program identifies the roles and responsibilities of appropriate staff and committees and delineates the relationships and channels of communication among them. The structure is comprehensive and embraces both clinical and nonclinical functions.

Table 6–1 Components of the Accreditation Decision-Making Process

Components		
Patient-Focused Functions	*Organizational Functions*	*Structures with Functions*
Patient rights and organizational ethics	Improvement of organization performance	Governance
Assessment of patients	Leadership	Management
Care of patients	Management of the care environment	Medical staff
Education	Design	Nursing
Continuum of care	Management of human resources	
	Management of information	
	Surveillance, prevention, and control of infection	

Source: Data from 1997 Comprehensive Accreditation Manual for Hospitals, Joint Commission on Accreditation of Healthcare Organizations.

The Zablocki VA Medical Center has developed an improvement of performance framework that promotes and directs a collaborative and systematic approach to performance activities to guide the design, measurement, assessment, and improvement of patient care and organization-wide functions. The structure of this organization is delineated in Figures 6–2 and 6–3. In the Zablocki model, the medical center director, associate director, and chief of staff (top management team) provide overall direction and coordination for all committee activities and maintain authority for the total quality improvement program. Quality improvement activities for clinical and non-clinical processes are governed by the top management team and division managers. All employees are encouraged to participate in performance improvement activities and are expected to support the guiding principles of the Medical Center.

In addition to the division-level quality improvement activities, various Medical Center–wide committees such as the Surgical Case and Invasive Procedure Committee and Blood Utilization Review Committee are appointed by the top management team and division managers. The Medical Center committees comprise multidisciplinary staff charged with responsibility for quality improvement issues that relate to those particular organization-wide functions. The division-level quality improvement and Medical Center–wide committees are responsible for designing and implementing a systematic process for monitoring and evaluating the quality and appropriateness of services, initiating actions when problems are identified, and assessing the effectiveness of those actions.

The CARE Section comprises CARE or quality improvement coordinators who are responsible for providing direction in implementation of the Medical Center quality, utilization and risk management, and safety and infection control programs. A CARE coordinator, assigned to each division, functions as a consultant and provides technical assistance and management oversight in support of division activities. The CARE coordinator provides consultation in areas such as measurement development, data collection and analysis, report writing, communication of findings, and implementation of actions. Another responsibility of each CARE coordinator is to coordinate collection and dissemination of quality, risk, utilization, safety, and infection control information. The CARE coordinator is a member of organization-wide committees or committees of the division to which he or she is assigned.

The establishment of quality improvement committees is not specifically mandated by the Joint Commission. However, a coordinated system providing for quality review and the effective implementation of corrective action is required, and quality improvement committees provide one method for accomplishing those functions. The structure of the system will vary among organizations.

The quality improvement reporting process is enhanced by a clear delineation of committee functions. The reporting system must be designed to accommodate the particular quality improvement organizational structure that exists within an organization. A description of the membership and purposes of two Zablocki Medical Center hospitalwide committees, given in Exhibits 6–1 and 6–2, serves as an illustration of committee structure designed to facilitate effective reporting. It also provides an example of an organizational context for the reporting systems described in the following section.

Reporting Systems

Issues of concern and relevancy in the evaluation of patient care services and maintenance of established standards may be identified through the following mechanisms:

- department/service/team quality improvement reports
- quality improvement subcommittee findings
- patient interviews or complaints

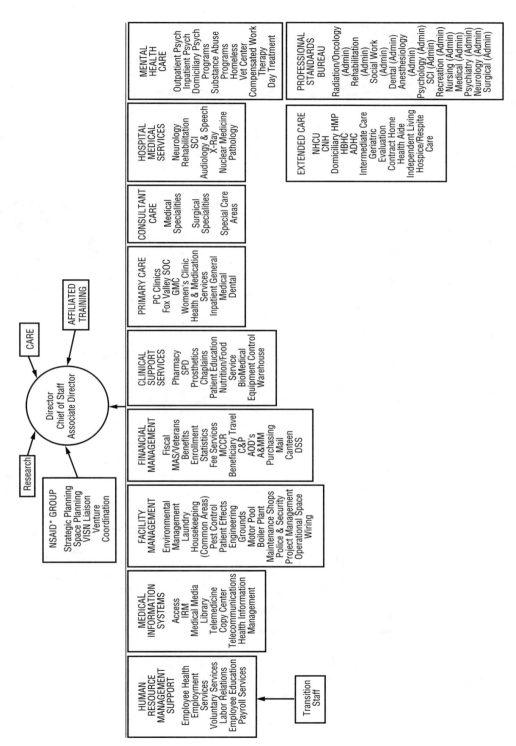

Figure 6–2 Courtesy of the Clement J. Zablocki VA Medical Center, 1996, Milwaukee, Wisconsin

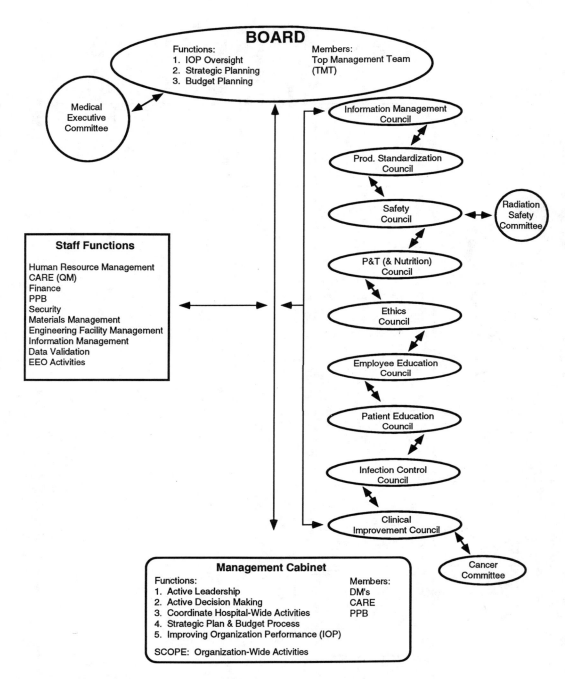

Figure 6–3 Courtesy of the Clement J. Zablocki VA Medical Center, 1996, Milwaukee, Wisconsin

Exhibit 6–1 Surgical Case and Invasive Procedures Committee

(1) Responsibility:

   (a) To establish and define a structured mechanism for a regular and objective evaluation and monitoring of all surgical and invasive procedures done in the Medical Center to ensure appropriateness and quality of these procedures.

   (b) To review regularly the justification, appropriateness and quality of all surgical and invasive procedures utilizing pre-established screening criteria and indicators. The review encompasses all tissue cases, all non-tissue cases including intravascular catheters, cases with non-diagnostic procedures done in all areas of the Medical Center, and autopsy cases.

   (c) To make recommendations to leadership regarding appropriate actions relating to discrepancies and problems identified during the regular reviews.

   (d) To work with CARE (Clinical Assessment and Risk Evaluation) Section in the implementation of quality improvement mechanisms concerning surgical and invasive procedures.

(2) Membership:

Chairman: Chief, Anatomic Pathology
Recorder: Secretary, Laboratory Service
Members: Chief, Surgical Service or designee
Chief, Urology Section or designee
Chief, Anesthesia Service or designee
Chief, Pulmonary Section or designee
Chief, GI Section or designee
Chief, Radiology Service or designee
Chief, Cardiology Section or designee
Chief, Spinal Cord Injury Service or designee
ACOS/Education
CARE Coordinator

Courtesy of the Clement J. Zablocki VA Medical Center, 1996, Milwaukee, Wisconsin.

Exhibit 6–2 Blood Utilization Review Committee

(1) Responsibility:

   (a) Transfusion practices are monitored to ensure that:

      1. They are in accordance with Professional Services Memorandum No. II-S, Blood Transfusions and Plasma Expanders, and

      2. They do not involve administration of inappropriate transfusions of blood or blood components and the proper documentation recorded.

   (b) Particular attention will be paid to packed cell usage.

   (c) Transfusion reactions will be reviewed: all investigations of blood transfusions will be in accordance with the procedures recommended in current editions of "Standards for Blood Banks and Transfusion Services" and "Technical Methods and Procedures" published by the AABB.

   (d) Minutes of the Committee will include all findings of reviews, conclusions, and actions taken as a result thereof.

continues

Exhibit 6–2 continued

(2) **Membership:**
Co-Chairman Chief, Hematology/Oncology Section, Medical Service
Co-Chairman Chief, Laboratory Service
Chief, Anesthesiology Service
Chief, Nursing Service
Representative, Nursing Service
Staff Physician, Surgical Service
Supervisor, Blood Bank (ad hoc)
(3) The Blood Utilization Committee will meet quarterly. Minutes will be distributed to all appropriate Division Managers and CARE Section in order to integrate with Quality Improvement Activities.

Source: Courtesy of the Clement J. Zablocki VA Medical Center, 1996, Milwaukee, Wisconsin.

- other organizational committee reports
- individual health care professionals
- satisfaction surveys
- occurrence screens
- length of stay reports
- tort claims
- incident reports
- drug and adverse reactions
- surgical/tissue/procedure reviews
- focused reviews
- medication usage reviews
- infection control reports
- mortality rate
- delinquent medical record review
- rate of nonacute patient days report
- unplanned admissions from ambulatory surgery
- return or readmission rates

Problems identified by these mechanisms can be effectively resolved through application of the quality improvement process only if pertinent documentation is comprehensive, accurate, and up-to-date. Each institution should consider developing forms for documentation and a system for communication of quality improvement information that applies to the characteristics and intricacies of its organization.

Information about specific reviews or evaluations may be documented in a narrative fashion or on a form specifically designed to accommodate such data. The use of a standardized form is highly recommended for the purpose of ensuring the consistency and quality of necessary information. General content areas may include the following:

- clinical indicator for care
- actual sample monitored
- clinical areas involved
- methodology
- findings
- conclusions
- recommendations
- actions
- follow-up
- effectiveness of actions
- person responsible

These content areas can be organized into formats such as those depicted in Exhibits 6–3, 6–4, and 6–5.

In addition to formal reviews of patient care problems, incident reports have relevancy to the quality improvement program. Incident reports consist of medication error reports; patient, staff, or visitor accident or injury reports; and miscellaneous incident reports such as those related to environmental hazards, theft, or property damage. These reports provide statistical information on which to base

Exhibit 6–3 Department/Service/Team Documentation of Quality Improvement Report

DATE:

PERFORMANCE MEASURE:

SAMPLE MEASURED:

MEASUREMENT:

SUMMARY OF FINDINGS (INCLUDE BENCHMARKED OR THRESHOLD DATA):

CONCLUSIONS:

RECOMMENDATIONS:

ACTIONS:

FOLLOW-UP (INCLUDE DATE AND SUMMARY):

EFFECTIVENESS OF ACTIONS:

Reported to: _____   Date: _____

Signature: _____   Date: _____

Source: Courtesy of the Clement J. Zablocki VA Medical Center, 1996, Milwaukee, Wisconsin.

Exhibit 6–4 Consultant Care Division Report Card

MISSION
Support Primary Care for the veteran patient by providing consultant Services that exceed expectations for Access, Quality and Cost-Effectiveness.
VISION
Recognized as a center for excellence in secondary, tertiary, and quaternary health care, education and research in the Department of Veterans Affairs Health Care System

Goals	Measures of Performance	Outcome											
		Jan	Feb	Mar	Apr	May	Jun	Jul	Aug	Sep	Oct	Nov	Dec
1. Cost effective care-appropriate utilization													
	Total surgical cases	241	207	250	229	233	238	214	219				
	***Ambulatory procedures	39.8	38.2	43.6	48.5	41.2	43.3	32.7	44.3				
	***Inpatient procedures	60.2	61.8	56.4	51.5	58.8	56.7	67.3	55.7				
2. Satisfy external reviews													
	***# Reviews passed by Peer Review	3	0	1	3	0	1	7	3				
3. Quality tertiary care													
	Surgical wound infection rate-% clean												
	***% clean	0.8%	2.1%	1.7%	1.7%	1.2%	0.5%	0.6%	1.3%				
	C-diff Index (# unique positive toxins/ # unique patient specimens)	18.2	19.7	13.9	15.7	16.6	13.1	15.4	16.7				
	Autopsy rate (%)	34.8	5.6	33.3	15.8	11.8	11.1	21.4	9.1%				
	Survival rate for code-4	29%	78%	55%	58%	45%	33%	50%	75%				
4. Timeliness of care													
	Surgical cancellation rate	6%	20%	15%	19%	20%	12%	11%	12%				
	***Avoidable cancellation rate for scheduled cases	0%	4%	7%	8%	9%	6%	6%	4%				

Courtesy of the Clement J. Zablocki VA Medical Center, 1996, Milwaukee, Wisconsin.

Exhibit 6–5 Report Card Data Sheet

Performance Measures	FY 97				Bench -marks	Actions
	1st Quarter	2nd Quarter	3rd Quarter	4th Quarter		
BDOC						
Acute Care						
Mental Health						
SCI						
Rehab						
Domiciliary						
NHCU						
Access Score						
% enrolled in primary care						
# specialty clinic visits						
Outpatient Surgery Rate						
Customer Satisfaction						
Internal						
External						
# Transfers						
# Congressionals						
Mandatory Education Rate						
Training Rate						
FTEE						
Payroll						
- Worked/Paid Hours						
- Unscheduled Time						
- Overtime						
- Fee Basis						
- Regular						
- Comp Time						

Courtesy of the Clement J. Zablocki VA Medical Center, 1996, Milwaukee, Wisconsin.

quality improvement efforts. All of these reports are reviewed monthly by the quality improvement coordinator for the purpose of identifying trends or patterns in the reported incidents. The identification of specific patterns may determine the need for a focused review or corrective action. Figure 6–4 is an example of a graph used to display monthly data on the frequency of patient falls. In relation to an organization's risk management program, incident reports provide valuable information to aid the safety committee in its efforts to prevent or reduce accidents. The incident report also provides useful documentation regarding corrective action taken to resolve a problem or improve a process.

Minutes of committee meetings are an essential component of a reporting system in a quality improvement program. Exhibit 6–6 displays a format for minutes that facilitates the communication of quality improvement activities. Circulation of quality improvement committee minutes among all concerned personnel provides an efficient and effective means of apprising the staff of the status of current quality improvement matters. Committee minutes serve to summarize data, document identified problems or processes, and advise of corrective action undertaken. A reporting system consisting of the timely distribution of quality improvement minutes that present a complete, but concise summary of pertinent quality improvement information in a clear and uniform format can form the basis for a comprehensive and cohesive hospitalwide quality improvement program.

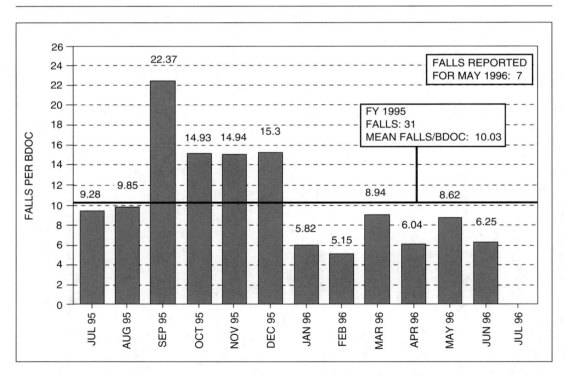

Figure 6–4 Ward 4C falls/bed days of care (BDOC) (7/95–7/96). Courtesy of the Clement J. Zablocki VA Medical Center, 1996, Milwaukee, Wisconsin.

Exhibit 6–6 Sample Agenda Format

I. Approval of minutes of previous meeting (date of previous meeting)

II. Old Business

    A. Follow-up reports regarding previous actions and recommendations

    B. Follow-up responses from committee referrals to other committees, departments, and individuals

    C. Other items of old business

III. New Business

    A. Performance improvement

        1. Benchmarking or statistical reports

        2. Ongoing monitoring

        3. Focused studies

        4. Other performance improvement activities related to committee function

        5. Performance improvement activities referred by other committees, departments, and individuals

        6. Reports from external sources

        7. Case review

    B. Oversight

        1. Policy, procedure, and criteria issues related to committee function

        2. Other oversight responsibilities

    C. Other items of new business

IV. Administrative report

V. Educational presentations

VI. Adjournment (time)

    A. Next meeting date, time and location

Source: Reprinted with permission from *Documenting Hospital Meetings*, 2nd ed., © 1996, Care Education Group Inc.

Presentation

Organizations have used various creative methods to display and communicate the success stories describing quality performance activities. A common method is the use of storyboards. Storyboards help advertise and showcase information. A storyboard is a way of summarizing a quality improvement report or improvement project using a minimal amount of text. Rather, it explains the whole process with the use of photographs, graphs, and displays of performance improvement tools. Storyboards also offer an opportunity to give recognition to individuals who contributed to the improvement process. An example of a model for a storyboard is displayed in Figure 6–5. Storyboards serve as an effective mechanism to keep others in the organization well informed of the performance improvement activities of the organization. For a sample storyboard, see Figure 28–3.

Slide presentations are another popular method used to communicate improvement information to a targeted audience. With the use of the latest presentation graphics software and innovative tools, performance improvement information can be converted easily from printed documentation into effective and

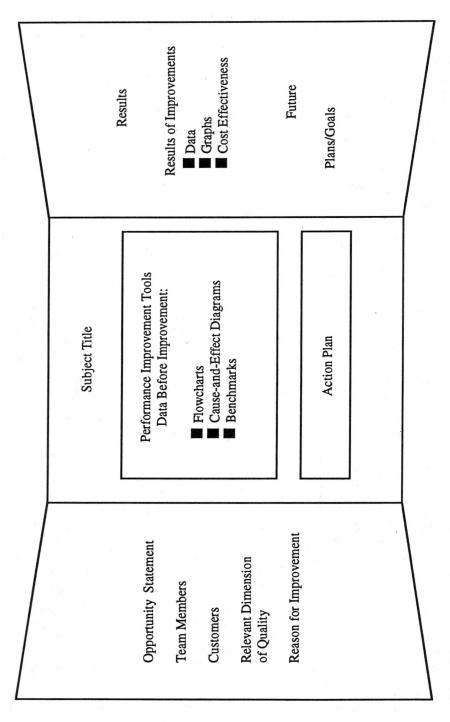

Figure 6–5 Model for storyboard. *Source:* Reprinted from Managing Hospital Quality, Risk, and Cost. Storyboards Showcase Performance Improvement, *QRC Advisor,* Vol. 12, No. 9, ©1996, Aspen Publishers, Inc.

attractive slides to quickly and easily create a professional-looking presentation. Slides can contain titles, text, graphs, drawn objects, shapes, clip art, drawn art, and visuals created with other applications. The latest software allows the user to create overhead slides, speakers notes, audience handouts, and an outline, all in a single presentation file. The software packages offer a myriad of possibilities for anyone who wants to create and use effective techniques to communicate information by visual presentation. When planning your slide presentation,

- Be concise.
- Use key phrases; eliminate unnecessary words.
- Make a single point with each slide.
- Remember the six-by-six rule: no more than six lines of type per slide and no more than six words per line.
- Do not cramp your slide.

Be creative and use a variety of different presentation techniques. Your goal is to catch the attention of the audience and communicate the highlights of quality improvement activities.

DISCLOSURE OF QUALITY MANAGEMENT RECORDS

Legal considerations concerning the disclosure of quality management records are complex and in a state of continual change. This complexity and flux underscore the need to obtain the assistance of legal counsel in the development of organizational documentation disclosure policy and when novel confidentiality issues arise (Strong, 1992). Nevertheless, a general knowledge of the basic law and ethical considerations relating to disclosure of quality management records is helpful.

The confidentiality of patient records is often discussed in terms of the physician–patient privilege. Awareness of this legal concept is important to all health care providers. However, in the early 1950s, a particular privilege relating specifically to peer review activities began to emerge.

Physician–Patient Privilege

The law of physician–patient privilege is a rule of evidence that provides a patient with the right to prevent disclosure of confidential communications or information obtained or disseminated for purposes of diagnosis or treatment. The privilege prohibits the physician and other health care providers from disclosing such information without the patient's consent (Strong, 1992).

The purpose of the rule is to avoid inhibition of the free flow of information between the patient and the health care provider that might result if the patient had to fear the potential for later disclosure of such information to third parties. This privilege may be waived by the patient and, in any event, does not ordinarily apply in legal proceedings in which the information relates to a condition that is an element of a patient's damage claim (Strong, 1992). Thus, in medical malpractice cases the physician–patient privilege generally does not apply.

Peer Review Privilege

In times past, hospitals enjoyed a limited degree of immunity from liability from patient claims. In recent decades, this immunity has been largely eroded and hospitals are now subject to claims based on a failure to adequately evaluate the quality of the medical care they provide. Quality review activity necessarily generates documentation that is, to some extent, critical of patient care performance. Therefore, a natural reluctance on the part of hospitals to be aggressive and candid in conducting such activities might be expected. Recognizing the public interest in encouraging quality management activities, governments sought to dispel such reluctance by enacting statutes establishing a privilege that protects peer review materials from disclosure (Rowland, 1988).

The District of Columbia and virtually every state have enacted peer review privilege legislation. In addition, federal and state courts have recognized a limited privilege in case law. Unfortunately, the law is not uniform and is subject to continual revision (Rowland, 1988). The privilege is subject to limitations and exceptions that vary depending on the jurisdiction and the context in which the issue arises.

Complicating matters, each state and the District of Columbia mandate by statute that hospitals report to state agencies information pertaining to the competence of medical staff. Furthermore, the federal Health Care Quality Improvement Act of 1986 requires all hospitals to report certain disciplinary actions pertaining to physician clinical privileges to the National Practitioner Data Bank and to their state boards of medical examiners. This law also provides limited immunity from damage claims (e.g., for defamation) that might arise out of peer review activities (Rothschild, 1993).

The peer review privilege was created to serve the valuable public policy interest of fostering vigorous quality management activity. It is, therefore, important that the hospital evaluate its policies and practices to ensure that the privilege is properly protected. The hospital's organizational structure, rules and regulations, staff bylaws, and procedural manuals should be reviewed with counsel and modified as needed to comport with the law of the applicable jurisdiction.

The rationale behind the development of the peer review privilege and the immunity from liability concerning peer review proceedings is the encouragement of frank and complete peer review activity by diminishing concerns about the exposure to liability that might otherwise result from such activity. The integrity of the National Practitioner Data Bank and its usefulness as a system for identifying deficient practitioners depends on accurate medical record reporting (Waller, Glasser, & Johnson, 1992).

Questions concerning disclosure of peer review documentation often arise in the con-

text of disciplinary proceedings or tort claims. Because of the unpleasant nature of such proceedings, there may be a tendency to moderate or exclude negative findings in quality improvement documentation at the expense of accuracy. Any such tendency should be resisted. The ultimate objective of quality improvement is to maximize the quality of patient care. That objective is not well served when the quality improvement process is dominated by risk aversion considerations that impair the accuracy of quality management documentation.

Aside from the legalities, basic ethical principles require sensitivity to the patient's reasonable expectations of confidentiality. In most instances, there is no need to specifically identify patients in quality improvement reports. The same care that is taken by the publishers of medical research to ensure patient anonymity can be taken with regard to quality improvement documentation with no detriment to its efficacy.

CONCLUSION

A successful quality improvement program depends on the clear delineation of lines of communication and responsibility as well as use of an effective reporting system. The documentation and communication of quality improvement activities involve the identification of problems, the specification of corrective action, and the identification of the individuals responsible for implementing these actions.

Quality improvement reports must be integrated into a network of communication among the appropriate people. The reporting system must be sensitive to patient confidentiality and information disclosure issues. Quality improvement reports are most effective when they are succinct, comprehensive, appropriately distributed, meaningful for the audience reviewing the information, and interesting.

REFERENCES

Carter, J.H., & Meridy, H. (1996). Making a performance improvement plan work. *The Joint Commission Journal on Quality Improvement, 22*(2), 104–113.

Health Care Quality Improvement Act § 11101 et seq., 42 U.S.C. (1986).

Joint Commission on Accreditation of Healthcare Organizations. (1996a). *1997 Accreditation manual for hospitals.* Oakbrook Terrace, IL: Author.

Joint Commission on Accreditation of Healthcare Organizations. (1996b). *Clinical performance data: A guide to interpretation.* Oakbrook Terrace, IL: Author.

Rothschild, I.S. (1993). The Health Care Quality Improvement Act and the National Practitioner Data Bank: Current issues and emerging legal and operational trends. In A.G. Gosfield (Ed.), *1993 health law handbook.* New York: Clark Boardman.

Rowland, H.S., & Rowland, B.L. (1996). *The manual of nursing quality assurance* (Vol. 1). Gaithersburg, MD: Aspen.

Rowland, J.M. (1988). Enforcing hospital responsibility through self-evaluation and review committee confidentiality. *Journal of Legal Medicine 9*(3).

Strong, J.W. (Ed.). (1992). *McCormick on evidence* (4th ed.). St. Paul, MN: West.

Waller, A.A., Glasser, D.L., & Johnson, T.A. (1992). Medical records: Current issues and emerging trends. In A.G. Gosfield (Ed.), *1992 health law handbook.* New York: Clark Boardman.

## CHAPTER 7

Evaluating Quality Improvement: Effectiveness and Cost

Carolyn H. Smeltzer and Ted Pfeiffer

CHAPTER OBJECTIVES

After completing the chapter, the reader will be able to

- describe the components of performance measurement
- judge an effective QI program
- evaluate deviation from desired performance
- distinguish between formative and summative evaluation
- use change theory as a framework for program evaluation

Nurse managers and other patient care leaders who hold responsibility for quality improvement (QI) programs are challenged to design, implement, and report on the effectiveness of their own programs to create a feedback loop and thus improve performance. The goal of QI is to optimize the allocation of clinical resources (achieving the greatest impact from increasingly scarce resources); yet, the term *quality* remains nebulous. Although perhaps one of the most frequently used terms in the health care environment, there is little universal agreement on the definition and operationalization of a clinical quality program. Regulators, professional organizations, payers, patients, and individuals each maintain their own definitions of *quality* and all too frequently assume that others share their view. Notwithstanding the general lack of consensus

on the specifics of what constitutes a high-quality patient care program, the common thread among all uses of the term *quality* seems to be an attempt to capture a satisfactory and constantly evolving system of delivering patient care.

Although the terminology surrounding quality has changed in the past and will likely continue to change, the fundamental principle of QI has operated as a fairly consistent process loop. To understand the loop, think of five steps: (1) setting standards, (2) measuring performance as it relates to such standards, (3) evaluating deviation from desired performance, (4) reporting performance or deviation, and (5) engaging in targeted action to close gaps between desired and observed performance levels. Understanding the quality loop makes evaluation of a QI program fairly straightforward. Quite simply, to evaluate the effectiveness of a QI program, the program should turn its evaluative light on itself and follow these general steps.

This chapter discusses the traditional role of the QI program as it has usually existed in hospitals as well as ideas for program evaluation at each one of the steps in the QI loop. The discussion demonstrates how the basic principles of continuous quality improvement may be applied to program evaluation efforts. The chapter also defines the formative and summative categories of evaluation and explains how they relate to the choices available when designing a QI program evaluation. To demonstrate that there is room for flexibility and creativity in the design of a QI program, the chapter also presents an alternative framework for program evaluation using the principles of change theory. Recognizing the ever-increasing pressure on organizations to operate cost consciously, the authors discuss the distinction between cost-benefit analysis versus cost-effectiveness as an essential component of the program evaluation.

UNDERSTANDING THE ORIGIN OF QI PROGRAMS

To understand the traditional role of QI programs, one must first understand the traditional role of regulatory agencies in the provision of health care. Accrediting organizations such as the Joint Commission on Accreditation of Healthcare Organizations exert enormous power over organizations in that their approval is necessary for an organization to receive reimbursement from government payers (the single largest payer category for most health care organizations). Even hospitals and other health care providers that do not operate with a profit motive must nevertheless pay attention to their own financial health ("If there's no money, there's no mission," goes the classic saying around many health care organizations affiliated with religious organizations). Thus, by holding the key to fiscal solvency, the approval of regulatory agencies is necessary to ensure the very survival of most organizations.

Given the enormous power held by regulators, QI programs have tended to evolve almost exclusively toward the goal of satisfying regulatory demands. Unfortunately, however, such exclusive focus on regulatory satisfaction may result in the inattention of a QI program to other critical stakeholders present in the organization's environment. Those stakeholders include physicians, private payer organizations, patients, and the community, each of which plays an important role in the fulfillment of the organization's mission. Yet, these critical stakeholders have at times been ignored in the myopic rush to anticipate and satisfy the QI demands of regulatory agencies.

RECOGNIZING THE ROLE OF QI IN A CHANGING ENVIRONMENT

Whereas power over the organization's success was once held almost exclusively by regulatory agencies, that power has now been diffused among many stakeholder groups with varied needs and interests. Although it was once sufficient to satisfy regulators, it is now the case that, in addition to regulatory compliance, the successful provider must satisfy a range of interested parties who approach the organization from a consumeristic point of view. The truly effective QI program recognizes the organization's need to satisfy the diverse interests of those parties and seeks to support such efforts.

Private payer organizations (insurance companies that pay on a fee-for-service basis and health maintenance organizations that contract for various services) are beginning to demand that organizations provide quantification of clinical effectiveness, a function that falls to the QI program. These same payers also expect clear proof that the organization has obtained satisfactory clinical outcomes. Unfortunately, however, one of the frustrations facing leaders in QI programs is the current lack of agreement among payer organizations and what constitutes appropriate clinical outcomes reporting. Until widely agreed-upon measures are in place, QI program directors must exercise their own judgment concerning clinical indicators, but also must remain alert to industry trends (most often communicated by professional publications). Perhaps most important, QI program directors must position their programs to be flexible and adaptable as definitions evolve regarding appropriate clinical outcomes reporting. The QI program director's best defense, therefore, may well be his or her understanding of the quality process as it applies to the evaluation of quality program effectiveness.

APPLYING THE QI PROCESS LOOP TO THE QI PROGRAM

Setting Standards

The QI Program articulates the value it seeks to add to the organization. Questions include, What tangible results has the program been designed to offer? What should be different or better about the organization as a result of the QI program?

The greatest challenge at this stage is *to be specific*. The truly effective QI program will clearly state the benefits it seeks to deliver as well as objective criteria for knowing when such criteria have been met. Review the following two fictional QI program performance standard statements and judge which is more truly effective in terms of setting performance standards.

Hospital A: Statement of QI Performance Standards

We will support our organization through timely tracking of key processes. Our commitment to quality will be met when all staff are committed to delivery of the highest quality patient care. We will know we are successful when every member of the staff provides appropriate care in a setting of caring and respect for the patient.

The quality program at Hospital A will work with all necessary parties to monitor the appropriateness and effectiveness of care, while ensuring that patient needs come first. We will strive to provide timely and accurate reporting to all key members of the organization and ensure that complete plans for correction are in place, where warranted.

Hospital B: Statement of QI Performance Standards

The success of Hospital B requires timely, specific evaluation of patient care outcomes; customer satisfaction (including internal customers); and performance of agreed-upon core processes. To that end, the QI program at

Hospital B will take monthly measurements of mortality rates, re-admission rates, and nosocomial infection rates on not less than 20 of those diagnosis-related groups that constitute the greatest volume of Hospital B's cases. In addition, the program will conduct surveys at least twice per year of the hospital's top three "customer" groups as identified by the Strategic Visioning Committee to assess those groups' perceptions of hospital performance. Criteria to be monitored in these surveys will include, but not be limited to, overall hospital performance; responsiveness to changing customer needs; value (as defined and perceived by the customers); and willingness to recommend Hospital B to others. Measurement and monitoring will also occur through quarterly measurement of error rates and turnaround times for at least 20 core processes as identified by Hospital B's chief operating officer.

Responsibility for the coordination and reporting of all QI functions will reside with the QI program staff under the direction of the QI program director. Wherever possible, however, responsibility for raw data collection will reside with the individuals with whom or units where the work being monitored is performed. The program's performance goal is that not fewer than 20% of *all* Hospital B employees will serve as participants in routine quality monitoring efforts as part of their usual job responsibilities.

All quality monitoring efforts will be reported publicly. The QI program staff will maintain bulletin boards at not fewer than five locations throughout the hospital on which it will display performance trends of the quality indicators listed previously. The bulletin boards will be updated no later than the 15th of each month with results through the end of the preceding calendar month.

Clearly, Hospital B has done the better job of establishing objective performance criteria for its QI program. Although there may not be anything outwardly objectionable in Hospital A's statement, it contains no clear pronouncement of standards for program success. During

Hospital B's self-evaluation, however, the program will be able to tell without question whether it succeeded in its intent. Notice that Hospital B has succeeded simply by articulating the who, what, when, where, and how of its QI program.

In many ways, this first step in the loop is the most difficult. It requires the participants in the QI program, and the organization as a whole, to come to concrete agreement on the role and outputs of the QI program. If program evaluation results in a finding that clear standards have not been set, there is no reason for the rest of the evaluation process to continue. Instead, attention should be directed to the essential task of defining the program and the value it seeks to create.

Measuring Performance

Because health care QI is a service function, and services are intangible, performance measurement can be especially tricky. Yet almost anything can be quantified somehow. The first challenge is to make sure that the measurement is the most direct possible reflection of performance on the criteria in question. One must construct an inquiry that ensures the usefulness of the data. Evaluating for this dimension is as easy as asking, Will this evaluation really tell us if we have performed well? Having considered the usefulness of the QI program inquiries, the still greater challenge is to ensure that the inquiry is unbiased.

Whereas *specificity* was the watchword in setting standards, the watchword for performance measurement is *objectivity*. Thus, the QI program evaluator should not be satisfied to merely test for the presence of QI measurement efforts, but should also assess the objectivity of those measurements. Narrative reports and commentary may be an appropriate component of performance measurement, but numerical measurements are far more likely to pass the test of objectivity. The evaluation process should therefore assess whether the program has gathered numerical data in the units identi-

fied in the initial standard-setting step. For example, in the fictional case of Hospital B, the statement of QI performance standards reads, in part, "not fewer than 20% of *all* Hospital B employees will serve as participants in routine quality monitoring efforts." Therefore, in assessing the quality of its own QI program, Hospital B must measure the actual number of employees who have played an active role in gathering QI-related data over the prior evaluation period. Toward the goal of objective measurement along this dimension, the evaluator may contact each department manager in the hospital and request the names of employees who participated in data collection. Alternatively, the evaluator might conduct a file review to identify names of individuals who submitted reports of performance data. The final tally would next be divided by the total number of hospital employees. The resulting percentage quantifies the actual performance of the program on this particular standard.

A balance must be achieved among the scope of the measurements, the speed with which the measures may be gathered or reported, and the frequency with which measures are taken. If the scope of measurement is too narrow, the purpose of objective measurement is defeated (i.e., it may be discounted as nonrepresentative). Yet, if the scope of measurement is too great, the time and other resources required to take the measures may be wasted, and the evaluation process slowed down in trying to cope with mountains of data. In evaluating itself, the quality program must also contemplate the speed with which it completes each cycle of the feedback loop as described at the beginning of this chapter. Because feedback is created for the purpose of changing behavior to close gaps between desired and actual performance, the timeliness of data is particularly important. If the data are "fresh," those individuals receiving feedback will be most likely to note the gaps and construct causal relationships (thus preparing recipients to take appropriate corrective action). However, the frequency with which the performance is measured should be determined in recognition that performance measurement incurs cost, and thus cannot be undertaken frivolously. The feedback loop must be engaged often enough to monitor changes in performance results, yet not so often that the organization lacks time to improve between cycles or that the costs of performance measurement begin to outweigh the benefits.

Involving Providers

Just as measurements regarding the quality of health care delivery should, whenever feasible, be taken by the providers who deliver the care, so too should QI staff participate in gathering program effectiveness data. Such structuring of data-gathering accountability reinforces the cultural value that everyone in the organization shares responsibility for quality. An additional benefit is that, when workers measure their own performance, feedback delays are virtually eliminated. Furthermore, the best measurements are those that are fact based (objective) as opposed to judgment based (subjective).

The bottom line of assessing the effectiveness of the QI program's measurement function is to determine if measurements are objective (cannot be influenced by the opinions of those accountable); timely; and completed by the individuals closest to the process being monitored. To the extent that the QI program evaluator designs the evaluation along these dimensions, the greater the richness of the evaluation and the greater the likely improvements.

Evaluating Deviation from Desired Performance

Because the QI program seeks to add value to the organization, it is appropriate for the program to not only measure performance, but also to articulate deviation from desired performance. The effective QI program will have the resources readily available to design deviation measurement right into its routine evaluation

process, and thus will improve the organization's overall efficiency by completing this step rather than merely passing uninterpreted performance measurements back to the organization.

The steps in the QI process loop are obviously interdependent. For the QI program director who has clearly identified objective standards of performance in an earlier step and who has gathered data in the same units of measurement (e.g., time, rates, and approval scales) as those identified in the standard, it now becomes a relatively simple matter to calculate deviation from desired performance.

Consider Hospital B's intent to realize not less than 20% participation in its QI efforts. Assume that, in measuring participation, the program evaluator discovers that 120 out of 950 employees played direct roles, yielding a participation rate of 13%. Thanks to the specificity of Hospital B's performance standard, and the objectivity of the measure, it is an easy matter to conclude that Hospital B simply did not meet its performance standard on this dimension of QI program effectiveness. Hospital B's program reports (and other documentation) should outrightly state the performance deviation of -7%. Recall that, when done correctly, setting standards (the first step) was the most difficult step in the loop. Conversely, evaluating deviation from desired performance ought to be the least complicated step in the process.

Reporting Performance and Deviations

Even the most comprehensive and efficient performance improvement program will not improve patient care if the evaluation findings are not clearly communicated to the organization. Therefore, when evaluating itself, the QI program must consider its commitment and performance related to ongoing communication of program findings. However, before designing a specific method for evaluating the communication efforts of the program, the evaluator should consider that communication carries a specific purpose in QI and that the purpose of the communications provides an excellent context for evaluation. Specifically, the evaluator must recall that QI data and performance gap analyses are communicated to change behavior in a way that will improve patient care (and other important process) outcomes. Communications efforts that merely send information out into the organization may result in behavioral changes, or they may carry no impact at all.

Instead of merely assessing whether results were distributed, a high-caliber program evaluation will assess the likelihood of whether the communications were performed in such a way to gain the organization's attention and commitment, so that changed behavior will most likely follow where warranted. High-impact communications are widely accessible, require little effort on the recipient's part, are easy to understand, and reflect trends in performance over time. Extra recognition should go to those programs that also include communication about appropriate corrective action for those dimensions on which performance is not meeting standards. These dimensions are those on which the communication efforts of the QI program should be evaluated.

Targeting Action to Close Performance Gaps

To complete the loop and improve QI program performance, the evaluation should consider whether the program design includes routine reevaluation (and revision) of its own performance standards. Because the process operates in a loop, and this step represents the completion of that loop, the same organizational difficulties will be experienced here as were encountered when the role and purpose of the program were originally agreed on in the first step. Once again, the organization is asked to take a hard look at itself to determine if it has made an honest commitment to a particular level of performance. One hopes that most QI programs will have found cause to celebrate fulfillment of their stated goals and objectives. For those organizations, there will only remain

the empowering task of determining how far to stretch their goals for the next period. Other organizations will not find good news in their self-evaluation results. Those organizations that say they value quality, but fail to deploy resources in such a way as to meet desired standards, will face the awkward choice of lowering standards or increasing the use of resources to ensure quality. Yet even when performance has not met expectations, the organization can take heart in having identified its shortcomings and given itself the opportunity to come to terms with its commitment to quality. The only scenario in which an organization can be said to have truly failed is when the organization simply chooses not to identify or address gaps in performance.

FORMATIVE AND SUMMATIVE EVALUATION

Even where the evaluative process is organized in recognition of the steps in the QI process loop, different categories of evaluative process may exist within each step. Program evaluation does not exist independently of the day-to-day operation of the QI program. Evaluation should be a continuous, ongoing process that permeates all phases of program planning, development, and implementation. When designed correctly, the QI program evaluation becomes a tool through which information regarding the strengths and weaknesses of the program is developed, thus enabling informed decisions about the future allocation of resources.

Two distinct types of evaluation exist, and their different roles should be well understood by the QI program evaluator. *Formative evaluation* considers the effectiveness with which the goals and objectives of the QI Program have been implemented. Because short-term objectives are continuously changing and because implementation of QI efforts is an evolving process, formative evaluation is an essential tool. The benefit of formative evaluation is its ability to provide information concerning whether any aspect of the program needs revision.

To understand the importance of formative evaluation, consider the importance of implementation in creating process improvement. Individuals and organizations often recognize, either through fact or feeling (fact being preferable), that their goals are not being achieved. With relative ease they may recognize the problem and underlying causes. They may even be able to design a way to correct the problem. All too frequently, however, a perfectly good solution fails to fix the problem because it is not implemented effectively. Implementation (or lack thereof) has been said to be "everything" in the overall success or failure of most QI efforts (Shortell, 1995). Understanding the critical nature of implementation should make the QI program evaluator especially interested in conducting formative reviews.

Summative evaluation considers the outcomes of the QI program. Typically, the summative evaluation would address measurement of the QI program's fulfillment of its overall goals. Because the QI program exists for the generic goal of improving patient care, a summative process evaluation would focus on patient outcomes and experiences.

One may consider the differences between formative and summative evaluations in the following terms: Formative evaluation reviews the performance of a program related to tactical implementation of programs (i.e., Did the program fulfill its plan?), whereas summative evaluation looks at the effectiveness of the program (i.e., Did the program fulfill its mission?).

CHANGE THEORY: AN ALTERNATE FRAMEWORK FOR PROGRAM EVALUATION

Although a clear understanding of the QI process loop is essential to the design of an effective evaluation process, and although the steps in the loop may provide an excellent framework for evaluation of program design,

program administrators can find other frameworks for evaluation design. One such opportunity comes from change theory, which provides a structural approach to understanding the generic process of change.

The ability to select change strategies and implement planned changes is an integral aspect of any QI program. It may seem obvious that the effective evaluation of a process that exists to create change is enhanced when the evaluator holds a clear conceptual framework as to how change occurs. Less obvious, but certainly reasonable, is the idea that a framework that seeks to model the steps in the change process may also serve as a framework for creation of a QI evaluative tool. Frameworks for change are not new, but may provide a deeper understanding of both the process of an effective QI program as well as the QI program evaluation.

Kurt Lewin (1962) has identified three stages in the change process along with six components of change. The three stages of change are

1. Unfreezing
2. Moving
3. Refreezing

During unfreezing, the discovery is made that change is desirable. During this stage, the individual is motivated to plan for and implement a change. In the moving stage, the actual change process occurs. In refreezing, the changed behavior is routinized until it becomes the established norm.

Lewin also has identified six components of change. These six components form the activity in which the changing entity (an individual or group) engages during the three stages of change:

1. Recognizing a needed change
2. Assessing the current situation
3. Identifying methods that will produce change
4. Planning for the change

5. Identifying the culture in which change is to occur
6. Creating the process of change itself

How might Lewin's three stages of change be matched to the design of a QI program evaluation? The first section of the evaluation might seek to discover the ability of the program to identify important issues. A key question to be answered is, To what extent did the members of the organization feel motivated to change based on data and analytical results uncovered and communicated through the QI program? That is, How effective was the QI program at unfreezing the organization? Using the second component of Lewin's framework, one might evaluate the QI program by asking, To what extent did change actually occur? At the most elementary level, the evaluation might measure the number of change efforts that resulted from the QI program. At the more abstract level, the evaluation might ask whether the desired changes (as designed in response to the unfreezing process) were implemented correctly and whether the implemented change achieved the desired results. (If those two dimensions of change evaluation sound familiar, it is because they represent the two types of evaluation, formative and summative, respectively.) The evaluator should seek to know the long-term continuity of the change: the refreezing of behavior. To do so, he or she could conduct longitudinal studies to revisit key behaviors and outcomes over time. The extent to which positive change has been reinforced, and thus continued, speaks to the overall effectiveness of the QI program.

COST-BENEFIT AND COST-EFFECTIVENESS ANALYSES

Resources used in conducting a program that monitors quality care must be evaluated in terms of their cost to the organization. Cost analysis considers all resources, including personnel time as well as materials, plus other contributions received from within and outside the organization. Both the use of resources and

the result of those expenditures must be evaluated (Knapf, 1982).

According to Knapf (1982), cost-benefit analysis and cost-effectiveness analysis require "two different methods of deciding between or among alternatives in order to arrive at a decision about the most advantageous use of available resources" (p. 427). Cost-benefit analysis requires both costs and benefits (in a service setting, benefits may be thought of as results) to be expressed in monetary terms. Of course, this method presents problems for the QI program evaluator. One may describe the benefits of an effective QI program in any number of ways, each presenting mind-boggling problems when it comes to assigning monetary value. Yet, as Knapf has pointed out, there is an alternative to monetary evaluation: cost-effectiveness analysis. Here, because it is not realistic to assign monetary benefits to program results, outcomes may be evaluated in a social context and by other nonpecuniary measures.

Unfortunately, too many organizations and individual health care providers assume that improved patient care necessarily requires additional cost. Even seasoned health care professionals often find it counterintuitive that reductions in cost can go hand-in-hand with improvements in quality. Yet hospitals and other provider organizations around the United States have found that precisely such win–win opportunities really do exist. For example, Wausau Hospital in Wausau, Wisconsin, recently undertook the challenge of reducing costs while maintaining or improving quality to patients and other "customer" groups. Among the hospital's many successes was the redesign of services provided in the Cardiac Catheterization Laboratory (Cath Lab), where a cross-functional team of staff and managers worked together to evaluate and redesign operations with a focus on hours of operation, staff scheduling, and employee skill levels. One type of analysis, called "staffing to demand," involved a study of patterns in the scheduling of procedures. The group discovered that, because of physicians' scheduling preferences, the Cath Lab was consistently underused on

Thursday afternoons. In response to that finding, the operating hours of the Cath Lab were reduced on Thursdays, thus enabling savings without compromising patient or physician access. As an overall result of the effort, not only did the Cath Lab team design benefit more than $155,000 in annual cost savings, but also identified 35 "service and quality metrics" expected to improve quality to six distinct "customer" groups (the Service Developer at the hospital led the Cath Lab redesign, and the director of quality management headed up the team that created the service and quality metrics cited as improved through redesign). Examples of service and quality metrics in Exhibits 7–1 and 7–2 may help focus the purpose and scope of the evaluation process.

The QI program evaluator's ability to measure the cost-benefit of and cost-effectiveness of the evaluation program is certain to improve with this more complete understanding of the relationship between costs and quality.

CONCLUSION

A QI program is only as effective as the data generated to instigate changes in behavior that lead to improved patient care outcomes, and the extent to which such data succeed in actually motivating such change. Evaluation of an effective QI program will reflect

- consideration that all steps of the QI loop are in place
- investigation that the QI program is comprehensive, well-coordinated, flexible, effective, and efficient in measuring well-defined goals
- an understanding of individuals' awareness of the underlying program concepts and mechanics
- a positive attitude as demonstrated by widespread involvement in the program and the resulting change process
- that management perceives QI data as an integral part of decision making
- improved patient care

An effective QI program evaluation tool will endow an organization with important benefits. By ensuring and maintaining a feedback loop, the evaluation process is critical to the maintenance of desired patient care outcomes and actually serves to create improvement. Having accomplished that, the program helps position the organization to thrive in the cur-

---

Exhibit 7–1 Developing Service Quality Metrics: How Do We Develop a QI Program That Recognizes "Customer" Needs?

Having identified the provider organization's primary customer groups, the QI program should seek to identify those factors each group deems most important and then develop means for measuring those factors. The following format offers a simple yet disciplined approach to creating quality metrics that can form the basis of a customer-focused QI program. The only limitation on the number of metrics that may be created for each customer group is the organization's willingness to measure and report the results.

The quality of service provided to _____
                                                                    (Customer group)

is evidenced by _____, which is measured by
                                          (Indicator)

_____ , who collect _____.
   (People closest to the indicator)   (Data)

Exhibit 7–2 Examples of Completed Service and Quality Metric Statements

---

"The quality of service provided to surgeons is evidenced by operating room (OR) turnover time, which is measured by surgical techs, who collect average time between surgeon's leaving the OR to time next patient is placed under anesthesia."

"The quality of service provided to payer organizations is evidenced by claim denials per incomplete information, which is measured by Accounts Receivable Clerks, who collect the rate of denied claims per thousand."

"Quality is in the eye of the beholder. Does your quality improvement (QI) program recognize that the provider organization's diverse constituent groups hold different perceptions of what factors indicate *quality*? Does the QI program recognize the diverse needs and values of the organization's varied "customers"? Who are the customers? They are

- patients (and their families)
- physicians
- payer organizations
- the community
- regulatory bodies
- employees (in their relationship with the institution)
- employees (in their relationship to each other)

"Thinking about customers and their diverse needs helps the QI program reach beyond the standard clinical and regulation-driven view of quality. A patient's judgment of the factors that indicate quality may include timeliness and completeness of communications regarding clinical condition, or cleanliness of the organization. On the other hand, a regulatory body may be interested in monitoring mortality and readmission rates. Each "customer" group has its own needs that are reflected in its view of quality. For each customer group listed, what are the top indicators of high-quality service? Can these be measured? How?

---

rent health care environment of significant change. It should be reassuring to the QI program evaluator to know that one of the few remaining certainties in the health care delivery system is that efforts to demonstrate the quality and effectiveness of patient care will likely increase in importance. Over time, as the QI program proves the presence of effective patient care practices, and has proven itself to be effective, employee job satisfaction is likely to increase, providing cause for celebration and recognition.

REFERENCES

Knapf, L. (1982). Applying cost-analysis techniques to nursing. *Nurse Health Care 3*(8), 427.

Lewin, K. (1962). Quasi-stationary social equilibria and the problem of permanent change. In E. Bennes & R. Chains (Eds.), *The planning of change*. New York: Holt, Rinehart & Winston.

Shortell, S.M. (1995). Assessing the evidence on CQI: Is the glass half empty or half full? [Special issue]. *Hospital & Health Services Administration, 40*(1).

SUGGESTED READING

D'Costa, A., & Sechrest, L. (1976). *Program evaluation concepts for health administrators*. Washington, DC: Association of University Programs in Health Administration.

Hopkins, J. (Ed.). (1990). Evaluating the QM program. *QRC Advisor, 7*(1), 1–8.

Kaye, R. (1983). Quality assurance—A strategy for planned change. In R.D. Luke & J. Krueger (Eds.), *Organization and change in health care quality assurance*. Gaithersburg, MD: Aspen.

Luke, R., & Wayne Boss, R. (1981). Barriers limiting the implementation of quality assurance programs. *Health Services Research, 16*(3), 305–314.

Michmich, M., Shortell, S., & Richardson, W. (1981). Program evaluation: Resource for decision making. *Health Care Management Review, 6*(3), 25–35.

Patton, M. (1980). *Qualitative evaluation methods*. Beverly Hills, CA: Sage.

Smeltzer, C.H. (1983). Organizing the search for excellence. *Nurse Management, 14*(6), 19–21.

Smeltzer, C.H., Feldman, B., & Rajki, K. (1983). Nursing quality assurance: A process not a tool. *Journal of Nursing Administration, 13*(1), 5–9.

Smeltzer, C.H., Hinshaw, A.S., & Feldman, B. (1987). The benefits of staff nurse involvement in monitoring the quality of patient care. *Journal of Nursing Quality Assurance, 1*(2), 1–7.

Warner, K., & Luce, B. (1982). *Cost benefit and cost effectiveness analysis in health care*. Ann Arbor, MI: Health Administration Press.

Wilson, C. (1984). Program evaluation: Theory, method and practice. In P. Schroeder & R. Maibusch (Eds.), *Nursing quality assurance: A unit based approach*. Gaithersburg, MD: Aspen.

## PART III

Processes Integral
to Improving Quality

## CHAPTER 8

The Customer: Perspectives and Expectations of Quality

Joann Genovich-Richards

CHAPTER OBJECTIVES

After completing this chapter, the reader will be able to

- describe two megatrends of accountability to customers
- define two characteristics inherent in customer–supplier relationships
- cite a variety of forces impacting consumer satisfaction surveys

When practitioners and scholars of the next millennium reflect on health care history, the last part of the 20th century will probably be recognized as the time when accountability to customers—internal and external—began to be measured, managed, and routinely reported, and consumers began to evolve into responsible partners who actively participated in health care maintenance and improvement processes. For the purpose of organizing this chapter, these two megatrends of accountability to customers and informed consumerism are discussed separately in terms of their roots, current manifestations, and possible evolution. In reality, they are interwoven, reinforcing each other; that they have occurred simultaneously is not coincidental.

Use of the terms *customer* and *consumer* warrant clarification. In this discussion, the *customer* is any recipient of a service or product. Therefore, in the organizational environment, the nursing staff is a customer of many day-to-

day systems including delivery of medications, results reporting of laboratory services, and so forth. Reciprocally, many organizations' departments are customers of nursing for information that initiates various support department processes. Each departmental area of the organization, at different times and for different activities, may be the supplier or the customer. Similarly, physicians are in both supplier and customer relationships with the organization.

Moving beyond organizational operations, the organization itself has important external customers. Increasingly, the revenue of an organization depends on the contracts negotiated with various managed care plans. In such situations, the organization is clearly a supplier, as are other care delivery sites (e.g., home care agencies and skilled nursing facilities), to the health plan. Of course, health plans themselves have customers, including the employers who agree to offer the health plan based on evaluations of cost, quality, and so on, and enrollees who can ultimately vote with their feet by leaving a health plan.

In addition to being categorized as *customers*, the enrollees of a health plan, patients of a hospital, clients of a primary care provider or home health agency, or residents in a skilled nursing facility—as well as their families or significant others—are *consumers*. Thus, consumers are a special category of customers who are the ultimate receivers of the services or products.

ACCOUNTABILITY TO CUSTOMERS

Both internal and external customer–supplier relationships share several major features. These features are discussed first, followed by a more in-depth discussion of the value purchasing phenomenon that is being primarily driven by the purchasers of health care. Although this phenomenon has most directly affected health care plans to date, it is expected that similar expectations will be applied to individual practitioners and care settings.

Customer–Supplier Relationships

Two defining characteristics have emerged for customer–supplier relationships in manufacturing industries over the past 15 years. First is the length of the relationship. Giving orders to the lowest cost bidder for only a limited project has given way to more deliberative evaluations of the cost and quality of potential suppliers and longer term contracting with the selected vendors. As part of the ongoing evaluation of suppliers, "scorecard" programs based on pricing, quality, and delivery are now commonplace (Desai, 1996). Second, as a result of the longer term relationships, there is a more open sharing of needs and information between organizations and their suppliers.

In many respects, dealing with external suppliers is the easy part. Few manufacturing and service organizations have a set of performance indicators that are parsimonious and reflect information about the internal production chain. One of the few is Federal Express, which daily produces widely shared summaries of aspects of the previous day's performance, generally based on timing between processing points. Health care settings lag behind other industries in this area, due largely to the customization of the health care product. It is hoped that when the next edition of this book is developed, there will be success stories from health care to relate on the topic of internal customer–supplier performance systems (see Chapter 5 for additional comments on how the

quality management system can at least partly provide relevant information).

Value Purchasing

At the core of value purchasing is the belief that health care can be improved and costs can be lowered. To date, the large national purchasers have been at the forefront of the accountability movement (Darling, 1995). However, these views are also shared by many providers and administrators, at least behind closed doors. As Sigmond (1995) noted,

> what the general public does not yet know is that almost all professional executives in the health care field will admit that, with strong community partnerships and coordination to reduce the fragmentation that characterizes the health care field, this nation can theoretically have better health care for all, and without any increase in expenditures at all. Many health care executives even agree privately that health status could be improved as health care expenditures are reduced substantially. (p. 6)

Because employers usually select insurance or health plans to offer their employees, the selection process is the point at which employers can offer the most leverage. To date, the most formal response to employers' search for information has come from the highly organized managed care systems, predominantly the health maintenance organizations (HMOs). Originally developed by the managed care trade associations, the National Committee on Quality Assurance (NCQA) is now an independent not-for-profit organization primarily involved with the accreditation of highly structured health plans. Many national employers and business coalitions are beginning to limit their offerings for HMOs to those accredited by NCQA or other accreditation bodies. Joint Commission on Accreditation of Healthcare Organizations and the Utilization Review Accreditation Commission have also begun to offer accreditation services designed to evaluate more loosely structured health services networks.

Beyond accreditation, the managed care field has been developing performance measures for various dimensions of plan performance. Where accreditation is only a subject of new information after several years (e.g., NCQA would review a fully accredited health plan again in 3 years), reports on performance measures can be required annually. The most widely recognized performance measurement set is the Health Plan Employer Data and Information Set (HEDIS). First developed by a group of employers and staff and group model HMOs, the effort has been under the auspices of NCQA beginning with the development of HEDIS 3.0. Part of the rationale behind HEDIS was to standardize the requests that came to the health plans for information from employers and their consultants, and to assure employers that an "apples to apples" analysis could be made in reviewing the proposals from various plans.

While HEDIS information for assessing health plan performance is used for Medicare, Medicaid, and commercially insured populations, each measure may or may not be applicable to each of these three populations.

HEDIS, 3.0 version, released in January 1997, addresses the eight domains from two kinds of measures—the Reporting set and the Testing set:

- satisfaction with the experience of care
- health plan stability
- use of services
- cost of care
- informed health care choices
- health plan descriptive information
- effectiveness of care
- access and availability of care

Performance measurement systems are also needed for traditional types of health insurance plans and the network models. To address this need for both private and public purchases as well as consumers, the Foundation for Accountability (FACCT) was formed in 1995 as an outgrowth of Paul Ellwood's Jackson Hole Group ("Care at HMO's To Be Rated by a New System," 1995). This is an important development to achieve a "level playing field" among insuring health plans. To some degree, HMOs have been most at risk and visible for scrutiny because they have clearly defined populations for which data can be provided (Genovich-Richards, 1995b). The FACCT initiative is also commendable for starting with reviews of the scientific knowledge base as the foundation for developing measures. As their first action, a series of papers on three population-level issues and eight clinical conditions was developed in 1996 (see Table 8–1 for listing), supported by funding from the Agency for Health Care Policy and Research (AHCPR).

"Trickle-Down" Accountability

To date, employers have placed the accountability demands on health plans. Over the next 10 years, it is reasonable to expect that similar demands will be placed on individual providers, hospitals, home care agencies, and other care settings. In some cases, purchasers will be directly interested in the performance information. Hospitals are of particular interest because of the high cost of inpatient care and the continued overbedding in most urban markets. Managed care plans will also become more interested in having a standardized set of expectations on which to base their selection of partners. Care settings will probably experience the same frustrations the managed care plans faced in responding to different demands for information, and thus will eagerly participate in consensus-building activities to develop the measures.

INFORMED CONSUMERISM

Informed consumerism, whether about health care, automobiles, fast food purchases, and so on, requires several events to occur

Table 8–1 AHCPR–Sponsored Papers for FACCT Performance Measures

Measurement Domain	Primary Author	Affiliation
Health status	Mark C. Hornbrook, PhD	Kaiser Permanente Center for Health Research, Portland, OR
Satisfaction	Allyson Ross Davies, PhD	Consultant, Newton, MA
Risk behaviors	Betsy L. Thompson, MD, MSPH	Centers for Disease Control and Prevention, Atlanta, GA
Asthma	Kevin B. Weiss, MD	Rush Presbyterian Center for Health Services Research, Chicago, IL
Cardiac risk factors/cardiovascular disease	Diane Orenstein, PhD	Centers for Disease Control and Prevention, Atlanta, GA
Depression	G. Richard Smith, MD	University of Arkansas for Medical Sciences, Center for Outcomes Research and Effectiveness, Little Rock, AR
Diabetes	Sheldon Greenfield, MD	New England Medical Center, Boston, MA
Low back pain	Dan Cherkin, PhD	Group Health Cooperative of Puget Sound, Center for Health Studies, Seattle, WA
Breast cancer	Patricia A. Gantz, PhD	UCLA Jonsson Comprehensive Cancer Center, Los Angeles, CA
Coronary artery disease	Daniel B. Mark, MD, MPH	Duke University Medical Center, Durham, NC
Arthritis	Lewis Kazis, ScD	VA Medical Center, Bedford, MA

within a relatively short time. First, comparative information about the class of products or services must be obtained, usually by an independent organization. The information may be obtained from the providers of the goods or services. Alternatively, the independent organization may acquire the products and test them independently. The information may also be obtained from surveys of individuals who have purchased the product or service.

Next, the information must be organized into meaningful displays and made available to the public though specialized publications or the general media. Examples of these activities for consumer products include publications such as *Consumer Reports,* evaluations by specialized firms such as surveys of automobiles, and media reports of which fast food restaurants have the healthiest selections. The process of information becoming available feeds an iterative cycle of educating the customer, improving the product and service, and refining the data-gathering and reporting processes.

The Evolving Business of Health Care Performance Reporting

As recently as the 1980s, a widely held belief in the health care field was that, unlike the concept of consumer sovereignty applicable to other commodities, consumers would be unable to evaluate their care (Feldstein, 1988). Three factors probably contributed to changing this view:

1. Health care itself changed into a frequently corporative commodity, with the entrée of for-profit health care delivery organizations accountable to their shareholders for stock performances on Wall Street.
2. Health care insurance shifted from a uniform set of predominantly hospital-related benefits covered by indemnity plans to a mosaic of models that covered routine preventive ambulatory care, home care, assisted living, and so forth. This product differentiation was encouraged with the passage of the Health Maintenance Organization Act in 1973, which mandated that employers with 25 or more employees had to offer an HMO option if there was a federally qualified HMO in their area. The market responded with an explosion of health plan products, producing the current "alphabet soup" of independent practice associations, preferred provider organizations, point-of-service plans, and so on.
3. Where employers once paid the full cost of an indemnity plan to all employees, rising costs resulted in the imposition of deductibles and copays so that employees became more price sensitive. Often employers now cover the full cost of a managed care option, or that option has the least out-of-pocket costs for the employee. If available at all, the premium indemnity plan may require high employee contributions through payroll deductions. The need for employee choice in selecting a health plan, in parallel with employer choice, opened the door to the current round of health care consumer reporting.

As performance measurement information has become available, purchasers, purchaser or provider coalitions, the health care industry, and the states have made an effort to make such information publicly available. Often the reporting products are referred to as "report cards," although "score cards," "performance profiles," and similar labels are emerging.

To date, many of the third-party reporting efforts have been based on HEDIS. The most systematic national effort involved 21 health care plans representing a broad spectrum of health care plan types, including point-of-service options and a third-party administration model (NCQA, 1995c). This effort also included a consumer survey conducted by an independent research firm. The State of Maryland Health Care Access and Cost Commission has undertaken a several-year implementation and evaluation effort to provide information on health plans to consumers (NCQA, 1995b). The commission's efforts will eventually include both consumer perceptions and provider perceptions of the plans obtained by surveys (State of Maryland, 1996).

Employers such as GTE and Xerox have begun to provide performance information to their employees at the time of open enrollment. A consumer magazine, *Health Pages,* is published in some large urban markets with support from local employers. Information, some independently obtained and some self-reported by the plans, is presented for local physicians, hospitals, and health plans, along with health education on various topics.

Consumer Satisfaction: What Have People Like Me Experienced?

As reviewed by Gold and Wooldridge (1995), surveys of consumer satisfaction are a recent addition to the health care landscape, being first piloted in the early 1970s. Consumer satisfaction as a specific component of health care reporting is a result of a variety of forces, including the widespread adoption of total quality management with its customer focus, increasingly assertive consumers, heightened competition, regulatory or accreditation requirements for satisfaction surveys and complaint management systems, and the increased evidence of relationships between satisfaction and quality of health care processes and outcomes (Schweikhart & Strasser, 1994). As an example of the relationships between satisfaction and quality of health care processes and outcomes, Weyrauch (1996) reported that, in a cross-sectional randomized telephone survey of more than 1,000 patients, those receiving their choice of provider for a visit had statistically different satisfaction scores in the more positive direction than patients who did not see their provider of choice. Similarly, Schauffler, Rodriguez, and Milstein (1996) reported on data collected from the 1994 Health Plan Value Check, conducted by the Pacific Business Group on Health; they found that patients who recalled that their physician or other health care professional discussed at least one health education topic in the past 3 years were more likely to be satisfied with their physician. This finding was consistent regardless of health insurance or plan.

As part of the iterative process of providing information, receiving feedback, and improving the information, a variety of organizations have recently supported focus groups with consumers (e.g., AHCPR and NCQA). One consistent theme from the focus groups was that they wanted performance information collected or verified by a third-party source, not obtained solely from the health plans. Another consistent theme was the high value consumers place on the consumer satisfaction reports. Although much of the performance information is only of interest at particular points in the life cycle (e.g., immunization rates are of interest if one has small children), the satisfaction information is easily understandable because most people have responded to such surveys and

tells the consumer what "people like me" have experienced.

There have been several public disclosures of consumer satisfaction in local communities. In 1995, the Minnesota Health Data Institute, a nonprofit public–private partnership, conducted a survey of 17,500 state residents on their perceptions of care in 46 health plans. Newspapers ran a 16-page, multicolored insert reporting the results. A series of town meetings was held across the state to discuss the survey project results. Similarly, in some markets, issues of *Health Pages* have provided results of independently conducted local consumer satisfaction surveys.

In recent years, the number of available satisfaction surveys has proliferated. Although each survey has its proponents, most tools have only been evaluated for reliability and validity by their developer. Because of strong proprietary interests, the development of the health care satisfaction field has not been known for its collegiality. Indeed, there has often been a strong "not invented here" orientation in terms of developers' assessments of their colleagues' efforts. To bring the development of surveys into the public domain and to advance the science base underpinning them, AHCPR has undertaken several recent initiatives. First, AHCPR contracted with the Research Triangle Institute to develop survey instruments for a variety of populations ready for validation and field testing (AHCPR, 1995). Table 8–2 summarizes the instruments and modules developed in this initiative, known as the Survey Design Project (SDP). One important feature of the SDP was cognitive testing with potential respondents to select items and response wordings. Table 8–3 summarizes the SDP cognitive testing phases. The development of many earlier surveys relied only on psychometric approaches to establish the items.

As a follow-up to the SDP, AHCPR is funding a 5-year (1995–2000) project entitled the Consumer Assessment of Health Plans Study (CAHPS) to consortia headed by Research Triangle Institute, the Rand Corporation, and

Table 8–2 SDP Surveys and Modules

Questionnaire (Mode)	Sample	Contents
Adult health care survey (mail and telephone)	Random sample of subscribers interviewed about their own most recent visit to a primary care or specialty provider	Coverage Subscriber's most recent visit Subscriber's overall care Full health plan assessment Reasons for "no care" module Subscriber/family characteristics
Child health care survey (mail and telephone)	Random sample of subscribing units containing covered children; covered children living elsewhere excluded by screening; person responsible for resident children's care interviewed about child with most recent "doctor's" visit	Coverage One child's most recent visit One child's overall care Children's health plan, limited assessment Reasons for "no care" module Subscriber/family characteristics
Hospital care survey (mail only)	Random sample of subscribing units experiencing a hospital stay; person hospitalized or responsible for patient care interviewed about most recent stay	Coverage Most recent hospital stay Overall hospital care Limited health plan assessment Subscriber/family characteristics
Mental health care survey (mail only)	Random sample of subscribing units experiencing a mental health service; patient or person responsible for patient care interviewed about most recent mental health service	Coverage Most recent mental health service Overall mental health care Limited health plan assessment Subscriber/family characteristics
Health plan disenrollment survey (mail only)	Random sample of individuals disenrolling from plan in past 12 months	Current coverage Reasons for disenrollment Subscriber/family characteristics
Module: Plan identification (mail only)	Individuals whose health plan is unknown	Name of plan *or* characteristics of current plan
Module: Facility identification (mail only)	Plan members whose facility is unknown	Name of main facility used

Harvard University. Four features distinguish the resulting CAHPS survey tool kit from existing consumer questionnaires:

1. Many existing instruments were designed to obtain information from consumers for use by plan administrators to identify needs for improvement or for marketing purposes. Although information obtained through the CAHPS instruments may be useful to

Table 8–3 SDP: Cognitive Testing

Pretest Round	Pretest Activity	Cognitive Research Goals
Round 1: Developing first draft materials	Intensive "think-aloud" interviews Cognitive appraisal analyses	Preliminary exploration of general measurement, design, and formatting issues Structured expert review of first draft questionnaire materials to identify potentially problematic questions and priority cognitive interview goals
Round 2: Testing first draft and developing second draft materials	Intensive "think-aloud" interviews Focus group interview	Testing and identification of revisions for question wordings, response wordings, response scales, and questionnaire formatting Exploration of general reactions to draft survey procedures and survey plans
Round 3: Testing second draft and developing third draft materials	Observation and debriefing interviews Intensive "think-aloud" interviews	Assessment of self-administration for high- and low-level readers and collection of additional information about item wordings, response scales, and questionnaire formatting Testing and identification of revisions for new questionnaires and questionnaire modules

these audiences, its primary purpose is to assist consumers—and purchasers acting on their behalf—to make more informed and appropriate selections of health plans and services.

2. Each survey item and response category in CAHPS will be evaluated through cognitive testing to ensure comprehension by people with lower levels of education or reading skills.

3. Rather than being limited to consumer satisfaction, CAHPS survey components allow assessment of a variety of plan and provider characteristics.

4. The tool kit will be designed for use with different types of consumers in diverse health care settings (e.g., the privately insured, Medicaid enrollees, enrollees in managed care plans, or fee-for-service plans).

The CAHPS tool kit will have two major sections. First, there will be a large set of *standard components*. Table 8–4 summarizes the standard survey contents. In addition, there will be a group of targeted components intended to address questions unique to specific populations. The planned targeted components include Medicaid enrollees, individuals with chronic conditions or disabilities, adults responsible for the health care of children, and disenrollees. It is anticipated that a draft of

Table 8–4 CAHPS Standard Survey Contents

Contents	Sets of Items
Enrollment	Benefits, coverage (including verification of current plan)
Cost	What, if anything, privately insured respondents pay toward premium
Plan administration	Paperwork, information provided about the plan/providers, customer service
Global evaluation	Overall ratings of care and of health insurance plan
Access	Access, availability of care, providers (including primary care doctor of other usual source of care)
Technical quality	Technical quality of care, including preventive care and wellness advice
Communication	Communication skills of provider, office staff; respect, patient involvement in decision making about care
Continuity	Continuity and coordination of care (from those respondents who have seen more than one provider in the past 6 months)
Use	Office visits, specialty care, hospitalization
Health status	Self-reported health status
Demographic information	Personal characteristics of respondent (age, gender, education)

many CAHPS components will be available for public use by early 1997, although the formal demonstration site evaluations will be undertaken over several subsequent years.[1]

Satisfaction Caveats

There are several reasons for concern about the health care industry's current fascination with surveys. First, citizens are being barraged with surveys from a wide variety of sources. Where surveys were once only conducted for research and generally performed by highly

esteemed research organizations, nearly every firm offering a product or service now solicits consumer feedback. Second, surveys have increasingly become a marketing tool. The best recent example was seen in the Republican presidential primaries of 1996 in which the use of "push-polls" became a subject of debate. As a consequence, response rates to surveys are declining.

Many organizations are in danger of a false sense of security from their satisfaction surveys. At management meetings, staff are pleased that only 5% to 15% of respondents are something other than satisfied. Often rationalizations are heard as to why that group cannot be satisfied. Alternatively, some individuals want to focus a large amount of resources on "finding" and "fixing" the concerns of this group. What often passes unnoticed is the limited percentage of respondents at the most positive end of the spectrum. Jones and Sasser's (1995) research suggests that many of the beliefs about satisfied customers are misguided: Satisfied customers defect. They

---

[1]For additional information about CAHPS, contact:
Christine Crofton
(e-mail address: ccrofton@po3.ahcpr.gov)
Charles Darby
(e-mail address: cdarby@ po3.ahcpr.gov)
Agency for Health Care Policy and Research
2101 E. Jefferson St.
Rockville, MD 20852
Telephone: 301-594-1352
Fax: 301-594-2155

specifically studied the hospital market along with other markets, using data from 10,000 surveys of patients treated at about 80 U.S. hospitals. A steep drop in loyalty occurred in the hospitals' markets for each drop in overall satisfaction. Summarizing the hospital analysis, Jones and Sasser (1995) stated,

> Nevertheless, most hospitals are still operating as if they had little effective competition. They continue to place little emphasis on patient satisfaction. One can speculate about the reasons. Perhaps their managers think that the centralization of purchasing power makes the health maintenance organizations and insurers, rather than individuals, the ones to please. Perhaps they think this centralization only raises the barriers that block dissatisfied patients from switching. If so, they may be in for a shock.

The lesson: Outstanding value must be consistently offered, as evidenced by the most positive response category. In addition, a company must also stay abreast of the changing external environment, particularly the innovations of competitors, to sustain customer loyalty. Given these caveats, what are some reasonable features for a health care delivery organization to include in its consumer satisfaction process?

Consumer Input and Feedback

Every individual who could use an organization's product or services can be classified into one of three types of consumers: a potential consumer, an existing consumer, or a former consumer. The strategies for the consumer satisfaction process must be tailored to each different group.

Potential Consumers

A neglected group by health care settings, potential consumers can be a source of new ideas for products and services. Health care settings have made few efforts to identify individuals in their service areas who have not used their facilities. One approach for identifying potential customers is to compare patients with address listings in specific city blocks. In most large metropolitan areas, there is usually a directory company that provides listings by county of each address on a specific block and the telephone number, if published (e.g., in Detroit, the service is called Bressers Cross-Index Directory Company). Public databases that provide geodemographic segmentation are also available, for example, PRIZM from Claritas Inc., and ClusterPlus from Donnelley Marketing Information Services (Rapp & Collins, 1996). Although labor intensive, this comparison of consumers who have used a facility and potential consumers can be done internally. Local marketing firms may also be able to provide this service.

Once a population of potential customers is identified, several steps can be pursued to obtain feedback from those individuals about where they have received such services in the past, what they liked about the experience, and *whether* they would be interested in information about your organization should the need for such services arise again. This feedback can be obtained by telephone interview, mail survey, or through focus groups. Of course, a follow-up tracking system needs to be implemented to find out if any of the individuals actually became consumers. When an individual becomes a consumer, a special effort should be made to acknowledge the new business and verify that it has been a positive experience.

Existing Consumers

Satisfaction surveys are the most popular vehicle for obtaining feedback from existing consumers. An effective strategy must be clearly developed for surveys to be worth the expense. Elements to consider include:

- How successful have the organization's survey efforts been to date? If responses are consistently less than 25% to 30%, a major reorganization of the satisfaction survey process should be undertaken.

- Are the organization's customers receiving multiple requests for feedback? Although it may be appropriate for clinical departments to receive some direct feedback, is there a way to stagger the specific surveys throughout the year?
- Is the organization participating in an externally conducted survey that periodically produces comparative data from local, regional, and national peers? Depending on the effectiveness of an organization's internal survey process, enrolling with one of the survey research firms for ongoing, annual, or every-other-year surveys could be a wise investment (Genovich-Richards, 1995a).

For hospitals, home care agencies, and so on, it is clear that existing customers are those who have been a patient. One of the interesting debates in the managed care part of the industry has been whether surveys should be of enrollees who received care (most of the existing surveys have some elements of satisfaction with providers and office staff as well as appointments) or of all enrollees, which would be particularly advantageous for determining if there are access problems. This debate has been partially resolved by the NCQA (1995a) Annual Member Health Care Survey, which specifies sampling of the entire enrolled population.

Debate has also occurred over whether to use telephone or mail surveys. The answer, in part, for any particular application may depend on the content of the survey. If the questions are only about satisfaction, telephone administration has some advantages, such as calling from an oversampling of the target population until a sufficient number of responses are obtained. However, if the survey contains information about health status or questions about clinical conditions, research has shown that respondents tend to answer those questions more positively by phone than on mail surveys (Ware, 1995).

In these days of dwindling response rates, multiple waves of survey approaches that combine mail and telephone may be needed to achieve a desirable response rate. Dillman (1978) proposed a five-wave design: (1) mailing of survey, (2) reminder postcard, (3) mailing of a second copy of the survey, (4) phone call reminder, and (5) telephone survey. Such a process can obtain response rates as high as 70%. Some survey projects have also included sending a letter before beginning the survey to alert people about who will be contacting them and the purpose.

Another way to promote customer loyalty is to involve customers in the design of products and services. One recent example of this approach was Ford's solicitation of input from members of Mustang Clubs for the redesign of the 1994 Mustang (Struebing, 1996). Customers have even critiqued design features by fax and e-mail.

Former Consumers

Identifying and approaching former consumers has not been attempted in health care. Of course, the best strategy is to prevent existing consumers from becoming former consumers! An important step in this regard is to have an ongoing process by which employees can identify unsatisfied consumers. Next, there needs to be a contact intervention used to, ideally, resolve the consumer's concern.

To identify consumers who have defected, the information systems staff can contact directly those individuals who would have been expected to have another contact with the organization in a reasonable period. To begin this process, it would be necessary to identify a list of diagnoses that would result in ongoing contact with the health system and a time frame for which a second contact would be expected (e.g., 1 year). The information systems staff would then need to produce a population of consumers who had been cared for with the diagnoses and had not reappeared during the designated intervals. The most delicate step would be contacting those individuals. One approach could be a phone call as a long-term follow-up on the individual's health and any current needs. If there were a negative experience that resulted in the person's electing to withdraw from contact, he or she would most likely tell the caller about the experience. Alternatively, the caller could probe whether the person would return to the organization if future care were needed. Clearly, the caller for such an intervention must be a highly trained and sensitive individual. The caller must also be able to take action within the system to address the identified concerns. A particular consumer may not return, but the goal is to resolve systemic problems that may be turning other current consumers into former consumers.

Consumer Surveys: Key Component for Many Outcome Measures

Consumer satisfaction is, of course, an important outcome measure. Consumers are also an important source of information on process measures. For example, consumers can report whether their blood pressure was taken at the last office visit. To capture relevant reports and satisfaction information before recollection of details deteriorates, many organizations are introducing point-of-service data collection systems. In these systems, a short survey is completed by the client on a computerized form so that it can be read on-site, correlated with other data about the visit, and integrated into the quality improvement process. The Harvard-Pilgrim Health Plan of Boston is using such a real-time system ("Real-Time Satisfaction Data," 1995). Point-of-service collection systems may eventually be used for internal quality improvement, whereas cross-sectional population surveys conducted by independent third parties may be used for external accountability.

In addition, results of surveys through which consumers report changes in health status and quality of well-being are increasingly being used as direct measures of outcomes. Such results are also being evaluated for use in risk adjustment and stratification of reporting for

performance measures. Many point-of-service data collection systems are also being developed to capture those types of consumer surveys.

To assist the field as a royalty-free distribution center for outcomes assessment systems in health care, the Medical Outcomes Trust was created in 1994. The Trust has an independently operating scientific advisory committee to establish standards for assessing the scientific quality of instruments and to recommend to the board instruments for distribution that have met the standards (Perrin, 1995). Exhibit 8–1 contains a list of currently approved instruments.[2]

Patient–Provider Shared Decision Making

Often in our society we speak of "rights and responsibilities." To the extent that it has been established that consumers have the "right" to information for selecting providers, health plans, and treatment options, the "responsibility" part of the bargain has also been strengthened. Increasingly, shared decision-making programs are used to consider the client's values and preferences, lifestyle, tolerance for discomfort or disfunction, and ability to cope with side effects of treatments. For example, Mulley, Mendoza, Rockefeller, and Staker (1996) and clinicians from the Medical Practices Evaluation Center at Massachusetts General Hospital accounted for a variety of patient preferences in their model for benign prostatetic hyperplasia. They found that patient preferences varied widely depending on the value given to the urinary dysfunction that started their search for an intervention, the prospect of sexual dysfunction that could result

---

[2] For additional information on available outcomes instruments, contact:

Lynn Paget, MPH
Director of Operations
Medical Outcomes Trust
20 Park Plaza, Suite 1014
Boston, MA 02116-4313
Telephone: 617-426-4046
Fax: 617-426-4131

Exhibit 8–1 Medical Outcomes Trust Approved Instruments

- Quality of Well-Being Scale
- SF-36 Health Survey United States (English)
- Sickness Impact Profile
- SF-12 Health Survey
- London Handicap Scale
- SF-36 Health Survey United Kingdom (English)
- SF-36 Health Survey Germany (German)
- SF-36 Health Survey Sweden (Swedish)

from an invasive procedure, and the probability of operative mortality for the individual.

Patient-generated measurement systems are being incorporated into a variety of chronic disease management approaches. Examples include home glucose monitoring for diabetic patients, blood pressure monitoring for hypertensive patients, peak expiratory flow rates for asthmatic patients, and progress with mobility for individuals undergoing physical therapy. Some clinicians are even using computer programs to transform the measurements and observations recorded at home into run charts that can be analyzed in terms of special cause and common cause variations with the client (Mulley et al., 1996).

Patient-generated measurements can be an important component of reengineered health care production methods. As an illustration of how practices are changing, Berwick (1996) shared the story of a four-year-old with asthma and the child's inner-city teenage mother whom he met while working as the pediatric triage doctor. In the past, such an encounter would have resulted in sending the child by ambulance to a hospital emergency room for admission. In this contemporary case, the mother produced a written record of the child's home nebulizer treatments for the past 24 hours, accompanied by the peak expiratory flow rate before and after each treatment, as well as a medication

history. The asthma outreach nurse was in the communication loop by cellular phone, and the allergy chief who knew the child also came to the triage area with a new medication during this episode. Rather than requiring a hospital admission, the child was home within several hours. As this example illustrates, a wide range of consumers can play an active role in their health care management. Therefore, it may be time to eliminate from our lexicon the concept of the *noncompliant patient*. Rather, *noncompliance* may be a sad commentary on the lack of creativity and inflexibility of the care providers to fully engage the consumer or understand the consumer's health preferences.

CONCLUSION

Accountability to customers will be a litmus test for organizational survival in the next millennium. It is important to remember that the babyboomer generation has been a discriminating purchaser on its passage through the lifecycle. That generation is just now reaching the age at which chronic conditions, health promotion, and so on are more personally relevant. Therefore, consumer perceptions about care, service, and satisfaction will become increasingly important components of a comprehensive quality management program.

REFERENCES

Agency for Health Care Policy and Research. (1995). *Design of a survey to monitor consumers' access to care, use of health services, health outcomes, and patient satisfaction.* (Contract No. 282-92-0045; prepared by Research Triangle Institute.)

Berwick, D. (1996). The year of "how": New systems for delivering health care. *Quality Connection, 5*(1), 1–4.

Care at HMO's to be rated by new system. *Wall Street Journal* (1995, Sept. 26).

Darling, H. (1995). Market reform: Large corporations lead the way. *Health Affairs, 14*(1), 122–124.

Desai, M.P. (1996). Implementing a supplier scorecard program. *Quality Progress, 29*(2), 73–75.

Dillman, D.A. (1978). *Mail and telephone surveys: The total design method.* New York: Wiley.

Feldstein, P.J. (1988). *Health care economics* (3rd ed.). New York: Wiley.

Genovich-Richards, J. (1995a). Designing quality management programs for today and tomorrow. In V. Kazandjian (Ed.), *The epidemiology of quality* (pp. 55–83). Gaithersburg, MD: Aspen.

Genovich-Richards, J. (1995b). Member satisfaction surveys: The next frontier. *Managed Care Quarterly, 3*(4), 1–9.

Gold, M., & Wooldridge, J. (1995). Surveying consumer satisfaction to assess managed care quality: Current practices. *Health Care Financing Review, 16*(4), 155–173.

Jones, T.O., & Sasser, W.E., Jr. (1995, November/December). Why satisfied customers defect. *Harvard Business Review,* 88–99.

Mulley, A., Mendoza, G., Rockefeller, R., & Staker, L. (1996). Involving patients in medical decision making. *Quality Connection, 5*(1), 5–7.

National Committee for Quality Assurance. (1995a). *Annual Member Health Care Survey manual 1.0.* Washington, DC: Author.

National Committee for Quality Assurance. (1995b). *Maryland HMO performance measurement pilot project.* Washington, DC: Author.

National Committee for Quality Assurance. (1995c). *Technical report: Report card pilot project.* Washington, DC: Author.

Perrin, E.B. (1995). SAC instrument review process. *Medical Outcomes Trust Bulletin, 3*(4), 1.

Rapp, S., & Collins, T. (1996). Special book bonus: The new maximarketing. *Success, 43*(3), 39–46.

Real-time satisfaction data stirs instant service changes. (1995). *Report on Quality Management, 2*(20), 5.

Schauffler, H.H., Rodriguez, T., & Milstein, A. (1996). Health education and patient satisfaction. *The Journal of Family Practice, 42*(1), 62–68.

Schweikhart, S.B., & Strasser, S. (1994). The effective use of patient satisfaction data. *Topics in Health Information Management, 15*(2), 49–60.

Sigmond, R.M. (1995). Back to the future: Partnerships and coordination for community health. *Frontiers of Health Services Management, 11*(4), 5–36.

State of Maryland. (1996, February). *HMO quality & performance evaluation system overview.* Baltimore: Health Care Access and Cost Commission.

Struebing, L. (1996). Customer loyalty: Playing for keeps. *Quality Progress, 28*(2), 25–30.

Ware, J.E. (1995). Data collection methods. *Medical Outcomes Trust Bulletin, 3*(1), 2.

Weyrauch, K.F. (1996). Does continuity of care increase HMO patients' satisfaction with physician performance? *Journal of the American Board of Family Practice, 9*(1), 31–36.

## CHAPTER 9

Integrating Risk Management, Utilization Management, and Quality Management: Maximizing Benefit through Integration

Barbara J. Youngberg and Diane R. Weber

CHAPTER OBJECTIVES

After completing this chapter, the reader will be able to

- trace the transformation of RM, UM, and QM over time
- identify RM, UM, and QM areas of interest and opportunities for integration
- discuss the emergence of new roles and relationships
- assess the degree to which an organization has integrated RM, UM, and QM
- describe strategies for integrating RM, UM, and QM

A HISTORICAL PERSPECTIVE

From the early 1970s to present, health care risk management (RM), quality management (QM), and utilization management (UM) programs have undergone profound transformation. Over time, they have become increasingly purposeful, demonstrating value-added benefit to hospitals facing managed care competition, cost containment, and a litigious environment. As a result, traditional RM, QM, and UM departments have developed into vital programs necessary for organizational survival.

As with many other departments or functions within health care organizations, the roles of professionals in these areas have evolved, taking on new, complex, and sometimes overlapping functions. Too often, opportunities to maximize the value of each of these disciplines has not been capitalized on because of the failure of one department to recognize what can be gained by better coordinating its activities with another. Although clearly specific functions may not lend themselves to integration, many functions, particularly those that identify quality problems and seek to resolve them, are ripe for improved integration and overlap.

Through its accreditation standards and survey process, the Joint Commission on Accreditation of Healthcare Organizations (the Joint Commission) assisted in the early development of RM, QM, and UM programs. Each program had been governed by a series of Joint Commission standards that addressed specific programmatic functions, reporting relationships, and outcomes. Early Joint Commission standards for QM and RM were prescriptive in nature, for example, mandating the use of the "10-step method" for quality assurance. In recent years, the Joint Commission standards have undergone modification to increase the flexibility with which organizations can demonstrate compliance, allowing more freedom to establish individualized programs and methods.

In the 1970s, the Joint Commission standards encouraged the integration of activities performed by then-called quality assurance and RM departments. A relationship designation does not appear in the current standards; however, QM-, UM-, and RM-related standards are all contained in the chapter, "Improving Organizational Performance." That chapter contains the standards addressing foundational aspects of quality programs institution-wide. Specific standards for RM and UM contained in this chapter are as follows:

- PI.3.2: the important processes or outcomes on which the hospital collects data include at least . . . PI.3.2.4 the appropriateness of admissions and hospital stays (utilization-management activities)
- PI.3.3: data on important processes and outcomes are also collected from PI.3.3.2 risk-management activities (Joint Commission, 1996).

In addition, the scoring guidelines for RM standard PI.3.3.2 also asks, "Do operational links to patient care and safety activities include the exchange of relevant information?" Many RM standards also appear in the Joint Commission accreditation manual chapter "Environment of Care." Effective management of the environment of care "includes using processes and activities to reduce and control environmental hazards and risks; prevent accidents and injuries; and maintain safe conditions for patients, visitors and staff" (p. 321).

MAJOR FUNCTIONS OF RM, QM, AND UM

Risk Management (RM)

RM "serves to prevent the loss of financial assets resulting from injury to patients, visitors, employees, independent medical staff, or from damage, theft, or loss of property. Risk manage-

ment also includes transfer of liability and insurance financing to cover unavoidable injuries or claims for damages" (University Hospital Consortium, 1994, p. 5). The responsibilities in the late 1970s focused primarily on the belief that injuries to patients were unavoidable and in need of quantifying and transferring—generally through the purchase of malpractice insurance. Once the insurance market tightened, the risk managers were forced to focus on behaviors or situations that give rise to risk. Modifying those situations and attempting to prevent injuries that give rise to claims or lawsuits was determined to be a more desirable approach. When this need for transition was identified, the RM professional changed from an insurance professional to a person who had some clinical or health care experience. Although there remained the need to financially insulate organizations from the types of injuries to patients that could not be anticipated, many organizations recognized that, of perhaps greater importance, was the identification of the underlying factors that give rise to risk, the modification of those exposures, and the subsequent reduction or elimination of those activities that in the past had given rise to patient injury or harm.

Although the health care manager's current functions and responsibilities may vary from organization to organization, generally the risk manager is responsible for risk financing and risk transfer—through the purchase of insurance or the management of self-insurance, loss control. This responsibility involves the management of claims and lawsuits arising from allegations of negligence as well as proactive RM, which involves the identification and management of situations within the organization that may give rise to patient injury or harm. It is this function that requires the highest level of integration with QM and UM.

Quality Management (QM)

In its early days, the department that handled quality monitoring activities was known as

Quality Assurance, but today's QM programs might have any one of a number of different names. The inconsistency in department names across organizations indicates the variation in programs, functions, and improvement processes used. A department called Clinical Process Improvement may be using a specific model of quality improvement. A Value Management department may have expanded its scope to address cost issues as well as quality issues. Clinical Resource Management units, also designed to reduce costs and length of stay while maintaining quality, are becoming more common. These units have emerged in response to competitive managed care contracting and the need to drive down costs. In larger facilities, clinical resource management units may have developed as a separate unit from any existing quality department. However, because of the overlapping functions, integration of efforts is indicated and seems to be underway.

Quality functions have also changed over time. Early quality assurance efforts focused on Joint Commission and other regulatory mandates such as indicator measurement, medical staff quality monitoring, peer review, blood utilization review, medical records review, drug usage evaluation, surgical case review, and infection control. Often, the attention was focused on compliance with these externally imposed mandates without any real measure of whether such compliance actually did enhance quality within a given organization. This need to achieve compliance often placed the quality assurance director at odds with others in the organization who resented the regulatory burdens imposed by external agencies, particularly when the mandates were not readily linked to what was actually occurring within the organization and with what needed to be done to improve the quality of the organization. In addition, many quality departments had shared responsibility for quality planning, medical staff credentialing, and board reporting with little attention paid to the integration of the information learned by each of the people or departments assuming partial responsibility for these functions. Today, many of these activities are still carried out by quality departments; however, the emphasis of their work may now be focused on other strategic priorities for the organization.

As continuous quality improvement (CQI) and total quality management (TQM) philosophies were instituted in hospitals in the 1980s, quality departments generally experienced one of two scenarios: they either led the effort to implement a new CQI/TQM program or were witness to the emergence of a separate CQI/TQM department. Over time, it appears as though hospitals, for cost-containment purposes or to reduce duplicative efforts, have pulled these separate departments together under a single quality umbrella. However, some organizations continue to have two or more independent quality efforts underway.

With the emergence of CQI, some departmental functions expanded to include CQI training, team facilitation, team leading, storyboard creation, and overall management of the CQI/TQM program. The emphasis on achieving standards compliance with the Joint Commission became less important, replaced by a focus on improvement for the sake of the patient or customer. Also in the late 1980s and in the 1990s, the demands for measurement of outcomes for reporting and comparison purposes increased. Quality departments were now involved in focused studies, outcomes studies, comparative database participation, severity of illness measurement, patient satisfaction, and benchmarking.

In today's managed care era, quality departments are more responsive than ever to the business needs of the organization, particularly as it seeks to compete with other local hospitals. The departments compile data for managed care contracting, report cards, and physician profiling. Often, they support efforts to reduce costs and improve operations efficiency through case management, pathway development and implementation, hospital reengineering, and clinical resource management. Others continue to strive for excellence in quality, conducting hospital evaluations using the Malcolm Baldrige National Health Care Quality Award criteria.

Utilization Management (UM)

UM is "the review of services delivered by a health care provider to determine whether, according to preestablished standards, the services were medically necessary" (University Hospital Consortium, 1994, p. 5). The origins of this department also date back to early Joint Commission mandates for monitoring the appropriate use of services. The major functions of this department are conducting inpatient and outpatient reviews; examining length-of-stay issues, payer contacts for precertification, and continued stays; responding to peer review organizations, preparing peer review organization denial appeals, and eliminating avoidable days. Some UM departments may have a shared responsibility in discharge planning or case management with other health care team members, such as nurses, physicians, and social workers.

Some organizations instituted a case management program to serve as an adjunct to UM or to entirely replace it. Performed by utilization review staff, registered nurses, or social workers, case management programs are designed to provide high-quality patient care in the most cost-effective way. Satinsky (1995) explained that case management "can cross provider lines and coordinate care rendered in multiple locations. It also can monitor quality and cost across a continuum of care, helping providers deal with the shifting of financial risk" (p. 2).

Emergence of New Roles

In the past few years, there have been significant changes to quality department responsibilities. Departmental roles have expanded, demonstrating utility beyond regulatory compliance to organizational survival. Major changes such as CQI/TQM and case management have occurred as a surprise—some departments did not appear ready to accept the challenge or delayed a reaction. In these situations, new departments were created in lieu of building on the existing related department. The success of all three functions increasingly relies on the ability to collect meaningful data and use the data to bring about needed change. Being able to continually measure the changes made and the impact they have on the achievement of organizational goals is equally important. Constant reassessment and improvement is part of the daily operation of all hospital departments that strive to stay ahead of their competitors.

Reporting Relationships

Similar to the variation in job responsibilities, reporting relationships also can vary greatly among organizations. When the reporting relationships allow for QM, RM, and UM to report to the same senior administrator in the organization, the ability to coordinate the flow of data and information is facilitated. This type of structure is not typical, however, because RM departments, which often play a large role in claims and financing decisions, often report to in-house legal counsel or to the chief financial officer, whereas QM and UM departments most frequently report to either a clinical administrator or the chief operating officer. The precise reporting relationship, though, is not as important as is the flow of information.

In the past, many quality departments fell within the oversight of the medical records department, nursing services, or ancillary services. Today, the majority of quality departments are part of a complex, interrelated set of hospitalwide functions that report directly to senior leadership in the organization or to a full-time physician leader. Many hospitals now have more than one "quality" department, a result of expanding needs for measurement and change and the increasing complexity of programs.

Areas of Common Interest to RM, QM, and UM

There is a large degree of commonality in functions, activities, and level of interest among the RM, QM, and UM departments. Hospitals should capitalize on this commonality of interest or purpose to determine if thorough integration of activities and operational improvements can be achieved. For example, risk managers, quality managers, and utilization review staff have a common interest in reviewing data regarding adverse events or other outcomes. Each individual may have a unique purpose for the data, but the data need is common nonetheless. Quality departments are historically rich with data on patient outcomes, appropriateness of procedures, blood utilization, medication use, and so forth. Infection control programs contain useful information about nosocomial infections and other surveillance activities that may also shed light on RM and UM issues. Several databases may exist within one organization, either alone or in combination with regional or national comparative data. The existence of these databases should be shared as a resource to departments that may need such information. Similarly, data needs from each area should be made known.

Risk managers have developed a visible role in dealing with capitation risk, which is of significant interest to UM and case management. The strategies undertaken and opportunities to minimize risk should be openly discussed between these departments. With managed care and capitation comes a stronger push for proactive discharge planning, some of which is happening before admission. Utilization managers and risk managers can jointly address capitation risk through discharge planning strategies and managed care utilization tracking. Automated systems for UM and case management may be capable of producing reports specific to managed care policies, enabling hospitals to monitor discordance with capitated reimbursements.

Retrospective analyses of length of stay and costs per case are common in hospitals, more recently conducted by "clinical resource management" units. These analyses may be similar to concurrent monitoring conducted by UM or case management departments. This overlap of responsibility signals an opportunity for shared, integrated efforts.

Although regulatory concerns are no longer of primary interest to RM, QM, or UM, regulatory compliance remains an absolute requirement for hospital operations. Any issue associated with licensure, accreditation, or other external inspection must be given due attention or the hospital will risk a loss of significant resources to reverse a larger problem. Often, the amount of resources required to reverse an accreditation or licensure problem is disproportionate to that required for proactive compliance, which otherwise would have prevented the problem. It is therefore advantageous to address regulations in a proactive manner to avoid costly, time-consuming repercussions that could be related to minor oversights of specific standards or requirements. Of particular concern are regulations related to medical staff credentialing, licensure, staff competency, safety, and environment of care.

As the RM, QM, and UM departments collaborate more fully, it is expected that more information will be shared among individuals and groups. The sharing of information must occur with full knowledge of the need to protect the confidentiality of this information, either through the Health Care Quality Improvement Act of 1986 or through the attorney–client privilege. Appendix 9–A is a checklist designed to help hospitals identify common interests across RM, QM, and UM departments and possible opportunities for collaboration or integration.

INTEGRATION OF RISK, QUALITY, AND UTILIZATION

Berwick and Nolan (1995) stated that "integration is optimizing the interactions among elements of a system to provide health services of high value to those the system serves" (p. 573). They explained that integration involves a redesign of products, services, and processes to better meet the customer needs while minimizing waste.

RM and QM Scenarios

Emergency Department

Consider how well the proactive RM and QM activities dovetail. In this scenario, the risk manager, following a review of claims occurring over the past 12 months, identifies the emergency department as an area of concern. Consistent in the allegations brought by potential plaintiffs are facts suggesting poor communication problems exist between emergency department staff and patients at the time of discharge. The risk manager arranges to perform a risk assessment in the emergency department, failing to know that quality audits have revealed that printed discharge instructions are outdated and inconsistently used. The department has already begun a quality project to identify methods for improving the discharge process. Following the risk assessment, the risk manager also identifies intradepartmental communication problems: lab and X-ray frequently take too long to report results and occasionally send incorrect information to the emergency department staff, which results in treatment problems. The scope of this problem, uncovered through an RM assessment, is so broad it cannot be solved by the risk manager; rather, resolution likely will involve a multidisciplinary approach. The risk manager can inform the group assessing the problem about the costs associated with claims brought by emergency department patients when the communication problems exist. QM staff can create a flowchart of the problems to help visualize why miscommunication between departments occurs. Furthermore, utilization review staff can provide information regarding how tests, if misordered or reordered, may affect reimbursement. The problems present implications for each professional, but cannot be fully understood, or solved, without input from everyone involved in the process.

Incident Reports

Another illustration to support integration is the chain of events that occurs upon completion of an incident report. Many different people review and handle the report, but their actions and responses may not be integrated within the organization. The claim may be so significant that the risk manager's first action is to engage defense counsel and begin to posture the case for an early settlement. The risk manager may be so engaged in this aspect of RM that he or she fails to advise QM that the incident arose in part because a piece of equipment was misused. Without this notification, the equipment remaining in service could continue to result in patient injuries.

The same may be true for patient outcome events tracked concurrently by utilization review personnel, which later also may be collected by QM staff. For example, a patient discharge to a more appropriate setting may be delayed because of a quality of care issue arising on the unit. The discharge delay could present the organization with a significant financial loss. The utilization review department acting alone might respond by implementing strategies to achieve an earlier discharge without considering the quality issues that may have caused the delay.

Securing Equipment

In another scenario, QM staff might retrospectively identify problems with securing equipment necessary for patient transfer but may not understand the financial impact of such a problem and, thus, may not focus sufficient attention on analyzing and solving the problem. Such activities are generally scattered throughout the hospital and individually addressed in departmental silos, where the full scope of the problem may not be appreciated. This fragmentation, which creates confusion and a lack of unified direction, inhibits the ability of an organization to develop fully integrated programs. Integration does not necessarily mean combining departments and centralizing activities. Although centralization can be useful in meeting organizational needs, facilitating teamwork, and controlling the efficiency of departmental processes, it may not be the best method for integrating functions, especially if only one or two activities need integration. Process teams, or groups working together to perform a process, may also emerge out of integration efforts, replacing activities formerly performed by specific departments. There are distinct advantages to a decentralized structure, such as departmental flexibility, customization, and responsiveness, which might be more beneficial if kept preserved (Berwick & Nolan, 1995).

Benefits of Integration

RM, QM, and UM department efforts are often fragmented. Each department may have its own forms, equipment, software, and methods for achieving tasks. Although some activities are similar, they are not well-coordinated across departments. There is tremendous variation in process across departments, and the quality of the information collected is not maximized. Through integration, new tools designed to integrate common functions may emerge to reduce redundant paperwork and the number of people analyzing the same problems without coordination. Integration ultimately will enhance the process of care.

Furthermore, integration might increase the effectiveness of department functions. Often, integration offers opportunities to execute tasks more quickly and with more satisfying results than before. For example, a concurrent-incident and event-reporting strategy implemented by RM and UM could result in more timely and comprehensive information, and could serve as an effective warning signal for potential claims. Also, integration may help consolidate resources across departments. Many organizations are being forced to assess staffing patterns and to reduce work force size.

Having staff in multiple departments collecting the same information is redundant and inefficient, preventing staff from doing other activities that might be more valuable to the organization. Therefore, integration should not only focus on increasing efficiency, but should identify opportunities to perform valuable functions that were not previously possible. For example, staff may discover ways to share databases or enhance data systems so that many users can use that information. Integration often focuses activities to better meet end users' needs for information. Integration efforts will help departmental members gain a more comprehensive understanding of each other's roles and the expected outputs of their work. As specific functions become better understood, opportunities to enhance and focus activities on intradepartmental priorities will become apparent.

Integration also can facilitate the effectiveness of reporting relationships. Through integration, reporting relationships may change to enhance the ability of each department to perform at its best. There may be value in creating dual reporting relationships for a single department when multiple and different functions are assigned to a department. For example, the risk manager may report to the chief financial officer regarding risk financing strategies, to legal counsel when handling litigation issues, and to the same senior administrator as the quality and utilization manager when addressing proactive RM strategies.

Relationship of Reengineering to Integration

With the financial constraints faced by many hospitals, the survival of an organization may depend on the integration of functions to minimize duplication of efforts and promote efficiency. Integration is one possible outcome of an effort to reengineer the processes of RM, UM, and QM. *Reengineering* is "the fundamental rethinking and radical redesign of business processes to achieve dramatic improvements in critical, contemporary measures of performance, such as cost, quality, services, and speed" (Hammer & Champy, 1993, p. 32).

Although many workers fear reengineering—equating it with job loss—the process appropriately focuses efforts on ways in which people can "work smarter and not harder," more fully understand their role and the respective roles of others, and become better at what they do. Reengineering helps to ensure that activities performed are directly aligned with the strategic goals of the organization.

How to Integrate

Integration requires cooperation and collaboration, most appropriately through a team of representatives from each department. Each department should communicate its major functions and corresponding procedures or work processes to the team. Tools such as flowcharts, process maps, or responsibility charts may be helpful in outlining these functions.

Identification of end users (customers) of the work of the department will be critical to clarifying for the team who needs what, why, and when. When discussing the use of quality and risk data, it will be important to ensure that the sharing of specific information is done in a manner to ensure its protection.

Once the departmental functions and activities are known, opportunities to integrate efforts such as data collection and reporting can ensue. To do so requires cooperation and fearlessness. What may result is a redesign of the actual structures of each department, focusing on linking the common activities of each. Teams are useful for discussing integration opportunities or establishing a single integrated function, such as a combined reporting format. For example, department managers may decide to eliminate duplication of incident reports, patient complaints regarding service, and various quality indicators. A temporary project team could be formed with the sole intent of creating a single reporting tool and associated procedure for reporting.

As RM, QM, and UM departments work together to communicate, collaborate, and integrate some of their functions, they will undoubtedly go through a variety of phases. Consider the integration of different departments akin to a business alliance or joint venture. Kanter (1994) identified five overlapping phases of successful business alliances. First, departments need to discover compatibility and identify common areas of interest. Second, departments need to develop plans for increased collaboration and integration. Third, once integration begins to occur, it may be discovered that each department had its own ideas of how the integration should work. During the fourth and fifth phases, attempts should be made to bridge the differences, facilitating the internal changes necessary to accommodate everyone's needs while achieving collaboration and true integration.

Integration of Data Collection Activities

One primary reason to support the integration of risk, quality, and utilization is to eliminate the fragmentation of data collection efforts, especially where like interests are apparent. Although each department may have its own reason for collecting various data, potential data users may span across the three areas, as well as other departments and individuals.

In its 1996 accreditation manual, the Joint Commission aptly described measurement as "the foundation of all performance improvement activities" (p. 250). Data are valuable commodities, requiring considerable staff time to collect and aggregate, yet are often underused. Each piece of information collected should have the potential to provide some value-added benefit to the organization. If it does not, measurement becomes a wasteful exercise.

Every health care organization needs to prioritize its measurement efforts according to selection criteria to appropriately address its unique data needs. For example, data that add value may be characterized as those that are used to evaluate and change practice patterns, proactively respond to risk concerns, and evaluate resource use.

Many problems can be associated with existing monitoring and information gathering: timeliness, complicated forms creating problems with missing data, little correlation between disparate data collection systems and databases, inadequate follow-up on issues, and a punitive process image. Elimination of wasteful data collection activities will permit more attention to the use of data to achieve improvements and meet specific organizational goals. Organizations will find that they can analyze and report data in a more sophisticated manner and focus their efforts on effective dissemination of information to the appropriate audiences.

Case Study: Bowman Gray/Baptist Hospital Medical Center

Bowman Gray/Baptist Hospital Medical Center is an 806-bed teaching hospital with more than 500 residents, more than 500 medical staff, and approximately 7,000 employees. The medical center is a tertiary referral center. The Risk Management and Quality Consulting departments at the hospital have worked together for more than 15 years to ensure operational efficiency in a variety of areas. Many functions have become integrated between the departments over time, such as incident reporting, data management, and patient complaint resolution. There are numerous customers common to both risk and quality who have benefited from integration efforts. Mutual customers include, but are not limited to, insurance companies, administrators, outside physicians and hospitals, physicians' office staff, hospital and medical committees, medical schools, medical staff, patients, vendors, lawyers, families, and visitors. QM and RM services are available to all areas of the health care–integrated delivery network enterprise, including affiliate hospitals, clinics, subacute

care, managed care companies, and affiliated physicians.

As depicted in the organizational chart (Figure 9–1), there are two separate directors for the Quality Consulting and Risk Management departments. Both directors report to the Vice President for Operations, who reports the activities of both departments to the board of trustees.

At the medical center, the Risk Management offices are located in close proximity to Quality Consulting and Utilization Review. The office space, designed by the department directors, presents an atmosphere that they believe facilitates the functional integration of RM and QM. There are no dividing walls between functions or departments. The two director offices share the same conference room. Department staff share the same break room, training center, and supply room.

The mission of the Quality Consulting department is to develop and provide the information necessary for customers to achieve their mission and the mission of the hospital. The vision of the department is to be recognized as a credible resource of vital information. Staff in the Quality Consulting department are responsible for medical staff quality, TQM, management consulting, quality consulting, and house staff quality. The activities of this department are overseen by and routinely reported to the Quality Improvement Committee.

The Risk Management department has three primary functions or sections: (1) the Safety/Security Section, (2) the Claims & Insurance Section, and (3) the Clinical Risk Management Section. The Safety Committee provides administrative oversight to the Safety/Security Section.

Evolution of Integration

The directors of Risk Management and Quality Consulting first began integration efforts almost 15 years ago. Faced with increasing work flow, limited staff, and budgetary constraints, they began to explore opportuni-

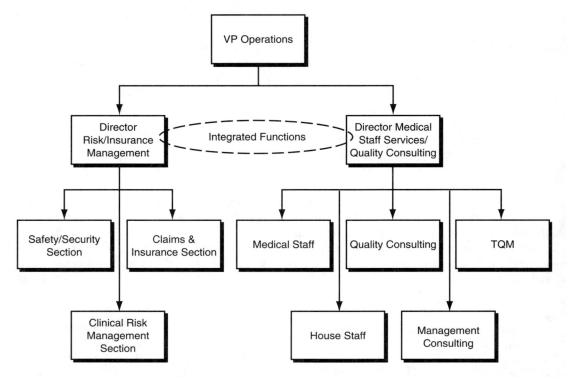

Figure 9–1 Risk Management/Quality Consulting integrated services. Courtesy of Bowman Gray/Baptist Hospital, Winston-Salem, North Carolina.

ties to increase efficiency while maintaining effectiveness. Based on the amount of routine communications that had been required to perform their respective functions in the past, it was apparent that the functions of risk and quality were connected.

The innovative decision to combine positions was therefore made out of necessity. Once the organizational need to integrate was identified, the directors began to create a situation to meet that need. They first defined the scope of both areas by function. They then compared the functions to find common areas or potential areas for integration. The directors also compared for separate areas/functions that did not overlap. Once the functions were understood, the directors developed a new common process to provide the services. They presented the proposed integration to senior leadership, who supported their decision.

Lessons Learned

Several lessons were learned from the integration experience. A foundation of interpersonal trust must be established for staff to be comfortable with integrating their work. Also, fear and ego can act as barriers to integration. "You have to leave your ego at the door," said the director of Risk Management (J. Smith, personal communication, April 2, 1996). Similarly, it is important to anticipate conflict, particularly when there is more than one leader involved. There is value to the combined strength of leaders, but because each individual is accustomed to handling problems and making decisions, this strength may sometimes slow the process. If, for example, there is total disagreement among decision makers, it may take longer to reach a compromise. Often, such conflict can result in a more beneficial decision well worth the discomfort of disagreement.

As staff worked toward integration, it was critical for them to recognize any areas of conflict and compromise for the benefit of the customers and the hospital. According to the director of Quality Consulting, "The hospital benefits because problems are solved with the best resources available between the two departments" (A.J. Koonts, personal communication, April 2, 1996).

The integration of Risk Management and Quality Consulting over time has resulted in innovation, increased productivity, decreased duplication, increased quality, and the successful leveraging of available resources. It has also resulted in the establishment of fail-safe systems for dealing with risk or quality issues. Each department director is comfortable responding to both risk and quality issues and is confident that consultations made by the other director are sound. Open lines of communication are maintained so that each director is kept informed of current issues.

Integrated Information Flow

An objective of the organization-wide plan for performance improvement is to integrate and coordinate data measurement systems for quality, utilization, and risk review. Integration of review activities begins with the process of information flow. The flow of quality improvement and RM-related information is depicted in Figure 9–2. The process begins with generic screen reports for quality and risk. Quality Consulting staff conduct concurrent chart reviews and enter the coded data into a quality consulting database. From this database, monthly generic screen reports are generated, reviewed, and disseminated to Risk Management.

If, during quality chart review, an RM issue is identified, the Risk Management department is notified by Quality Consulting staff. Staff in

Risk Management will check to see if the case is already in their database and, if not, the case is logged and an investigation is initiated.

When a QM or RM opportunity is identified, staff develop action plans in conjunction with other departments and clinicians as appropriate. Action plans are implemented and assessed for effectiveness. The information is reviewed by the Safety Committee and the Quality Improvement Committee, who provide feedback and recommendations. The board of trustees reviews the information annually.

Integrated Functions

Some of the functions integrated between the Quality Consulting and Risk Management departments included incident reporting, regulatory compliance, insurance plan, patient complaint resolution, generic screen integration, board reports, databank reporting, adverse actions against physicians, data management, resource integration, policy coordination, training, board orientation, reception area, and social events. Several of these functions are described as follows.

Incident Reporting. The Quality Consulting staff is responsible for reviewing patient records. When they come across an adverse event involving a patient, they are required to report this event through the Risk Management Incident Reporting System for investigation and follow-up.

Regulatory Compliance. Preparation for Joint Commission surveys is coordinated within the two departments.

Insurance Plan. Credentialing information is shared between departments if an issue surfaces that may warrant special attention from a legal perspective.

Quality/Risk Data. Quality Consulting collects and analyzes data for quality improvement activities that may lead to risk reduction or enhanced patient outcomes. In addition, the two departments share information on patient

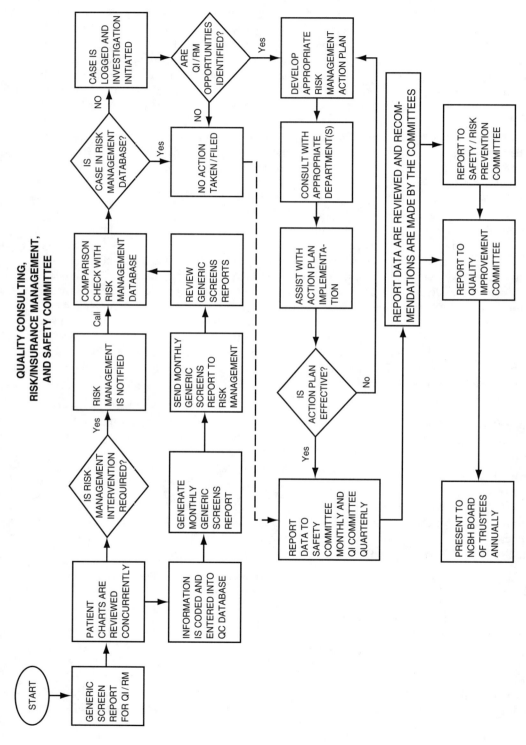

Figure 9–2 Quality improvement and RM information flowchart. Courtesy of Bowman Gray/Baptist Hospital, Winston-Salem, North Carolina.

complaints and coordinate responses to complaints from the medical staff.

Board Reports. Risk Management and Quality Consulting coordinate and produce seamless reports for the board of trustees.

Physician Events. Any time a physician is reported to the National Practitioner's Data Bank as having a claim settled in his or her name, there is coordination between the two departments. Similarly, any time official adverse action is taken against a physician, both departments are involved.

Policy Coordination. The two departments help coordinate the policies and procedures that affect the entire medical center, for example, the do-not-resuscitate policy and the informed consent policy. The departments cooperate to provide education to staff when these policies are implemented.

Training. The two departments have developed a common training program to ensure regulatory compliance and skill enhancement among departmental staff. Training sessions are scheduled every other month and a seminar is offered quarterly in a convenient setting. Required in-service programs include such topics as fire safety, disaster plan, and infection control. Sample optional in-service programs include competency review, employee appreciation day, and work group enhancement. These programs serve to promote camaraderie, cooperation, and team-building between the departments. The two departments also cooperate during the orientation and assignment of new board members.

Social Events. Employee Appreciation Day and other social events are scheduled so that employees from both departments are included and encouraged to attend.

Integrated Staffing

One staff member is responsible for coordinating the information systems and data management activities for the two departments.

The two departments also have combined reception area coverage. The receptionist for each area directs inquiries to the appropriate staff member.

Integrated Resources

The directors of both departments divide costs for equipment-related purchases, and have a long-standing agreement to share the equipment. For example, copy machines, fax machines, and other office supplies and equipment are purchased by both departments and used by both Risk Management and Quality Consulting staff. In addition, there is shared office space, a break room, and a beverage machine.

Future Plans

Integration is dynamic and is viewed as a continuous process at Bowman Gray/Baptist Hospital Medical Center. Integration opportunities will be used to maintain productivity, enhance information management, stay competitive, and improve quality. As with most integration efforts, departments will become "leaner and meaner" over time.

One planned activity is to conduct a comprehensive evaluation of the data collected by each area to identify opportunities to better manage the information. As information systems capabilities become more integrated and sophisticated, it will be possible to generate more reports without manual data collection.

According to the director of Risk Management, "What seemed like a common-sense way to get the work accomplished 15 years ago, today appears in books and comes from the mouths of management consultants as 'partnering,' 'seamless,' etc. I'm glad we didn't wait on the trend" (J. Smith, personal communication, April 2, 1996).

CONCLUSION

The roles, functions, and structures of QM, UM, and RM have undergone profound changes in recent years. Yet the benefits of these programs have become more evident and are viewed as necessary components of hospital operations.

The standards to maintain accreditation by the Joint Commission require organizations to establish and support quality, risk, and utilization functions. The Joint Commission standards are less prescriptive, permitting flexibility in the process and structure for achieving those functions. The major functions of RM include risk financing, risk transfer, loss control, and proactive RM. Proactive RM offers the highest potential for integration with quality and utilization functions.

The scope of QM functions varies from organization to organization. Functions have expanded to address issues necessary for competitive survival. Quality managers participate in benchmarking, outcomes studies, patient satisfaction, CQI/TQM, as well as traditional quality measurement activities. Accreditation preparation and standards compliance remains a function of many quality managers.

UM continues to be focused on the review of admissions and stays for appropriateness of care, although the efforts have become more rigorous and responsive to specific patient populations and managed care programs. Case management is a recent approach that complements, and, in some cases, replaces former UM strategies.

Many functions and activities are of common interest to RM, QM, and UM. At various levels of intensity, each department may have a vested interest in adverse events, outcomes, infection rates, databases, comparative data, capitation risk, proactive discharge planning, clinical resource analyses, accreditation, and length of stay.

Integration of RM, QM, or UM functions can be beneficial in that integration can reduce fragmentation of efforts, increase efficiency, increase effectiveness, consolidate resources, focus activities, and facilitate effective reporting relationships. However, integration requires communication among key individuals representing each department. There must be sufficient collaboration and cooperation to understand the functions, responsibilities, and opportunities for integration. The team must not lose sight of the end customers who receive services from each department.

Sample scenarios delineating opportunities for integration include cross-departmental process improvements, incident reporting, patient outcomes tracking, problem investigation, data collection, and use of databases. Successful integration of a variety of RM and QM functions has been achieved at Bowman Gray/ Baptist Hospital Medical Center, including incident reporting, regulatory compliance, insurance plan, patient complaint resolution, data management, and policy coordination.

As hospitals struggle financially to maintain a competitive position in the marketplace, it is critical that operational efficiencies be optimized. RM, QM, and UM departments should comprehensively evaluate the functions performed by each department, the procedures used, and the data collected and reported. Once identified, opportunities for integration of procedures, functions, or departments can then be maximized. Successful integration can result in such benefits as increased efficiency, cost savings, and increased effectiveness of programs. Through integration, departments can demonstrate their commitment to the overall success of the health care enterprise.

REFERENCES

Berwick, D., & Nolan, T. (1995). Cooperating for improvement. *Journal on Quality Improvement, 21*(11), 573.

Hammer, M., & Champy, J. (1993). *Reengineering the corporation.* New York: Harper Business.

Joint Commission on Accreditation of Healthcare Organizations. (1996). *Accreditation manual for hospitals.* Oakbrook Terrace, IL: Author.

Kanter, R. (1994). Collaborative advantage. *Harvard Business Review, 7–8,* 96–108.

Satinsky, M.A. (1995). *An executive guide to case management strategies.* Chicago, IL: American Hospital Publishing.

University Hospital Consortium. (1994). *Critical issues shaping medical practice.* Oak Brook, IL: Author.

United States Department of Commerce. (1993). Malcolm Baldrige National Quality Award 1994 Award Criteria. Gaithersburg, MD: National Institute of Standards and Technology.

APPENDIX 9–A

INTEGRATION/COLLABORATION OPPORTUNITY WORKSHEET
Common Interests of RM, QM, and UM

Directions: Using this form or a separate sheet, list the major functions performed by each department. Ask key representatives from each department to identify the functions that are of interest to them and to indicate their level of interest using the following scale. Place an asterisk (*) next to functions that have already been integrated. (The shaded boxes indicate functions that have historically been the responsibility of an individual department.)

Score:
0 = Of little interest
1 = Of some interest to this department
2 = Of moderate interest to this department
3 = Of high interest
* = Already integrated

Departmental Function	Risk	Quality	Utilization
Risk financing		—	—
Claims management		—	—
Workers' compensation		—	—
Safety management		—	—
Legal complaints and lawsuits		—	—
Incidents and events		—	—
Occurrence screens		—	—
Capitation risk		—	—
Patient rights		—	—
Discharge planning		—	—
Termination of third-party payment	—	—	
Advanced directives	—	—	
Clinical resource management	—	—	
Peer review organization denials and appeals	—	—	
Determine appropriateness of admission	—	—	
Determine appropriate service utilization	—	—	
Diagnosis-related group assignment/coding	—	—	
Case management	—	—	

continues

Departmental Function	Risk	Quality	Utilization
Licensure	—		—
Joint Commission accreditation	—		—
Credentialing	—		—
Reappointment	—		—
Staff competency	—		—
CQI/TQM program implementation	—		—
Quality indicators/outcomes measurement	—		—
Severity of illness measurement	—		—
External comparisons/benchmarking	—		—
Joint Commission teaching, preparation	—		—
Joint Commission-required measurement functions	—		—
Medical staff quality monitoring/peer review	—		—
Institution-wide quality planning	—		—
Clinical resource management	—		—
Pathways development and implementation	—		—
Operations improvement/reengineering	—		—
Infection control	—	—	—
Patient satisfaction	—	—	—
Managed care contracting	—	—	—
Report cards	—	—	—
Physician profiling	—	—	—
Other functions:	—	—	—
_____	—	—	—
_____	—	—	—
_____	—	—	—
_____	—	—	—
_____	—	—	—
_____	—	—	—
_____	—	—	—
_____	—	—	—
_____	—	—	—
_____	—	—	—

Scoring:

Add together the scores from *each respondent* and *average them for each function listed.*

- For scores = below 1, denotes little interest in integrating functions.
- For scores = 1–1.9, begin to share information about projects through courtesy copies and meeting minutes. Engage in casual conversation to regularly update departments about these activities.
- For scores = 2–2.9, discuss opportunities for increased communication, collaboration, and possible integration. Begin by discerning the specific interests with regard to the function(s). Consider simple strategies such as inviting a representative from another department to attend a meeting or join a committee.
- For scores = 3, explore opportunities for shared responsibility and integration of activities. Structure sessions designed to increase understanding of specific functions performed.

## CHAPTER 10

Legal Implications Inherent in Improving Quality

Tonia D. Aiken and Julia W. Aucoin

CHAPTER OBJECTIVES

After completing this chapter, the reader will be able to

- identify the various types of laws applicable to quality care and common types of violations of these laws
- describe standards of care and standards of practice used to determine negligence or malpractice
- discuss types of law governing quality practice
- describe legal issues of computerized documentation and confidentiality

Quality improvement is not only a buzzword for the late 1990s but has also become the focus for legal actions. As definitions vary, so do the legal implications of the quality movement. *Quality* became a household word with the advertisements of major automobile manufacturers. Since the consumerism movement of the 1980s, patients have demonstrated more comfort in demanding information and seeking alternatives. The quality movement has provided consumers with new avenues for inquiries as well as opportunities to examine flaws in their care. All regulatory state and federal agencies, voluntary accrediting bodies, and payers have specific expectations and mandates that also have legal implications for the provision of quality care.

RISK MANAGEMENT

The link between quality and the legal system begins in risk management. *Risk management* is the process through which potentially or actually harmful situations can be identified, improved, and resolved. When a harmful situation arises (or could arise), it should be identified by anyone who is aware of the possible consequences. It is incumbent on health care professionals to protect patients and staff from any harm that occurs out of negligence, poor systems and processes, and safety violations. A risk management department offers an objective response by skilled investigators to protect the interests of patients and the agency. The primary role of the department is to assist in the quality improvements process as well as limit exposure to unsafe situations.

Once a harmful situation is identified, then the risk management staff investigates causes for the situation, such as long-standing practices, lack of awareness of regulations, introduction of new practices by new staff, or lack of coordination of efforts by various departments. Each of these causes can create exposure to legal actions by astute consumers. A health care agency has the responsibility to orient and develop staff to follow consistent policies. Situations that create exposure can often be resolved by educating staff to policies and regulations. In the event a policy should be developed, then the health care agency should keep careful documentation to chronicle the process and track the policy distribution and subsequent education. Accreditation surveyors as well as trial attorneys can request records indicating how problems have been prevented or resolved. Two major sources leading to potentially harmful situations, that is, causing or contributing to a patient's death, serious injury, or serious illness, are unsafe technology and medication administration.

Safe Medical Devices

The Safe Medical Devices Act of 1990 (SMDA) was developed to protect consumers from unsafe technology. SMDA is intended to enforce the value of "doing no harm" by encouraging practitioners to voluntarily report information about medical devices that harm patients to the Food and Drug Administration (FDA) or the device's manufacturer (Hall, 1996). It provides an opportunity for reporting failures in medical equipment so that manufacturers can respond to needs for improvement. Even though equipment is tested before distribution, mechanical and operator errors can occur. Manufacturers are then accountable for correcting the problem properly. For example, a volumetric infusion pump that infuses fluid at more than the programmed rate would be removed from patient use, examined, and repaired. In the event of an assembly error or computer chip malfunction, the pump would be recalled and refitted to prevent further patient incident. The pump design would then be altered to prevent this problem in future versions of the pump—an improvement in quality control resulting in a decrease in patient injuries and potential lawsuits.

Adverse Drug Reactions

The FDA calls for the reporting of an *adverse drug reaction*, defined as any adverse change in a patient's condition that could be attributed to recognizable responses that could represent a minute portion of the population. Again, the intent is to note all unexpected responses to enable further investigation to occur and modifications to be made to the medications or medication administration processes so that harm will not occur and result in legal actions.

THE LAW

The value of doing good (beneficence) for the patient characterizes professional practice. Issues of quality care arise when the actual benefit of care provided is weighted against the burden, or potential for causing harm. Professionals assume a legal duty to care, and the law enforces that behavior. Laws are rules that are created to guide society and control or regulate individuals' actions and interactions. Various types of law governing practice include

- *Statutory laws*: the body of law created and enacted by federal, state, and local legislative branches
- *Constitutional laws*: laws and amendments guaranteeing individuals' rights such as freedom of speech and equal protection
- *Common laws*: created by judicial decisions rendered in the various courts
- *Administrative laws*: created by administrative agencies under the guidance of the executive branch of government

The Nurse Practice Act created the state boards of nursing as administrative agencies that in turn enforce nursing practice regulations. Disciplinary actions are usually presented to the boards before they are placed in the judicial system. Every state has a nurse practice act outlining violations that can end in the revocation of a license or in the suspension or limitation of practice. Nurses must be aware of what is included in the Nurse Practice Act to avoid potential disciplinary actions.

Common types of violations of which the nurse may be accused can include

- guilty of selling or attempting to sell, falsely obtaining, or furnishing any nursing diploma or license to practice as a registered nurse
- conviction of a crime or offense that demonstrates the nurse's inability to practice with the patient's health and safety in mind
- an entry plea of guilty of nolo contendere (no contest) to a criminal charge regardless of final dispositions of the criminal proceeding, including, but not limited to, expungement or nonadjudication
- unfit or incompetent by reason of negligence, habit, or other causes, including, but not limited to

1. failure to practice nursing in accordance with the legal standards of nursing practice
2. possession of a physical impairment or mental impairment that interferes with the judgment, skills, or abilities required for nursing practice
3. failure to use appropriate judgment in nursing practice
4. failure to exercise technical competence in carrying out nursing care
5. violation of patient information or knowledge
6. performance of procedures beyond the authorized scope of nursing
7. performance of duties and assumption of responsibilities when the nurse is incompetent or has not maintained the proper competency level
8. improper use of drugs, medical supplies, or patient's records
9. misappropriation of personal items of an individual or the agency
10. falsification of records
11. failure to act, or intentionally commit any act that adversely affects the patient's physical or psychosocial welfare, including but not limited to failing to practice in accordance with the federal Centers for Disease Control and Prevention recommendations for preventing the transmission of human immunodeficiency virus (HIV) and hepatitis B virus
12. delegation of nursing care, functions, tasks, or responsibilities to others contrary to regulations
13. leaving a nursing assignment without properly notifying appropriate personnel
14. failure to report, through the proper channels, facts known regarding incompetence, unethical, or illegal practice of any health care provider
15. failure to report when performing or participating in exposure-prone procedures and the nurse is known to be a carrier of the hepatitis B virus or HIV
16. violation of a rule or order by the board
17. violation of a state or federal law relating to the practice of professional nursing
18. violation of a state or federal narcotics or controlled substance law

- demonstration of actual or potential inability to practice nursing with reasonable skill and safety because of use of alcohol, drugs, or illness as a result of any mental or physical condition
- guilty of aiding or abetting anyone in the violation of any provisions of the act or the rules and regulations of the board
- mentally incompetent
- a denied, revoked, suspended, or otherwise restricted license to practice nursing or to practice in another health care field
- guilty of moral turpitude
- violation of any provisions of the Nurse Practice Act

All of the preceding violations demonstrate that the emphasis is on the quality and safety of the patient.

Criminal law provides guidance and protects people injured due to offenses against society and the public. Criminal law punishes or rehabilitates those who have hurt "society" rather than making the person "whole again" with a monetary award such as in a civil lawsuit. Criminal cases involving health care workers include crimes such as murder, rape, assault, and battery. Misdemeanors are considered lesser crimes and are generally punishable by fines of $1,000 or imprisonment for less than one year, or both, depending on the jurisdiction. Felonies are more serious crimes and carry harsher punishments, punishable by prison and even the death sentence, again depending on state laws. In many states, a felony conviction of a nurse can be grounds for denying, revoking, or suspending a nurse's license.

TORT LAW

Tort law deals with actions and the degree of intent present in the wrongdoer's act; it is a lawsuit in which the plaintiff (the patient) seeks to be monetarily compensated for damage that causes a *wrong*. Tort law encompasses both negligence and medical malpractice claims. If an individual intended the act, the wrong is classified as an *intentional tort*.

Intentional Torts

An *intentional tort* is a deliberate act that the person is reasonably certain will cause damage or injury as a result of his or her action. The types of intentional torts are:

- *assault*: occurs when one person causes another person to fear that he or she will be touched in an offensive or injurious manner, even if no touching actually occurs
- *battery*: the unpermitted touching of a person in an offensive or injurious manner; the allegations of medical battery are usually associated with a lack of informed consent (e.g., consent is given to remove the diseased left lung; however, the surgeon removes the healthy right lung); the patient can claim medical battery (an intentional tort) in addition to medical mal-

practice, which falls under tort law based on the theory of negligence
- *Breach of confidentiality*: an intrusion on the seclusion or private concerns of another; in the health care environment, the filming or videotaping of a person without his or her informed consent can be considered an intentional tort or intrusion if it is shared for purposes other than patient treatment; also, public disclosure of private facts about a patient invades that person's privacy; if false information is given to a third party that in some way damages the person economically or reputationwise, that action can result in a potential claim for *defamation* (also an intentional tort). *Oral defamation is slander; written defamation is libel.*

The release of information to the news media without the patient's permission is also a breach. Release of factual information about births or discharges usually does not violate a patient's privacy rights. Written policies must be developed so that all employees are aware of the rules and respond in a consistent manner to such situations.

Negligence (Malpractice)

The term *negligence* refers to a failure to act as an ordinary prudent person would do under similar circumstances with the same knowledge, experience, and expertise. The medical negligence or medical malpractice claims fall under the tort theory.

Four elements of negligence must be evident for a plaintiff (the person or entity suing) to have a successful outcome in a malpractice case. If the defendant (the person or entity sued) can prove that the elements are not met, then the plaintiff will not be successful. The elements are

1. *Duty owed to the patient*: The duty requires that the health care provider be reasonable in rendering care and maintaining the standard of care. The quality of care does not have to be the highest

level but must be reasonable under the circumstances.

2. *Breach of duty/breach of the standard of care*: The health care provider must follow the appropriate standards of care in effect at the time of the alleged act of malpractice.

3. *Proximate cause/causal connection*: A connection between the breach of duty or standard and the actual damages suffered by the plaintiff (injured party) must be apparent. If the health care provider has acted or failed to act or provide proper and timely treatment and causes injuries or damage to the patient, then there is proximate cause between the acts or omissions and injuries. Proximate cause can be thought of as a bridge linking the breach of duty to a patient's damages.

4. *Damages or injuries suffered by the patient*: The patient must sustain damages or injuries as a result of the breach of the standard of care by the health care provider. Damages fall into several categories. *General damages* are awarded for the plaintiff's pain and suffering caused by the defendant's acts. *Special damages* are based on the actual monetary losses, such as lost wages for the past, present, and future, and past, present, and future medical expenses.

Damages often alleged include pain and suffering; mental anguish; loss of chance of survival; disfigurement; past, present, and future medical expenses; past, present, and future lost wages; premature death; loss of nurturance; and loss of enjoyment of life. An example of medical negligence occurred in a case involving a 51-year-old female who experienced a drop in blood pressure and heart rate during back surgery. The defendants did not stabilize the patient until approximately 35 minutes later, which resulted in hypoxic encephalopathy. The patient died 6 weeks later, never recovering from the coma she lapsed into during the surgery. A $500,000 settlement was reached for wrongful death (*Marino v. Razza*, 1995).

STANDARDS OF CARE: TOOLS USED FOR QUALITY CONTROL

The *standard of care* or *standard of practice* is a measuring scale based on negligence and is used to determine what reasonable degree of skill, education, care, and diligence should be used by members with the same knowledge, experience, and background under similar circumstances. To decide whether the elements of negligence are evident in a malpractice claim, standards of care or standards of practice must be determined. What specific standards of care should have been applied or were applied in the particular situation at hand?

Standards of practice or standards of care come from many different sources. Sources include

- authoritative textbooks
- expert witnesses
- national specialty professional organizations
- state and federal agencies
- hospital or facility policies and procedures
- American Nurses' Association, American Medical Association, and so forth
- The Joint Commission, National Committee for Quality Assurance, National League for Nursing, and other voluntary accrediting bodies
- treatises and publications
- state statutes
- regulatory statutes
- bylaws
- rules and regulations
- job descriptions
- equipment instruction books
- nurse practice acts
- nurse practice guidelines

Exhibit 10–1 offers quality points to remember when drafting the standards.

Exhibit 10–1 Care or Practice Standards: Quality Points

- When drafting standards of care or standards of practice, it is important that you determine what is the national standard. Remember that, as a nurse, you are responsible for providing what is reasonable under the circumstances and not the highest level of care.
- Remember that standard of care testimony is routinely provided by expert witnesses in a medical or nursing negligence claim. In a disciplinary proceeding against a professional, standards of care may be assessed in terms of negligence, gross negligence, or incompetence.

CLINICAL PRACTICE GUIDELINES AND CLINICAL PATHWAYS

Using clinical practice guidelines, the health care provider must be careful not to elevate these guidelines to the level of standards of care. There are obvious legal implications if critical pathways are treated as guidelines versus standards. *Guidelines* are options that can be used; *standards* must be followed.

Four areas of practice in which quality control of care and treatment must be targeted are communication, treatment, medication, and monitoring. The following are common acts of omissions or commission within the four areas:

1. communication—failure to communicate in a timely fashion to other health care providers, failure to communicate the proper information, failure to communicate information to the proper person
2. treatment—failure to treat in a timely fashion, failure to properly treat, failure to treat in the appropriate manner according to the standards of care; an act of omission or commission can be a breach of the standard
3. medication—failure to administer properly; wrong site, wrong medication, wrong dosage, wrong technique; failure to recognize drug toxicity
4. monitoring—failure to properly monitor and report findings to the appropriate people, failure to monitor according to the standards of care, failure to act appropriately after evaluating the information obtained from monitoring

For example, in a case against a nursing home for the death of an 85-year-old, parties settled before a lawsuit was filed for $150,000 plus a waiver of a $14,000 debt for services rendered. Claims against the nursing home included

- failure to properly train its employees in the safe care of geriatric patients
- failure to prevent falls

The deceased patient had fractured her hip and suffered postsurgical complications (i.e., pneumonia) and expired approximately 3 months later (*Hooker v. Crystal*, 1995).

COMPUTERIZED DOCUMENTATION AND CONFIDENTIALITY

Owners of medical facilities and the administrators who manage them must determine ways to provide reasonable patient care in an environment that may not be conducive to the level of care needed. New ways are being recommended for managing and "creating" more quality time available for care and treatment needed by patients. One new method is computerized documentation. Automated charting can demonstrate if a practitioner follows a standard of care or critical pathway or fails to do so. With the development of software, consideration must be given to format, quality of the charting produced, location of the computer and the chart, education of the practitioners who are not computer literate, and costs.

With computerized charting, though, come concerns about the accuracy of documentation. Automated entries are clear and easily readable with specific times and dates for each entry. Some health care providers see this presentation as a benefit; others are concerned that times are "too exact" and may not properly depict what happened. Such concerns should be handled through education. Also, the facility attorney and risk managers should address potential problems with documentation pertaining to medical negligence claims, billing for reimbursement, and confidentiality.

Advantages and Disadvantages

Computer-based patient records offer advantages and disadvantages to maintaining health care records. Computerized documentation can be a quicker and easier method for recording patient information, thus allowing more hands-on patient time, increased morale, and limited paperwork. However, the easy availability and rapid transmission to other areas within an organization can lead to potential privacy violations. Other potential problems include the following:

- Information is sent to the wrong patient record.
- Information is seen by the wrong person.
- The place where the information is received is accessible to others who should not see such information.
- The information is improperly given or not given in a timely manner to the authorized individual who should receive the information.
- Digitized records are transmitted worldwide without a trace.
- Certain companies (e.g., life insurance companies) are allowed access to information about applicants, including medical history that can preclude the applicants from receiving services.
- Computer downtime will occur.
- Computers and software might be cost-prohibitive.

- Professional and paraprofessional staff will require education.
- Physicians may be reluctant to use computers.
- Practitioners may be reluctant to stop using "manual" worksheets.

To prevent leaks and quality problems, the organization must develop a method to determine who has access to the information. Also, a receipt or other tracking device placed in the patient's records can quickly lead to the perpetrator, who may be immediately terminated or prosecuted. Audit trails also act as deterrents.

The trend is to have a universal patient identifier that is assigned at birth or the first time a person has contact with the health care system and remains with the patient for life. A potential problem that may arise involves preventing direct linkage of the identifier with the patient, except by those individuals authorized to have that information. Policies and procedures must be developed to prevent incorrect information from being linked to an identifier. Methods must be designed to change incorrect data in a timely manner. A national health care database is a wonderful tool for preventing delays in determining past medical histories, allergies, reactions, and other valuable information that can increase the quality of care rendered to the patient. (Refer to Chapter 13 for greater detail regarding information systems.)

Computerized Documentation and Case Management

Case management of large patient specialty populations requires the use of computerized patient files. Computerized patient files allow easy access to valuable information and dates. Patient management and other valuable lists can be easily compiled and obtained. The use of computerized and customized patient and physician letters allows a rapid return of test results to the patient, family, and referring physician. Also, critical delays in information gathering are eliminated using computerized data. (Refer to Chapter 14 for greater detail regarding case management, clinical practice, and guidelines.)

PATIENT SELF-DETERMINATION ACT: QUALITY OF CARE AND QUALITY OF LIFE

A patient's autonomy—freedom to choose and act in one's own behalf—is a fundamental principle of the law. The *Patient Self-Determination Act (PSDA)*, part of the 1990 amendment to the Medicare law, is based on the principle of *informed consent*. A competent adult can consent to or refuse any invasive or noninvasive treatments or regimes directed to his or her body. The PSDA requires all federally funded institutions to inform patients of their right to prepare advance directives; this process is also mandated by the Joint Commission (1993).

Advanced directives include the *living will*, which is a legal document stating what health care treatment a patient will accept or refuse after the patient is no longer competent or able to make the decision. The state statutes will designate the conditions such as "terminal," "irreversible," or "in continual profound comatose state." The criteria determining when the living will becomes effective vary by state.

The *durable power of attorney*, or *health care proxy*, is a document that designates another person to make health care decisions for a person if he or she becomes incompetent or unable to make such decisions. The proxy does not have to be the spouse or next of kin. State statutes outline their requirements for executing and revoking the durable power of attorney and the living wills.

Informed consent is consent obtained from a patient or patient's legal representative or guardian after receiving the necessary informa-tion to determine whether to accept the type of care, treatment, or procedure offered. The elements of disclosure that must be made and discussed with the patient are

- the type of procedure or procedures to be performed
- the material risks and hazards inherent in the procedures
- the outcome expected
- available alternatives, if any
- consequences of no treatment

It is assumed that, after the patient has been given all the elements of disclosure, the patient has enough information to make an informed decision. With regard to children, informed consent is obtained after discussion with the parents unless the child is an emancipated minor. In that case, the child has the legal right to make decisions about his or her own health care. It is important that the health care provider realize that, to avoid any potential lawsuits with informed consent, all the elements of disclosure must be made. Exceptions are as follows:

- in an emergency situation
- if the health care provider or physician evokes a therapeutic privilege because he or she feels that to disclose the medical information may be medically contraindicated and may result in illness, emotional distress, psychological damage, or failure of the patient to seek and to receive the required life-saving treatment
- when the risk is obvious
- when the patient waives the right to receive the information

Exhibit 10–2 offers quality points regarding informed consent; Exhibit 10–3, regarding the PSDA; and Exhibit 10–4, regarding do-not-resuscitate (DNR) orders.

Exhibit 10–2 Informed Consent: Quality Points

- The physician is legally responsible for obtaining informed consent.
- The nurse who signs an informed consent witnesses the patient's signature only.
- It is important to understand that, as a nurse, if you assume a role of getting informed consent and there is an allegation of a lack of informed consent in a medical malpractice claim, you may be held to a higher level of standard in a court of law.
- If there is an exception to the duty to disclose, this exception must be documented in the informed consent sheet or in the progress notes or nurses' notes to protect the health care provider. Information that should be documented includes who was present during the discussions, what was specifically discussed, and what specific information was not related to the patient or family.
- If there is any question about the capacity of the patient to give consent, consult appropriate in-house legal counsel.

Exhibit 10–3 The Patient Self-Determination Act: Quality Points

- Be sure that the patient has had the opportunity to decide whether he or she wants an advance directive.
- Check to see if the patient has signed an advance directive or medical durable power of attorney or health care proxy. Have a copy of the advance directive and medical durable power of attorney on the chart so that all the health care providers know the wishes of the patient and the patient's family.
- Many times, a patient who is in a terminal or irreversible state decides he or she does not want any type of lifesaving treatment or procedures performed. However, the family members demand that the health care providers do everything possible to keep the patient alive, despite the patient's request in the living will. Such efforts may result in a quality of life the patient does not desire. To avoid any potential lawsuits by the patient, this conflict must be resolved as quickly as possible before the patient can no longer voice an opinion. Document that a living will and medical durable power of attorney exist and make those documents known to all health care providers caring for that patient.

Exhibit 10–4 Do-Not-Resuscitate Orders: Quality Points

- To be protected legally, the health care provider also needs a do-not-resuscitate order (DNR), which is separate and apart from the living will.
- Develop a DNR policy in your facility or institution.
- Be sure that all employees, physicians, and all independent contractors and agency nurses know what a DNR code means.
- If there is a question regarding DNR orders, contact the physician and in-house counsel.
- Monitor the health care providers to be sure there is no discrimination against a DNR patient.
- Document conversations, meetings, and questions regarding the DNR order.
- The DNR order must be reviewed and reordered. Facilities should have policies established.
- If your facility uses a "chemical code only" or "resuscitate but do not intubate" order, know what the orders mean. A policy should outline what such orders require.
- Quality improvement suggests that the staff be informed about the organizational policy regarding DNR. Situations that cannot be handled by the DNR policy should be forwarded to the ethics committee for further study or resolution.

CONCLUSION

The shared values of a society are the basis of their laws; society authorizes others to enforce the laws. Professional practice is governed by values: doing good by caring for the patient (beneficence); doing no harm to the patient (nonmaleficence); being fair to the patient and colleagues (justice); preserving the freedom of the patient and professional (autonomy); being loyal to the patient, telling the truth, and maintaining confidentiality.

The law controls potentially harmful behavior. It will either mandate (prescribe) that something must be done, or prohibit (proscribe) that something must *not* be done (Hall, 1996). The law is the legal minimum behavior and must be placed in a situational perspective. Professionals should act not only because something is mandated, but also because it is desired and achieves high quality care. Acting because it appears to be the mandate of the law may not be in the best interest of the patient or the professional.

REFERENCES

A new focus on advance directives. (1993). *Briefings on JCAHO*. July/August, pp. 10–11.

Hall, J. (1996). *Nursing: Ethics and law*. p. 184, Philadelphia: W.B. Saunders.

Patient Self-Determination Act. (1990). Public Law 101–508.

## CHAPTER 11

Improving Quality Care: An Ethical Imperative in a Time of Change

Mary Ellen Wurzbach

CHAPTER OBJECTIVES

After completing this chapter, the reader will be able to

- understand the relationship between quality improvement and bioethics
- assess an organization's readiness to develop a bioethics committee
- identify various roles assumed by the committee

The health care system is changing at an unprecedented rate. Networks of providers, hospitals, and insurance carriers abound in an ever-expanding association of diverse health care organizations. The ultimate goal of these networks is financial, that is, providing a profit for their shareholders.

Because the profit motive seems to be guiding the modern health care system much more than in the past, questions of ethics have arisen. For example, to whom are these new organizations responsible? Are they accountable for their actions? How does one preserve quality when cost-effectiveness is the desired end? Are efficiency, cost-effectiveness, and quality congruent goals?

This chapter describes the development of the current health care system, provides guidelines for the development of an organizational bioethics committee, and discusses ways to preserve an ethic of quality in a time of rapid change.

THE AGE OF REFORM

In 1970, the cost of health care was $60 billion; by 1996, $800 billion; and it is estimated that by 2000, costs will pass the trillion-dollar mark (Mohr, 1996; Morreim, 1985). Such unlimited growth has pushed health care payers, insurance companies, businesses, and the government to move from fee-for-service arrangements to managed care associations. Because many service organizations involve large alliances of providers and payers, the character of the system has changed from small business providers to large modern corporations. These corporations are characterized by centralized management, economy of service, and a wish to maximize market share (Mohr, 1996).

The entire climate of health care has changed from a service-oriented professional ethic to a more businesslike entrepreneurial ethic. Several nursing and medical observers have expressed concern about the rapid commercial changes of health care with their concomitant changes in the professional role. There is a belief that the possibility of providing appropriate care in such settings diminishes (Emanuel, 1995). The stage is set for the profit institutions, through mergers, organizational efficiency, and lower overhead, to control the health care system (Mohr, 1996).

The ethic of these merged systems is one of self-interest (Mohr, 1996). This ethic of self-interest means that the goal of the merged systems is to maximize profit, create wealth, and possibly create jobs. In a market economy, the universal principle is survival of the fittest. In such a health care "marketplace," the consumer may be at a disadvantage because the services provided are based on the uncontrolled principles of supply and demand.

Several concerns arise in an age of reform. For-profit health care organizations tend to provide more services than are necessary for the consumer, whereas health maintenance organizations tend to ration care. Thus, some organizations make money by overtreating and others by undertreating. Furthermore, patients must be educated consumers in a system where self-interest rules, yet few patients know enough about the system, their own needs, or the service provided to make educated decisions. In addition, the rise of all these large corporate entities raises the issue of monopoly control of health care (Mohr, 1996).

ETHICS: BUSINESS OR HEALTH CARE

A problem arises when one tries to combine a business ethic with a health care ethic. Businesses have far different standards than traditional health care organizations. Businesses value achievement of management goals, efficiency, product quality, and fair competition (Mariner, 1995). Several laudable ethical principles such as promise keeping, truthfulness, and fairness are accepted by the business community, but the purpose of these principles is to foster fair competition rather than quality health care (Mariner, 1995).

In addition, business practices are based on several assumptions that do not apply to health care. For example, in a business arrangement, it is assumed that both parties to the contract are of equal status; however, in health care, patients who sign health insurance contracts are less than equal (Mariner, 1995). In health care, the patient seldom has the knowledge, power, or motivation of the provider. In addition, both health care providers and businesses have fiduciary responsibilities but to different constituen-

cies: the business to its shareholders and the health care provider to the patient. Few patients understand or know what is in the health care contracts that they sign, whereas a business assumes full knowledge before making a contract or at least the ability to obtain such knowledge.

Several authors have described quality standards for the new health care system (Curtin, 1995; Mariner, 1995; Mohr, 1996; Wolf, 1994). Mohr (1996) suggested that, based on the social contract, health care has a responsibility to protect society's values. The values of society that are congruent with the values of health care are respect for people or autonomy, the right to self-determination, beneficence (doing good), and nonmaleficence (doing no harm). Justice also has been espoused in many forms by society.

Mariner (1995) has suggested that health care providers recognize both health care and business responsibilities and that organizational standards ought to reflect the values of society. Aroskar (1995) has recommended that health care maintain its sense of moral community with the principle of respect for people. She recognized, however, that ethics and the political process intersect.

DEVELOPMENT OF A BIOETHICS COMMITTEE

One method for maintaining quality within the institution is to develop a health care ethics committee. A health care ethics committee provides a forum for the practitioner to express ethical concerns and issues related to the organizational culture. It allows for the specification of values underlying health care. In addition, it may be used to develop a moral community within the organization.

Ethics committees have been a part of the health care system since 1984 (Edwards & Haddad, 1988). Many of these committees are multidisciplinary. The objectives of a health care ethics committee may be many and varied. Edwards and Haddad (1988) have suggested the following four objectives for nursing ethics committees, which could apply to all bioethics committees:

1. to assist the practitioner in assuming ethical responsibilities to make judgments as a professional who is effecting change
2. to influence the development of policies on health care standards within the professions and the institution
3. to serve as a resource to individual clinicians and managers whose responsibility for high-quality health care spans patients, families, and the community

4. to develop support within the system for health care practitioners' active participation in ethical decision making (p. 31)

Before developing an institutional bioethics committee, a multitude of questions must be addressed (Anderson, 1996; Edwards & Haddad, 1988; Mitchell, Uehlinger, & Owen, 1996; Ross, Bayley, Michel, & Pugh, 1986). Exhibit 11-1 presents a questionnaire to be used before setting up an organizational bioethics committee.

In addition, to answering the questions in Exhibit 11–1, the following suggestions might be helpful in the development of an interdisci-

---

Exhibit 11–1 Questionnaire for Assessing the Organizational Climate

Initial Questions	Yes	No	Comments
• Has a need been demonstrated for an interdisciplinary bioethics committee?			
• Do all the professions within the institution support the development of a bioethics committee?			
• Will all the professions (e.g., medicine, nursing, social services, therapies) be represented on the committee?			
• Does the administration of the organization support formation of a bioethics committee?			
• Do those initiating development of the committee have a clear idea of what they would like to accomplish?			
• Has a list of the ethical concerns most commonly faced by the practitioner in the institution been developed?			
• Has an ad hoc committee been set up to study the need for a bioethics committee?			
• Is there a bioethics study group already available to educate staff about the ethical issues?			
• Are educational programs relating to ethics and quality ongoing within the organization?			
• Is this a good time to begin developing the bioethics committee?			

continues

Exhibit 11–1 continued

Organizational Questions

- If this is a good time to set up a bioethics committee, what size will it be? _____

- What will be the goals, functions, and authority of the committee?

  _____

  _____

- Will the committee's function(s) be education, consultation and case review, and/or policy and guideline recommendation? _____

  _____

- What will be the primary focus of the committee:

Education?	Yes ___	No ___
Planning?	Yes ___	No ___
Guidance of staff?	Yes ___	No ___
Policy formation?	Yes ___	No ___
Case consultation?	Yes ___	No ___

- Will the committee make policy that is mandatory or develop guidelines that are not mandatory? _____

- How will the goals, functions, decisions, and authority of the committee be evaluated? _____

- What will be the membership requirements and how will members be selected? _____

- Will the committee include

Attorneys?	Yes ___	No ___
Consumers?	Yes ___	No ___
Professionals within the organization?	Yes ___	No ___
An ethics consultant?	Yes ___	No ___

- Where in the organizational chart will the committee appear? _____

- Are subcommittees of the overall committee necessary?   Yes ___   No ___
  If yes, describe _____

- How will new members be oriented to the committee? _____

- How will the staff of the organization, committee members, and the community be educated? _____

  _____

Legal/Ethical Questions

- How will records (e.g., minutes of meetings, goals, functions, policies, position papers, patients' health care records, case review records) be kept? _____

continues

Exhibit 11–1 continued

- Who should or should not be identified in the record:
  The patient?   Yes ___   No ___
  The person bringing the case to the committee's attention?   Yes ___   No ___
  Other: _____   Yes ___   No ___

- Will the patient be made aware of an ethics consultation about   Yes ___   No ___
  his/her case?

- Are case consultations voluntary and with the permission of the
  patient or surrogate decision maker?   Yes ___   No ___

- Who has access to committee records:
  Committee members?   Yes ___   No ___
  Patients?   Yes ___   No ___
  Families of patients?   Yes ___   No ___
  Nurses?   Yes ___   No ___
  Physicians of the organization?   Yes ___   No ___

- Will there be ethical guidelines for the committee regarding:
  Confidentiality?   Yes ___   No ___
  Privacy for the patient?   Yes ___   No ___
  Privacy for the professional?   Yes ___   No ___
  Informed consent to a case review?   Yes ___   No ___
  Respect for people?   Yes ___   No ___
  Other guidelines? Please describe._____

Case Review Questions

- What procedure will the committee follow to review cases? _____

- What will determine if a case is reviewed? _____

  Is there a mandatory review for some?   Yes ___   No ___
  Is review optional?   Yes ___   No ___

- Who may bring a case to the committee (e.g., staff members, the
  family, patients)? _____

- Who attends a case review? _____

- Who is informed that a case has been referred and who has access
  to the committee findings?_____

- Does the entire committee review a case?   Yes ___   No ___

- What happens at the conclusion of a case review?_____

continues

Exhibit 11–1 continued

• Will case reviews be		
Prospective?	Yes ___	No ___
Retrospective?	Yes ___	No ___
Both?	Yes ___	No ___
• Does the committee have access to legal counsel?	Yes ___	No ___

Quality Improvement Questions

• What mechanisms are in place for quality improvement? _____
  _____

• What are the mechanisms for changing policy in the organization? __
  _____

• Is the responsibility and accountability of practitioners for quality improvement clearly identified?	Yes ___	No ___
• Are communication avenues among practitioners, patients, families, and administration open?	Yes ___	No ___
Please describe these avenues. _____		
• Does the organization have a research committee that might undertake quality improvement projects?	Yes ___	No ___
• Will the bioethics committee be expected to do research?	Yes ___	No ___
• Are practitioners on the committee committed to the principles of bioethics and quality improvement?	Yes ___	No ___

plinary bioethics committee within the institution (Edwards & Haddad, 1988; Ross et al., 1986). For one, the committee ought to have wide representation from all clinical areas and levels of the organization. Clinical areas vary dramatically in the care provided, viewpoints about ethical issues, and appropriate action options. It is necessary to have as broad a representation of specialties and levels of the organization as possible to avoid factual mistakes or perceptual errors that might have been averted. The chair of the committee ought to be a morally and professionally credible person who has excellent interpersonal skills and a knowledge of ethics. Furthermore, the committee requires access to an ethicist or consultant who is an expert in both ethical theory and clinical practice.

Committee Rules

The ethics committee may be an educational as well as a planning and coordinating committee. The committee may provide educational workshops and in-service programs; these activities, which prepare staff for their roles, are a necessity and an integral part of the educational function of the ethics committee. The committee also may plan institutional changes based on the conclusions of particular cases brought before it, or coordinate the ethical efforts of the institution to preserve quality care.

In addition to its role as educator, the committee assumes the roles of supporter, decision maker, and consultant (Edwards & Haddad, 1988). The role of supporter cannot be overly stressed. The committee ought to be a visible affirmation of the support of colleagues for one another, including the support of management for staff and staff for management. Many of the committee's decisions may be controversial, with powerful people disagreeing in some cases. The administrative support necessary for the committee to be viable ought to be obtained. Many decisions will require the support of management for implementation; thus, management of the institution needs to be kept informed. Support is also necessary because many decisions may be poignant and may touch the committee deeply during the decision-making process.

The role of decision maker is probably the most difficult. In many cases, ethics committees are advisory, but if the committee makes mandated decisions, then clear deliberations, support for opposite viewpoints, and the courage of committee members are essential.

Consultant is the primary role an ethics committee may assume. Many of the committee's responses will involve suggestions, opinions, and clarification of the facts. As Edwards and Haddad (1988) have pointed out, the consultant will assist with "the decision-making process of identifying the ethical issue, the roles and responsibilities of those persons involved, the alternative courses of action, and the consequences of each action" (p. 31). The committee also provides time within the decision-making process to reflect on the process and the outcome of the committee's deliberation and action. The committee may decide that its role is advisory (consultative or educational), is that of decision maker, or as liaison between staff and patients. Whatever role is assumed, the committee's primary responsibility is ethical accountability in the form of quality preservation.

As a sounding board for staff concerns that may not have been addressed in the past, the committee must discern the differences between personnel issues and ethical issues and refer staff complaints to the appropriate personnel. Initially, committee members may need help discriminating between ethical dilemmas and other forms of conflict or communication fail-

ures. Once the dilemma has been identified and considered at a committee meeting, staff and managerial responsibilities for each possible action option are assigned. Assignment helps coordinate committee efforts (Edwards & Haddad, 1988).

An ethics committee maintains both the dignity of each patient and the integrity of the profession and the institution. Protecting the patient's dignity means promoting respect for people within the changing health care environment. Integrity means doing what one believes one ought to do. Because the health care system is changing so rapidly, many of the ethical dilemmas encountered may deal with organizational issues such as delegation, conflict between a patient's health care insurance policy and the necessary treatment, and end-of-life treatment decisions. The committee will be meeting its obligation to the staff, institution, patients, and society if it fosters a concerted effort to examine the health care issues, promotes the support to take action based on committee deliberations, and takes the time to reflect on the action taken and what might have been done differently.

The process for resolving bioethical dilemmas includes gathering and assessing the facts. This is probably the most important step because dilemmas frequently may be matters of fact rather than true dilemmas. Furthermore, this step identifies the conflicting values. For example, beneficence may be perceived as benign by one committee member but as a paternalistic restriction on the patient's autonomy by another member. Before the committee chooses an action option—frequently, only two solutions seem viable—it is suggested that the committee brainstorm to discuss all possible alternatives before drawing a conclusion. The committee would then implement the action option and reflect on it. Some questions Ross et al. (1986) have suggested the committee ask at this point are, What will be done about the conclusion of the committee? What steps will be taken to resolve the issue? Who will be responsible for following up? How should the decision be communicated to all parties voicing the concern? How will remaining concerns be handled? Is education related to the dilemma needed? Is a policy necessary to address similar concerns? What have we learned from this experience?

According to the American Hospital Association (Ross et al., 1986), the following are pitfalls in organizing an ethics committee:

- Lack of clarity about the committee's purpose—Many ethics committees are strictly educational. Case review may or may not be an essential part of the committee process. The committee must develop a clear reason for being.
- A focus purely on case consultation—Consultation may seem more exciting than education, when in reality the educational function might be more beneficial for an organization and its patients and staff.
- Insufficient member knowledge of ethics—The first responsibility of ethics committee members is to educate themselves. Frequently, members will have a deep and abiding interest in ethics, but no formal education in it. As Ross et al. (1986) have stated, "Taking any action before committee members feel competent may cause more harm than good" (p. 66).
- Great deal of enthusiasm, but little time—Plans may be made but never implemented. Enthusiasm must be contained and legitimate goals set.
- Domination—The committee may be dominated by a member or by the management of the organization. Reticent members may never express their feelings. Inadequate resources, committee function overlap, or failure to evaluate itself and its performance may also derail the committee.
- Legal ramifications—It would be well to consult an attorney or to have an attorney on the committee to consider issues such as the right to privacy of the patient and involved practitioner, confidentiality of records and committee minutes, criminal or civil liability, committee immunity from having its records brought into court, and discoverability. *Discoverability* involves evidence that may be procured by the attorneys of parties to a lawsuit while they are preparing their cases. The issue is whether the records or the participants at a committee meeting may be subpoenaed. Such legal issues should be addressed at the committee's inception because state laws differ.

ISSUES INHERENT IN LINKING ETHICS AND QUALITY IMPROVEMENT

The ethics committee holds great promise for an organization and for the development of quality improvement education within the organization; however, several authors have criticized bioethics committees. In discussing power and authority in ethics consultation, Agrich (1995) has suggested that the importance of judgment and discretion cannot be overemphasized in the process of ethical discourse and consultation. Judgment involves an awareness of relevant principles; paradigm cases; rules and regulations; the values of the people involved in a case; the details of the case; and the political, psychological, and social circumstances of the case.

Hayes (1995) has suggested that committee members need to have a current knowledge of the group process. He has expressed concerns about a lack of diversity among some bioethics committee members; the possibility of dominant people taking over the committee; and *groupthink*, which involves minimizing conflict, downplaying risks, limiting alternatives, and coercing committee members to reach consensus. His methods for minimizing group decision-making errors include maximizing diversity among committee members, screening members, providing in-depth education to the committee members, voting by ballot, and countering groupthink by using brainstorming. In addition, the committee needs to make a concerted effort to allow for the expression of doubts, concerns, objections, and alternative points of view.

Evaluation and Research

Singer, Pellegrino, and Siegler (1990) have recommended continuous ongoing evaluation of ethics committees. They have suggested that if ethics committees could teach professionals within the organization the aspects of ethical deliberation, committees might be less necessary.

Sugarman (1994) has suggested that ethics committees do research to support their normative function. He has recommended evaluation research of current committee activities, needs assessments that examine the quality of case consultations, and the use of research to make a contribution to clinical ethics. Some of the barriers to empirical research he identified are the subject matter that may not be easy to study, staff opposition, and conflicting responsibilities of the ethics committee members.

Organizational Issues

Several authors have explored the responsibility of health care organizations to maintain an ethical life over and above the practitioner's ethical life. Reiser (1994) suggested that the organization itself consider how organizational values affect the institution and the community to whom it is responsible. According to Reiser, the organization has an ethical commitment to its staff, patients, and the community at large. The organization must have vision and value statements and a method for connecting these stated values with the actions taken by the organization. Blake (1992) has recommended that the bioethics committee focus on education; the committee does not invent protocols for conduct, but gives voice to a community vision of bioethics.

Wolf (1994) pointed out that the development of an ethics of institutions is imperative if health care reform is to be compatible with health care ethics as currently practiced. Her additions to the current ethical climate would include the prohibition of financial incentives for health care practitioners, which deny patients potentially beneficial treatment, the obligation of health care institutions to support practitioners' capacity to fulfill their duties to patients, organizational support for practitioner advocacy for patients, fair procedures for challenges to organizational decisions, and processes for monitoring and continuously improving organizational ethical practice. The quality of an organization's ethics, ethical decision making, and subsequent behaviors directly affects financial viability of the organization.

CONCLUSION

During the 1980s, the definition of quality shifted from evaluation of the practitioner's competency or a review of the care process to determining the patient's benefits of care. Today, it is believed that a quality process does not necessarily translate into a quality outcome, nor is quantity of services always perceived as quality. In addition, many of the large health care companies contend that quality indicators are proprietary; therefore, preliminary data are not in the public domain (Priester, 1989).

Historically, quality care was based on two factors—credentialing and peer review—and responsibility for quality assurance used to be borne at the local level (Priester, 1989). Today, the patient and payer's perspectives can no longer be ignored. Patient satisfaction is one measure of quality, but the patient may attend to aspects of care other than quality, which makes basing care on patient satisfaction difficult.

New measures to determine quality need to be devised and implemented. An emphasis on quality might eliminate some major flaws of managed care and could help contain undertreatment and overtreatment. Informed consent to treatment or lack of treatment could be determined. Beneficence would be promoted and doing harm avoided.

Presently, health care is becoming increasingly businesslike. There is an emphasis on efficiency and cost-effectiveness, but at what price? Now, more than ever, it is important for health care practitioners to be vigilant in observing care to make certain it is quality care. Becoming involved in quality improvement studies and other forms of research will help maintain a standard of quality. If quality is compromised by short staffing, incompetent peers or subordinates, or denial of treatment or early discharge, the practitioner needs to voice concern. The bioethics committee may be one helpful mechanism for expressing those concerns.

REFERENCES

Agrich, G.J. (1995). Authority in ethics consultation. *Journal of Law, Medicine & Ethics, 23,* 273–283.

Anderson, C.A. (1996). Ethics committees and quality improvement: A necessary link. *Journal of Nursing Care Quality, 11*(1), 22–28.

Aroskar, M. (1995). Envisioning nursing as a moral community. *Nursing Outlook, 43*(3), 134–138.

Blake, D.C. (1992). The hospital ethics committee: Health care's moral conscience or white elephant. *Hastings Center Report, 22*(1), 6–11.

Curtin, L.L. (1995). Creating an ethical organization. *Nursing Management, 26*(9), 96–101.

Edwards, B.J., & Haddad, A.H. (1988). Establishing a nursing bioethics committee. *Journal of Nursing Administration, 18*(3), 30–33.

Emanuel, E.J. (1995). Medical ethics in the era of managed care: The need for institutional structures instead of principles for individual cases. *The Journal of Clinical Ethics, 5*(4), 335–338.

Hayes, G.J. (1995). Ethics committees: Group process concerns and the need for research. *Cambridge Quarterly of Healthcare Ethics, 4*(11), 83–91.

Mariner, W.K. (1995). Business vs. medical ethics: Conflicting standards for managed care. *Journal of Law, Medicine & Ethics, 23,* 236–246.

Mitchell, K., Uehlinger, K.C., & Owen, J. (1996). The synergistic relationship between ethics and quality improvement: Thriving in managed care. *Journal of Nursing Care Quality, 11*(1), 9–21.

Mohr, W.K. (1996). Ethics, nursing, and health care in the age of "reform." *N&HC: Perspectives on Community, 17*(1), 16–21.

Morreim, E.H. (1985). Cost containment: Issues of moral conflict and justice for physicians. *Theoretical Medicine, 6,* 257–279.

Priester, R. (1989). *Rethinking medical morality: The ethical implications of changes in health care organization, delivery, and financing.* Minneapolis: The Center for Biomedical Ethics.

Reiser, S.J. (1994). The ethical life of health care organizations. *Hastings Center Report, 24*(6), 28–35.

Ross, J.W., Bayley, C., Sr., Michel, V., & Pugh D. (1986). *Handbook for hospital ethics committees.* Chicago: American Hospital Association.

Singer, P.A., Pellegrino, E.D., & Siegler, M. (1990). Ethics committees and consultants. *The Journal of Clinical Ethics, 1*(4), 263–267.

Sugarman, J. (1994). Should ethics committees do research? *The Journal of Clinical Ethics, 5*(2), 121–125.

Wolf, S.M. (1994). Health care reform and the future of physician ethics. *Hastings Center Report, 24*(2), 28–41.

## CHAPTER 12

Linking Quality Improvement, Outcome Research, and Program Evaluation

Anna Marie Lieske

CHAPTER OBJECTIVES

After completing this chapter, the reader will be able to

- discuss various evaluation models
- describe the similarities between evaluation and outcomes research
- apply clinical evaluation and research processes to patient care practice

The evaluation procedures used in quality management and the research process are analogous, but, simultaneously, quite distinct. Both activities are integral elements of the health care professional's role, as evidenced by the continuing interest and involvement of organizations in evaluating determinants of quality patient care. On an increasingly frequent basis, health care organizations are defining these determinants through the research process. Applying the rigors associated with the research process transforms data into information that may have more credibility not only among professionals, but also among consumers who use such information to make health care choices. The more frequent references in both the professional and lay literature to the "best" hospital or the "best" doctor (Boosalis et al., 1993) clearly analyze data to draw conclusions about the quality and cost of health care and providers. This chapter explores the similarities and differences between evaluation and research to assist the reader in better

understanding how to apply these processes and to appreciate the appropriate application of each.

QUALITY MANAGEMENT PROCESS

Although numerous authors have defined quality in health care, perhaps the classic and most widely accepted definition is that provided by Donabedian (1988): *Quality of care* is "the ability to achieve desirable objectives using legitimate means." Health care systems or programs are developed and implemented such that the quality of care can be evaluated on an ongoing basis.

The major components of an ongoing evaluation of health care are

specification of criteria and standards of performance criteria, collection of accurate information about the quality of current performance, comparison with information on desired or acceptable standards of performance, analysis of the reasons for the differences between actual performance and desired standards of performance and determination of what needs to be done to eliminate these differences, adoption of the changes necessary to eliminate the differences between current performance and desired standards of performance, repeated collection of information to monitor the extent to which resolution of differences is taking place, and periodic iterations of these linked steps. (Committee on Nursing Home Regulation, Institute of Medicine, 1986, p. 60)

Although the specific terminology used to describe the evaluation process may change with time, the essential components remain the same. For example, the Joint Commission on the Accreditation of Healthcare Organizations (Joint Commission) refined a 10-step process developed in the late 1980s to the "Cycle for Improving Performance" described in *Clinical Performance Data: A Guide to Interpretation* (O'Leary, 1996). In the Cycle for Improving Performance, the evaluation process is divided into five major steps: (1) design, (2) measure, (3) assess, (4) improve, and (5) redesign. There is a high degree of correlation between these components and those of the Institute of Medicine as previously mentioned.

A characteristic of quality management that distinguishes it as an evaluative process is its focus on the judgment of merit or value. Bellinger (1976) has pointed out that *evaluation* is "the general process of judging the worthwhileness of some activity regardless of the method employed. This element of judgment is certainly consistent with the general usage of the term and should obviously serve as a foundation for assessing whether an activity is indeed evaluative in nature" (p. 115). In essence, quality management is the process of evaluation applied to the health care system and, more specifically, to the provision of health care services by the professional health care worker.

In the health care setting, the process of evaluation is most typically used to determine the effectiveness, efficiency, and quality of programs designed for specific patient populations. A *program* is "any unified set of services providing order to accomplish a certain group of related goals" (Stevens, 1978, p. 228). The objectives of a program play a crucial role in

the evaluation process because assessment data are based on reformulated objectives. Examples of patient programs include a diabetic teaching series or a self-help support group. Stevens (1978) has indicated that "programs also may be designed to meet the needs of staff members, e.g., a management training program or a clinical staff development program" (p. 228).

The evaluation process can also be used to determine the quality of sets of activities that are not formalized into a "program." Evaluations of specific health care practices as well as patient care outcomes belong in this category. A variety of models can be applied to determine the effectiveness of the structure or process of health care practices or patient outcome. Historically, health care evaluation has emphasized the assessment of structure, probably because of the ease of appraising characteristics associated with this variable. The emphasis on the evaluation of structure, however, is giving way to more outcome-based evaluation, as evidenced by the development of the Joint Commission's Indicator Measurement System (IMS). The IMS is a performance-based outcome measurement process that focuses on continuous improvement through comparative data analysis. Examples of outcome indicators that compose the IMS are mortality rates, complication rates, and patients' responses to specific therapeutic interventions.

EVALUATION MODELS

Systems Model

The systems model of evaluation encompasses the entire social unit, which includes inputs, activities (or processing), and outputs. Application of this model involves analysis of the interrelationships among these components. This model can be diagrammatically represented as follows (Isaac & Michael, 1982):

$$\text{Input} \longrightarrow \text{Processing} \longrightarrow \text{Output}$$
$$\uparrow \underline{\hspace{2cm}} \text{Feedback} \underline{\hspace{3cm}}$$

The compilation of a comprehensive database regarding the social unit under examination is required by this model. The information base should consist of an inventory of pertinent inputs, activities, and outputs.

Inputs include all variables that affect the operation of the social unit. Shortell and Richardson (1978) have identified the following inputs:

- program objectives
- financial resources
- personnel resources
- staffing patterns
- program sponsorship
- program characteristics (e.g., length, size, hours of service)
- characteristics of program participants (e.g., attitudes, motivation)

The authors pointed out that it is helpful to formulate a comprehensive listing of inputs "to ensure that nothing has been overlooked" (p. 31). However, it is usually only necessary "to select those inputs that are most likely to be under the program's control" (p. 31) for detailed examination.

The processing or activities component of this model refers to the manipulation of the inputs in relation to the achievement of the program objectives or goals. This component includes variables such as actual use of the services, perceptions about the services, adherence to established standards or policies, and interactions between clients and providers.

Outputs are based on program objectives and provide information with which to determine the value and effectiveness of the program. Outputs include both intended and unintended consequences of the program, for example, the measurements of a client's health status and changes in organizational structure or services.

The systems model provides a sound approach for evaluating the three dimensions of quality management—structure, process, and outcome. Holzemer (1980) suggested that the "systems evaluation of the quality of care delivered thus permits not only examination of patient outcomes but also may be utilized to assess the effects of the setting in which care is delivered and the actual delivery itself on the quality of care" (p. 33).

Goal Attainment

Another model, the goal attainment model or objectives approach, consists of four steps: (1) identifying program objectives, (2) elaborating on criteria to be used for determining the level of success, (3) measuring the level of success attained, and (4) recommending actions to facilitate the functioning of the program (Bellinger, 1976, p. 115). Because of the exclusive emphasis of the model on objectives, it is crucial that the objectives be reasonable, specific, and measurable. In the evaluation process, the objectives will become the measures of the degree of program success. One of the evaluator's tasks is to identify the indicators that are accurate measures of the degree of attainment of the objectives.

An obstacle encountered when using this model is the multiplicity of objectives usually associated with a program. Objectives emanate not only from the program under evaluation but also from the organization within which the program operates. In addition to these objectives, subobjectives may exist for the program as well as the organization. A critical step in the evaluation process is to place in rank order the objectives according to their importance in relation to the intended outcome of the program. This step provides direction to and delineates the evaluation process to decrease its complexity.

A limitation of the goal attainment model is its primary focus on outcomes. The assumption underlying this model is that if the objectives are attained, the process by which they are achieved is assumed to be functional. The use of formative as well as summative evaluations can have an influential effect on the conclusions formulated solely based on outcome-objective assessments. Isaac and Michael (1982) have explained two types of formative evaluations that can broaden and strengthen the goal attainment model. The first, *implementation evaluation*, "seeks out discrepancies between the plan and reality; keeps the program true to its design or modifies it appropriately" (Isaac & Michael, 1982, p. 2). The second, *progress evaluation*, "monitors indicators of progress toward the objectives; and makes mid-course corrections, as appropriate," and can be conducted concurrently with the implementation evaluation (Isaac & Michael, 1982, p. 2). Another benefit to inclusion of formative evaluations in the objectives-based approach is a potential cost savings. If the objectives cannot realistically be achieved, the organization can modify the program before the final evaluation.

The Evaluation Research Society developed program evaluation standards for the various evaluation models. The standards consist of six components: (1) formulation and negotiation, (2) structure and design, (3) data collection and preparation, (4) data analysis and interpretation, (5) communication and disclosure, and (6) utilization (Rossi, 1982, p. 11).

Plan–Do–Check–Act

Evaluation models typically found in health care are variations of the examples just discussed and include the Plan–Do–Check–Act (PDCA) cycle, the FOCUS-PDCA, and the previously mentioned Cycle for Improving Performance. These quality improvement models are used by groups for continuous improvement.

The PDCA cycle, which is a variation of the input–processing–output model, is defined as follows:

- Plan: Determine how an issue or potential improvement will be studied (what data will be collected to answer a defined question).
- Do: Implement the plan on a small scale.
- Check: Check the data or information gathered to analyze the effect of the action under study.

- Act: Implement the action or improvement and continue the process for further improvement.

Figure 12–1 illustrates the PDCA cycle.

FOCUS, as outlined in *An Integrated Approach to Medical Staff Performance Improvement* (Joint Commission, 1996), means

> **F**ind a process for improvement
>
> **O**rganize a team that knows the process
>
> **C**larify current knowledge of the process
>
> **U**nderstand causes of process variation; and
>
> **S**elect the process improvement. (p. 13)

The focus procedure immediately precedes implementation of the PDCA cycle. Both the PDCA model and the FOCUS-PDCA are examples of the influence of quality improvement concepts on the evaluation process. Characteristics of quality improvement that have affected the evaluation process are

- inclusion of those affected or involved in the evaluation process
- emphasis on work groups and group evaluation activities

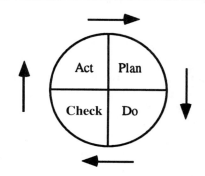

Figure 12–1 The PDCA cycle, developed by Walter Shewhart and widely taught by W. Edwards Deming, is useful in planning, testing, assessing, and implementing improvement actions.

- inclusion of tools such as fishbone diagrams, control charts, flowcharts, histograms, and Pareto charts to enhance an understanding of processes
- emphasis on continual change as compared with a snapshot or one-time assessment of a program or evaluation

THE RESEARCH PROCESS

Various authors have defined *research* slightly differently: "Systematic inquiry that uses orderly scientific methods to answer questions or solve problems" (Polit & Hungler, 1995, p. 621); "A systematic method for gaining new knowledge that can be verified and generalized beyond the sample studied" (Brink & Wood, 1978, p. 176); and "An activity whose purpose is to find a valid answer to some question that has been raised. The answers provide new knowledge to the world at large. It is a purposeful activity" (Abdellah & Levine, 1979, p. 703). Despite these variations, there are certain common elements. For one, research is characterized by the use of a scientific approach. Polit and Hungler (1995) defined the *scientific approach* as "a general set of orderly, disciplined procedures used to acquire dependable and useful information. The term research designates the application of this scientific approach" (p. 20). In addition, research is characterized by a systematic approach to the provision of new knowledge, which is used to expand or revise existing theories or develop original theories. Research is general in its focus; that is, its findings are not applicable to just one specific situation but to an extensive issue or problem.

Research has been categorized into two types: basic and applied. *Basic research* refers to the development of new knowledge for the purpose of formulating or refining theories. *Applied research* consists of the practical application of knowledge in everyday situations (Treece & Treece, 1982). Applied research may be confused with evaluation. However, despite similarities, they are distinct processes—evalu-

ation does not possess a scientific methodology, which is characteristic of both applied and basic research.

The research process consists of seven major steps and several substeps. Theory is an integral component of the research process. "Each of these stages is interrelated with theory in the sense that it is affected by it as well as affects it" (Nachmias & Nachmias, 1981, p. 22).

The first step in the research process is to select a topic and formulate this topic into a researchable question or problem. A substep involved in formulating a problem statement is to complete a comprehensive review of the literature, which provides an opportunity for the researcher to learn about previous studies on the topic and to develop a theoretical or conceptual framework. A theoretical framework provides an abstract structure for delineating the relationships between the variables under investigation.

Formulating a hypothesis is the second step in the research process. This step involves identifying the specific variables under investigation and formulating a statement that identifies the expected relationship between these variables. The hypothesis is more specific than the problem statement formulated in the first step. For example, the problem statement "Level of knowledge about diabetes is associated with adherence to a prescribed treatment regime" can be formulated into the hypothesis "Diabetic patients with higher levels of knowledge about diabetes exhibit significantly greater adherence to a prescribed treatment regime as compared with diabetic patients with lower levels of knowledge about diabetes." This hypothesis proposes the existence of a positive relationship between knowledge about diabetes and adherence to a prescribed treatment regime. The formulation of a hypothesis also involves the delineation of a study population and independent and dependent variables. The *independent variable*, also termed the experimental, treatment, or causal variable, is the variable manipulated by the researcher. In the example, level of knowledge, which is hypothesized to create greater adherence to a treatment regime, is the independent variable. The *dependent variable*, adherence to the treatment regime, is the variable the researcher hopes to explain or the variable on which manipulation of the independent variable exhibits its effect. Response variable or criterion variable are other terms for the dependent variable. "Problem statements represent the initial effort to give a research project direction; hypotheses represent a more formalized focus for the collection and interpretation of data" (Polit & Hungler, 1995, p. 43).

Selecting a research design, the third step in the research process, includes developing a planned approach to test the hypothesis. The following substeps compose selection of a research design:

1. Identify the approach (i.e., exploratory, descriptive, explanatory, historical, or experimental) to be used.
2. Identify the population and sample.
3. Select a specific method (e.g., survey, participant observation, projective tests, case study, or an experiment) for data collection.

The fourth step is to conduct a pilot study. The purpose of the pilot study is to identify weaknesses in the measurement tools and in the design itself. The pilot study provides the researcher with an opportunity to refine the study before its actual implementation to minimize the effects of unforeseen problems.

After necessary revisions are completed, the researcher begins data collection, the fifth step in the research process. The researcher collects information according to the predetermined plan. Adherence to the study design minimizes the potential for errors in this phase of the research process. Data collection involves gathering information from a sample that represents the total population under examination. Two methods for determining the sample are probability and nonprobability sampling. *Probability sampling*, which is most frequently associated with the research process, involves the random selection of a sample. *Random sampling* implies that every unit of a population has an equal chance of being selected as part of the sample. *Nonprobability sampling*, which is used both in the research and evaluation processes, does not ensure selection based on chance; therefore, it does not result in the degree of representativeness of the population as does probability sampling.

The sixth step, data analysis, involves a number of preliminary steps before the researcher can actually test the hypothesis. The researcher must initially categorize the data to facilitate statistical analysis. After scrutinizing the categorical data, he or she may put the data into tabular format to visually aid narrative explanations. The application of descriptive and inferential statistics may be necessary to further describe the data and clarify extant relationships.

One of the most important aspects of the research process involves interpreting the research findings. "By interpretation, we refer to the process of making sense of the results and of examining the implications of the findings within a broader context" (Polit & Hungler, 1995, p. 51). In addition to interpreting the results, the researcher must also formulate conclusions regarding their application to the hypothesis. The researcher then must generalize the results to other applicable situations.

The final step of the research process is to formulate recommendations for further study. The recommendations provide direction for future studies that may be designed to gain greater insight into the topic under investigation. The formulation of recommendations supports the cyclical nature of the research process. As Nachmias and Nachmias (1981) have pointed out, "The generalization ending one cycle is the beginning of the next cycle. This cyclic process continues indefinitely, reflecting the progress of a scientific discipline" (p. 23).

Communicating research findings facilitates the research process by fostering further investigations and advancing the scientific base of a discipline. Research findings may be communicated through presentations, reports, or journal articles. The most important aspect of this phase of research is not so much the vehicle for communication but the sharing of research findings with the appropriate audience.

DISTINGUISHING CHARACTERISTICS OF EVALUATION AND RESEARCH

The similarities in the evaluation and research processes include their value in improving health care, their systematic processes, and their need for support and resources to accomplish stated goals (Peters & Pearlson, 1989). The differences between evaluation and research include the goals of each. The primary intent of evaluation is to provide feedback about a product or service, whereas research is chiefly concerned with the generation of new knowledge for the purpose of developing or refining relevant theories. Evaluation is based on objectives and outcomes, whereas research is grounded in a theoretical framework. Despite these differences, evaluation and research both use a systematic approach to achieve their purposes. The principal difference between the two processes lies in their purposes. In distinguishing between evaluation and research, Stufflebeam (cited in Isaac & Michael, 1982) observed that the "purpose of evaluation is to improve, not prove" (p. 2). As this statement aptly indicates, evaluation involves the use of judgment, whereas research is based on the scientific method.

The outcomes of evaluation and research are distinct. The outcome of evaluation is the application of the decision-making process to effect changes in a specific program. The results and conclusions of the evaluation process are applicable only to the social unit assessed by the evaluator. In contrast to the specificity of the results obtained through evaluation, the findings of research are generalizable to comparable situations. The degree to which research results can be generalized depends on characteristics of the sample and the environment of the study. The extent of similarity between the sample and the target population determines the generalizability of the research findings. Factors present in the environment during the study may influence the results and, consequently, limit the degree of generalizability. The Hawthorne effect, one such factor, occurs when participants in a study change their behavior simply because they are aware of their involvement in a study. In such a case, the study results are applicable only to the research setting and cannot be generalized to other settings or situations.

Value plays a unique role in these two processes. The evaluation process totally embraces the concept of value in all phases. Indeed, the term *evaluation* is a derivative of *value*. Donabedian (1990) defined *quality* as "making a judgment on the goodness of healthcare" (p. 117) based on structure, process, and outcome variables. However, the role of value in research is limited solely to the selection of a topic for investigation. The researcher usually selects an investigation topic based on his or her interests, which are ultimately founded on personal values. The credibility of research can be jeopardized if the researcher allows values or feelings to interfere with the objective data collection and analysis.

The selection of a study topic in the evaluation process is predicated on the desires of individuals involved with a specific program. These desires result in the specification of a topic with accompanying objectives. The evaluator who may not have a voice in determining the topic of study must consider political influences that affect not only the program being studied, but also the evaluation process. Administrators, program participants (clients and employees), political figures, and constituents may have vested interests in the outcome of the evaluation. In comparison, the researcher is not limited to any topic. Rather, the researcher is totally responsible for identifying a subject based on, perhaps, interest or curiosity. Consequently, political influences should be nonexistent in research. Political influences in research are completely unacceptable because of their potentially detrimental impact on the scientific method of inquiry, which is based on the researcher's total objectivity.

Topic selection also determines the recipients of the final report. Evaluation reports are usually submitted to people internal to the organization and designated others. An evaluation report usually contains conclusions about the value of a program as well as recommendations for changes. It may even include a specific plan for the implementation of those recommendations. In contrast, research reports are communicated to members of the scientific community as well as the general public and can be general in scope. In addition to other components, the research report contains a discussion of the findings, theoretical and practical interpretations of the findings, conclusions, and recommendations for further study.

Although both processes use a systematic approach to achieve their purposes, distinctions exist in the specific methodologies used in evaluation and research. Evaluation methodology is based on the determination of the achievement of specific objectives. The research methodology is concerned with the testing of hypotheses to explain the relationships between variables. Consequently, the approaches used are different. Evaluation includes the collection of information based on the objectives, with little, if any, control of extraneous variables. The use of randomization is desirable, but not essential. Thus, replication of the evaluation findings is less likely. In contrast, the control of variables and the use of sampling techniques in the research process yields highly replicable results. Both methodologies may be similar in the use of descriptive and inferential statistics and scientific principles.

INTEGRATION OF EVALUATION AND RESEARCH

A theoretical integration of the evaluation and research processes has occurred in the establishment of the evaluation research discipline, which is a form of applied research. In evaluation research, the principles of research (i.e., the scientific method) are applied to the evaluation process. The purpose of evaluation research "is to measure the effects of a program against the goals it set out to accomplish as a means of contributing to subsequent decision-making about the program and improving future programming" (Weiss, 1972, p. 4). Weiss pointed out that "to measure the effects" refers to use of the research methodology in conjunction with evaluation. The definitional focus on future programming is consistent with both the research purpose of expansion of knowledge and the "social purpose of evaluation" (Weiss, 1972, pp. 4–5).

Figure 12–2 illustrates the theoretical domains of research and evaluation research. Each is a distinct discipline; however, overlapping functions and concepts exist in the area of evaluation research. In reality, the distinctions between the disciplines of evaluation and research are not quite as vivid as portrayed in Figure 12–2. This definitional dilemma was addressed by Norma Lang (1982): "Although the development of standardized instruments for use in quality assurance and selected controlled studies should be viewed as relevant research activity, quality assurance activities are not generally perceived as rigid, highly controlled studies. Rather, these activities are part of routine organizational and professional functions" (p. 2).

An example of how evaluation and research are integrated can be found in a recent article by O'Conner and others (1996). They reported that, in a multisite effort to improve coronary artery bypass graft outcomes, quality improvement techniques such as feedback of outcome data and training in continuous improvement techniques were used to achieve significant decreases in mortality rates. Exhibit 12–1 lists the interventions used to improve the mortality rates among participating hospitals. Clearly, these interventions are consistent with quality improvement activities. Yet, at the same time, research techniques such as development of a

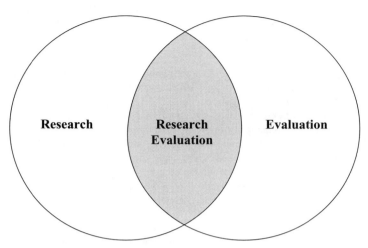

Figure 12–2 Research and evaluation domains

multivariate logistic regression model, comprehensive data collection, and the clear delineation of pretest and post-test measures were used to enhance the sophistication of the study. This example suggests that

- evaluation and research techniques can be used together in harmony
- the demarcation between evaluation and research (particularly applied research) is not always clear
- the application of techniques, typically used in research, to assess health care is more in demand because of the need to better measure outcomes

From a purely academic perspective, the characteristics of evaluation and research require distinction to appreciate the body of knowledge that helps to form each field of study. From an application standpoint, the nuances of each are important to understand how to effectively and accurately use the concepts. As the demand for well-grounded outcome data increases, research techniques will be used more frequently to evaluate health care practices. As this trend continues, the products of organizations such as the Agency for Health Care Policy and Research will continue to gain importance.

Exhibit 12–1 Reported Changes in Processes of Coronary Artery Bypass Graft Surgery Attributed to the Site Visit Program

Changes in the technical aspects of patient care
- Standardized postoperative management and implemented an extubation protocol
- Changed perfusion techniques such as reducing flows rather than turning off the pump when inducing hypotension before aortic clamping
- Decreased the number of preoperative coagulation tests
- Changed the type of prophylactic antibiotics to a less broad-spectrum version
- Changed myocardial preservation techniques; in general, there were increases in the use of warm cardioplegia and retrograde delivery of cardioplegic solutions

Changes in the processes and organization of inhospital care
- Developed and applied a standard set of postoperative care protocols and transfer orders
- Set up a critical pathway system with case managers on the patient care units
- Initiated a same-day admissions program
- Created multidisciplinary work groups to reexamine current clinical processes, such as preoperative screening, patient education, and postoperative transfer and discharge criteria
- Redesigned an existing operating room to accommodate a cardiopulmonary bypass pump to provide more timely care for patients requiring emergency cardiac surgery
- Changed the location of the cardiopulmonary bypass pump in the operating room and the position of the first assistant to increase ease of communication

Changes in personnel organization and training
- Changed to a dedicated operating room staff for the cardiac surgery program
- Hired a surgeon as a permanent first assistant
- Switched to the use of a one-perfusionist (rather than two) system and the use of checklists by the perfusionists
- Implemented a system for the cross-training of support staff to decrease problems with the transfer of patients from the postanesthesia recovery room to the intensive care unit

Changes in the methods of evaluating care and in making treatment decisions
- Implemented an enhanced internal review of all deaths, including detailed medical record review, assessment of cause of death, and discussion of patient care aspects by cardiologists, cardiac surgeons, nurses, perfusionists, and anesthesiologists
- Changed the time and organization of the cardiac catheterization conference to increase participation by cardiology and cardiac surgery staff
- Implemented a system to assess surgeon-to-surgeon variability in the use of resources

Source: Reprinted with permission from Journal of the American Medical Association, Vol. 275, No. 11, p. 845, Copyright 1996, American Medical Association.

REFERENCES

Abdellah, F.G., & Levine, E. (1979). *Better patient care through nursing research.* New York: Macmillan.

Bellinger, A. (1976). An examination of some issues pertinent to evaluation research and the assessment of health care quality. In *Issues in evaluation research.* Kansas City, MO: American Nurses' Association.

Boosalis, M. et al. (1993, January/February). Tracking "the best" hospitals. *Healthcare Forum Journal,* 53–57.

Brink, P., & Wood, M.J. (1978). *Basic steps in planning - nursing research.* North Scituate, MA: Duxbury Press.

Committee on Nursing Home Regulation, Institute of Medicine. (1986). *Improving the quality of care in nursing homes.* Washington, DC: National Academy Press.

Donabedian, A. (1988). Quality assessment and assurance: Unity of purpose, diversity of means. *Inquiry, 25*(1), 173–192.

Donabedian, A. (1990). Contributions of epidemiology to quality assessment & monitoring. *Infection Control & Hospital Epidemiology, 2*(3), 117–121.

Holzemer, W.L. (1980, March). Research and evaluation: An overview. *Quality Review Bulletin, 33.*

Isaac, S., & Michael, W.B. (1982). *Handbook in research evaluation.* San Diego: EDITS.

Joint Commission on Accreditation of Healthcare Organizations. (1996). *An integrated approach to medical staff performance improvement.* Oakbrook Terrace, IL: Author.

Lang, N.M. (1982, Spring). Introduction: Trends and issues in nursing quality assurance. In Nursing review: Criteria for evaluation and analysis of patient care. *Quality Review Bulletin, 2.*

Nachmias, D., & Nachmias, C. (1981). *Research methods in the social sciences.* New York: St. Martin's Press.

Nugent, W. (1996). Improving outcomes and reducing costs in cardiac surgery. *Quality Connection, 5*(2), 6–7.

O'Conner, G.T. (1996). A regional intervention to improve the hospital mortality associated with coronary artery bypass graft surgery. *Journal of the American Medical Association, 275*(11), 841–846.

O'Leary, M. (1996). *Clinical performance data: A guide to interpretation.* Oakbrook Terrace, IL: Joint Commission on Accreditation of Healthcare Organizations.

Peters, D.A., & Pearlson, J. (1989). Clinical evaluation: Research or quality assurance? *Journal of Nursing Quality Assurance, 3*(3), 1–6.

Polit, D., & Hungler, B. (1995). *Nursing research.* Philadelphia: Lippincott-Raven.

Rossi, P. (Ed.). (1982). Evaluation research society standards for program evaluation. *Standards for Evaluation Practice, 15,* 11.

Shortell, S.M., & Richardson, W.C. (1978). *Health program evaluation.* St. Louis, MO: C.V. Mosby.

Stevens, B.J. (1978). Program evaluation. In A.G. Rezler & B.J. Stevens (Eds.), *The nurse evaluator in education and service.* New York: McGraw-Hill.

Treece, W.T., & Treece, J.W. (1982). *Elements of research in nursing.* St. Louis, MO: C.V. Mosby.

## CHAPTER 13

Basic Tools for a Quality Improvement–Based Approach to Information System Selection and Implementation

Roy L. Simpson

CHAPTER OBJECTIVES

After completing this chapter, the reader will be able to:

- understand an organization's technological environment by conducting an inventory of various systems available in the organization
- detail useful guidelines necessary for understanding the process of selecting and managing technology for improving quality
- create a Quality Improvement Business Plan for an organization investing in technology

Entire books could be, and have been, written describing the endless variety of information systems available to health care providers. Meanwhile, the pace of technology continues to accelerate; today's hot technology trend may be tomorrow's tired news. How, then, can the concerned health care provider apply quality improvement (QI) principles to technology management? The answer lies not in dissecting the many different kinds of technology, but in understanding the *process* of selecting and managing that technology, no matter if it is a tried-and-true transaction system or a cutting-edge point-of-care bedside solution.

This chapter focuses on helping the health care provider make better information system planning, evaluation, and purchasing decisions. It details practical and pragmatic guidelines for action but steers away from theoretical discourse. After all, selection of the wrong kind of system or poor implementation of the right kind of system can subvert even the most carefully orchestrated QI program.

OVERVIEW: HOW TECHNOLOGY ENHANCES QI

QI programs work best when there are successful interrelationships among technology, strategy, and the organization. When all three are integrated, technology can enhance QI by supporting management behaviors such as

- Giving priority attention to patients and patient care: Beyond clinical systems that can assist clinicians with critical pathways and care protocols, information technology can also provide both microanalyses and macroanalyses of data on service satisfaction. Executives can use decision support systems or executive information systems to produce and interpret data to determine whether the organization is meeting its customers' requirements.
- Empowering rather than controlling staffs: In a QI environment, the manager's goal should be to find and correct problems in

the work process or environment, and not necessarily to continually check on the performances of individual staff members. For example, technology can help with tracking technology to improve supply management, staffing, and scheduling software to enhance floor performance, clinical information systems to implement patient-focused care, and so on.

- Identifying areas for improvement: Information technology systems can help QI managers spot problems or variances from standards more quickly and more accurately. For example, a critical path system can help the QI manager understand the particular problems associated with delivering a particular type of care.
- Containing costs: Technology captures and reports data, which is central to identifying areas where resources are being overconsumed or underconsumed. QI managers can take advantage of charge capture systems, quality assurance systems, decision support systems, and executive information systems to help them assess the cost of quality (and how costs can be contained without sacrificing quality).
- Benchmarking performance: Information technology can be used to benchmark both clinical and financial performances within the organization and across institutions.

IN THE BEGINNING: TAKING A BENEFITS-ORIENTED APPROACH

One of the biggest mistakes a health care manager can make is to buy a system without first thoroughly assessing current work flows and work processes. Yet, many departmental managers in particular continue to make this mistake. The following is a typical example of how a departmental or ancillary health care information system is selected and implemented: A system is purchased based on what features the department managers want and what costs are involved. Then the managers look at how the new system would fit into their current operations. They take some baseline measurements of efficiency and quality performance, identifying the benefits they think they can achieve with the system. They implement the system and then go back 6 or 8 months later for another benefit study to see if they have achieved any benefits.

There are significant problems with this approach, namely that work flows and work processes were only reviewed *after* the system was purchased. The best approach is to study processes and work flows significantly before even examining technology systems. Identify and state clearly what specific benefits are desired before approaching the Management Information System (MIS) manager or vendor. For example, a clearly stated benefit may be to "have x type of diagnostic test results reported at the nursing station within y hours of the test." Higher level benefits must also be stated clearly, for example, "nursing satisfaction (retention) improved by x percent, decreased lengths of stay, and reduced errors of omission." With a benefits management approach, QI managers look at how they are doing business today and assess the potential for change, which can vary greatly by institution.

For example, a QI manager at a community hospital with a large body of powerful voluntary physicians who exhibit little interest in automation would have little luck introducing a physician order entry system, no matter how persuasively or powerfully the manager could state the benefits. The potential for change in that kind of environment is limited. However, in an academic medical center, a QI manager could indeed push through a physician order entry system because the physician audience is captive and eager to comply. With this approach, before a request for proposal (RFP) is ever sent to a vendor or consultant, QI managers must spend the time to articulate operational weaknesses and opportunities and identify the benefits they want to achieve. Then, the system is selected to fit that vision rather than the other way around. Continuous benefits assessments should be integrated into all QI technology plans as an additional way to measure quality and performance. The emphasis here is on *continuous;* benefits, outcomes, and improvements should be continually reassessed; a benefits assessment is not a one-time approach.

QI managers should examine improvements and benefits derived from the system in relation to improvements to quality of care; savings in costs; improvements in productivity; and improvements in professionalism, recruitment, and retention. Although examining cost reductions or full-time equivalent savings is a significant way to assess benefits realized from the technology investment, it is also important to look at patient outcomes as a key part of benefits assessment. After all, in medical practice, for example, physicians will invest in a new computerized tomography (CT) scanner not because of the cost savings it represents (it usually does not represent any), but because of the improvements it can make to patient care. Because of the complex nature of realistic ben-

efits assessment, it is often advisable to work with a consultant who specializes in this area.

UNDERSTANDING THE EXISTING ENVIRONMENT: TAKING A SYSTEMS INVENTORY

Before QI managers can determine what type of system can help achieve the benefits desired, they must understand the kind of system they *can* have based on the commitments the organization has already made. For example, if a QI manager wants to purchase a multitasking, multiuser system but the institution has committed itself to maintaining mainframe operations for the next 5 years, then the manager will have to find a way to work within the current plans and limitations of the organization.

To begin, the QI manager must take a thorough inventory to find out what system is in place in the organization, what its limitations are, and into what direction it could lead. Ask the MIS department manager the questions found on the questionnaire in Exhibit 13–1.

Exhibit 13–1 Systems Inventory Questionnaire

1. What kind of systems are used in the following departments? Please either check appropriate circle or write in pertinent information.

Department	Personal Computer	Mainframe	Mini-computer	Workstation	Stand-alone	Networked	Integrated	User Capacity
Nursing	☐	☐	☐	☐	☐	☐	☐	☐
Radiology	☐	☐	☐	☐	☐	☐	☐	☐
Laboratory	☐	☐	☐	☐	☐	☐	☐	☐
Pharmacy	☐	☐	☐	☐	☐	☐	☐	☐
Dietary	☐	☐	☐	☐	☐	☐	☐	☐
Rehabilitation	☐	☐	☐	☐	☐	☐	☐	☐
Medical Records	☐	☐	☐	☐	☐	☐	☐	☐
Finance	☐	☐	☐	☐	☐	☐	☐	☐
Other	☐	☐	☐	☐	☐	☐	☐	☐

Other Pertinent Information_____

continues

Exhibit 13–1 continued

2. What is the architecture of your existing organization's information system (or series of systems)?

	Yes	No	Comments
• *Open?* (*Open* refers to the ability of the system to accept information from other internal and external systems, regardless of format.)	____	____	
• *Closed?* (Closed systems typically cannot accept data outside the limits of the system without using complicated and sometimes costly interface programs.)	____	____	
• *Proprietary?* (*Proprietary* means that it was uniquely built for your organization—it is not universally standard. Proprietary systems can offer greater features but can also create problems when there is a need to exchange information with other systems.)	____	____	

3. What kind of operating system is in use in the majority of the systems with which the system in question must link? Check all that apply and designate in which departments they predominate.

Operating System	*Departments*
☐ MS-DOS	_____
☐ MS-DOS with local area network (LAN) or wide area network (WAN)	_____
☐ Windows 95	_____
☐ OS2	_____
☐ UNIX	_____
☐ AIX	_____
☐ AS/400	_____
☐ DEC VAX	_____
☐ MVS/ESA (mainframe)	_____
☐ Others_____	_____
_____	_____

4. Who "owns" the source code (the programming code and its maintenance) for the majority of your hospital information system?

Source Code
☐   The vendor (monthly maintenance fee: $_____)
☐   Your MIS department (number of full-time equivalents required annually: _____)

ASSESSING SYSTEM BENEFITS

Once the QI manager conducts a thorough inventory of the current environment, he or she must evaluate or assess each system for its potential for meeting overall QI goals for the department in question. For example, if nursing processes are the focus for QIs, then the QI manager needs to interview each department head to determine how the department head's specific ancillary system interacts with nursing processes, how it interfaces with the nursing information system, and how it could benefit nursing if its potential was maximized. If individual meetings with department heads are not an option, a meeting with the specific vendors in question is a good alternative. Have the vendor (or vendors) specifically address the question, How can this system benefit nursing (or other departments in question) to improve patient care? Record the responses in Exhibit 13–2. A great deal of research time may be saved by going to the vendor.

By obtaining an understanding of how each departmental system works together to improve quality in a specific area, the QI manager is better able to get a holistic view of information system interaction. More important, the QI manager can get a clear sense of how each system *could* benefit a particular area of operation, expanding his or her horizons for managing the process.

UNDERSTANDING THE STRATEGIC PLAN OF THE INSTITUTION

Before investing time, energy, or money into any technology decision, QI managers must clearly understand the strategic plan of the larger institution. This understanding must encompass not only QI goals, but technology and future service directions and their overall effect on the organization.

In addition, there must be a strategic plan for the department in question. For example, if nursing is the focus, then it is advisable for nursing to also have a strategic plan that dovetails into the institutional plan. The QI manager should have access to all plans. To this end, the QI manager should ask the questions found in Exhibit 13–3.

CREATING A QI BUSINESS PLAN FOR THE TECHNOLOGY INVESTMENT

Should there be a QI business plan related to the purchase of technology? If the stakes are high (and they almost always are when an organization's information system is in question), then the answer is clearly *yes*. A business plan

Exhibit 13–2 Assessing System Benefits To Improve Patient Care

System/Department	How It **Benefits** Patient Care	How It **Could Benefit** Patient Care
Nursing		
Radiology		
Laboratory		
Pharmacy		
Nutrition		
Respiratory Therapy		
Physical Therapy		
Medical Records		
Finance		
Satellite Centers		

Exhibit 13–3 Examining the Strategic Plan

- Does the institution have a strategic plan? _____ If not, why not? _____
  Does the QI manager have a copy? _____ If not, why not? _____
- What is the mission of the organization? _____
- What are the long-range financial plans of the organization? _____
- What are its long-range product plans? _____
- What role will technology play in helping the organization achieve its goals and mission? _____
- Does the institution have a clearly stated goal or mission for quality improvements? How will achievement of those goals be determined? _____
- Does the organization have specific building plans? _____ Is it planning remote sites (or additional remote sites)? _____
- Does the organization have a

	Yes	No
Technology strategic vision?	_____	_____
What is it? _____		
Organization-wide system?	_____	_____
Why? _____		
Integrated system?	_____	_____
Why? _____		
Nonintegrated system?	_____	_____
Why? _____		
Proprietary solution versus vendor solution?	_____	_____
Why? _____		
Vendor solution?	_____	_____
Why? _____		

related to the technology investment in question helps clarify objectives, identify and articulate what is required in a system, prioritize the most important requirements, and "sell" the QI message to board members and other selection committee members. Most importantly, a business plan helps guide the selection to ensure a viable, cost-effective system that will meet the goals of QI.

Johnson's (1988) *The Nurse Executive's Business Plan Manual* is an excellent guide to creating a strategic plan. Although the manual is directed at helping nurse executives write

plans for creating new health care or nursing enterprises, many of the suggestions can be incorporated into a business plan for a specific technology investment. According to Johnson, a general outline should typically include the following components:

- Preliminaries
  1. Title page
  2. Contents
- Executive summary: The focus here is to encapsulate and "sell" the overall idea or vision of the proposed system. Emphasize

all the benefits and positive outcomes that are likely to be obtained if the hospital makes this particular investment. Potential challenges should also be articulated.

1. Purpose of plan: The overall objective should be addressed here. This section must clearly answer the question, Why should the institution make this investment?

2. Goals and strategies: Goals must be specific and quantifiable. It is not enough to say, for example, "The system will improve nursing productivity." Instead, set specific goals such as number of full-time equivalents, percentage of reduction of physician complaints, shortened lengths of stay, and so forth. Strategies must also be outlined in specific ways. What type of system is favored and why? What kind of support will be required and why?

3. Recommendations: Summarize the kind of system envisioned in use. Here is where the homework really pays off—one can be sure that recommendations for integration, bedside care, or any other advanced type of solution is solidly grounded in what the institution can afford and support within its current operating environment.

4. Conclusion: Summarize the overall proposition. Recap the problem and solution and how the type of system recommended will help achieve stated goals and also how it will dovetail with the larger strategic vision and plan of the institution.

- Introduction
  1. Statement of purpose: Articulate the exact purpose of the specific information system in question. What will it do for clinicians? Patients? Quality improvements? The organization as a whole?

  2. Mission definition: Define the mission for this particular technology investment or project. Be sure that it is consistent with the greater mission of the organization. For example, if the mission of the organization is to narrow its focus in for-profit areas, a system designed to improve the efficiency of services delivered to indigent patients is obviously misaligned.

- Environmental assessment
  1. Current environment: See the section *Assessing System Benefits* for guidelines. That section summarizes the kinds of systems the organization has already invested in, what their limitations are, and how they would "work and interact" with the type of system proposed.

  2. Competitor analysis: If possible, identify what kind of technology the competition is using and how this will affect the ability of the institution to meet its stated objectives and its ability to compete effectively in the marketplace.

- Operational and implementation plan
  1. Objectives: Review the overall objectives of the business or technology plan. Identify basic time lines as well as short- and long-term objectives. Include how staffing and facility resources would be used, changed, or consumed.

  2. Test sites: Identify where early implementations would occur. Identify those areas in which departments would be initially affected, and explain why they would be affected.

  3. Equipment needs: Identify and list the capital equipment required for the system—everything from additional telephones and telephone lines to the software peripheral devices required, such as printers, modems, or terminals.

  4. Staffing: Identify how the system will affect staffing during the early, middle, and late implementation stages. Identify the key players involved, such as systems manager, physician liaison, trainer, or support staff.

5. Time schedules: Include a time line with actual projected dates of when events would occur, from final selection to full implementation.
6. Costs: Identify and cost-out everything that you *imagine* might be incurred, including everything from the actual cost of the system to the added phone bills for the new lines. Include additional office furniture, additional staff, off-site and on-site training, and so on.
7. Evaluation and control: Establish how quality will be maintained before, during, and after transition as well as how you will evaluate whether goals are being met.
- Financial plan and schedules
To establish an adequate return on investment, identify the following:
1. staffing budget
2. expense budget
3. capital expenditures
4. miscellaneous expenditures, including additional training and support, if necessary

SELECTING AND PURCHASING TECHNOLOGY

Technology is growing so sophisticated so quickly; it seems as if just as one system gets implemented, it is replaced by yet another more "advanced" solution. Avoiding obsolescence is not easy in today's environment. Yet QI managers can protect their investments in technology. The key is doing their homework—studying current work flows and work processes and how they can be improved, understanding the current technology operating environment and how it will be affected, and reviewing the strategic vision for the entire technology project as a whole. The following are basic guidelines for selection.

Understand the current operating environment. QI managers should use the systems inventory questionnaire (see Exhibit 13–1) as a place to begin to grasp the technological environment in which the institution operates. They should demand that work flows and work processes be studied and chartered rigorously *before* the process of technology review gets seriously underway. QI managers should never discuss how technology could "change" operations until everybody involved understands how things are operating *now* and the benefits and disadvantages of each process.

Know the technology budget of the institution. It is best that QI managers understand budgetary limitations up front. Many a frustration can be avoided by looking squarely at not only the true commitment of the institution to technology (its "walk" rather than its "talk"), but at what can reasonably be afforded *today* as well as what could benefit the organization in the future. It is important to remember financial limits because it is easy to get seduced or distracted by exciting technology breakthroughs that are way beyond the current budgets of many institutions. Ignoring opportunities or capability to "add on" in the future may stifle the organization's future growth.

Be sure that there is adequate representation of frontline clinicians on the selection committee. Too often, a selection committee will be heavily represented by financial or administrative personnel, and too little by clinical staff. From the nursing point of view, the ideal representative is the clinical nurse specialist. If a patient care system is being reviewed, then it makes sense to have adequate representation from those personnel whose primary job is the day-to-day care of patients. Physician involvement is also important. Without physician involvement, even the most advanced and exciting health care information system will not meet its full potential.

Get and stay involved at the strategic planning level. QI managers should understand the strategic business plan of the institution and how and where QI fits in. Major technology decisions are made at the strategic planning level. By keeping a QI focus at every level of planning in the organization, it is easier to control the outcome.

Set specific objectives for process improvements. QI managers should chart all work flows that will be affected by the new technology and find out where the productivity gaps are. Furthermore, they should discover what clinicians do not like about existing technology. Managers should then set specific goals for process improvements by way of technology, for example, "The system should report x diagnostic test results at the nursing station within y minutes or hours of the test."

Understand the Request for Proposal (RFP). The RFP is a standard document that serves as a means to assess and compare how different vendors or consultants stack up to clearly identified goals, requirements, and standards. The RFP should

- introduce the vendor to the overall environment in the institution as well as the environment in which the system will be used
- identify general requirements for information to be supplied
- describe any performance bond or equivalent requirement
- state conditions of an equipment demonstration
- outline the method of financing
- specify training and orientation for the products
- cite evaluation criteria for evaluating proposals
- state the standards of performance that will be used in deciding system acceptability
- state specific hardware and software requirements

Use weighted values in the RFP. When ranking the needs and requirements in the RFP, QI managers should use weighted values and proper term definitions to identify general requirements. They must never assume that the vendors in question have an advanced understanding of clinical terms or of QI requirements (even if they claim otherwise). The use of weighted values, although imperfect, at least informs the vendor of the relative ranking of each requirement.

Demand veto power for the clinical representatives. Financial and administrative executives typically enjoy veto power, which is why there is such a preponderance of strong financial and administrative systems in most institutions. If clinical executives and representatives retain the right to say no if the system does not meet clinical requirements, the institution will save itself a great deal of frustration and lost expense later.

Determine how a system will affect staffs in terms of training and education. It is easy to underestimate the impact of a process change involving technology. The human resource time and effort—and, therefore, cost—that goes into a new system or system change can be astronomical, particularly if it was not anticipated or managed carefully. It is better to anticipate the time and effort up front than have to scramble to find the funds or the resources later.

Understand the fine print. QI managers must not abdicate contract negotiations to the MIS department. Rather, they should clarify issues such as warranties, intellectual property, maintenance agreements, maintenance fees and obligation, and upgrade management. Managers should obtain assistance from an objective consultant, if necessary.

ENSURING SUCCESS: MANAGING CULTURE CHANGES

Resistance to change can be one of the biggest stumbling blocks in the implementation of a new system. Even if a new system or process is undoubtedly a more effective way of operating, if it is not accepted by end-users, then it is doomed to mediocrity or outright failure. The bitter truth about information technology (not necessarily health care technology) is that 80% to 90% of business-critical systems projects fail. Studies have suggested that the problem is not necessarily technological—it is also social and behavioral. It is not just the systems that cause the problems, but it is also the people *using* the systems who are responsible for a large majority of the failures.

System sabotage can show up in the following subtle and not-so-subtle ways:

- Oral defamation: Degrading comments, jokes, and outright slander can diminish the success of a project before it even has a chance to work.
- Alleged inability to operate the system: Some end-users, despite hours of training, may show their displeasure at a perceived disruption by simply not doing things correctly.
- Data sabotage: It is rare, but it does happen. Some end-users may be so angry at the change in operations that they will outright sabotage data to make the new system look bad in the hope that things will go back to the "old ways" soon.
- End-users may refuse outright to use the system.

Fortunately, much can be done to avoid natural resistance to change or outright sabotage. QI managers must understand the reasons for resistance. Often resistance to change may mask deeper problems in the organization, related to morale or motivation. Resistance to a new technology change is often related to a fear of job loss. QI managers must be sensitive to the end-users' real fears that they will be replaced by computers.

Solicit "buy-ins" early in the process. QI managers must always include key individuals and constituencies (at different levels of the organization) early in the process. People are less likely to resist change if they feel a part of the process.

Audit current work flows. It is imperative not to automate inefficient work flows. Just because a process worked well under a manual system doesn't mean it should continue that

way under an automated system. Work flow reengineering is key—this is where frontline people should be involved most heavily. Most individuals, if given the chance, would love to have a voice in fixing inefficient or personally aggravating work flows that impede their own job performance. QI managers should involve key individuals in the work flow audits.

Assign change agents. Any new technology change should have a change "sponsor"—a high-level executive who understands the overall objectives, goals, and missions of an institution and can effectively articulate them to employees down the line. As important as the change sponsor is the "change agent"—a frontline individual who is charged with facilitating the introduction of new technology from the end-user's point of view. The change agent should be charged with

- "shadowing" nurses and other staff clinicians to determine actual information needs and likely usage of planned systems
- participating in system design to fit the system organizational structure, culture, and behavior
- facilitating user participation in the design activity to improve the system and acquire user buy-in
- assessing current work processes and creating new ones
- Planning the implementation and rollout, including education and training
- observing the new system in use and making changes

Based on these requirements, it is clear that change agents must be included in all aspects of the project from the very beginning—from work flow audits to implementation to observation during regular usage.

CONCLUSION

Choosing a QI-oriented health care organization information system obviously has tremendous ramifications for everyone providing patient care. The QI manager should understand that the process of evaluating, reviewing, selecting, and implementing a new system is complex and time-consuming (sometimes taking as long as 2 years). However, if enough time and care are spent in "doing one's homework" before an RFP is ever sent out—*before* the requirements of a system are even articulated—a great deal of time, frustration, and money can be saved.

REFERENCE

Johnson, J.E. (1988). *The nurse executive's business plan manual.* Gaithersburg, MD: Aspen Publishers, Inc.

Managing Quality through Outcome-Based Practice: CareMaps,® Case Management, and Variance Analysis

Maria Hill

CHAPTER OBJECTIVES

After completing this chapter, the reader will be able to

- describe the development of a variance management system
- discuss the development of CareMaps® and Case Management systems as collaborative strategies for achieving positive patient outcomes
- describe clinical concurrent and retrospective uses of variance for continually improving patient care

In the health care industry, *quality* is defined as the degree of excellence in care provision. Although many concepts and strategies are used to shape and determine quality care, including total quality management, continuous quality improvement, quality assessment, quality assurance, and quality control, it remains difficult to differentiate health care systems on the basis of quality care. Attention to the principles of quality occur within the organization itself in the quality department, state and federal government regulatory review agencies, and by the purchasers of health care. All purchasers are now pursuing both quality and value.

Value is the relationship between quality and cost. Payers are demanding high-quality ser-

vices with cost discounts. In a model of capitation, financial risk shifts to the provider, and there is a greater emphasis on health promotion, illness prevention, and condition/illness management. When disease strikes, the focus is the provision of necessary care at a reasonable cost. Because of these changing internal and external demands, health systems report that they are continuously developing, monitoring, communicating, and improving all aspects of patient care. It remains the job of providers to function *collaboratively* to differentiate and continually control and improve the quality of care delivered in the organization.

Despite this reported careful scrutiny of quality care, the concept of quality remains elusive. Quality studies have focused on criteria that reflect structure and process, but clinical outcomes have rarely been demonstrated. Traditionally, the elements captured have been nosocomial infections, fall rate, morbidity and mortality rates, and medication errors. These criteria alone do not highlight the relationship between clinical interventions and appropriate patient outcomes.

It is imperative that health care systems define quality, define the criteria to measure quality, and extend the time frame over which quality measures must be captured. In addition, it is important to consolidate traditional quality activities. Typically, an increasing number of quality elements are added without attention to continued value to the department and organization. Variance analysis can replace traditional department-based quality assurance studies. The CareMap® allows for the capture of multidisciplinary, quality data elements. Significant quality measures are placed on the CareMap® or preprinted variance sheets to eliminate redundant work, focus the effort of all disciplines, and create the opportunity for concurrent and retrospective variance review.

FACETS OF QUALITY

Donabedian (1980) identified three key categories within quality assessment and monitoring: structure, process, and outcome variables. *Structure* represents the stable attributes of the care setting including personnel, equipment, and the physical structure of the organization. *Process* includes the interventions performed by the health care team members and involves how skillfully these interventions are executed. *Outcome* is the change in the health status attributable to the care being assessed. Assessment of quality must include elements from all three categories.

With the advent of the prospective payment system and aggressive managed care, it was imperative to add *cost* as a key parameter to be measured over time. Each case type is evaluated as a business. The linchpins for the equilateral triangle are now *process*, *clinical outcomes*, and *cost*. Tracked are the variances or barriers that impede efficient management of patient care, additional costs associated with variance, as well as failure to meet identified patient outcomes (program effectiveness). Key process indicators, short- and long-term clinical outcomes, and cost are essential elements to track, monitor, and improve over time.

The core work of the multidisciplinary clinical teams and case managers is to continually reestablish the balance between cost, process, and clinical outcomes. Systems to effectively collect, collate, and report data must be developed to promptly feed data back to the team

or case manager. In turn, the data must be processed efficiently to change practice and maintain a balanced relationship among the three variables. The ultimate goal of the system is care management—to improve care little by little, all the time, with intimate involvement of the bedside clinicians at every step. In this manner, the team will maintain a competitive edge and continued commitment to value and service for the customer.

This chapter discusses the CareMap® and case management system as collaborative strategies for achieving positive outcomes. It defines *variance* and describes the operational issues affecting the success of variance management systems. The chapter also addresses the role of the collaborative group practice, the clinical (concurrent) uses of variance, the retrospective uses of variance for continuous quality improvement, the legal ramifications of variance collection and reporting, and the benefits of automation.

A CONCEPTUAL FRAMEWORK FOR VARIANCE

The CareMap® System

Because patient care is so complex—variable from patient to patient and inconsistent from practitioner to practitioner—it can be a challenge to guide the care delivery process. The goal of the CareMap® system is to manage the care delivered and outcomes achieved through a collaborative care process. The clinical path/CareMap® is a tool created and used by the multidisciplinary health care team to guide patient care. It replaces individual discipline plans of care, including the traditional nursing kardex.®

Zander (1991) defined the tool as a cause-and-effect grid that identifies expected patient or family and provider behaviors against a timeline for a case type (congestive heart failure [CHF], coronary artery bypass graft, insulin dependent diabetes) or otherwise defined homogeneous population (suicidal ideation, stage III wound, bereavement). The key components of a CareMap® tool include a (1) timeline, (2) an index of problems or issues with affiliated intermediate goals and short- and long-term outcome criteria, (3) a traditional critical pathway, and (4) a variance record. (The CareMap® actually mimics a GANTT or PERT project management chart, which maps time along the *x*-axis and actions against the *y*-axis.) Added to this traditional quality management tool are the standards of practice or the performance of interventions by all disciplines. This portion of the tool delineates the efficiency of the system and the cost associated with the work to be performed. The problem list and clinical outcomes depict the standard of patient care. This portion of the tool reflects the effectiveness of the system and the level of quality care achieved (Figure 14–1).

CareMap® Development

The CareMap® tool represents collaboration of clinicians from the disciplines and departments that have participated in authorship. Successful teams are often co-chaired by a physician and nurse. The team reviews current care and establishes the length of stay, categories within the timeline, a problem or issues list, clinical and cost outcomes to be achieved, and the essential components of care for every patient within the case type. The pathway components are developed following

- a review of the case type–specific literature
- practice guidelines and algorithms from appropriate professional societies
- standards of care from each relevant discipline
- clinical pathways from various institutions
- discussion regarding "best practice" by the clinical experts in the group
- managed care requirements for length of stay and resource utilization
- national, regional, and local length-of-stay, cost, and quality indicator data

The team must anticipate key potential complications related to treatment or to the specific disease condition and build interventions into the CareMap® to prevent the occurrence of potential complications. For example, the team

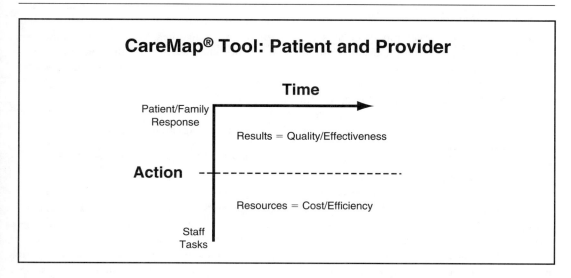

Figure 14–1 The CareMap® Tool. *Source:* Copyright © 1995, Center for Case Management, Inc.

must assess the potential for infection in the immunosuppressed chemotherapy patient and offer interventions to decrease exposure to infections, or risk assess the frail elderly patient presenting with pneumonia for nutritional depletion by taking a diet history and measuring serum albumin and skin turgor.

The team must also challenge traditional practice patterns, discussing the evidence for each major intervention. Evaluated are interventions based on

- tradition (the physician covers for a peer on the weekend, waiting for the primary physician to return to discharge a patient ready to go home)
- preference (chooses a brand name versus generic antibiotic, which is as effective in eradicating a patient's pneumonia)
- outdated practice (performs routine tracheal bronchial suctioning of the intubated patient every 2 hours)
- convenience (uses an expensive hip prosthetic device secondary to the relationship established with the device company sales representative and his or her assistance in the operating suite)

Accountability in Collaborative Care

CareMap® system development creates the need for the clinically expert team to continue to meet to develop action plans and to analyze and to respond to trends in variance data. In mature systems, the multidisciplinary health team evolves into a collaborative practice group. For such clinical groups, collaboration is an evolving process. It is a sophisticated developmental stage in the team-building process. The group must have mutual goals to which most members are committed, share in the vision to achieve the goals, experience mutual interdependence to accomplish their goals, identify individual discipline and group accountabilities, be willing to take risks to create new solutions to problems, and demonstrate mutual trust and respect. The group's goals are to prove efficient and effective care management, deliver the best possible service to patients and families, and demonstrate a system for performance improvement.

To clarify responsibility and authority, it is useful to identify the discipline(s) responsible for key interventions and accountable for each outcome within the CareMap.® Examples are as follows: Improve the comatose trauma patient's physiologic outcome through passive range-of-motion exercises to be performed by nursing and joint mobility by physical therapy on a scheduled basis, enhance patient or family coping by having nurses address anxiety in those patients who are experiencing a myocardial infarction, and improve the patient's functional status by having respiratory therapists assist chronic obstructive pulmonary disease patients to manage their activity–rest–sleep cycle with adjunctive use of bronchodilator therapy and peak flow management and to ambulate 10–25 feet before discharge from home care.

The clarification provided shifts the patient care team from passive care planning to strong care management. Team members know what to expect from each other, who to call on to assist when a patient falls off the pathway, and what discipline is to be evaluated regarding the achievement of specific patient outcomes. This system demands vigilant attention to patient and family outcomes, enhances the authority level for outcomes by each discipline, and fosters collaboration at both the patient's bedside and at the team level.

Variance Management System

Development of a Variance Management System

Variance has been defined as the fact, quality, or state of being variable (inconstant, changeable); difference, deviation, discrepancy, exception; not in agreement or accord. The Care-Map® defines the "norm;" the variance is then the exception to the norm. Variances are the exceptions or the unexpected events that occur during care delivery. Variance can occur from three categories: problem list, interventions, and patient or family outcomes. Variances can be positive or negative. Positive variances occur when an issue on the problem list does not apply to a patient; a patient is discharged earlier than the case type–projected length of stay; when select interventions are unnecessary, such as completion of a chest X-ray or administration of a scheduled pain medication; or when interventions can progress ahead of schedule, such as appropriately instructing a newly diagnosed diabetic patient on insulin injections, hypoglycemic reactions, and diet on the first home health visit. Negative variances occur when an intervention cannot be completed, when an outcome is not met within the identified time frame, and when additional interventions must be added to realize an outcome. Negative variances highlight lack of patient progress.

Because health care is so complex, variation is always present in care delivered, care received, and outcomes realized. Therefore, it is important to understand the goals of variance management. The goals in variance data collection are to identify and individualize the CareMap® to patient or family variances and to decrease system, clinician, and community variances. These goals are achievable if a vision and system for new knowledge and continual improvement are established.

Variance formalizes the evaluation phase of the patient's care plan. It relates the scientific method of care analysis directly to the care delivery process. Variance analysis provides caregivers with a mechanism to study variations in care and to identify ways to continually improve the processes and outcomes of direct patient care.

During development of a CareMap® system, it is imperative that the executive steering committee define variance; identify the goals of the variance system; and determine the type of variance information desired at a central, product line, and case type–level (e.g., pain management for the entire institution, smoking cessation for the cardiopulmonary product line, and ability to flex the knee at a 90-degree angle for post-knee replacement surgery). In addition, the steering committee must identify who will record variances, how variances will be collected and reported, what the process is for analyzing data and making recommendations to change practice, and how the system interfaces with quality assurance and quality improvement processes. The conceptual framework provides a way to evaluate the planned practice against the actual results (variance).

To achieve this conceptual framework within a health system, the steering committee must establish the variance infrastructure, categories of variables to be monitored, and number of variables to be monitored; design the variance tool; create guidelines for use; and determine the availability of resources to accomplish the work to meet system goals.

A salient operational issue that currently exists is the amount of data collected. Variance captured on 100% of the CareMap® (on all interventions, intermediate goals, and outcomes) creates voluminous data and has proven difficult to manage and analyze. In this situation, change in clinical practice based on variance data is not often made. Focusing variance data collection and analysis on a small list of *key* interventions, intermediate goals, and 100% of the outcomes per case type has proven more useful in a number of U.S. organizations. The directive regarding the number and case mix of variances comes from the executive committee. However, the collaborative group practices are responsible for identifying the key process and outcome indicators to monitor and are accountable for making appropriate practice changes based on variance analysis.

Shift to Outcome Management

A fundamental focus for the CareMap® group is the shift from task to outcome management. The outcomes to be depicted in the pathway include short- and long-term goals appropriate for the clinical case type. The out-

comes categories for ambulatory care identified by Benson (1992) are

- health status, which includes ability to function—ambulate 25 feet or the distance from the patient's bedroom to the bathroom, prepare meals, return to work for 8 hours per day
- patient's perceived quality of life
- disease-specific values, such as physiologic parameters, and biochemical and microbiologic laboratory values
- patient performance, including understanding of the disease and management plan, compliance with the plan, and absence of complications
- patient satisfaction with amenities, the art of care, and results of care

The team must determine the appropriate outcomes for acute care, home care, long-term care, and ambulatory care. In addition, it is essential to identify the intermediate goals that demonstrate progress to the outcomes. These intermediate goals serve as markers for continued patient progress. The team must then decide from which of the interventions, intermediate goals, and outcomes to capture variance. An example of a key intervention to track is time to extubation postcoronary artery bypass surgery. If extubation does not occur, the patient cannot move out of the intensive care unit and cannot begin the aggressive ambulation program on day 2 of the map. Failure to meet this first criterion has a cascading effect through all subsequent activities and creates a host of variances throughout the patient's stay. Luttman (1996) has called this the *"gateway"* variance concept. It is important for the team to highlight this variance and the causes, and measure the impact on care.

Understanding variance and the implications for continual quality improvement is imperative at a direct patient care and administrative level. Variances are derived from definitions of quality predetermined for a specific case type from the multidisciplinary author team. This process authenticates variance data collection

by the clinicians delivering bedside care. Also gained is team member support to review the aggregation of variance data. This team must review variance information for the patient case type(s). Two types of information should be provided: data on the effectiveness of the map and data on how well the plan is being followed or how often it is not followed, and why. This aggregated information makes trending and statistical analysis possible. The clinical experts must review practice, deciding what works, what is not working, and what improvements are required to achieve value and higher quality at a reasonable cost.

ISSUES IN VARIANCE SYSTEMS

It is important to address operational issues, analysis, and legal issues as variance management is established in health care systems. Variance systems are evolving nationally with solutions materializing to traditional problems.

Operational Issues

Operational issues include the ease of documenting variances. The CareMap® format typically does not incorporate all documentation related to patient care, most specifically the flowsheet and progress notes. In addition, for reasons related to risk management, many institutions keep the variance tool as a separate record, creating duplication of charting and, therefore, resistance to variance documentation. Integrity of variance data is at risk in many systems because of the cumbersome nature of the tools and their lack of integration into the documentation system, lack of participation of all disciplines in recording variance, and lack of timely feedback to clinicians of the variance results, which further decreases participation.

Organizations that fail to collect variance data are unable to demonstrate a continuous quality improvement process and are not realizing the key advantage to a CareMap® system. Simultaneously, institutions that have not carefully evaluated what data to collect become overwhelmed or gridlocked with data and are at risk for program failure. Voluminous variance data collected centrally can create an overwhelming situation in which the data are not analyzed and distributed to the CareMap® teams or bedside clinicians. The variance program typically erodes when this scenario occurs.

Documentation

To prevent erosion of this important care management system, it is essential for systems to integrate the CareMap® tool into the documentation system as the core of the patient medical record. In addition, the medical record must be reengineered with integration of the Care-Map,® flowsheets, and a multidisciplinary narrative or "lack of progress note" incorporated into the CareMap® document.

The design of this system lends itself to charting by exception, where exception equals variance. In the charting-by-exception philosophy, the caregiver is only required to document the problems, interventions, or outcomes that did not occur. When a variance occurs, it is recorded on a tracking form, which is used retrospectively for variance analysis and continuous quality improvement. The clinician completes the variance tracking form, identifying the date of the event, variance cause (source codes), action taken, variance resolution, and date (Exhibit 14–1). The caregiver also documents on the CareMap® the interventions required to reverse the negative variance, to reassign an unmet outcome to an appropriate time category, or to identify positive variances with outcomes met ahead of schedule. When these documentation systems are created, the accountability each discipline is to assume must be clarified.

Legal Issues

Another issue that must be addressed is the legal implication of using the CareMap® system. Many physicians express the fear that these tools represent cookbook medicine, that they eliminate the art of individualized patient care planning, and that they hold the physician

to a legal standard of care that may not be appropriate for all patients, especially if included as a permanent part of the medical record. In addition, nurses fear that adopting a charting-by-exception format will not legally protect them in a court of law, identifying the adage, "If it wasn't charted, it wasn't done."

The CareMap® represents a guideline for prudent practice for the patient case type. The CareMap® is designed to ensure that essential elements of care are addressed. The tool and the guidelines for the tool do not preclude necessary interventions when patients fail to progress or fall off the map. Nolin and Lang (1994) have raised two important points in their legal defense for CareMaps.® First, providers are held to practice guidelines, practice parameters, and standards of care already in existence from their professional organizations, Agency for Health Care Policy and Research, and so forth. Creating a CareMap® for a given organization encourages the clinicians to become aware of and evaluate the existing guidelines to develop the most appropriate guidelines possible for the patients cared for within the health system. Second, the CareMap® provides structure to the medical record, which currently looks like a disorganized "rat's nest" in the eyes of the jury. If the CareMap® guidelines are followed when a variance is recorded, and a well-orchestrated, prudent, multidisciplinary action plan is documented and reevaluated, the format will actually benefit the health care system in a litigation suit. The fundamental legal issue in the CareMap® system is that when patient or family variance occurs, it must be addressed in the medical record. In reality, this is not a new phenomenon and should be practiced whenever a patient varies from a guideline or standard of care.

Educational Requirements

Educational support is essential in all phases of program implementation and evaluation. The education must include principles and goals of clinical outcomes management, the role of

Exhibit 14–1 Example of a Variance Tracking Form

Date	Description	Prob	Path	Source	Action	Initials
			Variance Sheet CHF			
1-Feb	Son unavailable: out of town on business		8	A3	Ask ICU to call 2/2	AB
1-Feb	Afib O2 sat + 85% glucose 250 no Swan Ganz	5 1	. . 1	A1 A1 A1 B6	Transfer ICU Lasix, O2 6L Diabetic regime	CD
2-Feb	Unable to transfer to floor Afib	. 5		C9 . A1	Order to drop pt. to general care rate Benign	CD
2-Feb	Echo not done Hct 34, Hgb 13		2	C9	Schedule for Monday Begin FeSO4	CD
3-Feb	Unable to get home med delivery	6		D14	Provide pharmacy list to pt.	EF
3-Feb	Nutrition consult early		1	B7	Begin teaching	EF
4-Feb	Wt 135 Ankle edema	4 4		A1 A1	Continue Lasix Elevate feet Inc. ambulation Encourage rhythmic exercises in bed	EF
5-Feb	Complaining about CHF diet and doesn't want to make plans	6		A1 .	Arrange for VNA follow-up for 3 visits	GH
6-Feb	Requests nicotine patch			A2	Notify physician to order before she leaves. Call pharmacy to begin instruction	JK

Variance Source Codes

A   Patient/Family
  1 Condition
  2 Decision
  3 Availability
  4 Other

B   Clinician
  5 Order
  6 Decision
  7 Response Time
  8 Other

C Hospital
  9 Bed/Appt. Availability
  10 Info/Data Availability
  11 Other

D Community
  12 Placement/Home Care
  13 Transportation
  14 Other

Source: Copyright © 1992, The Center for Case Management, Inc.

each discipline in documenting on the CareMap® and variance tools, a review of guidelines for the use of those tools, and case reviews with variance monitoring and analysis to promote clinical decision making. Variance analysis should be viewed as the evaluative process demonstrating patient progress or lack of progress. If the patient fails to progress, the clinician must act on the situation immediately to promote patient recovery and to alert appropriate resources in a timely fashion. If the patient remains in significant variance for a prolonged period, a case review is held to determine the care plan and whether the CareMap® is a helpful tool. The team may decide to discontinue the case-specific map, based on the definition or criteria developed by the institution for falling off the pathway, and place the patient on a generic map. The follow-up on variance resolution is imperative and a step that is often unattended.

Variance management will only succeed under direct, active leadership. Ongoing formal and informal educational sessions should occur during a combination of small, organized, multidisciplinary, didactic groups; case reviews; grand rounds; just-in-time training during physician rounds; change-of-shift report; and staff meetings. In addition, each clinician's performance should be appraised on the person's ability to demonstrate clinical inquiry and patient management against clinical outcomes.

Concurrent Use of Variance in Clinical Practice

Another key operational issue is the inconsistent ability of caregivers to shift focus from tasks to outcomes management and to process variance information at the bedside; that is, alter the CareMap® in real time as necessary. The concept of variance is foreign to many bedside clinicians, and they struggle with what to record (i.e., variance from tasks, tasks and outcomes, tasks, intermediate goals and outcomes); how to record the information; deter-

mining what is causing the variance; and, most important, what corrective action to take with proactive reevaluation of the outcomes to be realized.

Retrospective Use of Variance

The ultimate benefit of the CareMap® system, along with variance analysis, is the ability to analyze patient populations and ensure continuous quality improvement. The groups must be able to discern which variances require action. According to Luttman (1996), variations in data occur because sample sizes by case type are traditionally small (less than 40 cases per quarter); because there typically is not independence between variance variables; and because trends are affected in health care systems by the resources available on nights, weekends, and holidays. Because of these complicating issues, a group could respond to variance data and make a change in practice data that does not improve overall outcomes. Therefore, it is essential to apply statistical methods to ensure significance of the variance before revising a CareMap.® This represents ongoing, action-based research.

For example, an orthopedic practice group discovered that the patients who underwent total hip replacement surgery on Monday had a shorter length of stay than those who underwent surgery on Thursday. Negative variance data demonstrated that the patients recovering in the hospital over the weekend did not receive physical therapy. A review of patient cases revealed that the patients were not adequately ambulated and instructed on hip precautions immediately postoperatively. Intensifying physical therapy services to patients on Monday did not enhance end outcomes. The team determined how changes had to be made so all patients would receive physical therapy in a timely manner.

The same group discovered that patients requiring total hip replacement who were seen by a case manager in their home preadmission had a shortened inpatient length of stay and subject report of greater satisfaction than did the patients not receiving this service. The case manager's primary mission was early identification of patients at risk for complications, education of the caretakers, and establishment of discharge resources needed in the home. The group practice is statistically evaluating the data to determine the impact of the case manager on cost and quality outcomes. In this case, the special cause for variance may be positive and prove desirable for the case manager to see every patient.

To this end, the collaborative practice groups must be given data in an organized, concise, and meaningful format. Samples of graphics displays for data analysis include variance reports generated on percentage of variance category (i.e., assessments, consults, tests or percentage of outcomes met), trend graphs for length of stay over time, or Pareto analysis of a variance category by case type (Figure 14–2). The goal is to generate reliable, simple, easily interpreted graphs and reports to enable the group to determine the significance of the identified problem and potential solutions.

CASE STUDIES

Percutaneous Transluminal Coronary Angiography *(PTCA) CareMap:*®
A Case Study

A CareMap® for PTCA was implemented on a telemetry unit in a midwestern hospital. With implementation of the map, patients were directly admitted to the telemetry unit, bypassing a traditional placement in the intensive care unit. On review of the variance data, 50% of the patients had experienced unrelieved pain postprocedure during the 24-hour length of stay. The clinical nurse specialist was assigned the task of reviewing the charts and nursing practice to determine the cause of the unrelieved pain. She discovered that staff were not differentiating pain due to discomfort with poor positioning versus pain due to dissection of the

vessel and a potential hemorrhage. The objective data were reported to the collaborative practice group, who created an action plan to educate staff on the pain assessment to be performed for the PTCA patient, the interventions to be instituted for the various types of pain described by the patient, and the guidelines to be followed for completing a pain variance on the tracking tool. Within 3 months, pain was identified as a variance in less than 5% of the patients who underwent a PTCA.

Continuum Management: Congestive Heart Failure Case Study

For a health care organization to become accountable for delivering high-quality care, it must partner with physicians to achieve cost and quality outcomes of care, develop Care-Maps,® assign case managers to each clinical product line, and develop tools and roles that span the continuum of care (Figure 14–3). The CareMap® tool provides the foundation for clinical programs of care that span the continuum and, with the depiction of short- and long-term clinical outcomes across the continuum, outcomes management and illness management are realized. For example, CareMaps® are being created for clinical/functional classifications of CHF, from health maintenance through acute exacerbations of failure, to home care, to health maintenance in the ambulatory care setting (Figure 14–4).

Case managers are assigned to the patient outliers, the complex patients whose care is difficult to manage on a map. Patients falling into Class IV of the New York Heart Association (NYHA) dyspnea at rest, increasing significantly with any physical activity, may meet the criteria for case management services. The focus of the case manager may be to arrange for dopamine or dobutamine drips in the home, educate the family on the potential risks of the delivery of these intravenous medications, create a CareMap® for home care agency staff, assist in obtaining financial funding for home care services, discuss advanced directives, re-

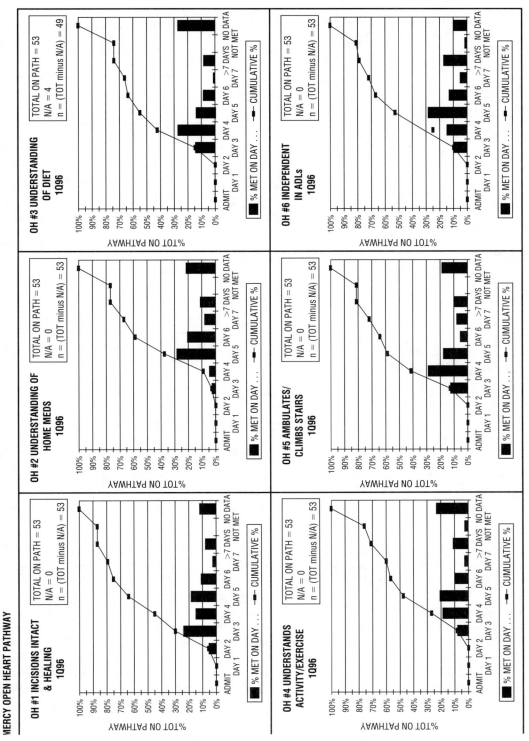

Figure 14–2 Example of a Pareto analysis of variance category by case type. Courtesy of Mercy Data Center 1996.

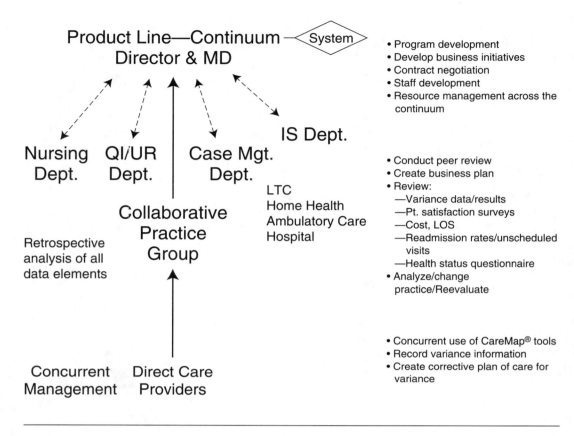

Figure 14–3 Product line structure for the continuum. *Source:* Copyright © 1996, The Center for Case Management, Inc., developed by M. Hill and S. Henry.

view the implications of waiting for a heart transplant, and assist the patient and family in meeting the patient's physical and emotional needs.

When building a CareMap® for CHF for NYHA Classes I–III, the team should incorporate appropriate material from the practice guideline developed by the Agency for Health Care Policy and Research on the use of ACE inhibitors and diuretic therapy, investigate appropriateness of prescribed digoxin, and focus on patient education to enhance self-care man-

agement. Also built into the map can be International Classification of Diseases-Ninth Revision (ICD-9) coding criteria to identify underlying etiology for CHF, NYHA score to determine severity of illness and inclusion or exclusion criteria for placement on the map, utilization review criteria used by local managed care organizations, checklist of cardiac risk factors to build an individualized patient plan of care, and follow-up activities. The collaborative group practice will then determine which CareMap® variables and patient satis-

Case Type: Congestive Heart Failure
- Underlying etiology _____
- Caregiver _____
- NYH Class _____

Causes of Variation:
Comorbidities
Ability of Caregiver ☐ ☐
Access to Services ☐ ☐
Cultural Diversity/Language ☐ ☐

Economic Issues ☐ ☐
Deconditioning ☐ ☐
Holiday/Special Events ☐ ☐
Support System ☐ ☐

Ambulatory Setting
(Preconditions, Case Find, Manage Risk)

Problem/Outcome

Alteration in Cardiac Output
- <20mmHg drop in orthostatic diastolic pulse pressure
- Weight stable
  <2 lb gain since last appt.
- Six-minute walk score stable
- Decreased episodes of acute CHF with hospitalization over 1 year
- Stable score on heart transplant survey

Knowledge Deficit
Patient and Caregiver re: Self-care Management

- Provides diet diary and states is monitoring ex.
- States medications on, schedule, key side effects
- Identifies who to call if wt. is <2lbs. in 24°/5 lbs.
- States and identifies exercise program

Interventions
- VS c̄ orthostatic BP
- Wt.
- Provide educational materials AHCPR Pt. Guide
- Review diary/calendar
- Schedule a follow-up appointment
- Communicate with cardiac rehab

Acute Care
(Stabilization)

Problem/Outcome

Decreased Cardiac Output/ Excess Fluid Volume
- Diastolic BP >80mmHg, Heart Rate and Rhythm stable
- Achieves target weight
- Patient reports improvement in dyspnea

Knowledge Deficit
Patient and Caregiver re: Self-care Management

- States ideal body weight
- Demonstrates how to weigh self, records weight in diary, knows who and when to call with ↑ weight.

Interventions
- VS q1° until stable then q4°
- Wt.
- Vasopressors & Lasix as indicated
- Labs, CXR
- Assess cardiovascular, neuro, GI, GU and pulmonary functional status
- Review survival skills for home management: diet, exercise, medications and weight diary

---

Home Care
(Managing Risk Managing Condition)

Problem/Outcome

Alteration in Cardiac Output
- Orthostatic BP and Heart Rate within normal limits for patient
- Maintains ideal body weight
- Patient denies significant changes in dyspnea and edema

Knowledge Deficit
Patient and Caregiver re: Self-care Management

- Creates and follows a plan to manage diet and exercise
- Weighs self on a daily basis
- Reports S & Sx of worsening failure
- States who to call with increased failure
- Keeps weight and sodium diary

Interventions
- VS c̄ orthostatic BP
- Assess ability to cope and to follow self-management plan
- Review patient's weight and sodium diaries and exercise plan
- Review pts. ability to manage self-administration of medication: *action – dosage – schedule – side effects*
- Review who will call for emergency

Figure 14-4 Sample CareMap® for congestive heart failure. *Source:* Copyright © 1996, The Center for Case Management, Inc., Developed by M. Hill.

faction and perceived quality of life tools to monitor to demonstrate the quality of the program for CHF patients across the health care system.

When integrated into the care delivery process, the CareMap® becomes a multidisciplinary documentation tool and is the core of the patient's medical record. Often the team develops a complementary set of physician orders that facilitate the interventions and treatments preprinted on the CareMap® itself. A patient version of the clinical pathway is also developed. The patient pathway serves as a strong educational tool and a contract between the patient or family and facility regarding the care activities to be accomplished by each party.

The CareMap® is used in daily practice as a micromanagement tool. Clinicians carefully manage and document care against the tool, highlighting variances and the associated plan of corrected action. During change-of-shift report, physician rounds, discharge planning rounds, and case conferences, the intermediate goals, discharge outcomes, and variances are the focus. In this manner, the CareMap® System is integrated into the fabric of the culture of the health organization, shifting the focus from task to vigilant management of outcomes, corrective actions for follow-up, and variance management (see Figure 14–4).

The CareMap® system becomes the vehicle for health care systems to demonstrate integration of clinical practice standards or guidelines into direct patient care; provide information on the outcomes management program at the case type, product line, and institutional levels; and provide evidence of a continuous quality improvement process. This system ultimately serves as the foundation through which quality of care is continually raised to a higher standard.

CASE MANAGEMENT

Case management is a complex phenomenon. Bower (1992) stated that "case management can simultaneously be described as a system, a role, a technology, a process and a service." In this chapter, it is referred to as a clinician or clinical group who oversees the plan of care across the episode or continuum (Figure 14–5). Not all patients require case management services. It is reserved for very complex cases, case types demonstrating high cost or high volume, patients repeatedly falling off a pathway, repeatedly admitted to acute care or with numerous unscheduled visits to ambulatory care, or presenting with great unmet socioeconomic needs. Fewer than 20% of patients cared for within a health system will require case management services. The goal of the case manager is to better manage care by predicting high-risk patient needs, intervening to prevent or decrease the number of acute exacerbations of the condition, and continuing to monitor the effect of the interventions over time.

Case management is often confused with *care management*. CareMap® tools can be used with both care coordination strategies; however, care management is a unit- or area-based model, whereas case management spans services across the episode or continuum of care. The case manager expedites services across traditional health care settings, transitioning with the patient and family.

Although many models for case management have emerged, coordination of care is the basic component of all models. Despite the multiple models and approaches to case management, the key defining characteristics include (Bower, 1995):

- Coordinating a patient or case type's care across the episode or continuum
- Ensuring and facilitating the achievement of quality and cost outcomes
- Negotiating, procuring, and coordinating services and resources needed by the patient and family
- Intervening at key points (and/or significant variance) for individual patients
- With the collaborative teams, addressing and resolving patterns in aggregate variances that have a negative quality–cost impact

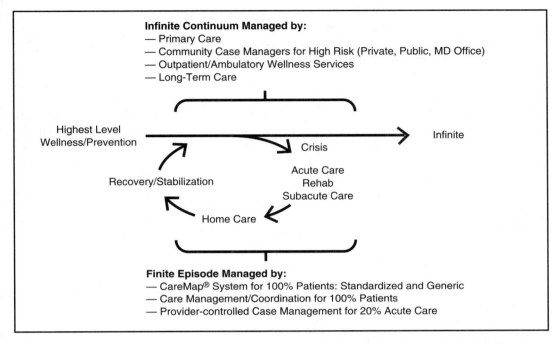

Infinite Continuum Managed by:
— Primary Care
— Community Case Managers for High Risk (Private, Public, MD Office)
— Outpatient/Ambulatory Wellness Services
— Long-Term Care

Highest Level Wellness/Prevention

Infinite

Crisis

Acute Care
Rehab
Subacute Care

Recovery/Stabilization

Home Care

Finite Episode Managed by:
— CareMap® System for 100% Patients: Standardized and Generic
— Care Management/Coordination for 100% Patients
— Provider-controlled Case Management for 20% Acute Care

Figure 14–5 Mapping and case management strategies for capitation. *Source:* Copyright © 1995, The Center for Case Management, Inc., Developed by K. Zander.

• Creating opportunities and systems to enhance outcomes

Once the goals for case management have been established within the health care system, a central steering committee's next step is to outline the details of the case manager's role. The primary responsibilities of the case manager should be synchronized with the program goals. The case manager role is multidimensional: expert clinical, administrative, managerial, and interpersonal skills are required. The case manager must

• effectively triage patients into the caseload
• develop a network of services within which to operate to achieve patient care outcomes
• establish a system for care coordination across each geographic location within the episode or continuum of care

• establish communication systems with physicians, other team members, payers, durable medical equipment companies, and community resources
• create methods to track patient care outcomes and cost through the health system (variance as indicated)
• evaluate the effect of case management services on a patient population
• appropriately discharge patients from the case management service

Case management is a powerful strategy to manage the care of complex patients or patient populations. When creating a case management position, it is important to outline the current flow of the patients through the health system, identify the needs and characteristics of the patient population, determine where in the care trajectory the case manager should intervene, and establish who should serve in the case management network. Case managers can develop tools to assist them in organizing their program of care; assist the collaborative practice group in highlighting the outliers requiring additional services; assist in compiling predictor variances requiring altered resources; and assist in summarizing clinical outcomes, readmissions, and costs realized by the individual patient and patient population. The case manager works closely with the collaborative practice group to enhance patient care programming.

FUTURE ISSUES

Physician–Organization Relationship

The economic environment is forcing integration of clinical and administrative services in the management of health care systems. To efficiently and effectively manage patient care, physicians, administrators, and community leaders must work together. Physicians have traditionally focused on effectiveness (quality) of the care delivered, access to the latest technology to accurately diagnose and cure disease, and program growth and development. Administrators have traditionally focused on decreasing resource use and capital investment or expenditures, gaining market share, and maintaining a profitable census. The two groups have not trusted each other because of their seemingly opposed missions and inability to effectively unite cost and quality outcomes. In the health systems that survive, physicians and health care administrators will create new partnerships, both groups coming together in a united effort to manage clinical and cost outcomes. These partnerships will have favorably negotiated financial incentives and clearly outlined accountabilities. A primary responsibility will be the development, active participation, and co-management of the collaborative practice groups. The goal is that patients receive the right care, by the right provider, at the right time, and at the right cost.

Data Management Specialists

The issues for the future are threefold. First, it is apparent that data management specialists will be essential members of the health care institution. Data management specialists will assist in the integration of data management systems, in data collation, and in the generation of reports and graphs, and will assist the clinical teams in statistical analysis of the data presented. The data management specialists will also assist the teams in collecting and managing data across the health care system. In addition, the specialists will assist the organization in reviewing data between the levels of care, that is, from the individual patient, case type, and product line and through the systemwide level, in eliminating redundant studies, in the monitoring of ineffective quality of care variables, and in consolidating expensive resources (Figure 14–6).

Automation

The development of computer systems to automate the entire CareMap® system could rectify the documentation struggles identified earlier in this chapter. When CareMaps® are built into an automated charting system, variance will be captured in real time and will no longer be a redundant effort. Creation of a forced-field screen would increase clinician compliance in recording and creating an action plan for the variance discovered. This would enhance the integrity and accuracy of data; potentially enhance interrater reliability by creating select, defined criteria; enhance retrieval of relevant clinical information for review; make data abstraction across the continuum immediately available for analysis and feedback; and make graphic display readily accessible for the collaborative team.

Systemwide Integration of Clinical Programs and Data

The last issue is to integrate variance analysis and the achievement of clinical outcome

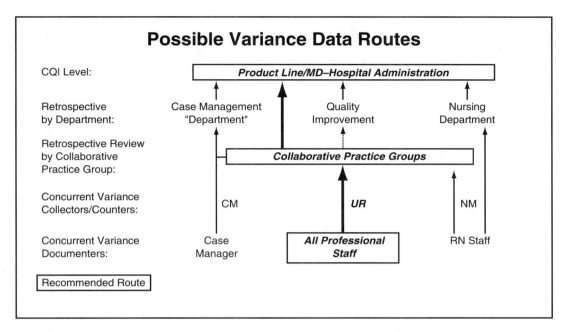

Figure 14–6 Possible variance data routes. *Source:* Copyright © 1992; Revised 1995, The Center for Case Management, Inc.

data and cost data by case type and product line across the health care system. This will allow practitioners and administrators to evaluate the effects of changes in practice in acute care on home care, long-term care, and in the ambulatory setting. The fundamental questions to be answered are, What preventive interventions make a difference and reduce risk? When and where in the health care continuum do additional resources actually add value for patients at risk for breast cancer? For diabetes? Where is care best provided for patients with CHF? By whom? For those chronically acute patient populations, case management will be essential. According to Zander (1996), in this clinical, continuum-based model of case management, the provider will actually be managing *risk* to health, described earlier as illness management. Case managers will be an essential member of the collaborative practice groups and will also require refined information systems to assist them in managing the clinical

and cost outcomes for the patients in their caseload.

CONCLUSION

CareMap® and variance management systems represent a process for concurrent patient care management, fostering enhanced clinical decision-making skills at the individual practitioner and collaborative team level. These systems allow for retrospective management at the aggregate case type level, with the potential to affect programmatic changes for the patient population. Individual clinicians are held accountable for the outcomes of care for individual patients, and the collaborative group practice is accountable for the clinical and financial outcomes of care at the case type and product line levels. When the collaborative practice becomes adept at interpretation of variance information and accurately integrates, interrupts, and uses variance analysis, cost and length-of-stay data, readmission rates, morbidity data, and patient satisfaction or perceived quality survey results to change practice, the quality of care is enhanced. This represents the scientific process:

practice→data→information→knowledge→change practice, demonstrating continuous quality improvement, that is, doing things better, little by little, all the time, at the direct patient care level.

REFERENCES

Benson, D. (1992). *Measuring outcomes in ambulatory care.* Chicago: American Hospital Association.

Bower, K. (1992). *Case management by nurses.* Washington, DC: American Nurses Association.

Bower, K. (1995). Case management designed for the care continuum. In K. Zander (Ed.), *Managing outcomes through collaborative care.* Chicago: American Hospital Association.

Donabedian, A. (1980). *Explorations in quality assessment and monitoring* (Vol. 1). Ann Arbor, MI: Health Administration Press.

Luttman, R. (1996). *How to design clinical pathway variance systems for continuous quality improvement: A layman's guide.* South Natick, MA: The Center for Case Management.

Nolin, C.E., & Lang, C.G. (1994). *An analysis of the use and effect of CareMap® tools in medical malpractice litigation.* South Natick, MA: The Center for Case Management.

Potter, P. (1995). The uses of variance. In K. Zander (Ed.), *Managing outcomes through collaborative care.* Chicago: American Hospital Association.

U.S. Department of Health and Human Services, Agency for Health Care Policy and Research (1994). *Clinical practice guideline no. 11: Heart failure: Evaluation and care of patients with left-ventricular systolic dysfunction.* Rockville, MD: Author.

Zander, K. (1991). CareMaps®: The core of cost/quality care. *The New Definition, 6*(3):1–3.

Zander, K. (1996). Evolving mapping and case management for capitation: Part III: Getting control of value. *The New Definition, 11*(2):1–2.

PART IV

Developing the Professional to Manage Quality

CHAPTER 15

Quality Improvement Teams and Teamwork

Lenard L. Parisi

CHAPTER OBJECTIVES

After completing this chapter, the reader will be able to

- describe the team development process
- compare differences between teams and committees
- discriminate varied roles and responsibilities of members comprising a team
- assess a team's effectiveness
- draft a code of conduct to guide team performance

In the health care version of the "learning organization," a significant amount of time must be spent building an individual's capacity to talk with others and to have meaningful conversations that can result in significant relationships. Given the complexity of health care organizations, in which people virtually speak different languages and perform unique functions, an even greater investment in skill building such as listening and inquiry techniques is critical. Physicians, for example, have been trained to know all the answers; real collegiality, learning to lead, and building relationships to create a larger community are innately foreign to their practice. The varied stakeholders in a health care organization—patients, physicians, third-party payers, all employees, and the community—must all be part of this skill-building process.

In the current health care environment in which the emphasis is on decreasing costs and demonstrating sustained quality of care, it becomes imperative for the health care team to eliminate barriers and work to improve systems and processes. Interdisciplinary collaboration among health care providers is essential to the delivery of high-quality care and positive patient outcomes. One highly regarded method for accomplishing professional collaboration in health care is the quality improvement team (QIT).

QITs are most commonly formed to evaluate and improve processes. The rationale for selecting a process for improvement and initiating a team varies across organizations. Recommendations for process improvement may come from the customer, senior management of the organization, regulatory agencies, payers, or accrediting bodies. Suggestions may also come from employees within the organization, who have identified an opportunity for improvement, based on their experience implementing a process.

TEAM DEVELOPMENT

A *team* is composed of a group of individuals who are involved in or affected by a problem or quality issue and who work together to solve a common problem. A team consists of a small number of people with complementary skills who are committed to a common purpose, a set of performance goals, and an approach for which they hold themselves mutually accountable.

Quality Improvement Teams Versus Committees

The development of a QIT for improving organizational performance has become common in health care. Before the development of QITs, committees were most often used to solve problems. There are, however, several important differences between teams and committees (Table 15–1).

QITs typically comprise members of the organization who implement or are involved in the process being studied (for improvement). Each member on the team has equal authority. Committees, in contrast, consist of members at similar levels of the organization who address changing tasks and goals. A QIT focuses on improving one process and is designed to "self-destruct" after recommending an improvement. The development of teams appropriate to examine, challenge, and improve the inherent processes involved in quality health care is critical.

Identification of Opportunities for Improvement

Regardless of how quality improvement projects are selected, there are common process problems that signal the need for improvement. One frequent problem is a lack of understanding of the process. This knowledge deficit is usually identified through a discussion with those individuals responsible for carrying out the process. Other indications that there are problems with a process are an increase in the number of errors, the addition of unnecessary steps to accomplish a task, and intentional deviations in practice.

Sometimes in organizations there is widespread variation in the implementation of a process. This symptom may also indicate that the process is not clearly defined. Consequently, the team must first identify the problem, then identify opportunities for improvement. These tasks might be accomplished more readily by identifying practice patterns and flowcharting the process.

When the opportunity presents to select a process for improvement, the team should consider one that affects customer satisfaction, can

---

Table 15–1 Differences between Teams and Committees

Team	Committee
• Shares leadership roles	• Has a strong, clearly focused leader
• Has limited members, usually 5–6	• Has unlimited members
• Provides individual and mutual accountability	• Provides individual accountability
• Members have a range of authority within the organization	• Members are at similar levels within the organization
• Is designed for short-term accomplishments	• Is ongoing
• Has defined goals	• Has changing goals
• Uses a scientific approach for process improvement	• Sometimes uses continuous quality improvement tools and techniques
• Recommends permanent solutions	• Often recommends quick fixes
• Measures performance directly by assessing collective work by-products	• Measures effectiveness indirectly by its influence on others

be commonly performed within the organization, is well defined, is not in transition, and will be considered important by most people within the organization. Such a process will ensure acceptance from the team members and result in a motivated and productive team.

Mission Statement

It is important that the goals and purpose of the QIT project be clear and well communicated to the team members and the organization. The written format for communicating this information to the organization is commonly known as a mission statement.

The *mission statement* is a narrative document that outlines the team's purpose, goals, and objectives. The mission statement of the QIT is derived from the original assignment given the team. This assignment typically will come from the referring source of the process. A mission statement that is clear will include the following components:

- a description of the process being studied
- the expected accomplishments of the team
- the team's goals and objectives
- the names of the team leader and facilitator
- the names of team members
- the limitations on resources
- the expected completion date of the project

In organizations in which several quality improvement teams function simultaneously, the mission statement is an excellent communication tool for registering the team with the senior-level committee responsible for prioritizing and selecting team projects. Having a mission statement will help avoid duplication by other teams who are trying to improve similar processes. It is advisable to distribute a copy of the mission statement to the team members before the first meeting. The document will communicate much of the information about the team and serve as a vehicle to stimulate discussion.

Engagement in the continuous quality improvement (CQI) process promotes management expectations of

- improved communication
- a focus on processes, not people
- a definition of customer(s)
- a change in the perception of the current job
- empowerment, that is, making decisions at the level closest to the problem
- support at all levels and functions
- the ability to identify problems and solutions
- team trust

Team expectations of management support include

- Released time for: training, meetings, data gathering, implementation, and monitoring and standardizing improvement
- clear, achievable, worthwhile projects
- honesty regarding parameters within which the team must operate
- all information needed to make informed decisions
- trust
- patience and empathy
- resources
- recognition and rewards

Team Membership

After clearly defining the team's mission, goals, expected outcomes, and the process to be studied, the most important task is to appropriately select team members. This requires careful consideration to ensure adequate representation of those involved in carrying out the process being studied. Four specific roles that enable a team to operate efficiently are: (1) team leader, (2) team facilitator, (3) team recorder, and (4) team members.

Team Leader

The *team leader* is empowered to coordinate organizational resources such as budget and training opportunities, and acts as a liaison between the team and management. The team leader is often selected by the organizational senior management team. The team leader's role is most important in setting the tone and direction of the team throughout the entire project. It is the team leader's responsibility to organize the team, write the mission statement, and select other team members. It is advisable that the team leader have knowledge of group dynamics, motivational theory, and CQI principles and techniques. The team leader coordinates the meetings, establishes the agenda, provides opportunities and CQI education to the team, and maintains all documentation related to the team's functioning, including minutes and reports. Given that the team leader is usually in a position of authority within the organization, it is important that he or she not dominate discussions during the meeting but, rather, allow team members to exchange ideas.

Team Facilitator

The *team facilitator*, or quality adviser, is an essential team member. The facilitator works closely with the team leader throughout the entire project, commenting on the team's progress and making recommendations about the team's functioning. The facilitator is the expert on quality improvement principles, usage of various CQI tools, and group process. It is the facilitator's responsibility to keep the team focused on the issues or tasks at hand and not to comment on the content of the discussion.

Team Recorder

The *team recorder* prepares all written documentation related to the team's functioning, including minutes and reports. The recorder maintains historical records of the team's activities.

Team Members

It is imperative that potential team members are selected based on their knowledge and expertise of the process being studied, not their job title or position in the organization. Such selection allows each team member to present his or her unique perspective on issues. Remember that those who carry out the process know it best.

The success of the QIT in accomplishing its goals and objectives depends on team membership. It is necessary to have adequate representation of all workers involved in the process on the team. Some experts recommend that a team consist of no more than five members. This number is extremely small and impractical given the size of many health care organizations. Teams have been reported to be successful with as many as 18 members. When it becomes necessary to limit team membership, consider selecting one representative from job categories or professions with similar functions. For example, if the process involves practitioners who interact with patients at the bedside, instead of including a respiratory therapist, physical therapist, and occupational therapist, select just one. The same principle holds true with other similar job functions (e.g., physician specialties).

Limiting membership does not exclude the team's need to seek the opinions of their peers and colleagues outside of the original team throughout the process. Not only does this discussion generate enthusiasm within the organization, it produces positive suggestions for change. The success of the QIT in accomplishing its goals and objectives depends on open and honest participation and a sharing of ideas.

THE FIRST TEAM MEETING

The first team meeting is important because it frequently sets the tone for future meetings. This initial meeting is the time to discuss group process. The agenda should include an overview of the commitment of the organization to CQI, team members' expectations, and a review of the mission statement and the proposed meeting schedule. Clarifying what is expected of the team members in the preliminary stages will help avoid misunderstandings later. The key to a successful first meeting is thoughtful planning.

Prior to the first meeting, a personal contact from the team leader places the team member at ease. This is also a good method for developing a rapport with each team member as well as an opportunity to clarify expectations of attendance and participation. Following verbal contact, send a written follow-up confirmation (agenda) identifying:

- date, place, meeting start and finish time
- purpose of meeting with a list of topic(s) to be covered
- person(s) responsible for topic to be discussed, if appropriate
- expected outcome(s)
- handouts members should read prior to meeting to enhance preparedness (mission statement, etc.)

The first meeting must be kept simple and provide an introduction to the team process. Encourage team members to introduce themselves and present any concerns they may have about their role on the team. All team members should participate in drafting a "Code of Conduct" or ground rules to guide how meetings should be conducted, how members will interact, and what kind of behavior is acceptable (Exhibit 15–1). This dialogue facilitates discussion and the opportunity for the team to learn about each other. It is also helpful to provide a directory listing the names of all team members, their organizational locations, and their telephone numbers. A directory will facilitate communication among the team members outside of the meetings. Expectations for meeting frequency and expected attendance must be clarified during the first meeting. Frequent meetings sustain the team's momentum and result in faster accomplishments and positive outcomes.

To be effective, individuals must have the ability to work within a team. The ability to communicate requires the following interpersonal skills: how to listen, how to speak, how to give and receive feedback, how to make decisions by consensus (group opinion or collective agreement), and how to manage conflict. Team members may periodically wish to assess their progress and ability to perform by using the team assessment form in Exhibit 15–2.

ANALYSIS OF A PROCESS FOR IMPROVEMENT

An important function of a QIT is to develop systems thinking and apply the scientific approach to exploring, clarifying, and improving a

---

Exhibit 15–1 Total Quality Management Code of Conduct

- Meetings will start and end on time.
- All members must contribute to team efforts.
- Members' opinions are respected; the right to disagree is upheld.
- Members must speak to be understood, *not* to win.
- Members should listen respectfully; do not interrupt, ridicule, or evaluate.
- Comments will be limited to the topic being discussed.
- Members should request clarification to understand rationale and data supporting statements.
- Conflict is merely a difference of opinion; it requires a team to consider all options or alternatives.
- All members, *not* just the leader, should manage conflict.

- Critique ideas, *not* people. *No* personal attacks will be permitted.
- Members should assume positive intent behind each other's motives and actions.
- The leader will share the leadership.
- Confidentiality of some information discussed in meetings must be respected.
- If members must miss a meeting, it is the absent person's responsibility to contact another member for "updating."
- Minutes from previous meetings and the agenda will be distributed to members before meeting.
- All team members are valued!
- Smoking is *not* permitted.

defined process. The team uses CQI principles and techniques to analyze and investigate underlying causes of problems within a process. This highly regarded approach may include implementation of any or all of the following CQI tools and techniques:

- *Brainstorming:* This technique facilitates problem identification and is used to generate as many ideas as possible in a short time.
- *Nominal group technique:* This technique is used for consensus building.

Exhibit 15–2   Team Assessment

Date: Team (ID/Name):

Directions: Please circle one appropriate response, from 1 to 6.

Part 1: Content

Question	All of the time			None of the time		
During the team meeting(s), did the team members						
• Come to the meeting prepared?	6	5	4	3	2	1
• Discuss the content of the meeting in a meaningful way, adding value to the subject?	6	5	4	3	2	1
• Meet the specified goals, outcomes, and objectives?	6	5	4	3	2	1
• Define the follow-up activities well?	6	5	4	3	2	1

Part 2: Process

Question	All of the time			None of the time		
During the team meeting(s), did the team members:						
• Participate equally?	6	5	4	3	2	1
• Meet the particular responsibilities of their roles?	6	5	4	3	2	1
• Create synergy?	6	5	4	3	2	1
• Openly express their opinions?	6	5	4	3	2	1
• Permit others to express themselves?	6	5	4	3	2	1
• Listen to others?	6	5	4	3	2	1

Reflections

Please write any additional comments about how the team meetings can be improved (use back of page if necessary)._____
_____ Thank you for your contribution.

Courtesy of Technicomp, Inc., 1991, Cleveland, Ohio.

- *Flowchart:* This tool allows the team to visualize the process it is studying step by step.
- *Pareto chart:* This tool quantitatively displays opportunities for improvement in descending bar graph format and allows the team to visually determine priorities.
- *Cause-and-effect diagram (fishbone/Ishakawa diagram):* This tool lists the variables contributing to a defined outcome, either positive or negative.
- *Control chart:* This line graph displays variations in a process over time and illustrates deviations from the mean.
- *Scatter diagram:* This tool allows the team to understand the relationship between two variables around a defined axis.

Refer to Chapter 16 for greater details and explanations of CQI tools and techniques.

This detailed analysis of a process will result in objective data that are based on sound rationale, are accepted by the team, and suggest solutions to resolve problems based on the data. Committees often make recommendations that are quick fixes because the composition of committee members does not always include those who are most familiar with the process being studied.

Troubleshooting a Stalled Team

Ongoing evaluation (see Exhibit 15–2) of the team's accomplishments is important because there may be times when the team reaches a barrier, and progress toward the desired outcome is delayed. This lack of progress may be related to

- an unclear mission statement
- poor member attendance at meetings or the substitution of a team member with an alternate
- unclear or unmeasurable team goals or a change in goals during the process
- dysfunctional group dynamics
- holidays and vacations

- personal obligations or job-related pressures
- meeting schedule, time, day, or place conflicts

If necessary, consider planning less frequent meetings. This does not mean, however, that team members will not have an assignment between meetings. The team leader must ensure that all team members have an interim assignment or task and that they completed it before the next scheduled meeting. When there are 3 weeks or more between meetings, it is imperative that the team leader follow up with team members to ensure that assignments are being completed. This follow-up will ensure more positive outcomes at the next meeting.

To resolve conflicts, all team members must

- acknowledge there is a problem
- take responsibility for reaching solutions
- listen carefully as all viewpoints are discussed
- focus on resolving conflict and making continued progress toward the team's goals
- agree on areas of agreement (or compromise) and disagreement (the leader/facilitator may repeat arguments on each side)
- agree to disagree

Evaluation of Team Accomplishments

It is imperative to monitor the progress of the team throughout the entire quality improvement process by measuring accomplishments against goals and objectives. Quality improvement tools such as flowcharts, Pareto charts, and control charts may be used to measure effectiveness. It is impressive for the team to demonstrate accomplishments by decreasing the steps in a flowchart, illustrate positive changes in targeted areas on a Pareto chart, or indicate evidence of statistical control on a control chart.

If the goal of the team was to implement a new process, a pilot study is suggested. The pilot study allows the team to "work the bugs out" of the process. It also allows for more controlled implementation with the support of team members. Following implementation, the pilot project must be evaluated at a predetermined time. Reconvening the team to evaluate the pilot project will also create the opportunity to discuss observations about the new process and make recommendations for improvement.

Disbanding the QIT

QITs are usually designed to be self-limiting. When the team has reached its goal and accomplished its objectives, it is time to consider disbanding. When considering bringing the team to a close, it is important not to overlook the powerful working relationships that have developed among team members and to sensitively help bring closure to these relationships as it relates to the project. This may be accomplished by preparing the team for the last meeting at least 4 weeks in advance. At this time, discuss any plans to reconvene the team at a later date to evaluate any new processes implemented. Planning a social event to acknowledge and celebrate everyone's hard work is an excellent method for bringing the team to closure. Perhaps their relationships will enhance individual members' networks and create opportunities for future team efforts. Invite key personnel from the organization to support the event.

The final team meeting requires as much planning as the first. This meeting may be used to present the final evaluation of the project and accomplishments to senior officers within the organization. Use the CQI tools and techniques that were implemented throughout the team process to demonstrate improvement. Be clear on any next steps to be accomplished or considered. If senior management attends, this may be an opportunity to gain consensus and obtain resources and a commitment to carry out the team's recommendations.

After the team process is completed, send thank you letters to team members, with a copy to their supervisors and human resources department file. This correspondence shows the appreciation of the organization, fosters good morale, and serves to document each employee's participation.

Celebration of Team Success

Celebrating the successes of the QIT provides the team with well-deserved recognition and sends a message to the organization that CQI is important. There are many ways in which to celebrate the team's accomplishments in addition to evaluation at the final meeting:

- Write an article for a professional journal and share the team's accomplishments with the health care community. Outline the process, methodology, and lessons learned as a result of the team's work.
- Write an article, describing the process improved, for the organizational newsletter. Include the names of the team members to promote organizational acceptance and generate enthusiasm for CQI.
- Display a storyboard within the organization in a commonly used location such as the cafeteria or lounge, or at a local or national conference. Using a storyboard is an excellent means for generating discussion with colleagues about the team's work, as well as for networking.
- Make a presentation of the team's accomplishments at grand rounds to provide those attending an opportunity to ask questions and gain insight into the team's work.
- Use standing committee meetings as an opportunity to promote the team's accomplishments.

There are many opportunities to celebrate and share information. Be creative and resourceful. CQI is contagious—share the team's success!

Successful process improvement and positive outcomes are a natural product of a well-planned, collaborative, and effectively functioning team. Appropriate selection of team members and correct application of CQI tools and techniques virtually will guarantee the team's success.

SUGGESTED READINGS

Joiner Associates. (1995a). *Introduction to the tools.* Madison, WI: Author.

Joiner Associates. (1995b). *The team memory jogger.* Madison, WI: Author.

Joint Commission on Accreditation of Healthcare Organizations. (1993). *Implementing quality improvement: A hospital leader's guide.* Oakbrook Terrace, IL: Author.

Katz, J., & Green, E. (1992). *Managing quality: A guide to monitoring and evaluating nursing services.* St. Louis, MO: Mosby-Year Book.

Katzenbach, J.R., & Smith, D.K. (1993). *The wisdom of teams: Creating a high performance organization.* New York: Harper Collins.

Parisi, L.L. (1993). Ten tips for initiating a QIT. *Nursing Quality Connection, 3*(2), 7.

Parisi, L.L. (1994a). Process improvement: Committee or team. *Nursing Quality Connection, 4*(2), 5.

Parisi, L.L. (1994b). Selecting the right quality improvement project. *Nursing Quality Connection, 4*(3), 2.

Parisi, L.L. (1995a). Celebrating the success of the quality improvement team. *Nursing Quality Connection, 5*(3), 31.

Parisi, L.L. (1995b). Clarifying the team's work: Writing a mission statement. *Nursing Quality Connection, 4*(4), 4.

Parisi, L.L. (1995c). Disbanding the quality improvement team. *Nursing Quality Connection, 5*(4), 42.

Parisi, L.L. (1995d). Planning your first quality improvement team meeting. *Nursing Quality Connection, 4*(6), 6.

Parisi, L.L. (1995e). Selecting quality improvement team members. *Nursing Quality Connection, 4*(5), 3.

Parisi, L.L. (1995f). When the quality improvement team stops functioning. *Nursing Quality Connection, 5*(2), 20.

Scholtes, P.R. (1988). *The team handbook.* Madison, WI: Joiner Associates.

Scholtes, P.R. (1995). Teams in the age of systems. *Quality Progress, 28*(12), 51–59.

Schroeder, P. Ed. (1993). *Improving quality and performance: Concepts, programs and techniques.* St. Louis, MO: Mosby-Year Book.

Swain, P.S. (1993). *A team approach: Quality of care in special care units.* St. Petersburg, FL: Paula Swain Seminars.

## CHAPTER 16

Using Statistical Process Control Tools in the Quality Process

Willa L. Fields and Dale Glaser

CHAPTER OBJECTIVES

After completing this chapter, the reader will be able to

- describe a variety of statistical process control tools to facilitate a team's decision-making process
- evaluate the usefulness of various tools in clinical situations

A multitude of quality improvement frameworks exist, each with their own specific steps, language, and processes. Each framework, though, shares common tools for arriving at a structured format for problem solving. Moreover, the tools within each framework serve in facilitating group decision making and progress, which furthers the current emphasis on decision making within a team context (Bucholz & Roth, 1987). Even though quality improvement methods were initially designed to be implemented within industrial settings, Deming (1986) accurately envisioned that those same improvement tools could readily be applied to the service sector, including health care. This chapter describes quality improvement tools that have been successful in improving patient care and organizational performance. Tools include brainstorming, multivoting, flowcharting, cause-and-effect diagrams, run charts, control charts, histograms, Pareto diagrams, and scatter diagrams. These tools can be used as part of a formal improvement team, or to support day-to-day management decision making.

BRAINSTORMING

Brainstorming is a group technique that generates new ideas and promotes creative thinking. Berk and Berk (1993) asserted that brainstorming can potentially provide "a checklist of target-rich value improvement areas" (pp. 197–198). Brainstorming can be done as either a structured or unstructured process and is particularly helpful in determining possible causes or solutions to a problem, planning steps to a project, or generating ideas that might be controversial. One caveat to brainstorming is that, although it provides a forum for novel ideas, it is not an unconditional substitute for data. Even though the ideas may wield a tenor of face validity, corroboration via valid and reliable data must still prevail.

Structured Brainstorming

Structured brainstorming follows specific norms and is particularly helpful when the subject is controversial and the meeting facilitator wants to encourage participation by all members. As most observers of group meetings will attest, it is common to detect a normal curve distribution for group participation: a few members dominate the conversation, a few add close to nothing, and the majority contribute moderately.

Given the emphasis on egalitarianism in structured brainstorming, dominant members are controlled and quiet members are encouraged to participate regardless of the qualitative nature of the content. Brainstorming "is the only tool that encourages quantity over quality" (Paulson, Wasik, Tarker, & Shumate, 1992, pp. 6–15).

A structured brainstorming session begins with a description of the purpose of the session and a review of brainstorming norms (Exhibit 16–1). It is helpful to write the norms on a flip chart and attach it on the wall for all to see throughout the session. Members are given a few minutes to jot their ideas down, and then each member takes a turn offering an idea. The meeting facilitator writes each suggestion on a flip chart so the ideas are visible to all. Participants are allowed only one idea per turn, and explanations for the idea are not given. If participants have no new ideas to offer at their turn, then they may "pass." Brainstorming stops when no new ideas come forward and everyone is passing. Once the brainstormed list is complete, discussion ensues about the merits of the ideas and what steps need to be taken next.

If the subject is controversial or volatile, anonymity of the ideas can be maintained by having the group members write their ideas on index cards. The cards are then given to the facilitator to transcribe onto a flip chart. This process is repeated until no new ideas come forward.

The absence of criticism, praise, or endorsement for the ideas as they are proffered is paramount for the success of brainstorming. New ideas are to be encouraged, not discouraged. Even subtle gesticulations and sundry nonverbal behaviors should be discouraged, as this may reduce the participation of the more timorous in the group and discourage creativity. Furthermore, the facilitator should encourage outrageous, even unconventional thinking. There is no wrong idea. Often, "hitchhiking" occurs, that is, one idea stimulates another.

Example

The housekeeping department in a large metropolitan hospital complained that needles and scalpels were being found in the linens and trash. Nursing complained that the sharps containers were overfull and not being emptied regularly. The situation was volatile, and the groups were blaming each other: "If the sharps containers were emptied regularly, we wouldn't have to dispose of this stuff in the trash"; "The physicians do it"; "The sharps containers are poorly located"; "Nurses don't care about what happens to the housekeeping staff," and so on. Using structured brainstorming, a group of physicians, nurses, and housekeepers identified why they thought needles and scalpels were found in the trash and linens. No ideas were allowed to be praised, criticized, dismissed, or endorsed. The purpose of the session was to identify all possible causes of sharps in the trash and linens, and later data would be collected to determine the frequency of proffered causes. In this way, no blame was attributed—sharps might be left on a tray after a procedure, and the person disposing the tray had no idea there was a sharp, and simply threw the entire tray in the trash. At the end of the session there was a comprehensive list, with few arguments, hard feelings, or blaming (Exhibit 16–2). The generated ideas were later organized into a fishbone diagram, and areas for data collection were agreed on through multivoting.

Exhibit 16–1 Brainstorming Norms

- Make contributions in turn.
- Present only one idea per turn.
- Do not provide explanations for ideas.
- Do not criticize, praise, or endorse ideas.
- Aim for large numbers of unconventional, imaginative, and even outrageous ideas.
- Pass if you do not have a new idea.

Unstructured Brainstorming

The primary difference between structured and unstructured brainstorming is that although structured brainstorming invites each member,

Exhibit 16–2 Brainstorming Results for Reasons Sharps Are Found in the Trash and Linens

- IV starts—2 needles needed—one accidentally in linens
- Lack of disciplinary action for noncompliance to proper disposal of sharps
- Part goes in sharps, part not; all in one bin (e.g., CVP insertion)
- Lack of way to monitor compliance to procedure for sharps disposal
- Needles—systems not used
- Opened tray and sharps not visible in bedside procedures
- Follow-up on incidents
- Clear safety policy and procedure standards
- Accountability for monitoring
- Person doing procedure does not clean up room; person who does clean does not know a sharp was used
- Where to put sharp plastics (e.g., IV tubing)
- Pushing drugs in codes without needle container available
- Training issues
- Who is responsible; unclear roles
- Unclear role definition of who checks for 3/4 full box
- Lack of knowledge of impact of not disposing correctly

- Unaware of consequences of misplacing sharps
- Lack of well-defined locations of sharps containers
- Sharps container full; what is full? Inconvenient
- Sharps container used for trash
- Trash can more convenient than sharps container
- Style of sharps container—lock out
- Position/location of sharps container
- Not enough needle boxes
- Not clear on what a "sharp" is
- Auto pilot—staff put sharps in regular trash automatically with other trash
- Unclear of what CNA, MD to put in box; varies by area and emergent nature of procedure
- Unclear expectation of role to empty sharps container
- Lack of knowledge of impact of not disposing correctly
- Accidental needles in trash and not searching trash for retrieval of sharp
- People who clean up room need to look for sharps in trays, etc.
- Inattentiveness

in turn, to provide an idea; unstructured brainstorming offers no such structure. Thus, anyone can contribute at any time. The unstructured format may be more advantageous when time is at a premium, thus, expediting the enumeration of ideas. The obvious pitfall is the potential for dominance by the more loquacious of the group; it does not take much for the session to degenerate into a cacophonous mess.

MULTIVOTING

Multivoting is a technique to quickly create consensus on choosing a few items from a long list. The list of choices, often generated through brainstorming, is numbered, and each member gets to vote multiple times, approximately one-fourth to one-third of the items on the list. The voting is done by a show of hands, and the items with the most votes are chosen. For example, if the original list has 30 items, each participant gets to vote 7 to 10 times. The more votes each participant has, the longer the process takes. Hatchet marks are made next to the item to represent a vote. Generally, a few items will have no votes, many items will have a few votes, and some items will be clear "winners" with most of the votes. Therefore, with limited debate, the group's preference is clear. Sometimes, the votes are scattered throughout the list with no clear group preferences. In this case, repeat multivoting with only those items that received at least two or three votes. Remember to limit the number of votes each participant has to no more than one-third of the items being voted on. If the new list has 20 items, then each participant has five to seven votes.

In the needle and scalpel example, participants wrote down the 10 numbers for the items they felt were high priority and warranted further data collection. The facilitator went item by item down the list and took a count of the hands/votes. In a relatively short time, the group identified which areas would be investigated further, with little discussion or arguing (Exhibit 16–3).

FLOWCHARTING

A *flowchart* is a graphic representation of the steps in a process such as admitting a patient to the hospital, ordering supplies, or scheduling an appointment. Once a problem area or quality improvement effort has been identified, one of the first steps needed is to construct a flowchart that describes the process (Berk & Berk, 1993).

Flowcharting uses universally accepted symbols to ease communication (Figure 16–1). These symbols identify procedural details such

---

Exhibit 16–3 Multivoting Results for Data Collection Priorities

### /	1 IV starts—2 needles needed— one accidentally in linens	//	17	Unaware of consequences of misplacing sharps
//	2 Lack of disciplinary action for non-compliance to proper disposal of sharps	### //	18	Lack of well-defined locations of sharps containers
	3 Part goes in sharps, part not; all in one bin (e.g., CVP insertion)		19	Sharps container full; what is full?
/	4 Lack of way to monitor compliance to procedure for sharps disposal	/	20	Inconvenient
			21	Sharps container used for trash
### ///	5 Needles—systems not used	### ### /	22	Trash can more convenient than sharps container
///	6 Opened tray and sharps not visible in bedside procedures	/	23	Style of sharps container—lock out
	7 Follow-up on incidents		24	Position/location of sharps container
	8 Clear safety policy and procedure standards	//	25	Not enough needle boxes
/	9 Accountability for monitoring	/	26	Not clear on what a "sharp" is
### ###	10 Person doing procedure does not clean up room; person who does clean does not know a sharp was used		27	Auto pilot—staff put sharps in regular trash automatically with other trash
//	11 Where to put sharp plastics (e.g., IV tubing)	/	28	Unclear of what CNA, MD to put in box; varies by area and emergent nature of procedure
###	12 Pushing drugs in codes without needle container available		29	Unclear expectation of role to empty sharps container
///	13 Training issues		30	Lack of knowledge of impact of not disposing correctly
/	14 Who is responsible; unclear roles		31	Accidental needles in trash and not searching trash for retrieval of sharp
### /	15 Unclear role definition of who checks for 3/4 full box	///	32	People who clean up room need to look for sharps in trays, etc.
	16 Lack of knowledge of impact of not disposing correctly		33	Inattentiveness

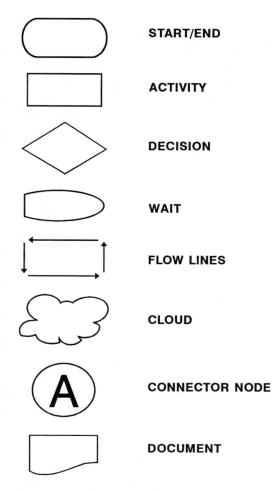

START/END

ACTIVITY

DECISION

WAIT

FLOW LINES

CLOUD

CONNECTOR NODE

DOCUMENT

Figure 16–1 Flowchart symbols

as start and end points, decision points, activity points, wait points, and clouds.

Flowcharting helps team members become knowledgeable about the entire process that affects the problem area. Thus, flowcharting ultimately serves to develop a common understanding of an overall process; uncover potential problems, bottlenecks, unnecessary steps, and rework loops or duplication of efforts; and guide a problem-solving discussion without directly observing the process. A flowchart provides a forum for discussing and formulating strategies geared to ameliorate inefficiencies in

the process. To couch it in a simplistic fashion, there is what may be euphemistically termed real work and non–real work. *Real work* is the minimal steps necessary to achieve a given output. However, frequently, additional steps may be needed to achieve a specific outcome, the causal nature possibly being due to incompetence, negligence, or lack of information. These additional steps exemplify rework or *non–real work*. A flowchart provides the background to investigate rework occurrences.

To ensure successful flowcharting, it is critical that the team be knowledgeable about the process at issue. Thus, if the process to be addressed involves a multidisciplinarian, multidepartmental effort, then representatives from each of the designated areas need to be part of the team. The assumption is that no single individual can be knowledgeable about the entire process; thus, the advantage of a diverse team becomes evident. For example, a continuous quality improvement project involving reduction in emergency room cardiac thrombolytic door-to-needle times may involve participants as diverse as emergency room physicians, nurses, admitting clerks, pharmacists, and transport staff. If the knowledge base about the process comes up lacking, then there are bound to be gaps in the flowcharting effort.

When the team first meets and agrees to focus their efforts in a specific process area, the flowcharting endeavor commences. First, there should be open discussion and consensus about the level of detail needed to define the process. A process may be a microcosm of another subprocess ad infinitum, so it is to the team's advantage to operationally define the specificity they choose to arrive at in constructing the flowchart. The team may agree to construct a general, high-level flowchart, with each activity potentially subsuming a wide array of processes; or they may isolate one specific process and arrive at an extensively detailed flowchart. Because this technique takes anywhere from two to four meetings, documentation should be on a transportable medium such as a flip chart or detachable notepads.

Given that constructing a flowchart can be a relatively time-consuming task, this process is served well by allotting a time limit to discussing any one specific step. The 5-minute rule is a productive rule of thumb: discussion regarding a particular step must not exceed 5 minutes without posting a symbol. If designating a symbol is problematic at this stage, then a cloud or a message is noted as a reminder to address this step at a later time.

Once the level of detail is agreed on, the group defines the first and last steps in the process. This provides a nice starting point to either work backward from the output or forward from the input. With one member facilitating the process, steps in the sequence are proposed and appropriately documented. Having too many clouds in the flowchart is a warning sign that not all of the key players are present. Once it is ascertained that the flowchart has been completed, it is reviewed in its totality to assess comprehensiveness and accuracy.

As the flowcharting process progresses, the facilitator encourages suggestions for improvement and potential intervention points. The flowchart process itself provides an opportunity for team members to juxtapose the actual process with what has been postulated as the ideal process. Points of discrepancies between the actual and ideal process can be discussed and noted as potential areas for data collection and subsequent intervention. Reviewing the flowchart also delineates where handoffs are occurring, either within or across departments, interdepartment work flows, rework loops, wait states, and points of measurement and decision making. Even though it is the collection of valid and reliable data that ultimately lends credence to what the primary problem areas may be in any designated process, the flowchart is designed to serve as a foundation to initiate problem identification efforts (Figures 16–2 and 16–3).

FISHBONE DIAGRAMS

A *fishbone diagram*, also called a cause-and-effect chart or Ishikawa diagram, is a visual display of causes of a problem. Information derived from flowcharting or brainstorming can serve as a springboard for deriving potential causes for problems. The overriding objective of fishbone diagrams is to organize and display theories about causes that may create a specific effect or problem. By focusing attention on a specific problem in a structured and systematic fashion, hypotheses and theories can be proposed.

The benefits of fishbone diagrams can be substantial. This technique allows constructive use of anecdotal evidence, encourages a balanced view of all possible causes, demonstrates the complexity and expansiveness of the problem, encourages scientific analysis, and can be helpful in guiding further inquiry and testing.

Assigning causality is always approached with caution, and, within the rigors of science, causation is made under conditions of random assignment, random selection, experimenter selection, and experimenter control (Keppel & Zedeck, 1989). Within the framework of quality improvement projects, experimental designs are rarely indicated, even though cause-and-effect analysis is a valuable adjunct to process improvement.

Cause-and-effect analysis entails constructing a skeletal structure, thus the name fishbone diagram, and designating major causal categories. Generically speaking, the categories may be what is called the 4 *M*s and a *P*: measurements, materials, methods, machines, and people. These categories are sufficiently broad and encompass most areas targeted for quality improvement efforts. Other causal categories may be tailored for specific problem areas (Exhibit 16–4).

To construct a fishbone diagram, begin with drawing a fish skeleton (Figure 16–4). Then write a clearly defined effect or symptom for which causes must be identified in the large box at the end of the horizontal line. Write the categories for the causes in the smaller boxes at the end of the oblique lines. Now fill in the diagram with causes under each of the major categories. If necessary, add subsidiary causes for

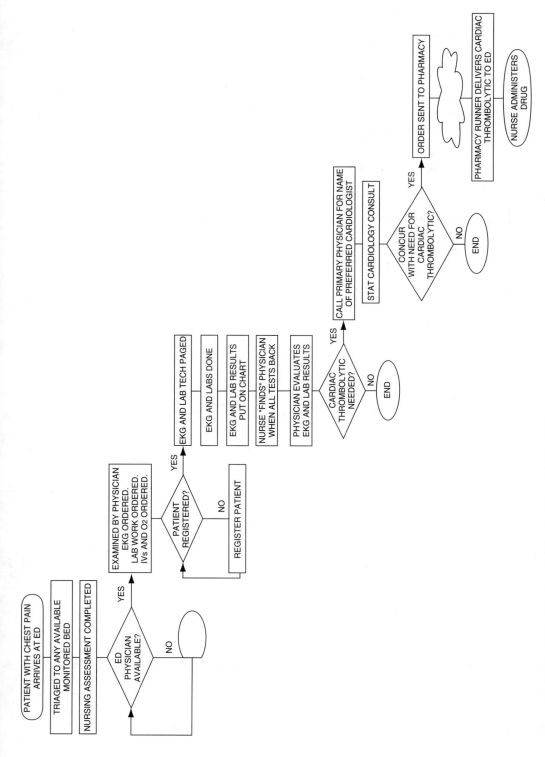

Figure 16-2 Original cardiac thrombolytic door-to-needle flowchart

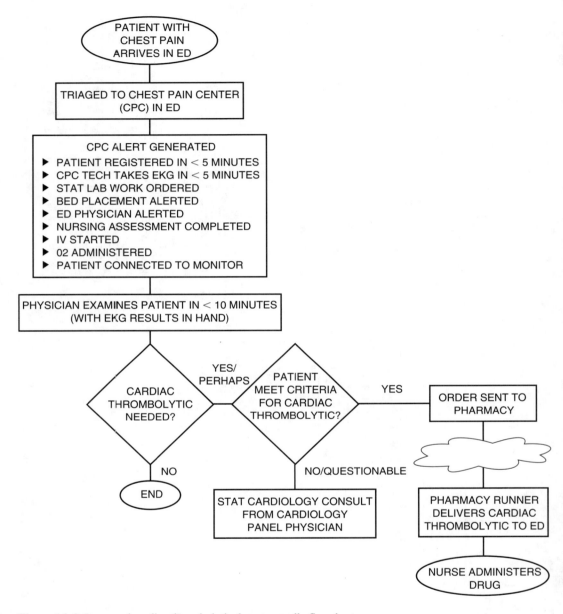

Figure 16–3 Improved cardiac thrombolytic door-to-needle flowchart

causes that have already been identified (Figure 16–5).

As with the other techniques, criticisms of novel but logical causal factors are overtly discouraged. Lengthy discourse over minutiae is

also suppressed. Once the diagram is completed, other quality improvement tools may be used. Multivoting may be used to prioritize problems or areas for data collection. Again, cause-and-effect analysis is only as effective as

Exhibit 16–4 Ws, Ms, Ps of Cause and Effect

What	Manpower	People
Why	Materials	Provisions (supplies)
When	Methods	Procedures
Where	Machines	Place (environment)
	Measures	Patrons (customers)

the logical input that is provided by the team members.

DATA ANALYSIS

A primary objective of quality improvement data analysis is to differentiate between common cause and special cause variation so appropriate improvement strategies can be formulated. *Common cause variation* is random and inherent in all processes. Data analysis is focused on all of the data. Remember, numbers do three things: increase, decrease, or remain the same. There is always a range of normal fluctuation in data, and that range is common cause variation. Improvement strategies for common cause variation are focused on identifying root causes and overhauling the work process. For example, cardiac door-to-needle times in one emergency room vary from 20 to 90 minutes randomly. The only way to decrease the overall, median rate of 47 minutes is to analyze the data from all patients, identify the root cause for the 47-minute median rate, and then improve the process.

Special cause variation is not random. Special cause variation is the result of special circumstances that cause some of the data to fall outside the range of normal fluctuation. Analysis is focused only on the data outside the normal range. Changes are made to prevent the special circumstances from recurring. Overhauling the entire process creates unnecessary

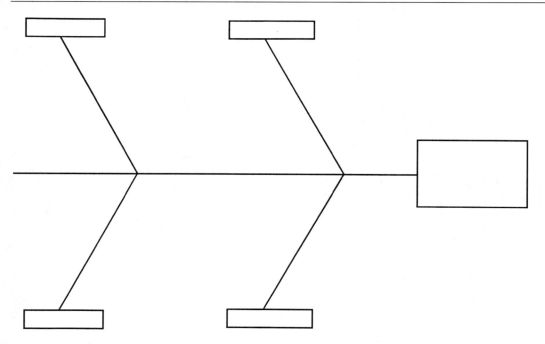

Figure 16–4 Fishbone diagram skeleton

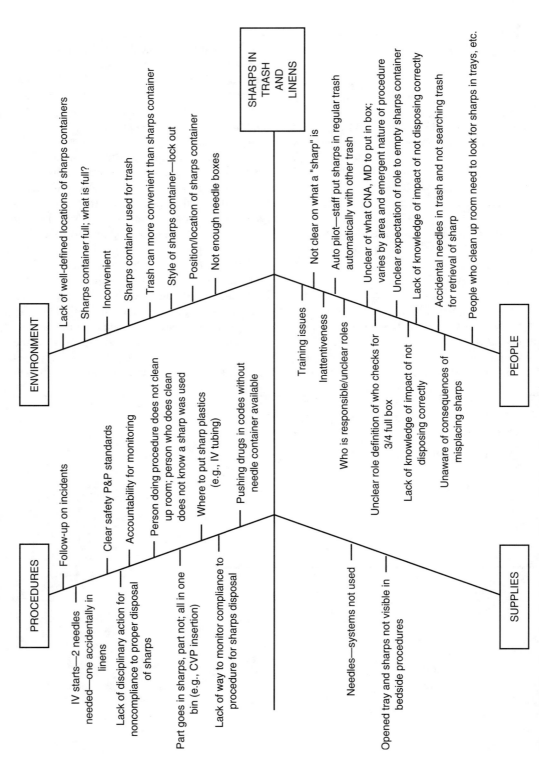

Figure 16–5 Needles and scalpels in trash and linens: Fishbone diagram

work and change if the overall performance is satisfactory. For example, the normal range for cardiac door-to-needle times in another emergency room is 15 to 45 minutes, with a median of 31 minutes. One cardiac door-to-needle time was 2 hours and 15 minutes. Embarking on a process improvement project to overhaul the entire process is inappropriate because the median and normal range of times is commendable. The improvement strategy is to determine what happened in the individual case that took 2 hours and 15 minutes. The objective is to prevent the special circumstances from recurring. Run charts and control charts are two tools that help differentiate common cause (random) and special cause (nonrandom) variation.

Run Charts

A *run chart* is a line graph that displays data over time and illustrates trends (Figure 16–6). The vertical axis represents the data value such as a frequency, time, or rate, and the horizontal axis represents the sequence of the measurement such as the day, month, or patient in order of occurrence. Data are plotted in the exact time occurrence and, generally, at least 15 data points are necessary to capture any patterns or trends. It is often difficult to determine if the variation is common cause or special cause with a run chart, and, hence, the need for control charts with statistically calculated control limits.

Control Charts

A *control chart* is a run chart with a mean or median line and a statistically calculated upper control limit (UCL) and lower control limit (LCL). Calculation of the UCL and LCL vary depending on the specific type of data; however, the two common control charts in health care are the individuals chart and the p chart (Fields & Siroky, 1994). Individuals charts are used when the data are individual measurements such as wait times, laboratory values, and other nonproportional frequencies. Two calculations are

needed to compute the control limits: the data mean $(\overline{X})$ and the median of the range between data points $(\widetilde{R})$. If there is wide variation in the data with outliers, the data mean will be skewed and should be substituted with the median. The formula for the UCL is $\overline{X} + (3.14 \cdot \widetilde{R})$ and the formula for the LCL is $\overline{X} - (3.14 \cdot \widetilde{R})$ (Table 16–1 and Figure 16–7).

The p chart is used when the data are proportional such as unplanned readmission rates, mortality rates, or percentage of patients on time. Two calculations are needed to compute the control limits: the mean of the proportions $(\overline{p})$ and the standard deviation of the proportion $(SD\overline{p})$. The formula for the UCL is $\overline{p} + (3 \cdot SD\overline{p})$ and the formula for the LCL is $\overline{p} - (3 \cdot SD\overline{p})$. The formula for the $SD\overline{p}$ is

$$\sqrt{\frac{\overline{p}(1 - \overline{p})}{\overline{n}}}$$

(Fields & Siroky, 1994; Table 16–2 and Figure 16–8).

Once the calculations are completed, horizontal lines for the mean or median, UCL and LCL are drawn and the control chart data can be analyzed. The UCL and LCL approximate three standard deviations above and below the mean or median. Data variation within the control limits is generally random and from variation inherent in the process with 99% confidence. Data outside the control limits are generally from special circumstances.

If all data are within the control limits, the process is considered to be in statistical control with only common cause variation (Fields & Siroky, 1994; Paulson et al., 1992). That does not mean performance is satisfactory. The question remains whether the overall average rate is acceptable. The questions to guide data analysis and focus improvement efforts in common cause variation include, What is common to all of the data? What caused this process to create this result? What needs to be changed to improve the process and outcome? In common cause variation, the strategy is geared toward eliminating those causes that are common to all of the data points. Day-to-day or

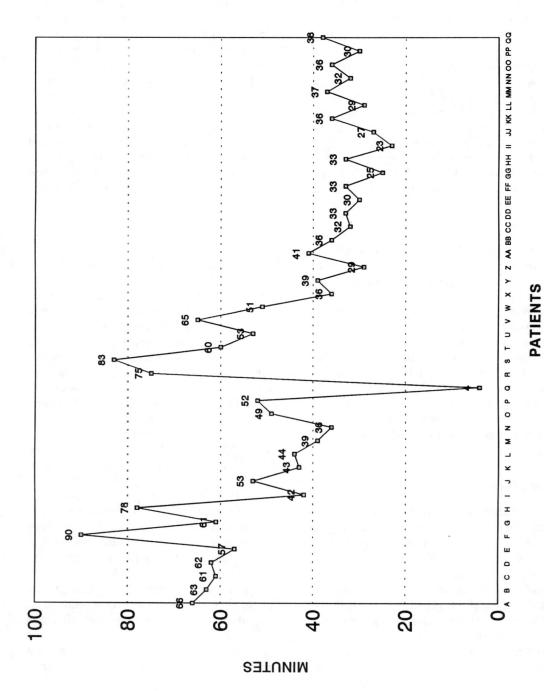

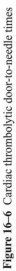

Figure 16–6 Cardiac thrombolytic door-to-needle times

Table 16–1 Calculations for Individuals Chart

Patient	Minutes	Range between Patients	Median of Ranges
A	65	—	1
B	63	2	1
C	61	2	1
D	62	1	2
E	57	5	2
F	90	33	3
G	61	29	3
H	78	17	3
I	42	36	3
J	53	11	3
K	43	10	4
L	44	1	4
M	39	5	4
N	36	3	5
O	49	13	5
P	52	3	5
Q	4	48	5
R	75	71	6
S	83	8	7
T	60	23	7 ←
U	53	7	8
V	65	12	• $\widetilde{R} = 8$
W	51	14	8
X	36	15	8
Y	39	3	8
Z	29	10	8
AA	41	12	9
BB	36	5	10
CC	32	4	10
DD	33	1	10
EE	30	3	11
FF	33	3	12
GG	25	8	12
HH	33	8	13
II	23	10	14
JJ	27	4	15
KK	36	9	17
LL	29	7	23
MM	37	8	29
NN	32	5	33
OO	36	4	36
PP	30	6	48
QQ	38	8	71

$$\overline{X} = 46.2$$

$$UCL = \overline{X} + (3.14 \cdot \widetilde{R}) \qquad LCL = \overline{X} - (3.14 \cdot \widetilde{R})$$
$$= 46.2 + (3.14 \cdot 8) \qquad\quad = 46.2 - (3.14 \cdot 8)$$
$$= 71.3 \qquad\qquad\qquad\quad = 21.1$$

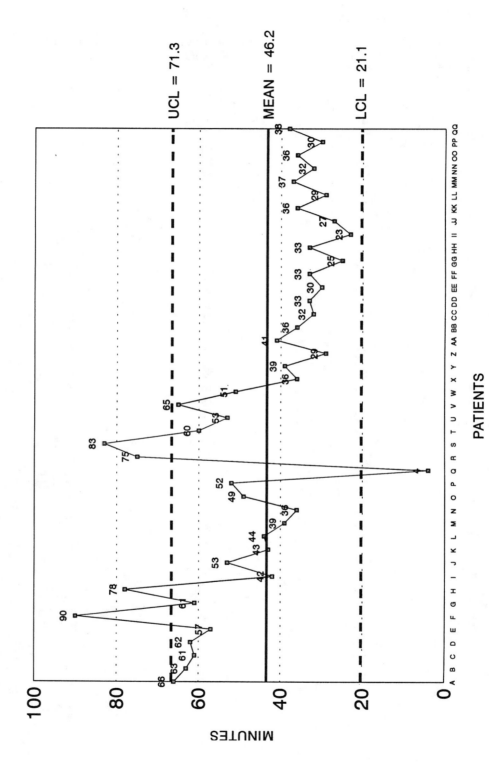

Figure 16–7 Individuals control chart

Table 16–2   Calculations for p Chart for Unplanned Readmissions

Month	Unplanned Readmissions	Hospital Discharges	Unplanned Readmission Rate (%)
J 95	54	2,455	2.2
F	69	2,405	2.9
M	93	2,525	3.7
A	88	2,721	3.2
M	89	2,555	3.5
J	104	2,588	4.0
J	110	2,736	4.0
A	95	2,677	3.5
S	88	2,760	3.2
O	108	2,534	4.3
N	92	2,486	3.7
D	118	2,563	4.6
J 96	104	2,576	4.0
F	91	2,560	3.6
M	89	2,493	3.6
A	80	2,469	3.2
M	97	2,685	3.6
J	93	2,554	3.6
J	86	2,612	3.3
A	87	2,454	3.5
S	86	2,581	3.3
		n = 2,571	p = 3.5%

$$SD\bar{p} = \sqrt{\frac{\bar{p}(100^* - \bar{p})}{\bar{n}}}$$

$$= \sqrt{\frac{3.5(100 - 3.5)}{2,571}}$$

$$= \sqrt{.1314}$$

$$= .36$$

$$UCL = \bar{p} + (3 \cdot SD\bar{p})$$

$$= 3.5 + (3 \cdot .36)$$

$$= 4.6$$

$$LCL = \bar{p} - (3 \cdot SD\bar{p})$$

$$= 3.5 - (3 \cdot .36)$$

$$= 2.4$$

*100 used because $\bar{p}$ is a percentage.

patient-to-patient variations are not meaningful. Pareto charts and scatter diagrams help further analyze common cause variation and direct areas for process improvement. As Deming (1986) has suggested: "Statistical control of a process is not an end in itself. Once statistical control is established, serious work to improve quality and economy of production can commence" (p. 354).

If there are data points outside the control limits, the process is not in statistical control and there is probably special cause variation. In this situation, the data outside the control limits are analyzed to determine what caused these specific results. Questions to help with this analysis include, What is special about this situation? What caused this value to be different? What happened to create this result this time?

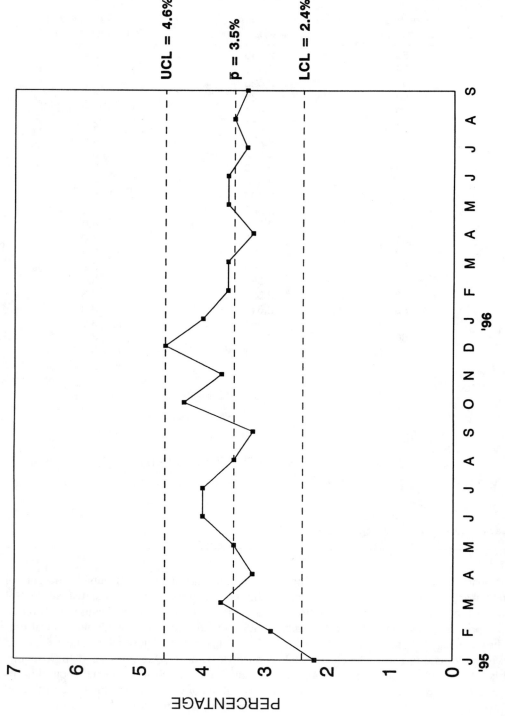

Figure 16–8 Unplanned readmissions p chart

Why is this value different from the others? Answers to these questions will help determine what needs to be prevented in the future.

Control chart analysis stimulates questions; it does not provide answers other than whether there is common cause or special cause variation. Control charts highlight areas for further investigation; they do not tell what the problem is or how to fix it. Control charts can illustrate if a process has changed. The process has changed if six or more consecutive data points increase, six or more consecutive data points decrease, or if eight or more successive data points are on the same side of the mean or median. Statistically, these data patterns occur only through process changes and not randomly. Therefore, the control chart displays a successful intervention or some change in the process. In Figure 16–7, the last 20 patients had door-to-needle times less than the mean. This pattern could not have occurred randomly, and is the result of a successful process improvement activity. It is now time to recalculate the control limits beginning with the first patient in the new process.

Histograms

A *histogram* is a bar chart that displays a graphical summary of the pattern and distribution of variation in a set of data. The length of each bar represents the frequency of the measurement. The order of the bars depends on what the histogram is illustrating. Figures 16–9 and 16–10 use the identical data, but the bars are arranged differently. Figure 16–9 highlights the wide variation across patient care units, whereas Figure 16–10 illustrates the units with the highest and lowest census and the gradual differences across units. Histograms are also used to summarize the frequency of various values such as wait times, laboratory values, or any other measurement in a sample. For example, Figure 16–11 graphically displays a summary of emergency unit patient stays in minutes. The histogram easily accents that, although the average stay is 191 minutes, most patients stay between 121 and 180 minutes, with hardly any patients staying longer than 361 minutes.

Pareto Charts

The Pareto chart, named after an Italian economist, is a bar chart that stratifies data by decreasing or increasing frequency and is grounded on the 80/20 rule. This rule maintains that 80% of the results are characteristically attributable to 20% of the causes (Berk & Berk, 1993). The Pareto chart ultimately ranks the importance of problems or conditions.

In health care, contributors to a problem might include services, items, process steps, time of day, day of week, people, complications, complaints, or resource use. For example, if one is interested in exploring the possible reasons for an unplanned readmission rate, a Pareto chart can be used to display stratified results of the patients included in the unplanned readmission sample, such as major diagnostic codes or types of unplanned readmissions (Figures 16–12 and 16–13).

The horizontal line represents the categories, such as major diagnostic codes, and the vertical line represents the frequency for each category. The curved line crossing the bars represents the cumulative percentage for each category. For example, in Figure 16–12 there are 164 cases who were readmitted for circulatory system problems. These 164 cases are 22% of the total sample of 752 patients. The 144 respiratory patients, when added to the circulatory patients, represent 41% of the total. This Pareto chart clearly demonstrates that more than 50% of the unplanned readmission patients are from three major diagnostic groups: circulatory, respiratory, and digestive. Figure 16–13 displays that the majority of the patients have chronic conditions and they are noncompliant with their treatment plans. Therefore, if the unplanned readmission rate is deemed an opportunity for improvement, then efforts should be directed toward chronic circulatory, respiratory, and digestive patients who are noncompliant. Focusing on ear, nose, and

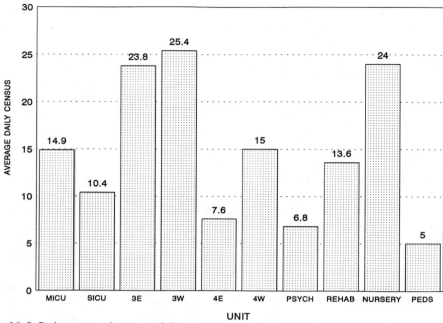

Figure 16–9 Patient care unit average daily census

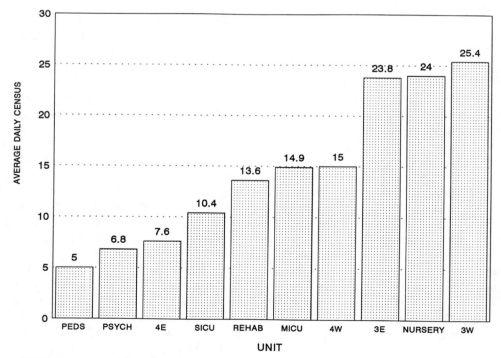

Figure 16–10 Patient care unit average daily census

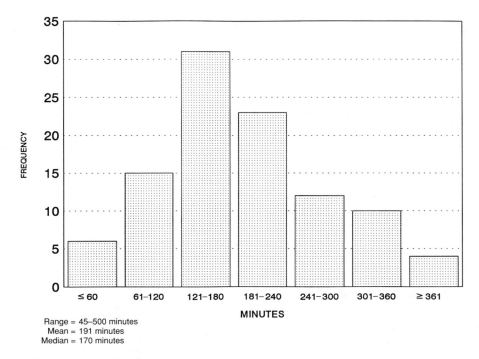

Range = 45–500 minutes
Mean = 191 minutes
Median = 170 minutes

Figure 16–11 Patient length of stay in emergency room

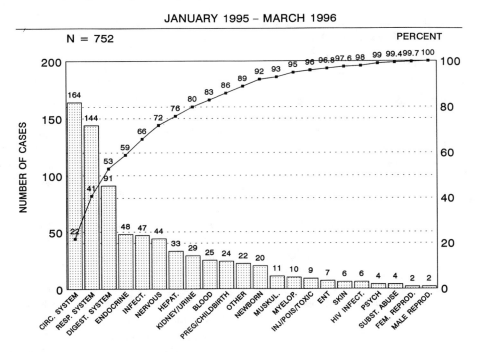

Figure 16–12 Unplanned readmissions by major diagnostic codes

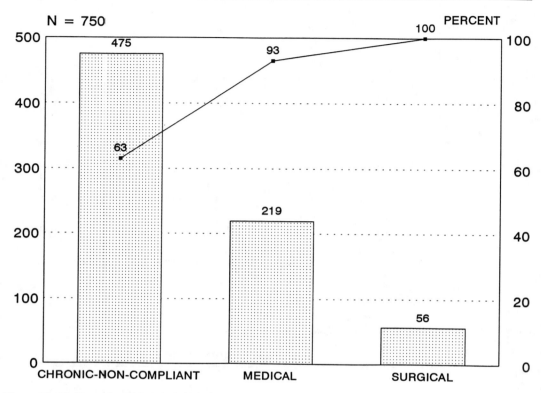

JANUARY 1995 – MARCH 1996.

Figure 16–13 Type of unplanned readmission

throat surgical patients will improve that category of patients, but because the number of patients in that group is small, the improvement efforts will have little effect on the overall unplanned readmission rate.

Scatter Diagram

A *scatter diagram* graphically represents the relationship between two variables. Many times we ask questions that invoke relationships among variables. What is the relationship between length of stay and charges? How are diet and cardiovascular reactivity associated? How do number of infections and number of staff nurses covary? Statistically speaking, the Pearson product–moment correlation coefficient (r) is used to calculate the relationship between two

variables (Heiman, 1996). The correlation coefficient (r) value can range from a $+1.0$ for a perfect, positive linear relationship, through 0.0 for no linear relationship, to a -1.0 for a perfect, negative linear relationship. A scatter diagram visually represents the Pearson product–moment correlation coefficient.

The data that serve as the foundation for analyzing a scatter diagram should be continuous in nature. Such variables may be time, speed, temperatures, or weights. Sometimes ordinal-level data such as a 5-point disagree-to-agree scale is used in a scatter diagram, but, mathematically, there can be problems and therefore a risk of misinterpretation exists.

In creating a scatter diagram, two continuous level variables are measured simultaneously, such as length of stay and charges. Enough paired data should be collected to sufficiently represent the spectrum of the data metric; otherwise one can run into a restriction in range difficulty (Nunnally, 1978). This occurs when the variability of one of the variables is constrained by biased sampling procedures. Graphically speaking, a horizontal and vertical axis are drawn, each representing one of the variables (Figure 16–14). Each of the paired data points is plotted in relation to the scales for both of the axes.

Once all of the paired data points have been plotted, the interpretation on the relationship of the variables commences. Variables that are positively related indicate that as one variable increases, the other also increases. Conversely, an inverse relationship is depicted by the increase of one variable with an attendant decrease of the other. If there is mass dispersion of the data points with no discernible pattern, a weak relationship is evident (see Figure 16–14). For example, in Figure 16–14, the scatter diagram with a negative relationship between length of stay and charges has paired data points in an upper left to lower right pattern. This pattern illustrates that, as length of stay increases, charges decrease. The closer the pattern is to a straight line, the more perfect the relationship is between the two variables of length of stay and charges. The scatter diagram with a positive relationship has paired data points in a lower left to upper right pattern, which illustrates that as length of stay increases, so do charges. The scatter diagram illustrating no relationship between length of stay and charges has a circular pattern.

However, just because a detectable pattern exists between two variables, it does not stipulate causation. Unfortunately, the boundaries between correlations and causation sometimes become blurred. For example, the conclusion that the number of years of education is associated with income slips into the conclusion that education will cause a person's income to increase. The conclusion that education will cause income to increase can only be verified with further statistical analysis within an experimental context. Hence, how one interprets the data, and ultimately articulates their interpretation, is critical if an unblemished picture of the data is to be accurately conveyed to staff and management.

CONCLUSION

This chapter has described common tools used in both formal quality improvement teams and management decision making. These tools assist with the effectiveness of group problem solving while minimizing interpersonal conflict. Used effectively, they help to create a continuous quality improvement culture in an organization.

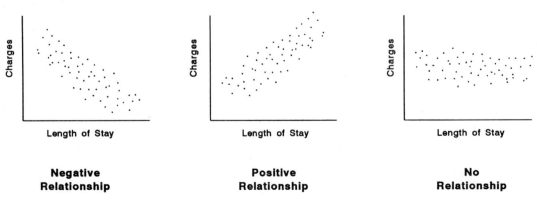

Figure 16–14 Scatter plot for length of stay and charges

REFERENCES

Berk, J., & Berk, S. (1993). *Total quality management: Implementing continuous improvement.* New York: Sterling Publishing.

Bucholz, S., & Roth, T. (1987). *Creating the high performance team.* New York: Wiley.

Deming, W.E. (1986). *Out of the crisis.* Cambridge, MA: MIT Press.

Fields, W.L., & Siroky, K.A. (1994). Converting data into information. *Journal of Nursing Care Quality, 8*(3), 1–11.

Heiman, G.W. (1996). *Basic statistics for the behavioral sciences* (2nd ed.). Boston: Houghton-Mifflin.

Keppel, G., & Zedeck, S. (1989). *Data analysis for research designs.* New York: W.H. Freeman.

Nunnally, J.C. (1978). *Psychometric theory* (2nd ed.). New York: McGraw-Hill.

Paulson, D., Wasik, J., Tarker, B., & Shumate, C. (1992). *Fundamentals of total quality leadership.* Department of the Navy: Navy Personnel Research and Development Center.

## CHAPTER 17

Preparing the Undergraduate Student and Faculty to Use Quality Improvement in Practice

Patricia Kelly-Heidenthal

CHAPTER OBJECTIVES

After completing this chapter, the reader will be able to:

- identify appropriate content for curricula using either an integrated approach or an individual course approach to teaching quality improvement
- conduct insightful self- and professional evaluations
- use several strategies to develop quality improvement knowledge and skills critical for students and faculties
- develop a master plan for evaluating a school or department

The authority for nursing, as with other professions, is based on a contract between society and the profession. Under the terms of this contract, members of the profession are expected to act responsibly and ensure quality. Inherent in this contract is the idea that every nurse is accountable for quality professional practice (Larson, 1992, p. 226). This accountability is essential if the needs of society are to be met.

Accountability applies to both nurse educators and registered nursing students at all three undergraduate levels—baccalaureate, diploma,

and associate degree. Early in the educational process, nursing educators lay the foundation for the development of student accountability for quality nursing practice. Faculty teach standards for quality and develop classroom and clinical strategies, including role modeling, to demonstrate accountability for monitoring and improving quality. This accountability will be further developed throughout the nurse's professional career.

CHARACTERISTICS OF THE EMERGING HEALTH CARE SYSTEM

The Pew Health Professions Commission, a national commission composed of nurses, physicians, and others concerned with health care, has identified that much of the U. S. health care industry has been transformed to systems of integrated care that combine primary, specialty, and hospital services. These integrated care systems strive to manage the care delivered to enrolled patient populations to reduce costs, enhance patient and consumer satisfaction, and improve health care outcomes.

The Pew Commission predicts that, by the year 2000, the American health care system, in general, will be (Pew Commission, 1995):

- **more managed** with better integration of services and financing
- **more accountable** to those who purchase and use health services

Note: The Editor wishes to acknowledge Elizabeth Larson, MSN, RN, Professor Emeritus, University of Wisconsin Oshkosh, who contributed this chapter to the first edition.

- **more aware** of and responsive to the needs of enrolled populations
- **more effective** in using fewer resources
- **more innovative and diverse** in how it provides for health
- **more inclusive** in how it defines health
- **more concerned** with education, prevention, and care management and less focused on treatment
- **more oriented** to improving the health of the entire population
- more reliant on outcome data and evidence

To deal with this health care system, the Pew Commission has identified a broad set of competencies that the Commission believes all health care professionals should master by the year 2005. These competencies broadly expand accountability for health care quality improvement for nursing and other health care providers. Nursing educators have begun to study these competencies as well as general health care trends to determine curriculum implications for broadening the quality improvement role of the nurse.

QUALITY IMPROVEMENT ROLE OF THE NURSE

The quality improvement role of the nurse builds on traditional nursing content and increasingly calls for nurses who are oriented to improving health care processes for customers in various settings. These customers include the patient, family, and community, as well as other health care departments and disciplines. Improving the health care process for these customers increasingly calls for such quality improvement knowledge and skills as

- developing awareness of cost-effective quality standards
- developing computer skills for managing information
- using statistical process control methods
- benchmarking, or comparing information against valid and reliable sources of information

- using structured problem-solving methods such as the Plan–Do–Check–Act (PDCA) method
- understanding the need for leadership commitment to improved cost-effective customer outcomes
- developing strategies to empower staff to work with a multidisciplinary team to improve all health care processes continuously
- developing the ability to evaluate customer outcomes from broad organization-wide and community-wide perspectives, in addition to traditional department- or discipline-specific perspectives

Some of this information may be new content for nursing education programs, and not all of it may be appropriate for the undergraduate nursing curriculum. This content for quality improvement, knowledge and skills, needs to be examined by faculty in all three types of registered nursing education programs (associate degree, diploma, and baccalaureate). All three of these programs should consider the inclusion of appropriate quality improvement knowledge and skills, in addition to traditional nursing content, in their curriculum design. The expanding quality improvement role of the nurse calls for this consideration.

Curriculum Design for Quality Improvement

When developing undergraduate curricula to prepare the student for the quality improvement role of the nurse, faculty will most probably use an integrated curriculum approach to quality improvement (Exhibit 17–1). A separate course on quality improvement can also be developed (Exhibit 17–2). These exhibits build on the sample curriculum, needs, and trends for health care education, quality improvement, and evaluation identified by Larson (1992); Gelmon and Baker (1995); Genovich-Richards (1989); Norman, Randall, and Hornsby (1990); Hoare, Burns, and Akerlund (1985); Johnson (1995); Reilly and Oermann (1992); Poirrier, Wills, Broussard, and

Exhibit 17–1 Integrated Approach to Quality Improvement

Introductory Courses
Level One and/or Two

- Roles
  - Nursing
  - Health care team
  - Patient as customer
  - Community as customer
- Components of quality
- Accountability, personal and professional
- Cost-effective quality care
- Values clarification
  - Quality
  - Health care
  - Nursing
  - Customer
  - Community
- Elements of quality improvement
  - Assessment of customer needs
  - Improvement of processes and outcomes
  - Structured problem solving
  - Report cards—benchmarks
  - Empowerment of the multidisciplinary team
  - Leadership responsibility
- Communication skills
- Standards of care
- Evaluation
  - Component of nursing process
- Need for personal and professional evaluation of self/peer/faculty
- Documentation
- Use of computers
- Agencies concerned with quality
  - American Nurses Association Model for Quality
  - Joint Commission on Accreditation of Healthcare Organizations
  - Federal and State regulators
  - Pew Health Care Commission
  - National League for Nursing
  - Agency for Health Care Policy and Research

Level Three

- Quality assurance versus quality improvement
- Quality improvement and the nursing process
- Structure, process, and outcome monitors
- Criteria development
- Professional, political, societal, and historical factors concerned with quality
- Nursing minimum data sets
- Uniform clinical data sets
- Clinical practice guidelines
- Personal and professional evaluation
- Use of power

Level Four

- Tools and methods to evaluate care
- Research and quality improvement—critique of studies
- Management information systems
- Retrospective/concurrent audits
- Risk management, utilization review
- Acuity systems
- Broad organization-wide and community-wide quality improvement versus department or discipline-specific quality improvement
- Multidisciplinary team building and empowerment
- Variation in health care
- Responsibility of professional leaders for quality improvement
- Change process
- Cost of quality
- Plan–Do–Check–Act method
- Storyboards
- Baldrige Health Care Quality Pilot Criteria 1995
- Development of methods to measure nursing interventions and outcomes
- Survey current practices in quality improvement, e.g., customer assessment tools, continuous process improvement, outcome monitors

Payne (1996); Headrick, Neuhauser, Melnikow, and Vanek (1991); Sposato (1994); Ackerman and Nash (1991); Best, Carswell, and Abbott (1990); the Pew Commission (1995); and the Malcolm Baldrige Health Care Pilot Criteria (1995). These exhibits are useful in faculty discussion of appropriate quality improvement content for various types of nursing curriculum.

Exhibit 17–2 Outline for Quality Improvement Course

Objectives
1. Discuss professional accountability for providing cost-effective quality nursing care.
2. Identify components of cost-effective quality.
3. Describe elements of quality improvement.
4. Discuss why quality improvement is needed.
5. Identify leaders in the quality improvement effort.
6. Describe management information systems for system-wide quality improvement efforts versus department-specific monitoring activities.
7. Demonstrate the knowledge, skills, and attitudes needed to participate in quality improvement activities in health care.
8. Participate in peer review and self-assessment activities.
9. Demonstrate an awareness of benchmarking and other current issues and practices in quality improvement.
10. Integrate critical thinking and evaluation of customer outcomes in all personal and professional activities.

Content

1. Accountability
   • Societal need for nursing care
   • Professional mandates
   • Personal and professional goals
2. Components of cost-effective quality
   • Need to define quality
   • Customer perspective
   • Access, clinical care processes, human aspects, outcomes, environment, function
   • Dimensions of quality, availability, accessibility, appropriateness, etc.
   • Cost-effective standards of quality
3. Elements of quality improvement
   • Customer needs assessment
   • Improvement of key processes and outcomes
   • Structured problem solving using Plan–Do–Check–Act (PDCA) method
   • Benchmarks
   • Statistical process control methods
   • Empowerment and strategies for increasing power
   • Multidisciplinary teams
   • Leadership responsibility for cost-effective quality outcomes
4. Factors influencing quality improvement
   • Customer definition—patient, family, community, multidisciplinary departments and disciplines
   • Legislation
   • Managed care for patient populations
   • Wennburg variation studies
   • Cost-effective care needs
   • High technology
   • Ethical issues
   • Management information systems
   • Process improvement

continues

Exhibit 17–2 continued

- System redesign
- Report cards
- Health care reimbursement—public and private insurance companies
5. Discussion of terms
    - Quality improvement, quality assessment, total quality management, continuous quality improvement, quality assurance, quality control
    - Criteria, standard, norms, objectives, indicators
    - Monitor, evaluate, assess, audit
    - Benchmarks
    - System-wide quality improvement versus department-specific monitoring
    - Data retrieval
    - Mission, vision, strategic planning
6. Gurus of Quality
    - Deming, Juran, Crosby, Ishikawa, Shewhart
    - Lange, Donabedian, Berwick
7. Standards
    - American Nurses' Association Model, National League for Nursing
    - Joint Commission on Accreditation of Healthcare Organizations
    - Federal and state regulations
8. Approaches to evaluating care
    - Structure, process, outcome indicators
    - Retrospective and concurrent review
    - Development of monitors
    - Tools for evaluating care
    - Report cards and benchmarking
    - Management information systems
    - Using data/technology/computers
    - Severity of illness acuity measures
    - Baldrige Health Care Pilot Criteria 1995
    - Uniform clinical data sets
    - Nursing intervention and outcome data sets
9. Skills needed in evaluation of care
    - Observation skills
    - Communication skills
    - Critical thinking
    - Change process
    - Self-evaluation
    - Peer review
    - Research ensuring reliable and valid data
    - Problem solving
    - Decision making
    - Conflict resolution
    - Power
    - Collaborative processes
    - Community/family/patient involvement

continues

Exhibit 17–2 continued

10. Approaches to improving practice
    • Implementing change
    • Motivating others
    • Lifelong learning
    • Leadership responsibility
    • Statistical process control
    • Plan–Do–Check–Act method
    • Reduction of variation
    • Agency for Health Care Policy and Research (AHCPR), Clinical Practice
    • Guidelines and Outcomes Research
    • Discipline-specific monitoring versus total outcome monitoring
11. Multidisiciplinary quality improvement teams
    • Empowerment and team building
    • National ICU study
12. Current activities
    • Risk management
    • Utilization review
    • Quality improvement
    • Storyboards
    • Credentialing

Faculty interested in quality improvement curriculum development may also want to observe future efforts of these organizations:

- National League for Nursing (NLN)
- American Association of Colleges of Nursing (AACN)
- Institute for Health Care Improvement (Boston)
- American Association of University Programs in Health Care Administration (Arlington, Virginia)

AACN is beginning a task force to review baccalaureate nursing education curriculum essentials, while the latter two groups have developed a curriculum guide for quality improvement education in health care (Gelmon & Baker, 1995).

Whether an integrated approach or a separate unit or course is developed, educators should consider whether integration of content throughout a curriculum introduces the risk that such content might be minimized or lost. They should take precautions to ensure inclusion of important curriculum content (Johnson, 1995). The other danger of developing a specific course or unit on quality improvement is that evaluation and quality improvement are addressed only in one nursing course and otherwise neglected. Whether faculty use an integrated approach or a separate unit or course, this content must be introduced early. This ensures that quality improvement becomes an integrated part of the student's learning experience, with classroom knowledge reinforced in the clinical lab and opportunities provided for the development of a quality improvement approach to personal and professional development.

Additionally, faculty may want to develop critical thinking strategies to assist the learner's quality improvement knowledge development. This will also lay the groundwork for progression from quality improvement novice to advanced beginner to competency to proficiency and finally, to expert, as a nursing student, and later as a registered nurse (Benner, 1984). Critical thinking cannot be developed in one course or through one clinical assignment. Development of this skill requires sustained learning activities over a period of time and teachers who in their interactions with learners encourage and support the critical thinking of students (Reilly & Oermann, 1992, p. 231). Some activities to develop personal and professional critical thinking and quality improvement skills are useful.

Personal and Professional Development of Quality Improvement

The ability to conduct realistic self- and professional evaluations, including participating in effective peer review, is an important behavior in the development of a professional nurse with critical thinking and quality improvement skills. Several activities that assist with this development might include (Larson, 1992, p. 230)

- Personal goal setting
- Professional goal setting

- Self-evaluation
- Patient interview
- Patient observation
- Criteria and indicator development
- Peer review exercises
- Chart audits
- Critiques of current quality improvement and research studies
- Attendance at quality improvement committee meetings
- Interviews of staff about role in quality improvement
- Development of a storyboard

Faculty and students can select tools from Exhibit 17–3, as well as refer to the references and suggested reading at the conclusion of this chapter, for a selection of readings to build knowledge and skills in some of these quality

Exhibit 17–3 Tools To Develop Student's Knowledge of Quality Improvement Activities

Personal and Professional Goal Setting (Exhibit 17–4)	Students learn to set and evaluate personal and professional goals as one step in personal quality improvement.
Peer/Self Evaluation (Exhibit 17–5)	Students develop and use quality improvement strategies for self- and peer evaluation.
Feedback Pitfalls (Exhibit 17–6)	This tool assists students and faculty to avoid common pitfalls in giving feedback (Larson, 1992).
Pain Monitor (Exhibit 17–7)	Students monitor patient satisfaction using tool developed from guidelines from Agency for Health Care Policy and Research (AHCPR) Clinical Practice Guidelines.
Plan–Do–Check–Act (PDCA) method (Exhibit 17–8)	Students apply problem solving for quality improvement using the PDCA method.
Staff Quick Quiz (Exhibit 17–9)	Students adapt nursing home quiz to interview agency staff regarding agency quality improvement needs.
Power Building (Exhibit 17–10)	This exercise builds student understanding of the role of power in improving quality.
Cost and Quality (Exhibit 17–11)	Students identify cost of delivering one nursing care standard.
Mission and Quality Improvement (Exhibit 17–12)	Students identify the relationship of mission to quality improvement monitors. SPC tools, benchmarking, and storyboards are highlighted.

improvement activities. Exhibit 17–4 illustrates a tool that is useful for personal and professional goal setting by students. The tool can be introduced early in the nursing curriculum and reviewed and revised regularly throughout to assist the student in goal setting for quality improvement.

Exhibit 17–5 illustrates a guideline and tool for peer and/or self evaluation activities. These tools are not used for grading, and data submitted in relation to a peer is not used by faculty to grade that peer (Larson, 1992). Exhibit 17–6 can be shared with students to help them avoid common pitfalls in giving peer feed-

Exhibit 17–4 Student Guideline for Personal and Professional Goal Setting

Identify goals in each area—evaluate and update on target date.

Personal	Target date	Evaluation
1.		
2.		
3.		
4.		
5.		

Professional/ Academic	Target date	Evaluation
1.		
2.		
3.		
4.		
5.		

Professional/ Career	Target date	Evaluation
1.		
2.		
3.		
4.		
5.		

Other	Target date	Evaluation
1.		
2.		
3.		
4.		
5.		

back. Faculty will also find these tips helpful in giving feedback to students. Exhibit 17–7 illustrates a quality improvement monitor that can be used by students to evaluate and improve the quality of pain management. This tool was developed using the Agency for Health Care Policy and Research (AHCPR) Clinical Practice Guideline for Pain Management.

Finally, for the more mature student, Exhibit 17–8 shows the use of the PDCA method as a structured problem-solving format for quality improvement. Exhibit 17–9 shows a tool for assessing organizationwide commitment to quality improvement. Exhibits 17–10, 17–11, and 17–12 help students explore the role of power in quality improvement as well as the cost of

---

Exhibit 17–5 Peer/Self Evaluation

OBJECTIVE
  Promote growth in professional autonomy.
  Improve quality of health care.
IMPLEMENTATION
  List 8–10 measurable criteria that indicate a quality patient outcome.
  Finalize criteria with peer—collect appropriate data.
  Evaluate self/peer, discuss, and complete form.
  No comments should be written that have not been discussed with peer.

TOOL FOR PEER/SELF EVALUATION

Evaluation Form   Student Name _____

_____ Self   Date _____

_____ Peer   Evaluator _____

Identify 8–10 criteria for outcome evaluation in the left column and complete the evaluation (self/peer).
RATING

	CRITERIA	S	U	COMMENTS
1.				
2.				
3.				
4.				
5.				
6.				
7.				
8.				
9.				
10.				

STRENGTHS

WEAKNESSES

AREA FOR QUALITY IMPROVEMENT

Exhibit 17–6 Common Pitfalls in Giving Feedback

PITFALLS	ALTERNATIVE ACTIONS
Labeling with value words: "You are a good thinker" or "you are a perfectionist"; "innovative"	Focus on behavior.
Using superlatives: "Excellent report."	Describe why.
Apologizing: "I hope you don't take this the wrong way" or "This is probably just me."	Describe the behavior.
Offering excuses: "You probably did this unconsciously"; "I know you would do this if you had more time."	Describe the behavior.
Giving mother advice: "You should believe in yourself."	Offer a specific suggestion.
Using generalities or being global: "Very good work."	Be specific—what was good?
Using the halo effect: "From knowing you, I know you would be good at whatever you do."	Be specific.
Talking down: "I couldn't do this better myself."	Use the criteria, standards, or established protocol for comparisons.
Using observations of others: "Someone said you didn't wash your hands."	Own your own data.
Using flowery language or obfuscating: "Your verbalizations were indicative of understanding the patient's condition."	State simply and clearly the behavior and what is being evaluated.
Preaching: "We must remember the patient is in the hospital for rest."	Avoid the supervisory attitude. Talk peer to peer.
Level of expectation too low: "Nice job of providing safety," meaning that the side rails were up.	Review criteria for level of performance and select critical criteria.
Rating rather than evaluating: "Good," "poor."	Use descriptor words for identifying level. Avoid value-laden words.

Courtesy of Elizabeth Larson, MSN, RN

quality and the relationship of quality improvement to the agency's mission. All these tools can be used by students and faculty to build understanding of quality improvement.

Faculty may want to consider if they will use these activities with students for formative or summative evaluation. Formative evaluation calls for ongoing quality improvement feedback and is generally considered less threatening. This can be especially helpful in the development of the autonomous practitioner. Students can be encouraged to ask themselves after each activ-

Exhibit 17–7 Continuous Quality Improvement—Monitoring Tool: Pain Management

---

Outcome Indicator: <u>Patients will verbalize their pain has been controlled.</u>

0–10   Numeric Pain Intensity Scale

0	1	2	3	4	5	6	7	8	9	10
No Pain				Moderate Pain				Worse Possible Pain		

Criteria

Using the scale above, please identify the following:

1. What is your current pain level?   _____
2. What is the worse pain level you have experienced since surgery?   _____
3. Was that pain brought under control?   _____
   How was it controlled?

   _____

   _____

4. When you received pain medication since surgery, what level on the pain scale was your pain after receiving the medication? _____
5. When you asked for pain medication, were you satisfied with the   Yes__   No__
   nurse's response?
6. Are you satisfied with your hospital stay?   Yes__   No__

Comments:

_____

_____

_____

_____

Patient Record Number _____   Date of Review _____

Type of Surgery _____   Date of Surgery _____

Surgeon's Name _____   Nurse Reviewer's Name _____

Name of analgesic received _____   Time since last dose _____

PCA Pump used   Yes__   No__

---

ity, "What are my strengths? My weaknesses? My quality improvement needs?"

Faculty Preparation for Quality Improvement

Faculty preparation for teaching quality improvement will include self study of content regarding quality, as outlined earlier in Exhibits 17–1 and 17–2. Faculty may also find it useful to participate on a hospital quality improvement committee. In addition, faculty serve as role models for quality improvement behavior by using tools for goal setting, evaluation, and quality improvement. When faculty share these quality improvement tools and how they are used with students, faculty demonstrate that they practice what they preach (Larson, 1992, p. 247). Van Arsdale and Hammons (1995) identify several findings from research that are useful in developing faculty evaluation systems (Exhibit 17–13). Other information faculty will

Exhibit 17–8 Plan–Do–Check–Act Method

1. Model for Quality Improvement—CIBEL
   - Customer definition of quality
   - Improvement of processes through better design of services and reduction in variation
   - Benchmark data using statistical process control, the PDCA method, and computers
   - Empowerment and multidisciplinary teamwork
   - Leadership for Continuous Quality Improvement

2. Keeping the CIBEL Model in mind, review the PDCA method
   (Schroeder, 1994, p. 8)
   A. This process specifies that one should:
      Plan
      - Identify one's customer groups
      - Define their unique needs and the characteristics of quality they hold most dear
      - Develop a product or service to meet these needs
      Do
      - Deliver the product or service
      Check
      - Continuously measure and analyze key aspects of quality
      - Contrast these data to customer needs and expectations. (Some suggest this step should be renamed "Study," yielding the PDSA approach.)
      Act
      - Refine/improve the system and product/service

3. Practice Session
   Plan
   A. Identify the type of setting you work in. What type of health care service do you provide to patients?
   B. Identify your customers in this setting and their needs. (circle both)
      a. External customers
         (1) Patients   good clinical outcomes and functional status
                                         low cost
                                         access
                                         satisfaction
         (2) Family   convenient visiting hours
                                         answers to questions
                                         follow-up care
         (3) Payers   reasonable charges, benchmark data with other agencies
         (4) Potential new staff   reputable institution
                                         good pay and working conditions
         (5) Community   access, network of services
         (6) Regulator   meet standards
         (7) Joint Commission   review functions
         (8) Other
      b. (1) Other units/departments   good working relationships
         (2) Physicians   good equipment
                                         helpful staff
         (3) Administrators   reimbursement/profit

continues

Exhibit 17–8 continued

>   (4) Other nurses   good working relationships
>   salary and benefits
>   (5) Other
>   C. Identify strategies you can use to further define your customer's needs (circle)
>   (surveys, questionnaires, focused discussion groups, community assessment, other).
>   D. Prioritize and identify one patient-related need of your customers.
>
> 4. **Do**
>   You are responsible for patient care in this setting and wish to deliver high-quality, cost-effective care to your customers. Identify the following:
>   A. Who will you appoint to the multidisciplinary quality improvement committee to work on this customer priority? (Review list of customers for committee membership ideas—identify 6–8 members.)
>   B. Describe how you will empower the team to improve care. Discuss budget.
>   C. The committee decides to develop a flowchart demonstrating the current process of patient care in your area. Do this now. Brainstorm steps of the current process first, then draw a flowchart.
>   D. The committee flowcharts how they want the future process to flow. Do this now.
>
> 5. **Check**
>   A. What indicator data should this committee begin to monitor and benchmark as a reflection of quality? (List examples.)
>   • Cost
>   • Clinical outcome
>   • Access
>   • Functional status
>   • Satisfaction
>   • Other
>   B. Identify one indicator. _____ How will you continuously measure and analyze this indicator using the following (be specific)?
>   • Computer
>   • Benchmark source
>   • Statistical process control method
>
> 6. **Act**
>   Later, if your data reveal no improvement in this one indicator, *brainstorm* what additional actions you will take.

find helpful in building quality improvement systems is outlined in the Summary of Faculty Quality Improvement Strategies (Exhibit 17–14).

Quality Improvement of the Education-Service Relationship

Since many of the student's experiences with quality improvement will occur in the clinical setting, it is useful to evaluate the relationship between the university and the clinical agency. Larson discusses a tool for faculty to evaluate the clinical agency (Exhibit 17–20). The tool could be modified slightly for use by students in evaluating the clinical agency (Larson, 1992). Larson also illustrates another tool for the clinical agency to evaluate faculty (Exhibit 17–21). These tools are intended to be used for formative, ongoing quality improvement feedback.

Exhibit 17–9 Staff Quick Quiz—CQI Inventory

Take a few moments to rate your nursing home on these 18 points. On the line before each statement, indicate the extent to which you agree with that statement. Use the following 5-point scale.

1	2	3	4	5
Strongly Disagree				Strongly Agree

1.___ The top administrators of our nursing home are committed to the improvement of quality in all aspects of our service (total management commitment to quality).

Take a few moments to rate your nursing home on these 18 points. On the line before each statement, indicate the extent to which you agree with that statement. Use the following 5-point scale.

1	2	3	4	5
Strongly Disagree				Strongly Agree

1.___ The top administrators of our nursing home are committed to the improvement of quality in all aspects of our service (total management commitment to quality).

2.___ Customers come first: our nursing home has a formal process we all follow to assess and meet customer needs and expectations fully (commitment to customer satisfaction).

3.___ Employee opinions and suggestions are encouraged and thoughtfully considered (participative management and empowerment).

4.___ Our nursing home consistently measures performance against established quality goals (quality measurement).

5.___ Quality standards have been established for all services and everyone knows what the standards are (quality standards).

6.___ Departments, units, or teams cooperate to meet common goals of our nursing home (total system integration).

7.___ Our nursing home encourages employees to use a team approach to solve problems that directly affect the quality or cost of their work (teamwork).

8.___ Management recognizes CQI as a way to achieve continuous improvement and keep our customers (continuous improvement).

9.___ Staff at our nursing home are encouraged to identify quality opportunities and bring them to the administration's attention (identification of quality opportunities).

10.___ Our nursing home adopts a rational approach to problem solving through observing, collecting, and analyzing data; generating potential solutions; and developing the best solution (problem solving).

11.___ Our nursing home has identified industry-best providers of critical work processes (benchmarking).

12.___ All employees participate for an average of 1 hour per week in ongoing training programs to reinforce and enhance their skills (training).

continues

Exhibit 17–9 continued

13.___ When problems occur, administration avoids quick-fix solutions and tries to understand the complete work process and determine causes of work problems to avoid recurrences (process orientation).

14.___ At our nursing home, quality is monitored at many steps during the work process. For example, in food service, quality is measured when food supplies are purchased, while food is prepared, before it is served, and after it is eaten by the resident (quality control).

15.___ Managers at our nursing home try to anticipate the effects of changes in laws, the community, and health care practices, and they develop ways to prevent those changes from having a negative impact on our home (proactive management).

16.___ Our nursing home is concerned with the cost *and* the quality of goods and services supplied by our vendors to ensure that it receives high quality goods (supplier quality assurance).

17.___ My supervisor and his or her superior have an open door policy that encourages staff to freely offer suggestions and opinions (internal communication).

18.___ Employees at our nursing home are recognized for good work performance (employee incentives and recognition).

Source: Reprinted with permission from C. Burczyk, P. Kelly-Heidenthal, and G. Falk, Measuring Your Nursing Home's Orientation to Quality, *Nursing Quality Connection*, Vol. 5, No. 4, pp. 38 and 45, 1996, St. Louis, Mosby-Year Book, Inc.

Exhibit 17–10 Exercise to Build Power

Objective

Develop knowledge and skills to continuously improve the quality of patient care.
1. Identify an interpersonal or organizational problem you have seen that interferes with quality nursing care in the clinical area.
2. Analyze this problem. Describe both the interpersonal and organizational factors that contribute to this problem.
3. Discuss elements of change theory that could be used to work on this problem.
4. Describe how developing collegiality and consulting with both nursing peers and other members of the health care team might assist with supporting you to solve the problem.
5. Discuss how you could seek administrative sponsorship from senior nurses to solve the problem.

Exhibit 17–11 Exercise to Build Understanding of Cost-Quality Relationship

---

Objective

1. Identify one nursing care standard.
2. Determine cost of delivering this nursing care standard.

Activity

1. Develop a nursing care standard for one selected element of nursing care or for one nursing diagnosis.
2. Identify the cost of delivering this nursing care. Consider nursing staffing cost, material cost, environmental costs, etc. Obtain your cost figures from your clinical agency, as directed by your faculty.

Exhibit 17–12 Mission and Quality Improvement

Objective

1. Describe the role of the mission of the nursing department or unit.
2. Identify the relationship of mission to quality improvement.

Activity

1. Describe the mission of your nursing department or nursing unit.
2. Identify five quality outcome indicators you could use to monitor this mission. Consider indicators of patient satisfaction, patient function, patient quality of life and caring, patient outcomes, cost, etc.
3. Discuss the use of one Statistical Process (SPC) tool to monitor this outcome and/or improve care if quality problems are identified (SPC tools include flowcharts, cause and effect charts, histograms, Pareto charts, run charts, control charts, and scattergrams).
4. Identify one source of benchmark information to compare with your monitoring results.

Optional

1. Monitor your five outcome indicators and work to improve any quality problems you find. Illustrate your problem-solving process using a storyboard.

Exhibit 17–13 Research Findings Re: Faculty Evaluation by Students

- Student evaluations should remain anonymous to be valid.
- Class size does not significantly affect how a student will rate teaching effectiveness.
- Students give higher ratings to faculty in difficult courses, for which they have to work hard.
- Student ratings of teaching performance are consistent with colleague ratings.
- Students rate teachers higher when they know the results may be considered in salary, tenure, or promotion considerations.
- Research and publications are not essential for good teaching as judged by students.
- An instructor's gender, age, teaching experience, and personality have little or no relationship to student ratings.
- Numerous studies have shown little or no relationship between a student's personality, age, gender, grade point average, or academic level and student's rating of teacher effectiveness.

Source: Reprinted with permission from P. Schroeder, *Improving Quality and Performance: Concepts, Programs, and Techniques*, p. 8, © 1994, St. Louis, Mosby-Year Book, Inc.

Exhibit 17–14 Summary of Faculty Quality Improvement Strategies

Exhibit 17–15	Purdue University Calumet Department of Nursing Hammond, IN	Master Plan for Evaluation
Exhibit 17–16	Cashin Tips (1996)	Tips for developing an effective faculty evaluation system
Exhibit 17–17	Larson (1992) Assessment of Teaching (Self/Peer)	This is a comprehensive tool that covers all dimensions of teaching. It may be used concurrently and/or retrospectively. This tool is designed to be used over an entire semester or year by faculty.
Exhibit 17–18	Larson (1992) Review of a class presentation (Self/Peer)	This tool allows for an evaluation of a single class presentation by faculty.
Exhibit 17–19	Student Review of a Class Larson (1992)	This tool to be used by students is for concurrent assessment of specific outcomes as perceived by students. The questions are intended to demonstrate to students the reciprocal roles of teacher–learner.

Exhibit 17–15 Purdue University Calumet—Department of Nursing—Master Plan for Evaluation

Evaluation Focus	Data Source and/or Method	Time Interval	Responsible Participants	Comments
CONTEXT EVALUATION				
Mission and Goals				
Department	Department Report	5 years	Department Head, PUC Academic Program Review Committee, VCAA, Chancellor	
Department/Programs	Purdue University and PUCalumet Mission Statements, Indiana Nurse Practice Act, ANA, NLN, Healthy People 2000	4 years	Faculty, Program Coordinators, Department	
Philosophies, Conceptual Frameworks	Purdue University and PUCalumet Mission Statements, Indiana Nurse Practice Act, ANA, NLN, Healthy People 2000	4 years	Faculty, Program Coordinators	
Enrollment Trends	National and regional trends, Indiana Task Force for Education, PUC Enrollment Management Committee	2 years	Program Coordinators, Department Head, SPS Dean	
Community Needs Consumer Expectations	Nursing Advisory Committee, Indiana Deans and Directors, Community Agencies	1 year	Program Coordinators, Department Head, SPS Dean, VCCA, Chancellor	
INPUT EVALUATION				
Faculty				
Development Activity Individual	Individual request, nature of program, available resources	Ongoing	Faculty member, Program Coordinators, Department Head	Includes conferences, seminars, workshops
Promotion	Individual promotion document, SPS Promotion and Tenure Guidelines	1 year	Faculty member, Primary Promotion Committee, Area Promotion Committee, Panel C. Board of Trustees	
Overall Activity	Annual Activity Report, Faculty Growth Contract, Management by Objectives	1 year	Faculty member, Program Coordinators, Department Head	

Resources

Sabbaticals	Individual request, eligibility guidelines, available resources	1 year	Faculty member, Department Head, SPS Dean, VCAA, Chancellor	
Research releases	Individual request, nature of study, available FTEs	Each semester	Faculty member, Research and Scholarly Activities Committee, Department Head	
Curriculum releases	Individual or department request, department need, available FTEs	Each semester	Department Head, Program Coordinator	
Special projects	Individual or department request, department need, available FTEs	Each semester	Department Head, Program Coordinator	
Travel funds	Annual budget and available departmental funds	Each semester	Faculty, Department Head, Program Coordinator	
Internal/external funding projects	Proposal, available FTEs	Each semester	Faculty, Department Head	
Performance Activity				
Teaching	Cafeteria Appraisal System, Student Evaluation of Faculty Form	Each semester	Students	Biennially for tenured faculty; faculty may use either method of evaluation
Teaching/curriculum contributions	Faculty Evaluation Form, Supervisor Evaluation Form	2 years alternating	Faculty	Biennially for tenured faculty. Faculty Evaluation Form used for both self and peer evaluation
Scholarly activity	Annual Activity Report, copies of work	1 year	Faculty, Program Coordinator, Department Head	
Service	Annual Activity Report	1 year	Faculty, Program Coordinator, Department Head	
Program Coordinators	Program Coordinator Evaluation Form	2 years	Faculty, Department Head	
Department Head	Department Head Evaluation Form	4 years	Department Faculty, SPS Dean VCAA	

continues

Exhibit 17-15 continued

Evaluation Focus	Data Source and/or Method	Interval Time	Responsible Participants	Comments
Program Coordinators	Program Coordinator Evaluation Form	2 years	Faculty, Department Head	
Department Head	Department Head Evaluation Form	4 years	Department Faculty, SPS Dean VCAA	
Teaching-Learning Resources				
Library	PUC Library Committee	1 year	Resource, Policy and Planning Committee	
Space	Faculty request	1 year	Resources, Policy and Planning Committee, Director of Learning Resource Center, Program Coordinators	
Audiovisual Computer hardware/software	Faculty request	Ongoing	Resource, Policy and Planning Committee, Director of Learning Resource Center, Program Coordinators	
Financial Resources				
Allocation	Annual budget	1 year (Jan)	Chancellor, VCCA, SPS Dean, Department Head, Program Coordinators	
	Biennial budget	2 years	Chancellor, VCCA, SPS Dean, Department Head, Program Coordinators	
	Current academic budget	1 year (spring)	Chancellor, VCCA, SPS Dean, Department Head, Program Coordinators	Evaluation Focus
Affiliating Agencies	Contracts, course evaluations, preceptor evaluations	Each semester	Students, Faculty, Course Coordinators, Program Coordinators, Department Head	
Students				
Characteristics (Admissions)	Individual program admissions requirements	AS-1 year BS, MS-ongoing	AS-Admissions Committee BS-Admissions Committee MS-Graduate Committee, Graduate School	

Enrollment trends	NLN, AACN enrollment and graduation reports	1 year	Admissions Committees, Program Coordinators, Department Head	
Retention	NLN, AACN enrollment and graduation reports	1 year	Curriculum Committees, Program Coordinators	
PROCESS EVALUATION				
<u>Curriculum</u>				
Course content Credit Allocation Sequencing Teaching-learning strategies	Syllabi, course evaluation, NLN accreditation criteria AS-NCLEX results BS, MS-End of Program Evaluations	1 year	Students, Faculty, Program Curriculum Committees, Department Curriculum Committee	
<u>Students</u>				
Academic Performance	Course objectives and requirements, grade summaries	Each semester	Faculty, Program Coordinators	
Progression	Academic records	Each Semester	Curriculum Committees, Graduate Committee, Advisors	
PRODUCT EVALUATION				
<u>Students</u>	AS-Course objectives, program objectives, NLN Diagnostic Readiness Test BS-End of Program evaluation, Written and Oral Communication Evaluation Ratings Scales, Therapeutic Intervention Project, Watson-Glaser Critical Thinking Appraisal MS-End of Program Evaluation, Paper and Presentation Evaluation Forms, Watson-Glaser Critical Thinking Appraisal	End of programs	Faculty, Program Curriculum Committees	
<u>Graduates</u>	AS-NCLEX reports BS, MS-Follow-up Studies—Student, supervisor, agency	4 times a year- 4 years	Faculty, Program Coordinators	Surveys 1997, 2001, etc., to coincide with University follow-up schedule

Courtesy of Purdue University Calumet, Department of Nursing, Hammond, Indiana.

Exhibit 17–16 Developing an Effective Faculty Evaluation System—Tips

1. The institution and the units within the institution must develop clear goals.
2. Decide on the purpose(s) data will be used for before any data are collected.
3. Use pilot programs when appropriate.
4. Significantly involve participants—especially campus leaders—in the development of the system.
5. Foster extensive open communication before, during, and after the adoption of the system.
6. Obtain support for the development of the system from the high-level administrators.
7. Ensure that the system is flexible.
8. Ensure that the system is legal.
9. Define major faculty responsibilities at the beginning of the evaluation period.
10. Define faculty *sub*responsibilities at the beginning of the evaluation period and determine their weighting.
11. Define the sources of data to be used to evaluate each subresponsibility at the *beginning* of the evaluation period.
12. Use *multiple* sources of data.
13. Ensure that the data/measures are *technically* acceptable, i.e., are reliable and valid.
14. *Specifically* define the criteria and the standards for each subresponsibility.
15. Train the evaluators to evaluate.
16. Train the supervisors in giving feedback.
17. Maintain *appropriate* confidentiality.
18. Reward *effective* performance.
19. *Combine* development with evaluation; have an on-campus consultant.
20. Review the system *periodically*.

Source: Reprinted with permission from Cashin, W.E. (1996), *Developing an Effective Faculty Evaluation System.* Idea Paper No. 33. Manhattan, KS: Kansas State University, Center for Faculty Evaluation and Development.

Exhibit 17–17 Assessment of Teaching (Self/Peer)

Faculty Member _____

Review   Self _____   Peer _____   Date _____

Directions: In assessing the quality of teaching, please use the following descriptive scale:

5 = almost always; 4 = often; 3 = usually (average); 2 = seldom; 1 = never; 0 = not applicable. Use the comments space for anecdotal statements, specific incidents, and/or behaviors you wish to describe in more detail. Use the blank spaces.

Criteria	Rating Scale						Explanatory Comments/Documentation
	5	4	3	2	1	0	
A. Knowledge							
1. Is my philosophy of teaching consistent with College of Nursing philosophy?							
2. Am I familiar with the total curriculum plan?							
3. Do I understand the relationship of my course(s) to total curriculum?							
4. Do I have current knowledge relating to clinical and class material?							
5. Do I have knowledge relating to clinical and class material?							
6. Have I clarified my own beliefs about students as learners?							
7. Have I defined my role and philosophy as a teacher?							
B. Planning/designing skills							
1. Am I prepared for course/level meetings?							
2. Do I collaborate with other peers?							
3. Do I share responsibility for preparation of course materials and exams?							

continues

Exhibit 17–17 continued

Criteria	Rating Scale 5	4	3	2	1	0	Explanatory Comments/Documentation
4. Do I share ideas for developing/updating course materials and learning activities?							
5. Do I facilitate ideas of others to implement changes to strengthen the course?							
6. Are my plans for activities and assignments consistent with course objectives and curriculum plans?							
7. Is planning done early enough to allow for use of resources and instructions to students?							
8. Is selection of content made on basis of "need to know" (critical performance indicators)?							
9. Do planned activities promote active learning?							
10. Is adequate time allowed for learning?							
11. Do I have adequate information about the learners (previous learning)?							
12. Do I do everything within my control to make the environment conducive to learning?							
13. Do I provide appropriate assignments/guidelines for students to prepare for classes and clinical?							
14. Do I build on previous learning of students?							
15. Do I take into consideration the differ							

16.					
17.					
C. Instructional skills/classroom setting					
1. Do I organize content and activities to meet course objectives and students' needs?					
2. Do I have a teaching plan? (See individual form.)					
3. Do I encourage students to think for themselves? How?					
4. Do I encourage questions and promote discussions?					
5. Do I explain terminology, theory, and abstract ideas clearly?					
6. Do I use teaching methods appropriate to content and objective?					
7. Do I speak clearly and at appropriate volume and speed (not at dictation rate)?					
8. Do I allow time for reflective thinking?					
9. Do I keep the focus of class on nursing? (Discuss why as well as how and interweave skills and rationale.)					
10. Do I use tactful/appropriate strategies to encourage quiet or reluctant students to participate?					

continues

Exhibit 17–17 continued

Criteria	5	4	3	2	1	0	Explanatory Comments/Documentation
11. Am I sensitive to nonverbal behavior?							
12. Do I use learner's questions/comments/experiences to illustrate content?							
13. Do I clarify ideas expressed by learners?							
14. Do I address group problems in a sensitive, positive manner?							
15. Do I use constructive methods to promote group activity and/or resolve differences?							
16. Do I structure class to allow for interactions, breaks, etc.?							
17. Do I plan for review, summaries?							
18. Do I make use of assigned materials (readings, etc.)?							
19.							
20.							
D. Instructional skills/clinical setting (in addition to components listed for classroom setting).							
1. Do I select and plan learning activities appropriate to the individual's needs?							
2. Do I provide opportunities for learners to plan and select their own learning activities?							
3. Do I correlate classroom material with clinical practice?							

4. Do I assist learners to develop their own goals?					
5. Do I assist learners to evaluate themselves objectively and honestly?					
6. Do I provide (or require) objectives for each learning activity?					
7. Do I balance direction giving with allowances for freedom when possible?					
8. Do I adhere to standards of performance for protection of patients' safety and rights?					
9.					
10.					
E. Evaluating skills					
1. Are test questions reflective of critical behavior ("need to know" information)?					
2. Do I have a test plan correlating evaluation techniques with objectives?					
3. Do I utilize appropriate criteria to evaluate students?					
4. Do I use formative and summative evaluation appropriately?					
5. Do I continually evaluate the progress of the group toward meeting goals?					
6. Do I continually evaluate my role in the group's progress or lack of progress?					

continues

Exhibit 17–17 continued

Criteria	Rating Scale 5	4	3	2	1	0	Explanatory Comments/Documentation
7. Do I give feedback in a positive manner?							
8. Do I accept responsibility for evaluating honestly?							
9. Am I tactful?							
10. Do I evaluate the effectiveness of activities and materials (e.g., class content, assignments, handout)?							
11. Do I seek information from appropriate sources to improve teaching?							
12.							
13.							
F. Interpersonal skills (peers/students/staff/administrators/clinical agency personnel/patients)							
1. Do I respect the confidentiality of information?							
2. Do I respect individuals' privacy and rights?							
3. Do I abide by group decisions in course/level matters?							
4. Do I demonstrate an interest in student activities?							
5. Do I demonstrate an interest in college and university matters?							
6. Am I conscientious in keeping appointments/time commitments?							

7. Am I willing to listen to others' opinions?											
8. Do I contribute to faculty deliberations?											
9. Do I give feedback to colleagues, staff, and others?											
10. Do I elicit suggestions from colleagues and staff?											
11. Do I demonstrate concern for the needs, rights, and individuality of people?											
12. Do I give recognition to the accomplishments of others?											
13. Am I reasonably accessible for consultations?											
14. Do I give credit when using material/ideas of others?											
15. Do I promote networking among students?											
16. Do I promote networking among faculty and clinical colleagues?											
17.											
18.											
G. Role modeling for students, peers, and public (scholarship, health, professionalism, appearance)											
1. Do I project a positive attitude toward nursing?											

continues

Exhibit 17–17 continued

Criteria	Rating Scale						Explanatory Comments/Documentation
	5	4	3	2	1	0	
2. Do I project a positive attitude toward the College of Nursing?							
3. Do I show evidence of having a breadth of knowledge?							
4. Am I well read in current nursing literature?							
5. Am I well read on current events?							
6. Do I practice positive health behaviors?							
7. Do I present a professional appearance in dress and demeanor?							
8. Do I articulate ideas clearly and grammatically?							
9. Do I seek ways to improve?							
10. Do I demonstrate an interest in improving the quality of teaching/nursing practice?							
11. Am I an active member of a professional organization?							
12. Do I attend conferences/seminars relevant to professional development?							
13. Do I demonstrate an awareness of ethical behavior in teaching and practice (e.g., respect confidentiality of information, respect, privacy, etc.)?							
14. Am I aware of legal issues in teaching and supervision?							

Courtesy of the University of Wisconsin, College of Nursing, Oshkosh, Wisconsin.

Exhibit 17–18 Classroom Presentation Review

Directions: The following items are general guidelines for review of a class presentation. For best results, the faculty being reviewed could indicate which particular areas should be emphasized (highlighted) in the review. A copy of the lesson plan, student assignment, and any handouts should be given to the reviewer prior to the class. In assessing the quality of teaching, please use the following descriptive scale: 5 = almost always; 4 = often; 3 = usually (average); 2 = seldom; 1 = never; 0 = not applicable. Use the comments space for anecdotal statements, specific incidents, and/or behaviors you wish to describe in more detail.

Faculty _____ Date & Time _____

Class Topic _____ Class Size _____

(Describe) _____

Method of Presentation:

Reviewer: Self _____ Peer _____

Criteria	Rating Scale						Explanatory Comments/Documentation
	5	4	3	2	1	0	
A. Content							
1. Identifies objectives and expected outcomes for class.							
2. Content consistent with objectives.							
3. Content related to previous learning/courses.							
4. Relevance to practice and importance is identified.							
5. Level of learner is considered in selection of content (evidence of previous assessment of learners' needs).							
6. Allows time for discussion of students' objectives for class experience.							
7. Relates content to nursing practice.							
8. Content is current and correct (consistent with research or accepted theory).							
9. Amount of content is appropriate for time allotment.							

continues

Exhibit 17–18 continued

Criteria	Rating Scale						Explanatory Comments/Documentation
	5	4	3	2	1	0	
10. Content selected on a basis of "need to know."							
B. Presentation							
1. Begins and ends class on time.							
2. Presents material in an organized manner.							
3. Emphasizes important concepts.							
4. Encourages student to participate/think/problem solve.							
5. Discourages rote learning and verbatim note taking.							
6. Summarizes at intervals.							
7. Responds to student questions in a helpful manner.							
8. Conveys interest in the topic and in helping students learn.							
9. Integrates knowledge from relevant fields.							
10. Assigned readings are used during discussion.							
C. Clarity of presentation							
1. Communicates clearly and audibly.							
2. Directions are specific and clear.							
3. Written materials are legible and organized.							
4. Audiovisuals are appropriate for content.							
5. Audiovisuals are clear and understandable.							

6. Teaching methods are appropriate for content. (Identify method.)								
7. Teaching methods are appropriate for content and promote involvement of learner (overheads readable, handouts used to avoid needless repetition).								
8. Learners are encouraged to be involved by a variety of techniques (cite examples).								
9. Speaks clearly and distinctly.								
D. Evaluation 1. Plans for and utilizes student feedback regarding understanding of concepts.								
2. Utilizes methods to evaluate the instructional methods.								
3. Evaluates audience perceptions and understanding of key points.								
4. Seeks feedback in regard to student understanding.								
E. Interpersonal skills 1. Responds to questions and comments tactfully and honestly.								
2. Shows genuine interest in students' comments.								
3. Maintains an environment conducive to learning.								

continues

Exhibit 17–18 continued

Criteria	Rating Scale						Explanatory Comments/Documentation
	5	4	3	2	1	0	
4. Communicates expectations of students clearly.							
5. Maintains a friendly yet professional demeanor.							
6. Is flexible and learner-responsive, within limits.							
7. Helps students relate and respond to one another.							
Summary Major Strengths: Suggestions for improvement/comments:							

Courtesy of the University of Wisconsin, College of Nursing, Oshkosh, Wisconsin.

Exhibit 17–19 Student Review of a Class

Directions: Please complete the review at the end of the class period. The faculty member will provide time for you to complete it. Your feedback will be helpful to the faculty member to continue to provide a worthwhile educational experience for you.

Presenter (Faculty) _____   Date and Time: _____

Method: _____ Lecture _____ Group Discussion _____ Other _____

Class Topic: _____ Class Size: _____ Reviewer (Student) _____

In order to do an effective evaluation of the teacher, you need to consider your own preparation for this class session. Please answer the following questions before completing the faculty evaluation on page 2.

A. I prepared for this class by:

B. What will you "always remember" from this class?

C. How has the class stimulated you to do more study?

Directions: In reviewing this class, please use the descriptive scale:
    5 = almost always; 4 = often; 3 = usually (average); 2 = seldom; 1 = never;
    0 = not applicable
    Use the comments space for anecdotal statements, specific incidents, and/or behaviors you wish to describe in more detail.

Rating Scale

Criteria	5	4	3	2	1	0	Explanatory Comments/ Documentation
1. I was able to follow the presentation.							
2. I could identify key points in the presentation.							
3. Content was meaningful to me.							
4. My thinking was stimulated by the questions/presentation.							
5. I could understand the presenter.							
6. I could see and read all the over-heads and other visual aids.							
7. I could apply the content to practice.							
8. I could relate material to some things I already know.							
9. The handouts helped me to under-stand the material.							
10. I thought the presenter was knowl-edgeable about the material.							
11. I thought the presenter was interested in helping me understand the material.							

Use the rest of this sheet to add any comments or suggestions. Please explain/clarify any questions rated 2 or below.

Courtesy of the University of Wisconsin, College of Nursing, Oshkosh, Wisconsin.

CONCLUSION

Accountability for quality improvement is a hallmark of the professional. Strategies to build knowledge of quality and quality improvement concepts must include theory building, classroom discussion, skill-building exercises, and exercises to strengthen a positive attitude and commitment to quality improvement practices, both personally and professionally. These practices will strengthen the student and faculty commitment to and accountability for quality.

Exhibit 17–20 Faculty Evaluation of Clinical Agency

NURSING EDUCATION/SERVICE INTERACTION GROUP EVALUATION OF CLINICAL AGENCY

Agency _____   Unit _____   Date _____

Directions:

Use the statements below to provide feedback to the service agency nurse. Comments should include specific examples when appropriate. Please use reverse side of page for additional comments.

Comments

Professionalism

1. Registered nurses serve as role models to nursing students.
2. Nursing personnel serve as resource persons to nursing students.
3. Professional behavior of nursing personnel enhances the public image of nursing.
4. Personal appearance of nursing personnel enhances the public image of nursing.
5. Nursing personnel display courtesy and respect to faculty and students.
6. Nursing personnel are available to assist faculty and students as needed.
7. Nursing personnel are supportive of faculty and students.

Communication

1. Agency contact person communicates with faculty to facilitate orientation.
2. Nursing personnel consistently maintain and utilize open lines of communication by:
   a. discussing concerns regarding student performance with faculty as appropriate
   b. informing students and faculty of change in patient care
   c. providing adequate time for feedback and exchange of information (i.e., shift report, patient care conferences, etc.)
   d. being receptive or open to students
3. Agency contact person communicates with faculty to obtain feedback following the clinical experience (i.e., exit interview).

continues

Exhibit 17–20 continued

	Comments

Teaching/Learning Process
1. Nursing personnel collaborate with faculty to support the teaching/learning process.
2. Policies/procedure manuals are
   a. accessible
   b. clearly written/understandable
   c. consistent with current practice
3. Nursing personnel consider input from faculty and/or students during the decision-making process regarding patient care.
4. The approval process for clinical projects is clearly defined and easily implemented.

Scheduling
1. Student clinical schedules are communicated to appropriate nursing personnel.
2. The patient population is appropriate for the learning experience.

Ancillary Services
1. Learning resources are accessible and contribute to the teaching/learning process.
2. Ancillary departments are cooperative and supportive of the students' learning experiences.
3. Opportunities are available for students and faculty to participate in educational activities offered by the agency (i.e., patient care conferences, inservice and continuing education).

1. What effect have agency and nursing personnel had on the teaching/learning process?

2. Are there any ethical concerns regarding nursing practice within the agency?

Faculty signature _____   Agency _____

Date: _____

Courtesy of the University of Wisconsin, College of Nursing, Oshkosh, Wisconsin.

Exhibit 17–21 Clinical Agency Evaluation of Faculty

NURSING EDUCATION/SERVICE INTERACTION GROUP EVALUATION
OF CLINICAL FACULTY MEMBER

Agency _____ Unit _____ Date _____

Directions:
Use the statements below to provide feedback to the clinical faculty member. Comments should include specific examples when appropriate. Please use reverse side of page for additional comments.

Comments

Professionalism
1. Demonstrates knowledge of nursing care appropriate to patients/clients/residents.
2. Demonstrates appropriate role model for the college.
3. Professional behavior of faculty enhances the public image of nursing.
4. Personal appearance of faculty enhances the public image of nursing.
5. Displays courtesy and respect to nursing staff and students.
6. Demonstrates respect for the rights of patients/clients/residents.
7. Resolves problem situations by using an objective problem-solving approach.

Communication
1. Orients staff to the learning needs of students.
2. Communicates with staff to promote both quality education and patient care.
3. Reports to appropriate staff regarding changes or problems.
4. Makes assignments promptly and in accordance with unit/agency expectations.
5. Consults nursing staff, as appropriate, regarding nursing care assignments.
6. Follows correct channels of communication.
7. Shares expertise and/or resources to promote the professional development of nursing personnel.

Supervision of Students
1. Orients students to agency in preparation for the clinical experience.
2. Provides guidance to students.
3. Follows agency policies and procedures.

continues

Exhibit 17–21 continued

1. What effect have these students and this faculty member had on the quality of nursing care on this unit/agency?
2. What other effects have these students and this faculty member had on this unit/agency?
3. Are there any ethical concerns about the appropriateness of assignments?

Date _____

Agency/Unit _____

Agency Staff Signature _____

Source: Courtesy of the University of Wisconsin, College of Nursing, Oshkosh, Wisconsin.

REFERENCES

Ackerman, F., & Nash, D. (1991, June). Teaching the tenets of quality: A survey of medical schools & programs in health administration. *Quality Review Bulletin,* 201–203.

Benner, P. (1984). From novice to expert: Excellence and power in clinical nursing practice. Menlo Park, CA: Addison-Wesley.

Best, M., Carswell, R., &. Abbott, S. (1990). Self-evaluation for nursing students. *Nursing Outlook, 38*(4), 172–177.

Cashin, W.E. (1996). Developing an effective faculty evaluation system (Idea Paper No. 33). Manhattan, KS: Center for Faculty Evaluation and Development Newsletter, Kansas State University, Division of Continuing Education.

Gelmon, S.B., & Baker, G.R. (1995, Winter). Incorporating quality improvement in the health administration curriculum. *The Journal of Health Administration Education, 13*(1), 91–107.

Genovich-Richards, J. (1989, December). Evolving quality management through curriculum offerings. *Quality Review Bulletin,* 366–368.

Headrick, L., Neuhauser, D., Melnikow, J., & Vanek, J. (1991, August). Introducing quality improvement thinking to medical students: The Cleveland Asthma Project. *Quality Review Bulletin,* 254–260.

Hoare, C., Burns, M., & Akerlund, K. (1985, March). The perceived training needs of quality assurance professionals in eight eastern states. *Quality Review Bulletin,* 87–92.

Johnson, J. (1995). Curricular trends in accredited generic baccalaureate nursing programs across the United States. *Journal of Nursing Education, 34*(2), 53–60.

Larson, E. (1992). Teaching quality assurance: The undergraduate student/faculty experience. In C. Meisenheimer (Ed.), *Improving quality: A guide to effective programs* (pp. 226–259). Gaithersburg, MD: Aspen.

Malcolm Baldrige National Quality Award, Health Care Pilot Criteria. (1995). *National Institute of Standards and Technology.* Gaithersburg, MD: Author.

Norman, D., Randall, R., & Hornsby, B. (1990, September). Critical features of a curriculum in health care quality & resource management. *Quality Review Bulletin,* 317–336.

The Pew Health Professions Commission, NCFS Center for the Health Professions. (1995). *The third report of the Pew Health Professions Commission: Critical challenges: Revitalizing the health professions for the twenty-first century.* San Francisco: Author.

Poirrier, G., Wills, E., Broussard, P., & Payne, R. (1996). Nursing information systems: Applications in nursing curricula. *Nursing Educator, 21*(1), 18–22.

Reilly, D., & Oermann, M. (1992). *Clinical teaching in nursing education* (2nd ed.), New York: National League for Nursing.

Sposato, C. (1994). Guidelines for a curriculum in healthcare quality & resource management. *Journal of Healthcare Quality, 16*(1), 4–13.

Van Arsdale, S., & Hammons, J. (1995). Myths & misconceptions about student ratings of college faculty: Separating fact from fiction. *Nursing Outlook, 43*(1), 33–36.

SUGGESTED READING

Agency for Health Care Policy and Research. (1994). *Clinical practice guidelines.* Silver Spring, MD: Author.

Aronow, D., & Coltin, K. (1993). Information technology applications in quality assurance & quality improvement, Part II. *Journal on Quality Improvement, 9*(10), 465–477.

deTornyay, R. (1992). Reconsidering nursing education: The report of the Pew Health Professions Commission. *Journal of Nursing Education, 31*(7), 296–301.Gorman, S., & Clark, N. (1986). Power & effective nursing practice. *Nursing Outlook, 34*(3), 129–134.

Dieneman, J. (1992). CQI in nursing. Washington, DC: American Nurses Association.

Evenson, B. (1990). Teaching quality assurance. *Nurse Educator, 5*(2), 8–12.

Fields, W., & Siroky, K. (1994). Converting data into information. *Journal of Nursing Care Quarterly, 8*(3), 1–11.

Gaucher, E., & Coffey, R. (1993). Total quality in healthcare. San Francisco: Jossey-Bass.

Goal/QPC. (1994). *Memory Jogger II.* Metheren, MA: Goal/QPC.

Jones, G., & Wakefield, B. (1991). Including nursing students in an agency quality assurance program. *Journal of Nursing Quality Assurance, 5*(2), 77–80.

Kaluzny, A. (1995). Extending quality assurance improvement beyond the health care provider. *Journal on Quality Improvement. 21*(1), 40–41.

Katz, J., & Green, E. (1992). Managing quality. St. Louis, MO: C.V. Mosby.

Kirk, R. (1992). The big picture: Total quality management & continuous quality improvement. *Journal of Nursing Administration, 22*(4), 24–31.

Lawler, T., & Rose, M. (1987). Professionalism: A comparison among generic, baccalaureate, ADN, and RN/BSN nurses. *Nurse Educator, 12*(3), 19–22.

McCloskey, J., & Bulechek, G. (1994). Standardizing the language for nursing treatments: An overview of the issues. *Nursing Outlook, 42*(2), 70–75.

Nelson, E., Batalden, P., Plume, S., Mihevc, N., & Swartz, W. (1995). Report cards or instrument panels: Who needs what? *Journal on Quality Improvement, 21*(4), 155–171.

Nelson, E., Larson, C., Hays, R., Nelson, S., Ward, D., & Batalden, P. (1992, September). The physician & employee judgement system: Reliability & validity of a hospital measurement system. *Quarterly Review Bulletin, 309*–314.

Northrop, C. (1990). A student experience in quality assurance. *Journal of Nursing Education, 29,* 375–377.

Schroeder, P. (1994). *Improving quality & performance.* St. Louis, MO: C.V. Mosby.

Shortell, S., Zimmerman, J., Gillies, R., Duffy, J., Devers, K., Rousseau, D., & Knaus, W. (1992, May). Continuously improving patient care: Practical lessons & an assessment tool from the national ICU study. *Quarterly Review Bulletin, 150*–155.

Wakefield, B., McCloskey, J., & Bulechek, G. (1995). Nursing interventions classification: A standardized language for nursing care. *Journal of Healthcare Quality, 17*(4), 26–33.

Wennberg, J., Freeman, J., & Culp, W. (1987). Are hospital services rationed in New Haven or over-utilized in Boston? *Lancet, 1,* 1185–1189.

Werley, H. (1991). The nursing minimum data set: Abstraction tool for standardized, comparable, essential data. *American Journal of Public Health 81,* 421–426.

Williams, A., & Perkins, S. (1995). Identifying nursing outcome indicators. *Journal of Healthcare Quality, 17*(2), 6–33.

Wink, D. (1995). The effective clinical conference. *Nursing Outlook, 43*(1), 29–32.

## CHAPTER 18

Graduate Preparation for Managing Quality in Practice in the 21st Century

June A. Schmele and Kathryn L. Clark

CHAPTER OBJECTIVES

After completing this chapter, the reader will be able to

- describe how the graduate student must be prepared for managing quality in the 21st century
- identify necessary competencies for quality professionals to practice
- differentiate between integration vs. specialization of QI content in graduate curricula
- discuss the barriers to integration of QI principles into the curriculum

Preparation at a graduate level is essential if the field of quality management is to respond to the needs of our times. It is vital that those in leadership roles acquire the skills, knowledge, and abilities needed to respond to the providers' and the consumers' demands for quality. As early as 1988, Kibbee acknowledged the need for professionals working in this area to have a vigorous and systematic educational program. In 1991, quality management experts such as Norman, Randall, and Hornsby (1990) emphasized the growing need for strong academic preparation at the graduate level so that leaders would be prepared to offer the desired level of quality management skills. The current and continuous upheaval in the health care system calls for even greater leadership competencies to maintain a desirable level of quality.

The purpose of this chapter is to describe how the graduate student will prepare for managing quality in the 21st century. Through a review of the literature, personal communications with experts, and our own experiences in the field of quality, the following three questions will be discussed:

1. What must graduates know in order to manage quality?
2. How will graduates learn to use quality improvement (QI) in practice?
3. How will educators evaluate graduate competencies in QI?

It is recognized that there are semantic differences in the quality jargon of the present day. For purposes of consistency in this chapter, the term *quality management* (QM) will refer to the broad, encompassing, total organizational leadership philosophy of quality. *Quality improvement* (QI) will refer to techniques, tools, and methodologies used within the organization to monitor and improve quality processes.

WHAT MUST GRADUATES KNOW TO MANAGE QUALITY?

Clearly, health care organizations expect that the graduates who will be assuming leadership positions will have knowledge of QM concepts as well as the ability to implement them in various types of dynamic nontraditional settings.

The rapid changes occurring in the health care delivery system have influenced QM. This in turn directs the formulation of role competencies and the preparation of health care professionals.

Evolution of Health Care Delivery

In the health care field today, two primary issues facing health care leaders are the cost of doing business and the quality of the health care that is provided. Of those issues, both the literature and reports of consumers' and providers' experiences in the delivery and reimbursement system make it quite clear that the driving force is cost. Special attention and expertise are required if quality is to retain its rightful emphasis. Through the application of QI principles, both the cost and the quality of care can be addressed. Millions of dollars of the cost of health care can be cut by doing the right things the right way at the right time. These same principles will respond to the public's demand for quality of care.

Changes in health care delivery have resulted in increasing multidisciplinarity and interdisciplinarity in nontraditional settings. Some examples of emerging multidisciplinary or interdisciplinary models of care delivery include managed care, case management, collaborative practice, and product line management.

Just as the health care delivery system is undergoing rapid changes, so are the approaches to the management of quality. In 1990, Lomas described three changes in the approach to improve quality:

1. integrating quality management into every work process that takes place in an organization, as opposed to isolating the tasks of quality assurance
2. focusing more on health outcomes than on individual provider competence
3. paying more attention to the establishment of explicit practice guidelines rather than simply using implicit judgments

These recommendations are still timely and offer broad guidelines for the development of QM expertise.

In 1992, the Joint Commission on Accreditation of Healthcare Organizations (the Joint Commission) began a carefully planned transition to standards that emphasized continuous quality improvement (CQI). The main focus shifted to process improvement, with emphasis being placed upon those processes that are important to patient care. The shift in focus was further emphasized by the change in the *Accreditation Manual's* chapter title "Quality Assurance," to "Quality Assessment and Improvement." Organizational performance focused standards promoted cross-departmental attention to quality and emphasized interdepartmental review of care and services. In fact, the new direction was further emphasized by the integration of specialty or unit standards into organizational standards for improved organizational performance. This change in focus was described in the chapter entitled "Improving Organizational Performance," which was published in 1994. It further described the essential activities that an organization may choose in its approach to QI (Patterson, 1996). Under the new standards, the quality professional is no longer the only person accountable for quality; all those providing leadership in health care organizations are accountable as well.

Evolution of Roles

Congruent with health care delivery system changes, roles of the quality professional are also changing and evolving. The quality assurance (QA) professionals of the past were frequently in isolated positions and focused on monitoring of quality indicators and other regulatory matters. In 1996, MacRoberts and Schmele described a major redefinition of the role of the quality professional in terms of a focus on the total practice environment. These new quality process experts serve as coaches, facilitators, and consultants. Current roles carry such titles as director of CQI/case management, manager of clinical/quality management, and performance improvement coordinator. Though some of the accountabilities in these roles seem to be those of traditional QA, others include QI as well. For example, one health maintenance organization (HMO) described the current QM role as managing quality outcomes by tracking and trending utilization statistics and by implementing CQI. Many health care organizations require the ability to work with multidisciplinary and interdisciplinary quality/process improvement teams. According to MacRoberts and Schmele (1996), graduate-level knowledge is necessary in these roles, including knowledge of information management, organizational behavior, systems theory, and change process theory. In addition, superb communication and problem-solving skills are vital.

The need for graduate preparation as a requisite for leadership positions is well accepted in health care. The study of the science of quality will continue to be of primary significance and a necessary component of academic preparation of health care administrators. It is increasingly important that candidates for administration and managerial positions in health care possess the knowledge to manage quality in their organizational unit and to assess and revise processes that link their unit with others. For example, some managerial positions currently described in the literature view in-depth knowledge of CQI and an ability to work closely with other disciplines as essential. Batalden (1993) pointed out that all leadership positions require knowledge and application of QI principles. He recommended that because QI is the primary job of every individual in the organization, these abilities should be a requirement of all roles.

Although written several years ago, Fair's (1989) article on quality education is very applicable to the competencies required in today's graduate education. She described the need for course work that would prepare practi-

tioners to manage problems that reach beyond the traditional clinical and management boundaries. She contended that one primary education component is the ability to use reasoning skills to derive creative solutions to complex problems. This attribute will be expected of today's graduates as they enter the health care system.

Identified Competencies for Quality Practitioners

In addition to the need for QM and QI preparation for all health care roles, there also exists a need for quality specialists. For purposes of this chapter, this role will be identified as that of *quality practitioner.* Bleich (1996) described this specialty role as that of consultant, motivator, educator, and systems designer. He envisioned the role as transitional, assisting management and staff in the creation of an environment of continuous quality, and posited that as the QI culture matured, the need for the specialist role might no longer exist. The body of knowledge that such a specialist would need to facilitate the cultural change would include clinical outcomes, patient satisfaction, measurement, informatics, systems design, strategic planning, conflict management, and statistical analysis.

A comprehensive needs assessment survey done by Norman et al. (1990) identified perceived curricular components necessary for the preparation of quality professionals. This study was conducted by the University of Houston and the University of Texas, endorsed by the National Association of Quality Assurance Professionals (NAQAP), and approved by the American College of Healthcare Executives. A three-round Delphi approach was used to survey representative samples from three of the stakeholders who were perceived to be appropriate to make informed decisions about curricular requirements for the field of quality professionals. The sample consisted of 250 quality professionals, 250 hospital administrators, and 250 directors of health care administration programs. The study was grounded in social cognition theory, which supports the idea that a key process in organizational change is cognitive restructuring based on a sound assessment of instructional needs. The major curricular areas that were used as a basis for the study were adapted from the competency outline of NAQAP. Broad areas of knowledge and skill that were perceived to be most important were quality program design, standards and regulation, management, and finance. Priority learning needs for quality practitioners were management information systems, risk management, and quantitative methods. Norman et al. (1990) strongly emphasized that higher education is lacking in programs that prepare professionals to meet rapidly evolving QM needs. Their recommendations include the incorporation of the study findings into a thoughtfully developed curriculum derived from the theoretical principles of instructional design.

QI Education for Health Services Leaders

The Association of University Programs in Health Administration (AUPHA) has also identified QI as central to the educational preparation of health services leaders. Over a 4-year period (1989–1992), AUPHA addressed the development of teaching materials and QI research initiatives through a project funded by The Pew Charitable Trusts. One of the project outcomes was the recognition that with the movement from QA to QI, as well as the shift from acute hospital care to other settings, an adaptation of health administration curriculum is called for to incorporate current thinking in QI.

The Institute for Healthcare Improvement (IHI) provided funds to AUPHA for the development by Gelmon and Baker (1994) of *A Quality Improvement Teaching Resource Guide*. This guide recognized QI as a strong integrating theme for health administration curriculum and emphasized the need to include QI theory and application in health care administration curriculum. It synthesizes key compo-

nents of quality improvement and quality management, provides useful methods to help with curriculum planning and design/redesign, and includes sample syllabi from multiple quality courses. Because this is a classic and seminal guide to the academic teaching of QI, we will rely heavily on its content here.

Responding to the need to provide systematically a thorough QM education for health administrators, Gelmon and Baker formulated the following goals for their book.

- To offer QI/QM concepts, sample syllabi and course objectives, and other resources in a compendium that was both comprehensive and accessible
- To develop a reference that was usable in various organizational settings that offered different approaches to incorporating QI into current curricula and that assisted in the development of new materials
- To disseminate to health administration programs, other interested health sciences, and related disciplines a synthesis of experience with QI education from various academic settings
- To inspire educators in health administration programs with the concept of QI as a management system and a leadership philosophy

Gelmon and Baker (1994) organized the extensive body of knowledge related to QI and QM into a framework of primary QI concepts (see Figure 18–1). Recognizing that curriculum structure and organizational setting may place constraints on how many of the concepts can be offered to the graduate student, they provided a matrix to demonstrate the level of emphasis that certain concepts and tools would require (see Exhibit 18–1). A second matrix provided by Gelmon and Baker relates key QI content and tools to curriculum content areas that have been defined as essential by the Accrediting Commission on Education for Health Services Administration (ACEHSA; see Exhibit 18–2).

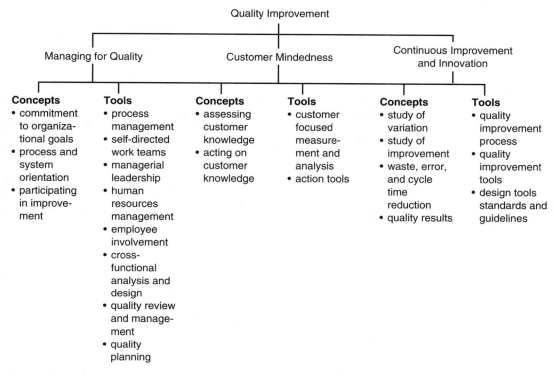

Figure 18–1 A model of quality improvement. *Source:* Reprinted with permission from S.B. Gelmon and G.R. Baker, *A Quality Improvement Teaching Resource Guide*, p. 32, ©1994, AUPHA/IHI.

Gelmon and Baker (1994) also offered five broad learning objectives that establish consistency for curriculum development:

1. To apply QI theories, concepts, and tools when addressing the improvement of health care quality
2. To identify the roles and accountabilities of all health system managers, professionals, and employees in the improvement of quality of care
3. To include both the organizational and the individual processes necessary for continuous improvement and innovation
4. To be customer focused and to create and improve services that meet the needs of the customer
5. To improve quality through the analysis and application of organizational and individual change strategies

By establishing an organizing framework and by identifying key QI educational components that need to be incorporated into curriculum, Gelmon and Baker's guide serves as a comprehensive resource to educators. It recognizes different ways in which QI is taught and provides several approaches, usable in a variety of organizational settings, for building QI concepts and strategies into existing curricula and developing new materials. *A Quality Improvement Teaching Resource Guide* is highly recommended for faculty who are responsible for teaching QI content. According to Baker

Exhibit 18–1 A Quality Function Development Matrix

	Process Management	Self-Directed Work Teams	Managerial Leadership	Human Resource Management	Employee Involvement	Cross-Functional Analysis and Design	Design of Products and Services	Quality Review and Management	Quality Planning	Customer-Driven Management	Process Improvement	Standards for Excellence	Benchmarking	Relationship Management	SQC SPC JIT
Commitment to organizational goals		●	●	●	■	■	■	●	●	●				●	
Process and system orientation	●	●	■			■	■	■			●	■	■		●
Value-adding participation		●	●	●	●	■					■				
Customer knowledge		■			■	●	●			●			●	●	
Customer needs and expectations		■	■			●	●			●	■	■	●	●	
Quality results	●			■				●	●	●	●	●	●		●
Variations/study of variation	●	■		■		■	■	●	●	●	●		■		●
Waste, error, and cycle time reduction	●	●		■		●	●	●	●	●	●	●	■	■	●

Note: ● = major coverage; concept application taught in depth. ■ = minor coverage; assumed knowledge.
Source: Reprinted with permission from S.B. Gelmon and G.R. Baker, *A Quality Improvement Teaching Resource Guide*, p. 45, ©1994, AUPHA/IHI.

Exhibit 18–2 Matrix of Core Concepts and ACEHSA Content Areas

	Commitment to Organizational Goals	Process and System Orientation	Participation	Assessing Customer Knowledge	Acting on Customer Knowledge	Study of Variation	Waste, Error, Cycle Time Reduction	Quality Results	Study of Improvement
Health system overview	●	●		●				■	■
Planning and evaluation	■	●	■	●	●	■	■	●	●
Policy and regulation		■		■	■			■	●
Human resource management	■		●	■	■				■
Information management	■	●	■	●	■	■	■	●	■
Quantitative methods, statistics, epidemiology		●	■	●		●	●	●	
Organizational behavior and management	●	■	●	■	●	■	●	■	●
Health care finance and economics	■	■		●	■	●	■		
Values and ethics	●		●	●	■		■	■	■
Core quality course	●	●	●	●	●	●	●	●	●

Note: ● = major coverage; concept application taught in depth. ■ = minor coverage; assumed knowledge/used as tool.
Source: Reprinted with permission from S.B. Gelmon and G.R. Baker, *A Quality Improvement Teaching Resource Guide,* p. 49, ©1994, AUPHA/IHI.

(personal communication, April 1996), a second teaching guide, entitled Assessment in a QI framework, focuses on specific teaching tools and ideas. (Both resources are available from the AUPHA.)

HOW WILL GRADUATES LEARN TO USE QI IN PRACTICE?

As the health care industry gains experience with QI, the need for educational strategies increases. Just as major health care corporations adapt educational strategies from nonhealth industries to develop training materials for their internal staff, universities are becoming creative in developing graduate curriculum strategies.

Integration versus Specialization

A review of current literature and a telephone survey of graduate faculty showed that some universities offer distinct QI courses, whereas others attempt to integrate QI concepts into all graduate courses. As Reublinger (1989) pointed out, and as personal communications with several nursing faculty across the nation and our own experience indicate, there is a trend away from offering special courses on QM and toward the integration of QM into all graduate nursing courses. In contrast, Meisenheimer (personal communication, April 23, 1996) described a trend more toward separate courses, especially in colleges of business.

Gelmon and Baker (1994) suggested that in planning and redesigning curricula, consideration be given to where QI concepts could fit, such as introductory courses, core courses, cross-disciplinary courses, and experiential learning through field placements. They also emphasized that if efforts are made to integrate QI concepts, those concepts should not just be "inserted" into other courses. Rather, methods for successful integration include

1. using QI tools in core courses
2. reinforcing QI concepts across all programs and departments

3. developing student and faculty QI teams for addressing process improvement
4. identifying practice sites that are making significant progress in QI

At this time, there is a lack of evidence to support the superiority of integrated content over specialized content or vice versa. It would seem appropriate to use either or both approaches depending upon program outcome objectives.

QM Content Integration

One example of integration of QI into the curriculum can be found at the School of Nursing of the University of Michigan at Ann Arbor. Dr. Dick Redmon, director of the division of nursing and health systems programs (personal communication, April 8, 1996) stated that QI concepts and tools are integrated throughout their curriculum and that there is no specialty QI course at the undergraduate, graduate, or doctoral level. For example, in courses on human resource management, the concept of QI teams is discussed, including the formation, management, and fiscal implications of such teams. To integrate QI successfully and ensure that the graduate is able to apply QI in practice, the university works very closely with the University of Michigan Medical Center, which subscribes to QI as a vital leadership philosophy. The medical center's need for graduates who can apply QI concepts has contributed to the collaborative effort of the medical center and the School of Nursing. Leaders of these programs believe in the QI philosophy and in their responsibility to teach it; thus faculty QI education is provided by medical center leaders who also teach introductory courses for the graduate students.

Steps taken by the university to integrate QI concepts into the curriculum have included

1. recognizing that graduates need to be able to apply QI principles in practice
2. preparing the nursing faculty to teach QI through a series of workshops provided by medical center QI leaders

3. analyzing all levels of curriculum (undergraduate, graduate, and doctoral) for integration of QI concepts and tools into all courses
4. including opportunities during student clinicals for the students to participate in QI activities and to apply QI tools
5. applying QI concepts to processes that are integral to the faculty and are in need of improvement

Redmon emphasized the final step as being of primary importance: not until the faculty was able to apply QI concepts and see benefits of process improvement did they place the necessary emphasis on teaching QI concepts. One example of a successful process improvement was the improvement of the grant application process, to which many of the faculty could relate. The faculty team's process revision was obvious evidence to the faculty that QI works. This practice experience added value to QI concepts and assisted the faculty in enhancing the integration of QI concepts into their courses. Role modeling, on the part of faculty, is a powerful tool for teaching the QI process.

QM Specialization

An example of a separate QM course taught through the collaborative efforts of academia and service was described by Verhey and Haw (1994). The course, entitled "Quality Management," prepares the health care professional for participation in QI activities and for using QI principles in practice. The graduate-level course is offered by the San Francisco State University Department of Nursing and is the result of a partnership between the university and over 80 clinical agencies. It is offered to graduate students and to practicing nurses in the community. It is aimed at building a solid QM knowledge base, including the skills needed by the practicing professional when actively participating in QM activities. The course objectives illustrate the integration of service and academia and incorporate concepts

that are applicable to the nurse in such roles as clinician, educator, manager, and quality practitioner. The application of QM principles to specific patient populations and to selected settings contributes to the preparation of a graduate who can apply QM principles in practice. The students spend at least 10 weeks developing and implementing a proposed QM program in their assigned clinical agency. Course content includes such concepts as

- quality definitions and QM trends
- models and tools of CQI
- regulatory and accreditation standards
- developing a QM program in a health care agency
- developing structure, process, and outcome standards
- developing tools and data collection methods for monitoring
- analyzing data and developing action plans
- documenting and reporting improvement
- evaluating effectiveness of agency programs

The work of Verhey and Haw (1994) will provide the reader with ideas upon which faculty may build.

Additional rich resources are provided by Gelmon and Baker (1994), including over 30 sample QI course syllabi and descriptions. These syllabi were submitted by faculty from a variety of university departments, including health administration, health systems management, health policy and administration, and business administration. Table 18–1 includes a convenience sample of QI syllabi being offered by university departments.

Application of QI Principles in the Academic Setting

Whether resources in the academic setting allow distinct QI courses to be offered or whether integration of QI concepts into curriculum is the selected strategy, a key to teach-

Table 18–1 Sample Syllabi from Courses on Quality

University	Department	Title	Description	Comments
University of Michigan	Nursing	N652: Synthesis of Theory and Practice in Nursing Administration	"This integrative seminar provides an opportunity for critical examination of issues and problems related to the efficient and effective administration of resources for patient-care delivery. Contemporary problems in nursing administration provide a framework in which alternatives for more effective delivery of nursing care are emphasized. The case study method is employed to illustrate ill-defined complex problems from actual organizational situations. A wide range of organizational issues is considered, with particular emphasis on the management of planned change in relation to improving quality within a constraining economic environment."[a]	Katherine Jones, RN, PhD, FAAN, Associate Professor and course instructor (personal communication; March 15, 1996), states that use of case studies offers graduate students an opportunity to apply QI concepts to real-life situations.
University of Oklahoma Health Sciences Center	Nursing and Health Administration and Policy	N5990-710 and HAP 6940-709: Total Quality Management in Health Care	"An interdisciplinarity lecture course focusing on the concept and implementation of Total Quality Management and the use of related measurement tools in health care settings."[b]	This course was developed and offered by the author Dr. Schmele and by Dr. Al-Assaf of the Health Administration and Policy Dept. It was available through both the schools of nursing and HAP, and its one offering had graduate students from both the departments attend.

University of Oklahoma	Health Administration and Policy	HAP 5883: Healthcare Quality Management	"An introduction to the process of Quality Improvement in health care organizations. Different criteria and guidelines for implementing total quality management and the continuous quality improvement process are discussed. Differentiation will be attempted between quality assurance and quality management."[c]	
University of Michigan	Public Health Management and Policy	HMP 683: Quality of Care	"Focuses on the concepts and practices of quality of care assessment, control and improvement in health care delivery settings. It is designed to provide students with an in-depth understanding of basic concepts and frameworks and of their applicability and relevance in specific situations. In addition, the course seeks to cover the major approaches to quality of care assessment, improvement, and control currently in use in the health care field."[d]	Course instructor Dr. Leon Wyszewianski (personal communication, March 18, 1996) states that graduate students from the Public Health, Nursing, and Pharmacy departments attend the course and that it focuses on issues that arise when trying to change physician practice or trying to deal with accreditation. The course requires a background in hospital operations and a knowledge of Medicare and Medicaid.

continues

Table 18–1 continued

University	Department	Title	Description	Comments
Johns Hopkins University	Hygiene and Public Health	Quality Assurance Management Methods for Developing Countries	"To provide a thorough grounding in the principles and practice of Quality Assurance Management for those who have or will have responsibility for health systems in developing countries. Through informal talks in a seminar setting, exercises to develop competencies in selected QA methods, and a series of case studies, participants will work through a systematic process for closing the gap between what should be accomplished with presently available resources and what actually takes place with health care efforts in most of the developing world. Included is the importance of a genuine team approach in the face of a generally authoritarian tradition; recognition of the entire community as the customer requiring an active participatory approach; [and] the introduction of measurement-based methods for problem identification and solving."[e]	Course faculty Dr. Al-Assaf (personal communication, February 27, 1996) stated that participants included graduate students and various other individuals from the United States and other countries.
University of Toronto	Health Administration	CHL 3202: Quality Assessment and Continuous Improvement in Health Care	"The quality of health care and the effective use of health care resources are fundamental issues for health care organizations. While most health care organizations have developed quality review processes and utilization management programs, these have had only limited impact in improving health care. At the same time, many believe that the increasing financial constraint experienced by health care organizations will decrease the quality of care and that efforts to respond to this constraint by	

controlling the use of health care services may proscribe professional autonomy and adversely affect health outcomes. In this course, students will study a new approach to quality measurement and quality improvement developed from U.S. industrial quality efforts, refined by Japanese corporations, and now being applied by health care organizations in Canada and the U.S. Often referred to as Continuous Quality Improvement (CQI) or Total Quality Management (TQM), this approach focuses on the improvement of care delivery and supportive processes in health care organizations and the development of customer knowledge as the key to more effective health care."[f]

[a]University of Michigan School of Nursing, Winter 1996 (N652: Synthesis of Theory and Practice in Nursing Administration). Course Outline.
[b]University of Oklahoma Health Sciences Center, 1994.(HAP 6940-709 or N5990-710: Total Quality Management). Course Syllabus.
[c]University of Oklahoma College of Public Health, Health Administration and Policy Department, 1995 (HAP 5883: Healthcare Quality Management). Course Outline.
[d]University of Michigan School of Public Health, Department of Health Management and Policy, 1995 (HMP 683: Quality of Care). Course Syllabus.
[e]Johns Hopkins University School of Hygiene and Public Health, Departments of International Health and Health Policy and Management, Baltimore and the Center for Human Services, Bethesda, 1995. (Quality Assurance Management Methods for Developing Countries). Course Syllabus.
[f]S.B. Gelmon & G.R. Baker, 1994. *A Quality Improvement Teaching Resource Guide*, pp. 88–89.

ing QI successfully is that QI also be applied to processes in the academic setting. This has been substantiated in the practice setting. Reublinger (1989) argued that the involvement of academia is vital to integrate theory into practice. Only when the leadership of the organization places value on QI concepts and a cultural change occurs do faculty and staff in that setting find opportunities to get involved in improving processes.

Fair (1989) contended that to integrate quality into organizations, recognition of the following essential principles is vital:

1. Quality is an organizational goal.
2. Quality is as important as the financial bottom line.
3. Quality and the assessment of quality should focus on improvement opportunities.
4. Quality will increasingly be redefined as resources are more constrained.

When QI is a leadership philosophy and is practiced every day, it becomes integrated into the belief system of the faculty. The integration of QI concepts relies heavily upon the culture of the organization, whether it is an academic or a practice setting. Only when the culture supports QI beliefs do those working in that setting place value on QI. The University of Michigan model discussed earlier integrates QI concepts into the faculty thought processes and offers a strategy that has been successful in practice.

Batalden (1993) described four questions that may be useful in an organization's transformation toward a quality leadership philosophy. Those questions, if applied to an academic setting, provide insight to the process of providing education and assist with the process of infiltrating QI thinking into the organization:

1. Who are the "customers" of academia? Who benefits from what is produced?
2. What processes are the staff and faculty involved in as they do their work?
3. What steps are involved in the processes of work?
4. How can the waste, complexity, and rework that may be involved in those processes be reduced?

When work can be seen in this new way, the entire organization will benefit.

Barriers to Integration of QI Principles into the Curriculum

Time constraints are frequently given as a reason by faculty for not successfully integrating QI concepts into a curriculum (Patterson, personal communication, April 22, 1996). A second barrier is a lack of QI faculty knowledge. For example, in a survey, graduate faculty at the University of Oklahoma College of Nursing suggested that efforts to integrate quality concepts would be more successful if standard definitions and curriculum guidelines were available to them. It is understandable that if QI knowledge is not basic, and is not being used in an academic setting, faculty are not likely to use it in their teaching.

A third major barrier is the identification of clinical sites that practice the principles of QI. Many health care organizations are focused on reengineering and cost reduction without using QI concepts to accomplish those efforts. Baker (personal communication, April 22, 1996) suggested that if organizations were to recognize that one of the outcomes of QI is cost reduction, QI initiatives would again become a priority and would be seen as the principle that can lead an organization through this era of reengineering.

It is recognized that positive incentives for faculty involvement in QI may be lacking. Reward systems for faculty are often based on solitary accomplishments such as grant awards or publishing endeavors rather than on carefully cultivated interdisciplinary QI efforts. Because QI requires interdisciplinary approaches, it is important that academic leaders support and encourage such collaboration.

HOW WILL EDUCATORS EVALUATE GRADUATE COMPETENCIES IN QI?

An important aspect of the teaching and learning of QM concepts and techniques is the evaluation of the objectives. It is important to look at structure, process, and outcome objectives of individual sessions, courses, and programs.

Meisenheimer (personal communication, April 23, 1996) recommended a straightforward evaluation technique for classes. She suggested that students answer three succinct questions after each class (faculty members may wish to reflect on the same questions):

1. How did I prepare for today's class?
2. What did I learn that will be useful in my future practice?
3. What still needs clarification?

This brief evaluation is also used by various QI "teams" at the end of each team meeting, and it provides information that assists in improving the process of holding a meeting. This technique is quite transferable to classes and will provide feedback to the faculty to be used as formative evaluation data.

Another student data source may be student self-reports. For example, in a purposive sample of graduate students at the University of Oklahoma College of Nursing (OUCN), the following survey questions were asked:

1. In what courses throughout your graduate program did you find quality of care integrated into the course?
2. In what ways was quality of care integrated into the courses mentioned above?
3. How should quality of care be taught (integrated into other courses or as a separate course)?

A small and sketchy student response rate was attributed to timing late in the semester when other priorities were high. The majority of the respondents recommended that the topic of quality be integrated into several courses. One student pondered over whether it was realistic to teach about quality within the tumultuous money-driven health care environment when caregivers are struggling to provide even the basic necessities to patients.

A mail evaluative survey was conducted on former OUCN master's-prepared nurses graduating between 1993 and 1995. A one-time mail-out to 110 graduates yielded a 37% return rate. In this survey of seasoned graduates, the following questions were asked:

1. During your graduate nursing program, did you take a separate course on quality of care?
2. If you did take a separate course, have you found it useful in your practice?
3. If you did not take a separate course, was quality of care integrated into any of your other courses? If so, which courses?
4. If quality of care was integrated into other courses, have you found the concepts taught to be useful in your practice?
5. How have you used the concepts of quality of care in your nursing practice?
6. How would you recommend that quality of care be taught?

A small minority implied that there was only minimal opportunity to consider quality of care in their patient care work environment. However, the majority offered much more enthusiastic and descriptive responses. Only a few of the respondents had taken a special QM course; it was not a program requirement. Most graduates readily identified courses in which QM was integrated and substantiated the importance of its inclusion, especially as it related to application in practice. Most respondents placed heavy emphasis on the use of concepts of quality in their professional practice environment. Respondents offered elaborate feedback about how "quality of care" could be taught in the graduate academic setting. Serendipitously, this probably points out that they view the study of quality as a high priority and that they themselves have experienced a need for greater preparation in this subject. In general, respondents recommended that the quality learning experience include at least the following:

- definitions
- concepts
- objectives
- measurements
- collaboration
- TQM/CQI
- multidisciplinarity
- linkage with cost
- linkage with ethics
- application in practice
- program development

The majority of respondents agreed that the teaching of quality should be integrated throughout the curriculum on a continuous basis. They also emphasized the need to begin this process at the undergraduate level.

Although their focus was on upper level courses, Gelmon and Baker (1994) described a viewpoint similar to the students', emphasizing that QI concepts be reinforced across all program levels. They did not specifically address tools with which to evaluate the learning of students, but they emphasized the relationship between academia and practice in ensuring that QI would become a leadership philosophy in both settings.

Ideally, the best measure of effective teaching of quality management would be the evidence in practice of the maintenance of standards of quality in specific patient care programs or individualized patient care situa-

tions. Because this is the subject of this entire book, we will defer this discussion to later chapters.

FUTURE CHALLENGES AND DIRECTIONS

Many products, including education, are market driven. As the market's focus changes, so must academia change in its "product," the graduate. As outcome becomes the focus as well as the measurement tool for appropriateness of care, should not outcome be the guide for preparing the graduate? Should we not plan QI education around aggregate outcome data? Lomas (1990) described the use of outcome data to identify education needs of practitioners and to target training for providers. Patterson (personal communication, April 22, 1996) suggested that as practice settings are using clinical pathways to manage care and to measure outcomes, so academia also needs to identify ways to focus on outcome as a curriculum guide. One of the challenges will be to use outcome-based information systems that provide timely information to academia that will facilitate rapid responses to the changes in practice.

Will graduate-level QI preparation be adequate to face the challenges of the 21st century? According to Starck, Duffy, and Vogler (1993), the preparation of future clinical leaders may require even a practice-focused doctoral curriculum. Patterson (personal communication, April 22, 1996) described postgraduate and even postdoctoral residency programs that are available at the University of Pennsylvania and the University of Laverne in Laverne, California. These courses offer a formalized QI practicum to prepare future health care leaders.

As cost-effectiveness is the driving force in today's health care market, and as QI is recognized as resulting in cost savings, QI courses will need to focus on such major concepts as resource allocation, utilization, and evaluation of health care delivery systems. Dr. Katherine Jones, Associate Professor at the University of Michigan School of Nursing (personal communication, March 15, 1996), described such a course at the University of Michigan ("Synthesis of Theory and Practice in Nursing Administration" [N652]).

In the international scene, there are those who suggest that the teaching of quality management needs to begin very early in the learning sequence. For example, the Ecole Primaire Mixte de Montreuil, a French primary school in Versailles, has been successfully using the Deming philosophy for 2 years, according to Dr. Al-Assaf at the University of Oklahoma School of Health, Administration, and Policy (personal communication, February 27, 1996). It is reasonable to speculate that doing the right thing at the right time in the right way could become a strong value even at such an early age. One might speculate that this could offer a foundation for quality even at a societal level in the 21st century.

REFERENCES

Batalden, P.B. (1993). Organizationwide quality improvement in health care. In A.F. Al-Assaf & J. A. Schmele (Eds.), *The textbook of total quality in healthcare* (pp. 70–72). Delray Beach, FL: St. Lucie.

Bleich, M.R. (1996). Leadership and development of the quality professional. In J.A. Schmele (Ed.), *Quality management in nursing and health care* (pp. 343–354). Albany, NY: Delmar.

Fair, P.A. (1989). Today's students, tomorrow's leaders: Learning about quality. *Journal of Quality Assurance, 11*(4), 30–32, 44.

Gelmon, S.B., & Baker, G.R. (1994). *A quality improvement teaching resource guide.* Arlington, VA: Association of University Programs in Health Administration.

Gelmon, S.B., & Regan, J.T. (1996). *Assessment in a quality improvement framework: A sourcebook for health administration education.* Arlington, VA: The Association of University Programs in Health Administration.

Kibbee, P. (1988). An emerging professional: The quality assurance nurse. *Journal of Nursing Administration, 18,* 30–33.

Lomas, J. (1990). Quality assurance and effectiveness in health care: An overview [Editorial]. *Quality Assurance in Health Care, 2*(1), 5–12.

MacRoberts, M., & Schmele, J.A. (1996). Redefinition of quality-management roles in a time of shifting paradigms. In J.A. Schmele (Ed.), *Quality management in nursing and health care* (pp. 539–550). Albany, NY: Delmar.

Norman, D.K., Randall, R.S., & Hornsby, B.J. (1990). Critical features of a curriculum in health care quality and resource management. *Quality Review Bulletin, 16,* 317–336.

Patterson, C.H. (1996). The Joint Commission and organization performance improvement. In J.A. Schmele (Ed.), *Quality management in nursing and health care* (pp. 295–308). Albany, NY: Delmar.

Reublinger, V. (1989). The emerging professional: The quality assurance nurse. *Journal of Nursing Administration, 18*(4), 30–38.

Starck, P.L., Duffy, M.E., & Vogler, R. (1993). Developing a nursing doctorate for the 21st century. *Journal of Professional Nursing, 9*(4), 212–219.

Verhey, M.P., & Haw, M.A. (1994). Teaching quality management in a nursing graduate program: A collaborative university-agency quality team. *Journal of Nursing Care Quality, 8*(4), 48–54.

## CHAPTER 19

A Continuous Quality Improvement Program: Developing the Employee

Traci L. Raether

CHAPTER OBJECTIVES

After completing this chapter, the reader will be able to

- explain the relationship between a caring curriculum model and the CQI "Learning Wave" program
- develop a QI curriculum for employees
- use the "Spider Diagram" as a CQI measurement tool

Education is the cornerstone to the survival of a health care organization. Regulatory compliance, escalating health care costs, and consumerism are challenging organizations to change the way they operate. Organizations must provide services differently, with the needs of the customers—internal and external—being the driving force. The implementation of continuous quality improvement (CQI) is the means to meet the fiscal expectations of third-party payers and customers receiving services without sacrificing quality. To respond to the expectations of customers in the new customer-focused paradigm, a fundamental shift in an organization's culture is required. CQI education for all employees, front line and management, is the key to accomplishing the culture shift needed in health care organizations. All employees need to be educated in the new quality philosophy, team development, and the techniques required to monitor and improve quality.

The teaching methodology used in a CQI educational program is important due to the difficulty of integrating new knowledge into practice in the workplace. The Caring Curriculum, developed by Bevis and Watson (1989), addresses the need to change from traditional teaching/learning models to a new paradigm of teachers and students interacting so they have an opportunity to learn from each other. This interaction demonstrates the new relationships needed to change the "way work has always been done" in the workplace. The premises of the Caring Curriculum reflect the application of CQI principles in the workplace. Only when all staff are educated in CQI principles, in a way that demonstrates the expectation of the new paradigm of customer-centered health care, will the culture shift be accomplished to ensure the organization's survival in the marketplace.

ORGANIZATIONAL CULTURE SHIFT

Organizational culture is defined as the values and beliefs held by members of the organization that govern their behavior. A CQI educational program must address the need to depart from traditional values and beliefs and identify the rationale for adopting new values and beliefs that are customer centered. The new culture must emphasize how a work group shapes behavior via trust, information sharing, and adaptiveness (Maddox, 1992).

Development of a quality culture, in which the quality of service is the overriding goal, requires that employees receive information and education related to teamwork, communication, problem-solving skills, departmental interdependence, decision making, and methods of data collection and analysis. Education must be provided to all employees to provide the organization with a solid foundation. Every employee within the organization must have a common CQI knowledge base and the feeling of being included in the organization's mission for the culture to be transformed from the traditional health care environment to the desired customer-centered environment. Emphasis on the elimination of non-value-added work, duplication of work, and rework must be included in the educational program. The goal of every employee to perform work processes right the first time will be essential to the success of the organization.

Health care providers must recognize and accept that consumers have specific expectations of desired services and will choose a provider that will meet or exceed those expectations. This means all organizations must be aware of their customers and the services they expect. Instead of responding to the customer in the traditional fragmented departmental manner, a more effective means of meeting customer needs is to work together as a team. Milakovich (1991) viewed the institution in the new culture of total quality health care as an "interconnected network of interdependent processes, linked laterally, over time, through a network of cooperating (internal and external) suppliers and customers" (p. 12). This process must be allowed to develop from within the organization and must not be imposed from the top down. All employees must be included in the development of a new culture because all processes in the facility are subject to continuous improvement. The adaptation to a quality organization necessitates a paradigm shift from the traditional management model of top-down authority and clear chains of command to an inverted triangular approach with a customer

focus, flexibility, and employee involvement in decision making.

CQI EDUCATION FOR ALL EMPLOYEES

The importance of education to the successful implementation of CQI must not be underestimated. Everyone in an organization needs CQI education to form the foundation of knowledge on which all other developments and improvements are built. Quality improvement efforts begin with the education of each member of the organization. All employees, including managers and front-line employees, must participate in the educational program to facilitate the adoption of a customer-centered culture where all employees work together to deliver high-quality services to the customers. According to Kirk (1992), throughout a quality organization, managers and empowered employees create the systems and processes that will efficiently, effectively, and predictably produce and ensure the best possible clinical service and satisfaction outcomes. Quality management is an excellent way to handle business, with every facet of the business working toward a common goal of providing the best possible services at the lowest achievable cost. Using a total quality management (TQM) philosophy, customer-centered care requires a cross-functional team approach. By developing an efficient and effective labor base, an organization can provide a valuable service to the customer.

Gopalakrishnan and McIntyre (1992) stated that any education should take place during regular paid time. The focus of education should be on learning by doing. Education should address real working conditions and problems. According to Crosby (1980), investment in the education of employees and rewards for teamwork actually save money in the long run by (a) increasing productivity, (b) reducing waste and rework for corrections, and (c) increasing profitability through positive comments to potential customers by satisfied customers. Crosby emphasized changing the organizational culture to expect quality rather than merely the meeting of specifications. This change in organizational culture requires a shift to the use of TQM/CQI principles in the workplace.

Learning activities in a CQI educational program should be developed using the strong sense of support students enjoy from each other to enhance knowledge acquisition, thus encouraging camaraderie rather than competition among students. This sense of being responsible for one's own learning as well as that of one's classmate can transfer into practice such that students will willingly share their knowledge in a caring way with others, rather than selfishly withholding their knowledge from peers (Nelms, 1990).

Education is critical not only to each individual but to the productivity and competitive advantage of companies and the community as a whole. The employer's interest in learning tailored to the workplace, in contrast to more general academic preparation, stems from the fact that on-the-job learning directly supports the employer's organizational culture and strategic goals. Such education occurs in the context of the employees working as a team, encouraging efficiency in the work group. In addition, employer-based education occurs in the context of the employer's strategy, products, and market niche, thereby encouraging new efficiencies, quality improvements, and innovations. Employers increasingly depend on the skills of all their employees for improvements in efficiency, quality, and customer service and for the development of new applications for existing products and services (Carnevalle, 1989).

TEACHING METHODOLOGY: A CARING CURRICULUM

The teaching methodology used in the development and implementation of a CQI educational program needs to support the changes desired in an organization's culture. This will assist the participants of the educational program in applying their new knowledge in the workplace. The use of the Caring Curriculum (Bevis & Watson, 1989) in a CQI educational program reflects the implementation of CQI principles applied in the workplace. The implementation of CQI in the workplace stresses that interactions between front-line employees and management and effective communication between departments are necessary to meet or exceed customer expectations. Likewise, the Caring Curriculum principles recognize the importance of the students' interaction with each other as well as with the teacher. All employees in a CQI workplace are of equal importance. Each individual has a role to fulfill to provide service to the customer; no role is more significant than another. In a learning situation, the teacher and students alike make discoveries from their interactions.

The Caring Curriculum is designed to enable participants to be more responsive to societal needs and individual customer needs, to be more creative and more capable of critical thinking, and to bring scholarly approaches to customers' problems and issues. These outcomes are also desired by the organization implementing the CQI educational program. The application of the Caring Curriculum principles helps to accomplish what has been difficult or impossible with the traditional educational model. Its alternative paradigm of learning encourages interaction between participants and allows for the internalization of knowledge by experiential learning. The premises of the Caring Curriculum as a new model for learning represent the crux of the new paradigm; they sum up the values, methods, models, and mission of the humanist educative model.

Although the Caring Curriculum model offers no rules and no real road maps, it does offer some guidelines. It offers possibilities for teachers and employees to collaborate as individuals and as professionals providing health care. It offers the opportunity to make learning a lived experience that is analyzed, reflected upon, synthesized, and understood. It offers alliances instead of opposition. It allows freedom for individuality, creativity, style, and multiple ways of knowing. It legitimizes intuition, caring, and morality. The use of the Caring Curriculum promotes the application of new CQI knowledge to an employee's job.

THE "LEARNING WAVE": THE CQI EDUCATIONAL PROGRAM AT EVERGREEN RETIREMENT COMMUNITY

Evergreen Retirement Community (ERC) is a not-for-profit continuing-care retirement community that provides an array of living options for senior citizens ranging from independent cooperative housing, homes, and apartments to assisted-living arrangements and a skilled nursing home. ERC serves nearly 290 residents and provides employment to approximately 245 staff.

The Learning Wave is a 30-hour CQI educational program with specific learning objectives (Exhibit 19–1). All Evergreen employees are required to participate in a Learning Wave. The duration of the program is either 6 or 7 weeks, depending on the length and frequency of weekly sessions and related homework. The employee must attend at least five of the six educational sessions to "graduate" (Exhibit 19–2). Staff from nursing, social services, dietary, laundry, buildings and grounds, rehab services, housekeeping, clerical services, business office, and administration are represented in each Learning Wave. During a 2-year period, the Learning Wave is conducted for all employees. All employees are paid for their time and replaced on their department work schedules to allow participation in the program. The quality resources director leads/teaches the educational program.

The following 11 key topics are included in the educational program: (a) paradigms; (b) Evergreen's mission, vision, and values; (c) team-building skills; (d) CQI principles; (e) methods of decision making; (f) internal and external customers; (g) data collection methods; (h) the process flowchart; (i) problem-

---

Exhibit 19–1 The Learning Wave Objectives

Upon completion of CQI educational sessions, participants will:

- understand Evergreen's mission, vision, values, and quality improvement model.
- understand the role of Evergreen's Quality Council and the Quality Resources Director.
- understand the need for organizational change.
- define our internal and external customers and explore various ways to assess and meet their needs.
- readily communicate CQI principles to others.
- communicate in an effective manner with all customers: residents, family members, other employees, and suppliers.
- function as effective team members.
- discover the effectiveness of teamwork.
- understand "empowerment."
- utilize a problem-solving process to address issues and concerns.
- utilize CQI tools to perform data-based decision making.
- recognize the interdepartmental cooperation necessary to provide high-quality service to our customers.
- define the roles and processes of an effective meeting.
- verbalize an understanding of how to apply CQI principles in their job.

Courtesy of Evergreen Retirement Community, Inc., Quality Resources Department, Oshkosh, Wisconsin.

Exhibit 19–2 Learning Wave Curriculum

Session 1 (8 Hours)
Welcome, Name Tags, Data Gathering, and
  Agenda Review
Discussion of Paradigms
Review Objectives of the Course and Set Ground
  Rules
Discuss "Why CQI at Evergreen"
Discuss Role of the Quality Council and Quality
  Resources Director
Quality Council Definition of Quality and
  Mission Statement
Evergreen Vision, Mission Statement, and
  Values (Presented by CEO)
Evergreen Quality Improvement Model
Lunch
Evergreen Bingo: Get-Acquainted Exercise
Core Concepts of CQI
Perception Exercise: How Many Squares?
Small-Group Exercise To Demonstrate Group
  Effectiveness
Brainstorming and Affinity Diagram of
  Improvement Opportunities
Identification of Project Team Topics
Program Evaluation

Session 2 (4 Hours)
Agenda Review
Meeting Minute Information
Discussion of "The Quality Gurus"
Discussion of Consensus Decision Making and
  Other Decision-Making Methods
Review Information on "Customers" and
  Homework Assignment
Teams for Excellence Tape #8: Interpersonal
  Skills
Discuss Communication Skills
Small Groups for Project Teamwork
Program Evaluation

Session 3 (4 Hours)
Agenda Review
Discussion of Teams
Teams for Excellence Tape #4: Conducting a
  Meeting

Information on Meetings: Roles and the
  Process
Small Groups for Project Teamwork
Large-Group Discussion of Project Teams
Program Evaluation

Session 4 (4 Hours)
Agenda Review
Warm-Up: Brainteasers
Empowerment Information from *ZAPP! The
  Lightning of Empowerment*
Teams for Excellence Tape #6: Technical
  Requirements of Teams
Large-Group Activity: Cause-and-Effect
  Diagram
Small Groups for Project Teamwork
Program Evaluation

Session 5 (4 Hours)
Agenda Review
Warm-Up
Discuss Problem Solving, PDCA Cycle, and
  Quality Tools (i.e., Run Charts)
Group Activity: Process Flow Diagrams
Small Groups for Project Teamwork
Large-Group Discussion of Project Team
  Progress
Video: Application of Quality Principles in a
  Variety of Organizations
Program Evaluation

Session 6 (6 Hours)
Agenda Review
Teams for Excellence Tape #10: Achieving
  Team Excellence
CQI Concept Application in the "Real
  World"
Small Groups for Project Teamwork
Group Discussion of Project Team Outcomes
Lunch (Provided by Evergreen) and Group
  Picture
Graduation Ceremony
Program Evaluation

Courtesy of Evergreen Retirement Community, Inc., Quality Resources Department, Oshkosh, Wisconsin.

solving skills; (j) interpersonal skills; and (k) empowerment (see Spider Diagram, Figure 19–1).

Scheduling the Learning Wave/Cross-Functional Participation

The program must be scheduled at least 2 months in advance so that managers will have an opportunity to plan for scheduling changes to accommodate staff's participation in the educational program. During the past year, the quality resources director conducted eight "learning waves" sessions with approximately 30 participants each for a total of 240 employees. To ensure cross-functional participation, all departments, including professional and paraprofessional staff, were represented in one of the eight sessions.

Communication with Participants Prior to Session 1

All participants receive a memo outlining the class schedule, time-keeping instructions, dress requirements, educational objectives, and a list of participant names. It is important to give participants as much information as possible to create an exciting and comfortable experience for them. Many staff have not had an opportunity to attend education within the workplace, especially on new topics such as CQI, and this can create anxiety. To alleviate staff anxiety, advance information about program expectations and common questions asked is very helpful.

Using the Caring Curriculum Conceptual Framework

In the Caring Curriculum, as well as in a CQI educational program, it is important to respond to the participants' needs. Experiential learning can be achieved by providing participants with an opportunity to apply concepts in "real-life" situations versus focusing only on content. It is more important that the participants understand and be able to apply key concepts to their jobs than that they have a lot of information that they are unable to use. The principles of CQI value "teamwork" and the importance of sharing individual viewpoints when evaluating a system within the organization. The Caring Curriculum also values the sharing of individual paradigms to promote experiential learning among participants.

The Caring Curriculum is designed to enable participants to

> be more responsive to societal needs, more successful in humanizing the highly technical milieus of health care, more caring and compassionate, more insightful about ethical and moral issues, more creative, more capable of critical thinking, and better able to bring scholarly approaches to client problems and issues and to advocate ethical positions on behalf of clients. (Bevis & Watson, 1989, p. 1)

A caring curriculum must liberate both students and faculty from the authoritarian restraints of empiricist/behaviorist models as represented by specified behavioral objectives and teacher roles and functions necessitated by these objectives; the course objectives of the Learning Wave are written in terms of the participants' expectations. Each participant is responsible for deciding to what degree the course objectives affected him or her personally. The curriculum does not include any tests or other required achievement measurements.

Congruent with CQI, the Caring Curriculum acknowledges students as equal partners in the educational enterprise and restructures the way teachers and students relate to each other; the educational program is based on the principle of empowerment. The teacher of the session makes it clear to the participants that there are no experts in the areas discussed and that the "teacher" and participants are learning together.

Bevis and Watson (1989) defined curriculum as interactions between and among students and teachers with the intent that learning take place. Throughout the educational sessions, the teacher of the Learning Wave frequently encourages group discussions about new CQI information and the relationship of this information to the participant's responsibilities in the organization. The interaction between cross-functional project teams' participants in the educational program also provides an opportunity for them to recognize the interrelatedness of their roles in providing service to customers. A discussion evolves about identification of internal and external customers and what it means to the participants—the appreciation that each member plays an essential role within the organization to meet the customer's expectations.

Participants discuss pertinent issues in their work area and solve problems with the group on ways to improve processes by using CQI principles. To engage the learner, various methods of presentating information are used throughout the Learning Wave sessions, including small- and large-group discussions, games, teamwork, role playing, videos, guest speakers, and handouts to reinforce key concepts, as well as an exercise to explain the concept of "paradigms" and discussion of how they apply to the participant's perception of the world. The integration of a different learning structure actively engages the learner (Bevis & Watson, 1989).

Classroom Setting

The classroom is decorated festively with streamers and balloons to help create a fun and comfortable atmosphere to decrease staff anxiety, create interest, and encourage participation in the program. This atmosphere also helps staff to experience and understand "paradigms" and "paradigm shifts" that are discussed on the first day of the program. The classroom is arranged in a large horseshoe so that all participants can see each other as well as the presentation media. Large name tags are displayed on the tables so staff who are unfamiliar with each other may learn the names of their coworkers. Casual dress is encouraged to allow participants to feel comfortable.

Program Highlights

Considerations

The first day of the educational program is crucial to the success of the entire program. It is important to share information at the first session to give all participants a common understanding of the quality principles and also to emphasize that CQI education is important to the organization and to them as employees of the organization. The festive atmosphere and meals supplied on the first day not only lighten the mood of staff but also let the staff know they are valued. The CEO's presentation of ERC's vision, mission, and values in all Learning Waves is essential to demonstrate top leadership commitment to the educational program and the implementation of CQI within the workplace.

The most important question to be asked throughout the program is "How do the things that we have learned apply to our job?" Significant time is spent in open dialogue on participants' questions, comments, and feelings about what they have learned so they can take something back to their job. Project team reports on data used and outcomes are shared and celebrated with the large group. A special graduation luncheon is served to all participants. It is important to celebrate the commitment of each participant to the program and the relationships that have developed through the educational process. A group picture is taken and published in the organization's newsletters. A formal graduation ceremony is held at which all participants receive a gold QUALITY pin and are given the opportunity to share their feelings with their peers on what they have learned.

Concepts

Paradigms are discussed to provide an understanding of the culture shift of doing work differently versus adding additional tasks to the work currently being done. It is also very important to identify the external factors to the organization that are creating a need for change, including consumerism, regulatory requirements, and the rapidly changing health care delivery system. The relationship of these variables to the survival of an organization must be made clear.

Principles of empowerment are discussed with the class. The plan-do-check-act (PDCA) cycle for process improvement, problem solving, and decision making is discussed, including the steps involved in each segment of the cycle and appropriate quality tools to be used. A discussion of teams is presented to broaden the participants' understanding of the team approach to problem solving. A discussion of the roles of people within a team is critical to participants' understanding that being an active team member is important to the team's success or failure. A list of responsibilities of each role of an Evergreen team is distributed to all participants.

Texts

One of several resources used in developing the discussion of paradigms is Stephen Covey's *Seven Habits of Highly Effective People* (1989). The Technicomp *Teams for Excellence* video series provides another teaching medium for necessary discussion topics. Participants are given a copy of the book *ZAPP! The Lightning of Empowerment* by Byham and Cox (1988) to read as homework. Reading this book gives participants a real-world example of the culture shift from the traditional way of doing work to the new paradigm of empowerment and shared decision making.

Quality Tools

Formal *brainstorming* techniques are taught and then used by the participants to identify possible improvement opportunities within the organization. The *affinity diagram* process is introduced, and the participants group the improvement opportunities into like categories. After the affinity diagram is completed, the participants choose six pertinent and cross-functional improvement opportunities to be worked on during the project team portion of the educational program. Another quality tool, the *cause-and-effect diagram*, is introduced. To apply this concept, all participants provide input in drawing a simple cause-and-effect diagram to show what causes people to be late for work. A review of quality tools used by teams in decision making is conducted. Examples of *run charts* showing time-series data are shared with the group. Interactively, the entire group does a *process flow diagram*—first as individuals, then as small teams—to present to the large group to show how different groups perceive processes.

Project Teams

Throughout the Learning Wave, the participants are involved in project team processes to enable them to apply new CQI concepts as they are being learned. The project teams meet for one hour per session. Team members focus on using "real" data, gaining practical application of the principles learned, and team building. The "team process" experience is more important than the project outcomes. From the third session through the final session of the educational program, the project teams share their individual learning experiences and progress with the rest of the Learning Wave participants.

PROGRAM EVALUATION

Measurement of the effectiveness of a CQI educational program was essential to assess whether the goal of becoming a customer-centered culture had been achieved and whether the large financial investment the organization was making in providing all employees with educational programs was worthwhile to the organization and the employees. The effectiveness was evaluated with a pre-post evaluation research design by identifying and comparing participants' perception of their knowledge of the 11 components of the CQI educational program prior to and immediately following the educational program.

Sample Description

The sample for this study included 52 participants of two Learning Waves representing all departments within the organization: social services, buildings and grounds, dining services, public relations, administration, business office, rehab services, nursing, housekeeping, and laundry. Data from a sample of 43 (83%) subjects participating in the first and second Learning Waves were compiled for analysis purposes.

Data Collection Instrument

The spider diagram (Figure 19–1), a CQI measurement tool, was used to represent the participants' perception of their current level of knowledge in relationship to actual content of the program and what needed to be accomplished (Fox Valley Technical College Quality Academy, 1993). The participants plotted their perceived level of knowledge of the 11 components of the Learning Wave on an ordinal scale ranging from 0 to 8 on the spider diagram prior to and immediately following the program. Zero was interpreted as no knowledge of the concept, 4 as a moderate understanding of the concept, and 8 as a thorough understanding of the concept.

The 11 components of the Learning Wave were (a) paradigms; (b) the organization's mission, vision, and values; (c) team-building skills; (d) CQI principles; (e) methods of decision making; (f) internal and external customers; (g) data collection methods; (h) the process flowchart; (i) problem-solving skills; (j) interpersonal skills; and (k) empowerment. Each component had a range of 0 to 8 for the participant to identify his or her perceived level of knowledge. The lower the mean score

(closer to 0), the less knowledge the participants perceived they possessed. Conversely, the higher the mean score (closer to 8), the more knowledge the participants perceived they possessed.

Findings

Despite the relatively small ($N = 43$) number of participants, the findings did have significant implications for ERC and its employees.

As shown in Table 19–1, for all 11 components of the Learning Wave, the participants' perception of knowledge following the Learning Wave was higher (shaded area) than their perception of knowledge prior to the program. The data indicated that significant knowledge was gained during the Learning Wave for all 11 components, with each component at the $p = .000$ level of significance. The reliability of the instrument was determined by conducting a Cronbach's alpha test on the data. The Cronbach's alpha result of the preprogram data was .92; the postprogram data also had an alpha of .92.

The larger standard deviation prior to the program indicated more variance, which may be attributed to the participants' limited knowledge of the components. The decrease in standard deviation after the program indicated less variance than before the program and may indicate an increase in their understanding of the program components, increased comfort with the 11 components of the Learning Wave, and more congruence between the participants, leading to increased team effectiveness. Team solidarity resulting from a more congruent knowledge base was evident from the qualitative data.

Qualitative data were gathered from open-ended questions on surveys distributed prior to and immediately following the Learning Wave (Table 19–2).

Eighteen (42%) participants were unable to give examples of CQI application on the job prior to the Learning Wave. Those who did respond most frequently cited examples related

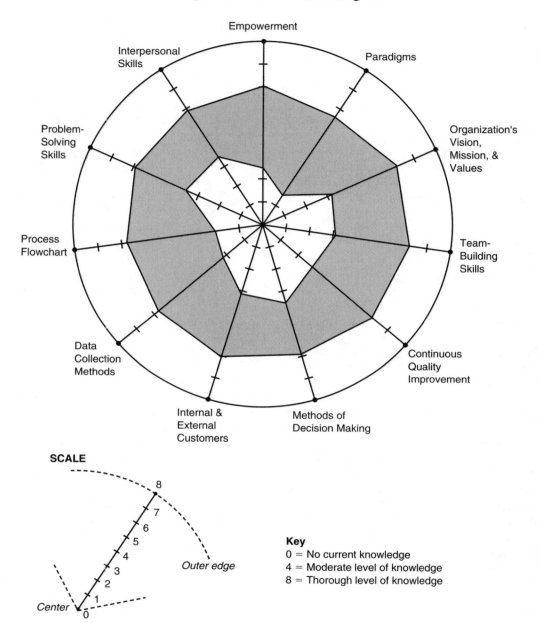

Figure 19–1 Spider diagram.

Table 19–1 Participants' Perception of Knowledge of the Learning Wave Components before and after the CQI Educational Program as Indicated by the Spider Diagram

Component	Before Program		After Program	
	Mean	SD	Mean	SD
Paradigms	1.4	2.3	5.3	1.9
Organizational vision	3.1	2.2	6.2	1.6
Team building	3.1	2.1	6.3	1.7
CQI	2.9	2.4	6.1	1.6
Decision making	3.8	2.3	6.0	1.6
Customers	3.1	2.6	6.3	1.8
Data collection	2.2	2.4	5.7	1.8
Process flowchart	1.8	2.4	5.6	1.7
Problem solving	3.7	2.3	5.9	1.4
Interpersonal skills	3.5	2.5	5.8	1.5
Empowerment	2.8	2.8	6.0	1.7

Table 19–2 Behaviors Identified by Participants before and Immediately after the CQI Educational Program

Component	Before the Program	Immediately and 1 Month after the Program
Paradigms	(No responses)	It's really up to me to make changes, not just to complain
Organizational vision, mission	(No responses)	Heightened awareness of everyone's value and participation in all phases of operation
Team-building skills	Using agendas and schedule facilitator/recorder for monthly meetings	Using meeting guidelines for weekly contact with other staff Working together as team to do job more effectively within and among departments Learned more about leading a team and defining goals Using teamwork to get things done on time and the right way Trust is vitally important
CQI	Used CQI techniques without realizing it	Practicing more communication Less critical of other departments due to a better understanding of their jobs

continues

Table 19–2 continued

Component	Before the Program	Immediately and 1 Month after the Program
		Promptly responding to customer requests and following through when matter can't be resolved at that time (PT charges)
		Addressing issues, not people
Data collection	(No responses)	Problems are solved more easily when others' ideas are shared
Process flowchart	(No responses)	Approaching problem by brainstorming
Problem solving	(No responses)	Trying to view problems and concerns as improvement opportunities Working with residents to solve problems Called together an interdisciplinary team to assist in problem solving
Interpersonal skills	Giving positive feedback to other staff Keep in mind other person's feelings and opinions Greeting residents by name	Giving coworkers choices and listening to their ideas for improvement Using an approach with family to defuse anger and solve a problem Listening more for detail than I used to (hearing the deeper meaning) Accepting constructive criticism better than I used to
Empowerment	Communicated concerns about residents to supervisor to resolve issue	Switched from loose sheets on clipboard to 3-ring binder to eliminate curled pages Redesigned calendar on unit for easier readability for residents and staff As manager, I involve staff with planning, budget issues, and problem solving Front-line staff solved a staffing problem without supervisor Less reluctant to voice an opinion More likely to do something that I saw needed to be done More willing to propose input to manager on possible solutions without the predisposition that I would be ignored

to interpersonal skills, meeting skills, and empowerment in decision making. Participants commented:

- "Others who have been through the Learning Wave are practicing more communication."
- "I give positive feedback to others who help me."
- "We prepare an agenda, have a schedule indicating the facilitator and recorder on a regular basis, and share responsibility of bringing up discussion items."

Immediately following the Learning Wave, five (12%) participants were unable to provide examples of CQI application on the job. Over half of the responses described behavior changes on the job based on new CQI knowledge. Other responses described knowledge gained as a result of the Learning Wave:

- "I have been more likely to do something that I saw needed to be done. I have also been more willing to propose input to managers on possible solutions."
- "Instead of going to a manager with problems, we all solve them on our own. We make sure the shift is covered on the schedule."
- "This has brought to my attention the effort and commitment an employee needs to make in order to make the workplace better for everyone. It's really up to me to make changes, not just to complain."
- "I take time and give full attention when other staff or customers are speaking to me. I promptly respond to customer requests and follow through when the matter can't be solved at that time."
- "I address issues and not people."
- "It proved to me that anyone, regardless of position, department, shift, etc., can form a group."

The most frequent responses from participants prior to the Learning Wave about their expectations of the training were learning what CQI is, learning how departments function

together, meeting employees from other departments, discovering better ways to provide quality care for the residents, and learning how to be a better employee. One participant wrote that a goal of the training would be to "understand how my department as well as the organization as a whole can work together better." For another participant, the goal was "to work more as a unit making decisions rather than working as independent individuals." No negative comments were written by the participants.

Identifying expectations of the Learning Wave provided insight for the teacher to meet the needs of the participants. The expectations identified by the participants prior to the Learning Wave were congruent with the 11 components included in the Learning Wave. This congruence reinforced the premise that implementing a CQI educational program could enhance employees' ability to do good work as indicated by their desire to perform efficiently and effectively to meet or exceed the customer needs.

LESSONS LEARNED

After conducting eight Learning Waves in our organization, we have learned several valuable lessons. Our experiences have validated some of our assumptions but have changed or modified our thinking in other areas. Each time it is presented, the Learning Wave content changes for various reasons. The positive responses shared by the participants have indicated not only the achievement of the course objectives but also participants' internalization of the objectives into their daily work life. These results support the use of the Caring Curriculum when planning an education program to maximize experiential learning. Evaluative comments from the participants are integrated to improve the Learning Wave.

We have noted that the culture within the organization is shifting. Some of the concepts taught during the first Learning Wave have become a part of daily operations and do not need to be formally taught but merely to be mentioned as a part of the implementation of CQI. Different teaching methods are implemented when participants struggle to understand the information presented. As time goes on, there is more information in the literature about quality in health care. This up-to-date information is shared as it appears. In different areas of our quality initiative, procedures are being developed that are shared with the participants.

All staff must participate in the Learning Wave together. Initially, managers had completed 16 hours of CQI education 18 months prior to the first Learning Wave. The management team in our organization decided not to participate with front-line staff in the Learning Wave because they felt their presence would inhibit front-line staff participation in the group. Because of the initial education, the management team also felt they knew CQI and did not have to attend any more education. By the third Learning Wave, however, front-line staff asked why managers were not in the Learning Waves. After reevaluation, managers became participants in the Learning Wave. The CEO and the board of directors chairperson also participated in a Learning Wave. This was received positively by staff and showed the commitment of top management to the CQI process.

Management must have a good understanding of CQI principles and their application before front-line staff begin their participation in a CQI educational program. Managers need to support and guide staff as they apply the new concepts in their daily work. *The Team Handbook* (Sholtes 1988) was used as a framework for an advanced management educational program. Managers need to develop "coaching" skills in the following areas: interpersonal skills, problem solving, conflict resolution, team building, and the use of quality tools and data in decision making.

It is important to provide additional CQI education and support for staff as they complete a Learning Wave. Graduates of the early Learning Waves were outnumbered by staff who had not yet participated in the program. This situation created some conflict in the workplace. To address the transition from the "old paradigm" to the "new paradigm," the quality resources director scheduled periodic meetings for Learning Wave graduates. Additional information on CQI principles was presented, and time was spent on discussing different approaches in applying CQI principles to one's job. Staff were engaged in informal conversation to identify their specific needs, and others in the group offered suggestions to help coworkers resolve the challenges identified.

CONCLUSION

The implementation of the Learning Wave is the first step. The next step is the integration of CQI information into practice in daily operations. Overcoming "the way we've always done it" mentality is the biggest challenge of all and requires the efforts of all staff to be achieved.

A common misconception of the implementation of CQI is that it will replace traditional quality assurance (QA). The truth is, CQI and QA need to be merged to provide the most benefit to the resident and the organization. The outcomes and the measurement of the attainment of those outcomes must be recognized by all staff. When performance is not meeting the expectations of the customers and/or regulatory agencies, quality improvement principles should be applied. The involvement of all staff, including the frontline worker, is integral to the success of this process. Organizations must accept the responsibility of maintaining or providing superior service in the marketplace.

One way of communicating the level of service that is being provided within the organization is to develop and continually monitor quality indicators on key performance outcomes. The use of quality indicators will enhance an organization's ability to meet the certification requirements of organizations such as the Joint Commission on Accreditation of Healthcare Organizations. This is significant as we move toward the future and merge with other health care organizations to provide services as a partner in a managed-care-environment.

REFERENCES

Bevis, E.O., & Watson, J. (1989). *Toward a caring curriculum: A new pedagogy for nursing.* New York: National League for Nursing.

Byham, W.C., & Cox, J. (1988). *Zapp! The lightning of empowerment.* New York: Ballantine.

Carnevalle, A.P. (1989, February). The learning enterprise. *Training and Development Journal,* 26–33.

Covey, S.R. (1989). *The seven habits of highly effective people.* New York: Simon & Schuster.

Crosby, P. (1980). *Quality is free.* New York: New American Library.

Fox Valley Technical College Quality Academy. (1993, October). *Continuous quality improvement tools.* Paper prepared for the Annual Quality Conference, Appleton, WI.

Gopalakrishnan, K.N., & McIntyre, B.E. (1992, April). Hurdles to quality health care. *Quality Progress,* 93–95.

Kirk, R. (1992). The big picture: Total quality management and continuous quality improvement. *Journal of Nursing Administration, 22*(4), 24–31.

Maddox, P.J. (1992). Successful implementation of a CQI process. In J. Dienemann (Ed.), *Continuous quality improvement in nursing* (pp. 115–124). Washington, DC: American Nurses Publications.

Milakovich, M.E. (1991). Creating a total quality health care environment. *Health Care Management Review, 16*(2), 9–20.

Nelms, T.P. (1990). The lived experience of nursing education: A phenomenological study. In M. Leininger & J. Watson (Eds.), *The caring imperative in education* (pp. 285–297). New York: National League for Nursing.

Scholtes, P.R., et al. (1988). *The team handbook.* Madison, WI.

Technicomp, Inc. (1991). *Teams for excellence video series.* Cleveland, OH.

## PART V

Applying Quality Improvement in Various Clinical Settings

CHAPTER 20

Improving Quality in Ambulatory Care

Judith M. Bulau

CHAPTER OBJECTIVES

After completing this chapter, the reader will be able to

- address the components of a QI Plan for an Ambulatory Care Setting
- describe a QI problem-solving process
- compare four methods for assessing patient care

Ambulatory health care organizations face significant challenges as they experience competitive demands to demonstrate their delivery of high-quality, safe services in a cost-effective manner. The continually changing health care environment confronts ambulatory health care providers with economic, political, and legal pressures to balance escalating costs without sacrificing quality and safety.

ELEMENTS OF THE QUALITY IMPROVEMENT PLAN

The ability of an ambulatory health care organization to address quality health care issues primarily depends on a collaborative partnership between management and staff. The organization's administrative staff's commitment and support for its quality improvement program ensures a successful program. An effective program that has management support is guided by (a) a comprehensive writ-

ten plan and (b) a method for evaluating the effectiveness of the program. The plan describes how people in the organization implement the quality improvement program to improve the performance continually (what is done and how well it is done) of health care systems and processes. It ensures that a planned, systematic approach is used and defines expectations for quality improvement activities. An example of a quality improvement plan is shown in Exhibit 20–1.

The quality improvement plan should address the following areas:

- administrative control
- mission statement
- philosophy
- objectives
- scope
- quality improvement committee
- quality improvement project teams
- continuous quality improvement (CQI) activities
- special quality improvement studies
- confidentiality policy for quality improvement information
- documentation methods for quality improvement activities
- system for communicating quality improvement information
- method for evaluating effectiveness of quality improvement program

Exhibit 20–1 Ambulatory Health Care Organization Quality Improvement Plan

---

Administrative Control

The ambulatory health care organization's Board of Directors is ultimately responsible for the quality of ambulatory health care services delivered. The President of the ambulatory health care organization is responsible for the overall quality improvement program. The Administrator of the ambulatory health care organization is responsible for establishing the quality improvement program. The Quality Improvement Manager is responsible for the operations of the quality improvement program. The ambulatory health care staff are responsible for conducting quality improvement activities according to the organization's quality improvement program. Communication of quality improvement information occurs according to the organizational structure.

Mission Statement

The mission of the ambulatory health care organization is to provide for the quality, safe, and cost-effective delivery of ambulatory health care services to individuals in need of those services. The ambulatory health care organization's Board of Directors and administrative staff are committed to the provision of ambulatory health care services that are guided by a quality improvement program in order to ensure that the delivered services constitute quality, safe, and cost-effective services for patients.

Philosophy

Quality improvement activities are guided by the overall philosophy of the ambulatory health care organization. The adoption of the appropriate philosophical approach in providing quality ambulatory health care services is based on the following basic assumptions:

1. The maintenance and realization of the full potential of human life are supreme values.
2. Humans possess a unique hierarchy of needs, as defined by Maslow:
    a. physiological needs
    b. safety needs
    c. belongingness and love needs
    d. self-esteem needs
    e. self-actualization needs
3. Humans search for meaning in personal life experiences.
4. Humans make choices and decisions based on their individual beliefs and values.
5. Humans exert personal control over their lives in making such choices and decisions.

The philosophy of the ambulatory health care organization, based on these assumptions, stipulates that each ambulatory health care patient:

1. desires ambulatory health care services that promote the patient's value of life by:
    a. minimizing negative patient illness and disability outcomes
    b. maximizing potential patient level-of-independence outcomes
    c. restoring, maintaining, and promoting patient health
2. possesses unique physiological, safety, psychological, self-esteem, and self-actualization needs that require consideration in the patient's plan of ambulatory health care
3. searches for meaning in the personal life experiences surrounding the patient's illness or disability
4. makes choices and decisions about the provision of ambulatory health care services relative to the patient's self-defined unique needs and according to the patient's personal beliefs and values
5. exerts personal control over the patient's personal life in collaborating with ambulatory health care staff members regarding the provision of services

continues

Exhibit 20–1 continued

In support of the ambulatory health care organization's philosophy, the provider is dedicated to the provision of comprehensive quality patient-centered and patient family-centered ambulatory health care that is focused on the patient's unique physiological, safety, psychological, self-esteem, and self-actualization needs. The provider is committed to the provision of ambulatory health care services that will assist the patient in searching for meaning in the personal life experiences surrounding the patient's illness or disability; to make choices and decisions about the provision of ambulatory health care services based on the patient's self-defined unique needs; and to collaborate actively with the ambulatory health care provider staff and other health care providers regarding the provision of ambulatory health care services. The ambulatory health care provider is also dedicated to the provision of ambulatory health care education to the patient, the patient's family, and the community.

Objectives

The ambulatory health care organization implements quality improvement activities to achieve the following objectives:

1. To develop, implement, and evaluate standards to measure medical, nursing, and therapy practice and delivery of ambulatory health care services
2. To develop, implement, and evaluate effective quality improvement activities according to the ambulatory health care organization's mission statement, philosophy, and objectives
3. To develop effective systems for problem assessment, identification, selection, study, corrective action, monitoring, evaluation, and reassessment of nursing/interdisciplinary team practice and ambulatory health care services
4. To provide focus and direction for quality improvement activities
5. To develop effective verbal/written information systems to communicate quality improvement activity outcomes to appropriate individuals and committees
6. To provide educational opportunities for all ambulatory health care staff members to increase their knowledge and participation in quality improvement activities
7. To correlate the findings of quality improvement activities with the content of ambulatory health care staff continuing-education programs
8. To encourage input and participation of all ambulatory health care staff relative to quality improvement activities
9. To coordinate and integrate the ambulatory health care organization's interdepartmental/ intradepartmental quality improvement activities with the organization's overall quality improvement activities
10. To ensure administrative commitment and support for quality improvement activities

Scope

The scope of the quality improvement program includes all of the services provided by the ambulatory health care organization, such as medical; nursing; physical, occupational, and speech therapy; and nutrition, pharmacy, laboratory, and radiology services.

Quality Improvement Committee

The Ambulatory Health Care Quality Improvement Committee consists of:

1. Administrator
2. Medical Director

continues

Exhibit 20–1 continued

   3. Nursing Manager
   4. Quality Improvement Manager
   5. two ambulatory health care registered nurses
   6. two ambulatory health care licensed practical nurses
   7. two ambulatory health care assistants
   8. interdisciplinary team members/ancillary support services staff
   9. physical therapist
 10. occupational therapist
 11. speech therapist
 12. dietitian
 13. pharmacist
 14. laboratory technician
 15. radiology technician
 16. Financial Manager

Quality Improvement Project Teams

Quality improvement project teams are responsible for applying the quality improvement problem-solving process once projects have been defined and selected. Each project team reports to the Quality Improvement Committee.

Quality Improvement Activities

Quality improvement activities are established by developing, implementing, and evaluating:

1. quality improvement program
2. quality improvement policies and procedures
3. continuous quality improvement activities: problem assessment, identification, selection, and study; corrective action; monitoring; evaluation; and reassessment
4. special quality improvement activities: study topic selection; data collection, analysis, and interpretation; conclusions; and recommendations
5. confidentiality of quality improvement information
6. administrative policies and procedures
7. clinical policies and procedures

Approval

The ambulatory health care organization's quality improvement program as outlined in this plan is approved and will become effective on (*Date quality improvement program will be effective*).

_____

Signature of President   Date of Signature

_____

Signature of Board of Directors Representative   Date of Signature

Source: Adapted from J.M. Bulau, *Quality Assurance Policies and Procedures for Ambulatory Health Care,* pp. 116–117, © 1990, Aspen Publishers, Inc.

Meeting the Goals of the Quality Improvement Plan

Once the plan has been developed, policies and procedures are established to implement it. Two important types of policies and procedures are those specifying administrative domains and linkages and those specifying CQI activities.

Administrative Domains and Linkages

The administrative component of the plan consists of guidelines specifying lines of communication among the health care organization's governing body and administrative staff and lines of authority for the delegation of responsibility concerning quality improvement activities. The quality improvement organizational chart in Figure 20–1 and the chart showing responsibility and authority for quality improvement tasks in Exhibit 20–2 are examples of such guidelines.

CQI Activities

Exhibit 20–3 shows a sample policy and procedures statement for CQI activities. This statement reflects the purposes of quality improvement activities to

- ensure delivery of high-quality ambulatory health care to all patients
- continuously monitor problems with delivery of high-quality ambulatory health care
- monitor performance of organizational systems and processes
- monitor health care trends that warrant study, particularly in relationship to quality of care
- continuously monitor diagnoses and clinical procedures and treatments that demonstrate significant risk for complications, frequency of occurrence, and adverse health outcomes
- continuously monitor problems potentially producing adverse patient outcomes
- identify problems for special quality improvement studies

An example of a form that can assist ambulatory health care staff in monitoring and documenting CQI activities according to the policy and procedure requirements is shown in Exhibit 20–4.

Complementary Policies and Procedures

Additional policy and procedure statements complement the CQI activities policy and procedure statement, making it easier to implement. For example, accountability for engaging in CQI activities may be encouraged by incorporating practice standards.

Health Care Standards

A policy and procedure statement that discusses the use of standards in the quality improvement program provides a framework for CQI activities. These are standards of patient care and clinical practice for nurses and interdisciplinary team/ancillary support services staff.

The actual standards being used can accompany the standards policy and procedure statement as an exhibit, or their sources can be listed for easy reference by ambulatory health care staff. This provides staff with current health care standards that assist them to be accountable for their clinical practice and patient care outcomes. Examples of standards that may be supplements to the standards policy and procedure statement are the American Medical Association Principles of Medical Ethics (Exhibit 20–5) and the American Nurses Association Standards for Nursing Practice (Exhibit 20–6).

Quality Improvement Problem-Solving Process

Other policy and procedure statements that complement a CQI activities policy and procedure statement are related to the type of problem-solving process used in quality improvement activities.

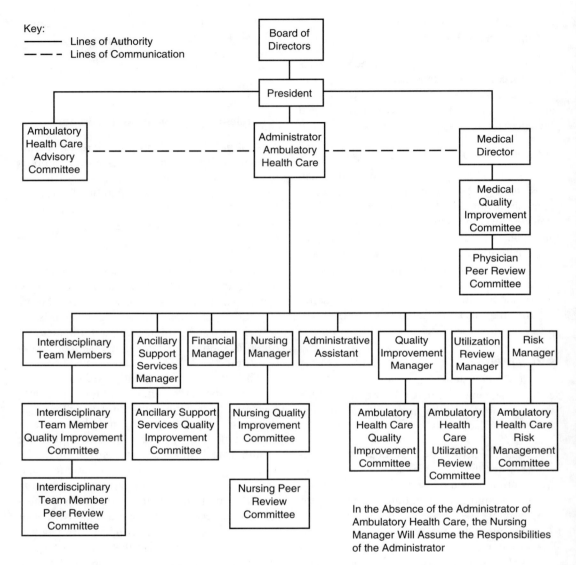

Figure 20–1 Quality improvement organizational chart. *Source:* Adapted from J.M. Bulau, *Quality Assurance Policies and Procedures for Ambulatory Health Care,* p. 15, © 1990, Aspen Publishers, Inc.

The process for solving problems includes problem assessment, identification, selection, study, corrective action, monitoring, evaluation, and reassessment as shown in Exhibit 20–7. Policy and procedure statements can be written for areas of problem assessment, problem identification, and program evaluation that enhance the CQI activities policy and procedure statement.

Problem Assessment

A policy and procedure statement covering problem assessment helps staff to assess a problem's impact on patient care and clinical

Exhibit 20–2 Responsibility and Authority for Quality Improvement Tasks

Quality Improvement Tasks	QI Committee		Organization Administration	
	Responsibility	*Authority*	*Responsibility*	*Authority*
Review data sources			x	x
Identify areas needing improvement	x	x		
Prioritize areas needing improvement			x	x
Investigate potential problems			x	x
Recommend corrective action			x	x
Implement corrective action			x	x
Recommend monitoring activities			x	x
Implement monitoring activities			x	x
Document impact on patient care and/or clinical performance			x	x
Assess results of monitoring activities	x	x		
Recommend further corrective action if initial action was not effective	x	x		
Implement further corrective action if initial action was not effective			x	
Report impact on patient care and/or clinical performance	x	x	x	x

Source: Adapted from J.M. Bulau, *Quality Assurance Policies and Procedures for Ambulatory Health Care*, p. 14, © 1990, Aspen Publishers, Inc.

Exhibit 20–3 Example of Continuous Quality Improvement Activity Policy and Procedure Statement

---

AMBULATORY HEALTH CARE ORGANIZATION
QUALITY IMPROVEMENT
POLICY AND PROCEDURE
1011

Subject: <u>Continuous Quality Improvement Activities</u>_____

Drafted by: _____   Date drafted: _____

Revised by: _____   Date revised: _____

Approved by: _____   Date approved: _____

Supersedes date: _____   Page #: _____

Date effective: _____   Page: _____ of _____

POLICY

The ambulatory health care organization conducts continuous quality improvement activities.

PURPOSE

1. To ensure quality of ambulatory health care to all patients.
2. To monitor continuously problems with delivery of quality health care.
3. To monitor health care trends that warrant study, particularly in relationship to quality of care.
4. To monitor continuously diagnoses and clinical procedures and treatments that demonstrate significant risk for complications, frequency of occurrence, and adverse health outcomes.
5. To monitor continuously problems that have potentially adverse patient outcomes.
6. To identify problems for special quality improvement studies.

PROCEDURE

1. An available, accessible, and appropriate data collection and retrieval system is maintained to support continuous quality improvement activities.
2. Specific quality improvement steps are used for continuous quality improvement activities, which incorporate the following:

   a. problem assessment
   b. problem identification
   c. problem selection
   d. problem study
   e. problem corrective action
   f. problem monitoring
   g. problem evaluation
   h. problem reassessment

3. Continuous quality improvement activities:

   a. are integrated with special quality improvement studies, as necessary
   b. address health care trends that warrant study, particularly in relationship to quality of care
   c. address diagnoses, treatments, and procedures that demonstrate significant risk for complications, frequency of occurrence, and adverse health outcomes
   d. address improved delivery of health care services that has a positive impact on patient care and/or clinical practice.

4. Ambulatory health care organization nursing, interdisciplinary team, and ancillary support services staff members:

   a. document continuous quality improvement activities on a Problem Identification Form (see Exhibit 1029-1)
   b. submit the completed Problem Identification Form to the appro-

continues

Exhibit 20–3 continued

priate nursing/interdisciplinary team/ancillary support services management staff member

5. The nursing/interdisciplinary team/ancillary support services management staff member:
   a. reviews the completed Problem Identification Form
   b. initiates a Continuous Quality Improvement Activity Form (see Exhibit 1011-1)
   c. submits the reviewed Problem Identification Form and the Continuous Quality Improvement Activity Form to the Administrator of Ambulatory Health Care

6. The Administrator of Ambulatory Health Care:
   a. reviews the submitted Problem Identification Form and the Continuous Quality Improvement Activity Form
   b. submits the reviewed Continuous Quality Improvement Activity Form to the Quality Improvement Manager
   c. presents information regarding continuous quality improvement activities to the President and Board of Directors of the ambulatory health care organization

7. The Quality Improvement Manager:
   a. reviews the submitted Continuous Quality Improvement Activity Form
   b. presents the Continuous Quality Improvement Activity Form to the Ambulatory Health Care Quality Improvement (AHCQI) Committee
   c. monitors quality improvement activities using a Quality Improvement Activities Monitoring Log (see Exhibit 1011-2)

8. The AHCQI Committee:
   a. reviews information regarding the continuous quality improvement activity

   b. makes recommendations relative to the continuous quality improvement activity, as appropriate
   c. presents information regarding the continuous quality improvement activity to the ambulatory health care organization's Ambulatory Health Care Advisory Committee

9. The ambulatory health care organization's Ambulatory Health Care Advisory Committee:
   a. reviews information regarding the continuous quality improvement activity
   b. makes recommendations relative to the continuous quality improvement activity, as appropriate
   c. presents information regarding recommendations for the continuous quality improvement activity to the Administrator of Ambulatory Health Care

10. The President and Board of Directors of the ambulatory health care organization:
    a. review information regarding continuous quality improvement activities
    b. make recommendations relative to continuous quality improvement activities

11. Continuous quality improvement activities are communicated to individuals, as appropriate, according to Policy and Procedure 1010: Confidentiality of Quality Improvement Information, and Policy and Procedure 1001: Administrative Control.

12. The completed Problem Identification Form and the Continuous Quality Improvement Activity Form are filed in the ambulatory health care organization's Problem Identification and Continuous Quality Improvement Activity administrative files.

Source: Adapted from J.M. Bulau, *Quality Assurance Policies and Procedures for Ambulatory Health Care,* pp. 60–61, © 1990, Aspen Publishers, Inc.

Exhibit 20–4 Continuous Quality Improvement Activity Form

AMBULATORY HEALTH CARE ORGANIZATION
CONTINUOUS QUALITY IMPROVEMENT ACTIVITY

Following Section To Be Completed by Manager Initiating Quality Improvement Activity

Date of Problem Identification Review	Date Quality Improvement Activity Implemented

Quality Improvement Activity Approach
(please check [✓] one)
❑ Structure ❑ Process ❑ Outcome

Quality Improvement Activity Time Frame
❑ Prospective ❑ Concurrent ❑ Retrospective

Reason(s) Quality Improvement Activity Selected and Warranted (please check [✓] one or more)
❑ Health care trends' relationship to quality of care
❑ Diagnoses, treatments, and procedures demonstrate actual/potential adverse health care outcomes
❑ Diagnoses, treatments, and procedures demonstrate significant risk for complications
❑ Adverse diagnoses, treatments, and procedures demonstrate significant frequency of occurrence
❑ Improvement in delivery of health care would have a positive impact on patient care and/or clinical practice
❑ Benefits for patient care and/or clinical practices worthy of cost expenditures for quality improvement study
❑ Probability exists that adequate resources exist to achieve completion of quality improvement activity

Identified Problem (please describe only *one* problem per form)

Criteria Used for Problem Identification, e.g., from Standard, Policy, and Procedure, Patient Bill of Rights, Code of Ethics

Cause of Identified Problem

Corrective Action Objective(s) (please include information regarding who, what, when, where, and how)

Description of Expected Outcome(s) after Corrective Action Implemented

Implementation Date of Corrective Action	Projected Evaluation Date of Implemented Corrective Action

Name of Individual Responsible for Implementation of Corrective Action

Description of Actual Outcome(s) after Corrective Action Implemented, Including Relevant Statistical Data (please attach supporting information, as appropriate)

---

continues

Exhibit 20–4 continued

Description Regarding Impact of Quality Improvement Activity on Patient Ambulatory Health Care and/or Clinical Practice

---

Manager's Evaluation Regarding Resolution of Problem As Result of Quality Improvement Activity (please check [✓] one)
❑ Identified Problem Resolved
❑ Identified Problem Not Resolved

Manager's Recommendation Regarding Disposition of Quality Improvement Activity (please check [✓] one)
❑ Discontinue quality improvement activity
❑ Continue quality improvement activity for interval problem assessment
❑ Continue quality improvement activity for constant problem assessment

---

Signature of Manager	Date of Signature

Following Section To Be Completed by AHCQI Committee Chairperson

Date of AHCQI Committee Review of Quality Improvement Activity

---

Description Regarding Impact of Quality Improvement Activity on Patient Ambulatory Health Care and/or Clinical Practice

---

AHCQI Committee Evaluation Regarding Resolution of Problem As Result of Quality Improvement Activity (please check [✓] one)
❑ Identified Problem Resolved
❑ Identified Problem Not Resolved

AHCQI Committee Recommendation Regarding Disposition of Quality Improvement Activity (please check [✓] one)
❑ Discontinue quality improvement activity
❑ Continue quality improvement activity for interval problem assessment
❑ Continue quality improvement activity for constant problem assessment

---

Signature of ACHQI Committee Chairperson	Date of Signature

Following Section To Be Completed by Ambulatory Health Care Advisory Committee

Ambulatory Health Care Advisory Committee Evaluation Regarding Resolution of Problem As Result of Quality Improvement Activity (please check [✓] one)
❑ Identified Problem Resolved
❑ Identified Problem Not Resolved

Ambulatory Health Care Advisory Committee Recommendation Regarding Disposition of Quality Improvement Activity (please check [✓] one)
❑ Discontinue quality improvement activity
❑ Continue quality improvement activity for interval problem assessment
❑ Continue quality improvement activity for constant problem assessment

---

Signature of Ambulatory Health Care Advisory Committee Chairperson	Date of Signature

continues

Exhibit 20–4 continued

Following Section To Be Completed by Administrator of Ambulatory Health Care

Ambulatory Health Care Advisory Committee Recommendation Regarding Disposition of Quality Improvement Activity (please check [✓] one)

❏ Approved and Referred   ❏ Not Approved (please explain) _____
   to Quality Improvement   _____
   Manager for Disposition   _____

Signature of Administrator of Ambulatory Health Care	Date of Signature

---

Following Section To Be Completed by Quality Improvement Manager

Disposition of Quality Improvement Activity per Administrator of Ambulatory Health Care Approval (please check [✓] one)

❏ Discontinued; Manager Notified   ❏ Continued for Interval   ❏ Continued for Constant Problem
                                     Problem Assessment;   Assessment; Manager Notified
                                     Manager Notified

Date Quality Improvement Activity:

___ Discontinued   ___ Continued for Interval Problem   ___ Continued for Constant Problem
                        Assessment; New Continuous   Assessment; New Continuous Quality
                        Quality Improvement Activity   Improvement Activity Form Initiated for
                        Form Initiated for Completion   Completion by Appropriate Manager
                        by Appropriate Manager

Signature of Quality Improvement Manager	Date of Signature

Source: Adapted from J.M. Bulau, *Quality Assurance Policies and Procedures for Ambulatory Health Care*, pp. 62–64, © 1990, Aspen Publishers, Inc.

Exhibit 20–5 American Medical Association Principles of Medical Ethics

---

AMERICAN MEDICAL ASSOCIATION
PRINCIPLES OF MEDICAL ETHICS

PREAMBLE:

The medical profession has long subscribed to a body of ethical statements developed primarily for the benefit of the patient. As a member of this profession, a physician must recognize responsibility not only to patients, but also to society, to other health professionals, and to self. The following Principles adopted by the American Medical Association are not laws, but standards of conduct which define the essentials of honorable behavior for the physician.

   I. A physician shall be dedicated to providing competent medical service with compassion and respect for human dignity.

  II. A physician shall deal honestly with patients and colleagues, and strive to expose those physicians deficient in character or competence, or who engage in fraud or deception.

 III. A physician shall respect the law and also recognize a responsibility to seek changes in those requirements which are contrary to the best interests of the patient.

---

continues

Exhibit 20–5 continued

IV. A physician shall respect the rights of patients, of colleagues, and of other health professionals, and shall safeguard patient confidences within the constraints of the law.

V. A physician shall continue to study, apply and advance scientific knowledge, make relevant information available to patients, colleagues, and the public, obtain consultation, and use the talents of other health professionals when indicated.

VI. A physician shall, in the provision of appropriate patient care, except in emergencies, be free to choose whom to serve, with whom to associate, and the environment in which to provide medical services.

VII. A physician shall recognize a responsibility to participate in activities contributing to an improved community.

Source: Reprinted with permission from *Principles of Medical Ethics*, American Medical Association.

Exhibit 20–6 American Nurses Association Standards for Nursing Practice

Standard I.

The collection of data about the health status of the client/patient is systematic and continuous. The data are accessible, communicated, and recorded.

Standard II.

Nursing diagnoses are derived from health status data.

Standard III.

The plan of nursing care includes goals derived from the nursing diagnoses.

Standard IV.

The plan of nursing care includes priorities and the prescribed nursing approaches or measures to achieve the goals derived from the nursing diagnoses.

Standard V.

Nursing actions provide for client/patient participation in health capabilities.

Standard VI.

Nursing actions assist the client/patient to maximize his health capabilities.

Standard VII.

Health planning agencies must identify needs of populations and address the development and orderly growth of health care services provided in the home.

Standard VIII.

A national health policy should support research to develop innovative and forward directions for health care at home.

Standard IX.

A national health policy should recognize and reaffirm the individual's responsibility for his own health and should acknowledge the home as the primary site for health care.

Source: Reprinted with permission from *Standards of Nursing Practice*, pp. 1–4, ©1973, American Nurses Association.

Exhibit 20–7 Problem-Solving Process Used in Quality Improvement Activities

Problem assessment:	Problems are monitored and assessed for identification and selection as a quality improvement activity.
Problem identification:	Problems are identified for possible selection as a quality improvement activity.
Problem selection:	Identified problems are selected for study relative to their impact on patient care and clinical practice.
Problem study:	Selected problems are studied relative to their impact on patient care and clinical practice.
Problem corrective action:	Corrective action is developed and implemented based on study outcomes.
Problem monitoring:	Implemented corrective action is monitored on an ongoing basis.
Problem evaluation:	Monitored corrective action is evaluated for effectiveness in problem resolution.
Problem reassessment:	Actual/apparent resolved problems are reassessed as necessary.

practice and to determine its scope, type, characteristics, complexity, and prevalence. An example of a problem assessment policy and procedure statement is shown in Exhibit 20–8.

Just as the CQI activities policy and procedure statement has complementary policies and procedures, the problem assessment policy and procedure statement may also have policies and procedures that support it. For example, policy and procedure statements for reviews of patient care structure, process, and outcome and reviews of clinical indicators related to patient care provide direction to staff in assessing problems as a part of CQI activities.

Review of Patient Medical Care. One method for assessing problems consists of conducting retrospective outcome-oriented reviews of patient medical care. A policy and procedure statement can be established directing physicians to conduct reviews to

- assess patient outcomes against established patient outcome standards
- determine appropriateness of ambulatory health care services
- determine adequacy of patient medical care
- determine effectiveness of patient medical care process and outcomes

- identify problems with continuity of patient medical care
- monitor performance of organizational systems and processes
- implement quality improvement activities for resolution of identified patient medical care problems
- ensure peer review of patient medical care
- ensure that established policies and procedures are followed in the provision of ambulatory health care services

An example of an outcome auditing and criteria system that is useful for conducting these reviews is shown in Exhibit 20–9.

Review of Patient Nursing Care. Another method of problem assessment is process- and/or outcome-oriented reviews of patient nursing care. The purpose of these reviews can be defined in a policy and procedure statement as follows:

- to assess patient process/outcomes against established patient processes/outcome standards
- to determine appropriateness of ambulatory health care services
- to determine adequacy of patient nursing care

Exhibit 20–8 Sample Problem Assessment Policy and Procedure Statement

---

**AMBULATORY HEALTH CARE ORGANIZATION
QUALITY IMPROVEMENT
POLICY AND PROCEDURE
1025**

Subject: <u>Problem Assessment</u>

Drafted by: _____   Date drafted: _____

Revised by: _____   Date revised: _____

Approved by: _____   Date approved: _____

Supersedes date: _____   Page #: _____

Date effective: _____   Page: _____ of _____

POLICY

Problems are monitored and assessed for identification and selection as a quality improvement activity.

PURPOSE

1. To assess problem's impact on patient care and clinical practice.
2. To determine problem's existence, scope, type, characteristics, complexity, and prevalence.

PROCEDURE

1. Multiple internal/external data sources are organized to monitor and assess ambulatory health care services for quality of health care problems relative to:
   a. problem's relationship to quality of delivered care
   b. problem's prevalence that would warrant correction
   c. problem's propensity to be resolved
   d. benefit to patient care that would result from resolving problem versus the cost of assessing and resolving problem
2. Problems are assessed for identification and selection through utilization of:
   a. internal data sources, which include but are not limited to the following:

(1) patient clinical records
(2) patient accident/incident reports
(3) medication error reports
(4) infection control reports
(5) Patient Concerns Form (see Policy and Procedure 2010: Patient Concerns, and Exhibit 2010-1)
(6) patient letters and/or comments regarding ambulatory health care services
(7) Patient Evaluation of Ambulatory Health Care Services Form (see Exhibit 2011-1)
(8) ambulatory health care staff and interdisciplinary team/ancillary support services staff member credentials
(9) Problem Identification Form (see Exhibit 1029-1)
(10) Continuous Quality Improvement Activity Form (see Exhibit 1011-1)
(11) ambulatory health care staff orientation, inservice, and continuing education records
(12) interdepartmental and intradepartmental committee meeting minutes
(13) formal group meetings
(14) informal group meetings:
   (a) lunch
   (b) breaks

continues

Exhibit 20–8 continued

(c) any gathering where two or more persons are communicating
(15) patient case conferences
(16) mortality reports
(17) utilization review reports
(18) drug utilization review reports
(19) blood utilization review reports
(20) surgical case review reports
(21) medical record review reports
(22) pharmacy and therapeutics evaluation reports
(23) structure, process, and outcome study data
(24) accreditation/licensure/certification survey reports
(25) PSRO/PRO data
(26) patient classification data
(27) research studies
(28) ambulatory health care standards
(29) personnel records
(30) financial reports
(31) quality improvement suggestion box
(32) personal knowledge/expertise
(33) personal experience
(34) other data relating directly or indirectly to patient ambulatory health care
b. external data sources, which include but are not limited to the following:
(1) professional organizations
(2) regulatory agencies
(3) review agencies
(4) cost review agencies
(5) third party payers
(6) literature
(7) local, state, and national PSRO profiles
(8) National Center for Health Statistics reports
(9) Department of Public Health reports

(10) data routinely collected from other ambulatory health care providers
(11) diagnostic and surgical procedure indices
(12) continuing education conferences
(13) professional conferences
c. valid and relevant structure, process, and outcome of patient care/clinical practice criteria that:
(1) are developed to define the focus for monitoring and assessing quality of health care problems
(2) are appropriately implemented to monitor and assess quality of health care problems
(3) include objective and measurable statements
d. prospective, concurrent, and retrospective monitoring activities that are appropriately implemented to assess quality of health care problems
e. appropriate study sample that:
(1) is representative of the assessed problem
(2) has adequate number of representative cases with which to study problem
(3) has sufficient quality of representative cases with which to study problem
(4) can be studied with adequate resources in a cost-effective manner
3. Problem assessment information is documented on a Continuous Quality Improvement Activity Form.
4. Problem assessment information is communicated to individuals, as appropriate, according to Policy and Procedure 1010: Confidentiality of Quality Improvement Information, and Policy and Procedure 1001: Administrative Control.

Source: Adapted from J.M. Bulau, *Quality Assurance Policies and Procedures for Ambulatory Health Care*, pp. 102–103, © 1990, Aspen Publishers, Inc.

Exhibit 20–9 Example of Outcome Auditing and Criteria System

SCREENING QUESTIONS
DIABETIC ACIDOSIS

PT. NAME _____   CLINIC _____

PT. ID NO. _____   BIRTHDATE _____ SEX _____ AGE ____

EFF. DATE OF HMO ENROLLMENT _____   PRIM. M.D. _____

HOSP. _____   ADM. DATE _____ DISCH. DATE _____

CONSULTANT _____

PRIM. DX. _____

SEC. DX. _____

SURG. PROCEDURES _____

CODES: 250.1, 250.2, 250.3, 251

DEFINITION: All hospitalizations for diabetic acidosis with lab reports indicating blood sugar > 250 mg./dl, arterial ph ≤ 7.30 or venous CO_2 < 12 and ketonuria or ketonemia.

DATA TO BE COLLECTED REGARDING OUTPATIENT CARE:	**YES**	**NO**
1. Was there a physician visit related to this diagnosis outside the hospital within 10 days prior to admission? (s = same day) Date _____	____	____
2. Was patient seen in ER within 10 days prior to admission? (s = same day) Date _____	____	____
3. Was there telephone contact related to this diagnosis within 10 days prior to admission (s = same day) Date _____	____	____
4. Was diagnosis of ketoacidosis made more than 24 hours prior to admission?	____	____
5. Was patient a known diabetic?	____	____
6. Was there a history of any of the following within 10 days prior to admission? If yes, circle: a) infection; b) change in diet; c) trauma	____	____
7. Was there a history of any of the following within 10 days prior to admission? If yes, circle: a) weight loss; b) abdominal pain; c) polyuria; d) dehydration	____	____
8. Was patient on insulin prior to admission?	____	____
9. Was patient seen in outpatient setting for diabetes in last 6 months? Date last seen _____	____	____
10. Were blood sugars monitored by patient or clinic within 30 days prior to admission? (s = same day) Date _____	____	____
11. Was patient on home glucose monitoring or had they been instructed in glucose monitoring?	____	____
12. Was there follow-up care within 10 days after discharge? If yes, circle where it occurred: a) clinic; b) nursing home; c) home health care; d) other _____	____	____
13. Was there evidence of patient noncompliance with treatment plan (e.g., drugs, diet, follow-up visits)? If so, comment _____	____	____
14. Was there a readmission or mortality within 30 days after admission? Date _____ Diagnosis _____	____	____
15. Were there other admissions related to this diagnosis within 6 months before or after this admission? Date(s) _____ Diagnosis _____	____	____

❑ Check if comments on back.

---

continues

Exhibit 20–9 continued

INSTRUCTIONS

"Primary M.D." is the physician who had seen the patient most frequently during the preceding year.

"Consultant(s)" are the one or more physicians, other than the primary care physician, seen either before hospitalization or during preceding year.

Record "yes" or "no" answers from information in either inpatient or outpatient record.

When Emergency Room (ER) is used, the term includes both hospital ER and urgent care clinics outside of hospitals.

When a question asks whether there was a documented history or symptom, record "yes" if there is documentation in chart to answer question in the affirmative; or "no" if there is documentation in chart to answer question in the negative or absence of data requested by the question.

Comments:

continues

Exhibit 20–9 continued

REVIEW CRITERIA
DIABETIC ACIDOSIS

Computer review of answers to screening questions will identify cases with a high likelihood for problems in ambulatory care in the following categories:

1. **DELAYED DIAGNOSIS**
   - *a. 1 = Yes (not s)   physician visit
     - 5 = Yes   patient known diabetic
     - 4 = No   diagnosis not made more than 24 hours prior to admission
       - and one of the following
     - 6 = Yes   infection, change in diet, trauma
     - 7 = Yes   weight loss, abdominal pain, polyuria, dehydration
   - *b. 2 = Yes (not s)   ER visit
     - 5 = Yes   patient known diabetic
     - 4 = No   diagnosis not made more than 24 hours prior to admission
       - and one of the following
     - 6 = Yes   infection, change in diet, trauma
     - 7 = Yes   weight loss, abdominal pain, polyuria, dehydration

2. **DELAYED ACCESS**
   - *a. 3 = Yes (not s)   telephone contact related to diagnosis
       - and one of the following
     - 7 = Yes   diagnosis of weight loss, abdominal pain, polyuria,
     - 6 = Yes   dehydration
       - and   infection, change in diet, trauma
     - 1 = No   no physician visit

3. **INADEQUATE SCREENING/MONITORING**
   - a. 5 = Yes   known diabetic
     - 9 = No   patient not seen in 6 months
   - b. 8 = Yes   patient on insulin
     - 10 = No   blood sugar not monitored in 30 days

4. **DELAYED/INADEQUATE TREATMENT**
   - *a. 4 = Yes   diagnosis made greater than 24 hours prior to admission

5. **INADEQUATE WORKUP/EVALUATION**
   - *a. 1 = Yes (not s) or   physician visit or
     - 2 = Yes (not s)   ER visit
     - 5 = Yes   patient known diabetic
       - and one of the following
     - 7 = Yes   weight loss, abdominal pain, polyuria, dehydration
     - 6 = Yes   infection, change in diet, trauma
       - and one of the following
     - 11 = No (not s)   no home monitoring or instruction in monitoring
     - 13 = No   compliant patient

6. **INADEQUATE MANAGEMENT**
   - *a. 15 = Yes   patient hospitalized for DKA within 6 months before or
     - 11 = No   after admission
       -      no home monitoring or instruction in monitoring

continues

Exhibit 20–9 continued

7. **INADEQUATE FOLLOW-UP**
   a. 12 = No   no follow-up in 10 days
8. **PATIENT COMPLIANCE**
   a. 13 = Yes   evidence of member noncompliance
9. **UNFAVORABLE OUTCOME**
   *a. 14 = Yes   patient readmitted or died within 30 days
10. **DOCUMENTATION**
   a. 6 = No   no documentation of infection, change in diet, trauma
   b. 7 = No   no documentation of weight loss, abdominal pain, etc.
11. **STATISTICAL ANALYSIS**
   # of cases with ER visits within 10 days prior to admission
*Charts needing physician review.

Source: Reprinted with permission from *The Minnesota Project,* © 1987, Group Health Plan Inc., HMO Minnesota, and Share Health Plan.

- to identify problems with patient nursing care, process, and outcomes
- to identify problems with continuity of patient nursing care
- to monitor performance of organizational systems and processes
- to implement quality improvement activities for resolution of identified patient nursing care problems
- to ensure peer review of patient nursing care
- to ensure that established policies and procedures are followed in the provision of ambulatory health care services

Examples of forms that may assist staff in implementing process- or outcome-oriented reviews of patient nursing care policy and procedure statements are found in Exhibits 20–10 and 20–11.

Review of Patient Diagnosis or Category. A third method for assessing problems is process- or outcome-oriented reviews of a specific patient diagnosis or category. Again, a policy and procedure statement can be written to reflect that ambulatory health care staff and interdisciplinary team members conduct these reviews to

- assess the patient care delivery process

- assess patient outcomes against established patient outcomes standards
- assess patient diagnoses and categories having high potential for quality-of-care problems
- identify both individual and collective care problems and patterns
- monitor performance of organizational systems and processes
- determine adequacy of patient care
- determine effectiveness of patient care
- identify problems with continuity of care

A sample audit tool developed from a policy and procedure statement for assessing problems via review of patient diagnosis or category policy and procedure is shown in Exhibit 20–12.

Review of Individual Patient Care. Finally, problem assessment may occur through process-oriented review of individual patient care. A policy and procedure statement can guide ambulatory health care staff and interdisciplinary team members as they do these reviews to

- determine adequacy of patient care
- determine appropriateness of continuing ambulatory health care for patients
- identify problems with patient care

Exhibit 20–10 Form for Process-Oriented Review of Patient Nursing Care Plans

AMBULATORY HEALTH CARE ORGANIZATION
PROCESS-ORIENTED REVIEW OF PATIENT NURSING CARE PLANS

Nursing Diagnosis To Be Reviewed	Clinical Record Number	Dates of Reporting Period	Date of Review

PLANNED NURSING ORDER	DATE NURSING ORDER PLANNED	NURSING ORDER IMPLEMENTED APPROPRIATELY			DATE NURSING ORDER IMPLEMENTED	COMMENTS
		YES	NO	WHY NOT?		

Signature of Individual Completing This Form	Date of Signature

Source: Reprinted from J.M. Bulau, *Quality Assurance Policies and Procedures for Ambulatory Health Care,* p. 232, ©1990, Aspen Publishers, Inc.

Exhibit 20–11 Form for Outcome-Oriented Review of Patient Nursing Care Plans

AMBULATORY HEALTH CARE ORGANIZATION
OUTCOME-ORIENTED REVIEW OF PATIENT NURSING CARE PLANS

Nursing Diagnosis To Be Reviewed	Clinical Record Number	Dates of Reporting Period	Date of Review

PATIENT OUTCOMES EXPECTED	DATE PATIENT OUTCOME TO BE ACHIEVED	DATE INSTRUCTION GIVEN FOR ACTUALLY ACHIEVING PATIENT OUTCOME	PATIENT OUTCOME ACHIEVED			DATE PATIENT OUTCOME ACTUALLY ACHIEVED	COMMENTS
			YES	NO	WHY NOT?		

Signature of Individual Completing This Form	Date of Signature

Source: Reprinted from J.M. Bulau, *Quality Assurance Policies and Procedures for Ambulatory Health Care,* p. 233, ©1990, Aspen Publishers, Inc.

- monitor performance of organizational systems and processes
- ensure peer review of patient care
- ensure that established policies and procedures are followed in the provision of ambulatory health care services
- meet clinical record review requirements

The same sample audit tool shown in Exhibit 20–12 may be used for this method of problem assessment.

Review of Clinical Indicators. Establishing clinical indicators aids in assessing problems with delivery of patient care. Guidelines for establishing clinical indicators to evaluate important aspects of care are shown in Exhibit 20–13. Sample indicators for ambulatory health care are shown in Exhibit 20–14. A worksheet for collecting data related to clinical indicators is given in Exhibit 20–15. A summary sheet that helps in comparing the worksheet data to the thresholds for evaluation is shown in Exhibit 20–16.

Exhibit 20–12 Sample Audit Tool for Assessing Care Problems by Review of a Specific Patient Diagnosis or Category

Criterion	Exception(s)	Standard	Met	Met by Exception	Not Met	Comments	Instructions to Auditor
1.							Where data are to be found in the record
2.							
3.							
4.							

Courtesy of St. Michael Hospital, © 1980, Milwaukee, Wisconsin.

Exhibit 20–13 Guidelines for Establishing Clinical Indicators

- Describe scope of patient care to provide a basis for identifying those aspects of care that will be the focus of monitoring and evaluation.
- Identify important aspects of patient care to focus monitoring and evaluation on those areas with the greatest impact on quality care.
- Identify objective measurable objectives for each important aspect of patient care that will help direct attention to potential problems or opportunities to improve care.
- Establish thresholds for each indicator that define the level or point at which intensive evaluation of patient care is required.
- Collect and organize information to facilitate comparison with the thresholds for evaluation.
- Identify problem areas and refer them to quality improvement for further evaluation.
- Continue to monitor patient care using clinical indicators.

Source: Reprinted with permission from *Compendium of Clinical Indicators,* © 1990, University Hospital Consortium.

Exhibit 20–14 Sample Ambulatory Health Care Indicators

- Waiting periods for scheduling appointments
- Waiting periods in an outpatient area to see a provider
- Waiting periods for obtaining a referral to another provider
- Follow-up on patients who fail to keep appointments
- Adverse patient outcomes resulting from:
    1. complications
    2. diagnostic or therapeutic treatment, including invasive procedures
    3. use of pharmaceuticals
    4. use of blood or blood products
- Adverse patient outcomes resulting from failure to appropriately and adequately diagnose and provide therapeutic treatment
- Follow-up on patients informing them of abnormal diagnostic test results that were not available during the ambulatory health care visit
- Selected studies of diagnoses that may have a high risk for adverse outcomes
- Unexpected or unplanned ambulatory health care visits for problems associated with most recent visit
- Unexpected or unplanned emergency department visits for problems associated with last ambulatory health care visit
- Hospital admissions that are unexpected, unplanned, or done on an emergency basis for problems associated with last ambulatory health care visit
- Patients' refusal to undergo diagnostic or therapeutic treatment, noncompliance with the medical care plan, or leaving the treatment area against medical advice
- Patient incidents/accidents in ambulatory health care area
- Patient dispositions from ambulatory health care
- Patient transfers from ambulatory health care to another provider
- Patients requiring emergency resuscitation in ambulatory health care area
- Patient deaths in ambulatory health care area
- Patient satisfaction surveys
- Patient verbal/written complaints, comments, or questions
- Selected studies of ambulatory health care documentation, including informed consent
- Clinical evaluation of ambulatory health care professionals
- Financial decisions/incentives that adversely affect delivery of ambulatory health care
- Current ambulatory health care claims alleging medical malpractice
- Regulatory and accrediting agency guidelines for ambulatory health care

Source: Reprinted with permission from J.M. Bulau, *H.C. Report,* p. 6, ©1992, St. Paul Fire and Marine Insurance Company.

Exhibit 20–15 Sample Worksheet for Collecting Data on Clinical Indicators

To complete this worksheet, select a group of clinical indicators you wish to review. Write in those clinical indicators in the blanks below. Then select a sample of patient care records (related to the clinical indicators being reviewed) and write in the record identification numbers in the boxes provided. Next, check each patient record to see if it contains the clinical indicators listed. Check the "Yes," "No," or "N/A" columns accordingly. Make duplicate copies of this worksheet if you are working with more records than the number of spaces provided. When you have finished with your review, summarize your findings on Summary Sheet #4 that follows this worksheet.

Clinical Indicators	ID#			ID#			ID#			ID#			ID#			ID#			Total Number		
	Yes	No	N/A	Yes	No	N/A	Yes	No	N/A	Yes	No	N/A	Yes	No	N/A	Yes	No	N/A	Yes	No	N/A

COMMENTS

SIGNATURE OF REVIEWER   DATE OF SIGNATURE

Exhibit 20–16 Sample Summary Sheet to Compare Worksheet Data to Thresholds for Evaluation

Please write in the clinical indicators you have chosen in the blanks where indicated. Next, choose related thresholds that you use to indicate when corrective action is required. Write in these thresholds in the blank spaces provided. See completed Compliance Worksheet for totals of the "Yes" and "No" columns. Enter these totals below for each item. Enter the total number of patient care records reviewed in the "Sample Size" column. Divide the total number of "Yes" responses by the sample size and enter the percentage in the "% Rate of Occurrence" column. Identify problem areas, take corrective action, and reevaluate.

Date This Form Completed				Dates of Reporting Period		
Clinical Indicator	Threshold for Action	Total Number of Responses		Sample Size	% Rate of Occurrence (Total No. of "Yes" Responses/Sample Size)	Comments
		Yes	No			
Total						

Signature of Individual Completing This Form	Date of Signature

Source: Reprinted with permission from *Risk Prescription,* ©1995, St. Paul Fire and Marine Insurance Company.

Once the cumulative data reach the threshold for evaluation, for any clinical indicator, patient care can be reviewed to evaluate whether a problem exists. Guidelines for reviewing patient care are depicted in Exhibit 20–17. The Continuous Quality Improvement Activity Form in Exhibit 20–4 can be used for this review.

Problem Identification

The second step in the problem-solving process is problem identification. Problems are identified for possible monitoring via quality improvement activities according to their impact on patient care and clinical practice. Providing a problem identification policy and procedure statement, such as the example in Exhibit 20–18, directs ambulatory health care staff in how to properly identify problems. A problem identification form, such as the one shown in Exhibit 20–19, can be written to provide further help to staff.

Program Evaluation

It is critically important also to devise a process for evaluating the quality improvement program to determine how well the plan has served to accomplish the organization's goals for high-quality and safe patient care. The evaluation method reveals the extent to which the quality improvement program is appropriate, adequate, effective, and efficient. In the example of an evaluation policy and procedure statement (Exhibit 20–20), the purpose of evaluation is defined as follows:

- to assess the extent to which the ambulatory health care provider's quality improvement activities are appropriate, available, and adequate
- to identify unnecessary duplicate quality improvement activities
- to ensure coordination and integration of quality improvement activities
- to determine if quality improvement goals are being met
- to ensure that the quality improvement program is consistent with internal and external legal and third-party payer requirements

Exhibit 20–21 provides an example of an evaluation form that can be used by ambulatory health care staff to assess an organization's quality improvement program. As the form suggests, the areas to be evaluated include at least the following:

- mission statement
- philosophy
- objectives
- administrative control
- scope of quality improvement activities
- standards
- CQI activities
- special quality improvement studies
- communication of quality improvement results
- education
- quality improvement policies and procedures
- organization
- medical services quality improvement activities
- nursing services quality improvement activities
- therapy services quality improvement activities
- ancillary support services quality improvement activities
- other quality improvement activities
- coordination of quality improvement activities

ENSURING HIGH-QUALITY, SAFE, AND COST-EFFECTIVE HEALTH CARE

The emergence of quality health care concerns with increasing health care costs has created a challenging opportunity for the ambulatory health care industry. This opportunity consists of the sharing of individual and collective expertise, experience, and leadership for the refinement of ambulatory health care quality improvement programs and activities. Ultimately, this may help realize the dream of providing high-quality, safe, and cost-effective health care to every individual who needs it.

Exhibit 20–17 Guidelines for Reviewing Patient Care

- Evaluate patient care when the cumulative data reach the threshold for evaluation to determine whether a problem exists.
- Identify possible trends, patterns of performance, and causes of any problems or methods by which patient care or performance may be improved.
- Take corrective action to solve problems or improve patient care.
- Assess and document effectiveness of corrective action. If further actions are necessary to solve a problem, take them and assess their effectiveness.
- Communicate and report findings from and conclusions of monitoring and evaluation, including corrective action taken to solve problems and improve patient care through the established channels of communication.

Source: Reprinted with permission from *Compendium of Clinical Indicators* © 1990, University Hospital Consortium.

Exhibit 20–18 Example of Problem Identification Policy and Procedure Statement

**AMBULATORY HEALTH CARE ORGANIZATION
QUALITY IMPROVEMENT
POLICY AND PROCEDURE
1028**

Subject: <u>Problem Identification</u>

Drafted by: _____	Date drafted: _____
Revised by: _____	Date revised: _____
Approved by: _____	Date approved: _____
Supersedes date: _____	Page #: _____
Date effective: _____	Page: ____ of _____

POLICY

Problems are identified for possible selection as a quality improvement activity.

PURPOSE

To select problems for quality improvement activities according to their impact on patient care and clinical practice.

PROCEDURE

1. Problems are identified for possible selection as a quality improvement activity after they have been assessed according to Policy and Procedure 1025: Problem Assessment.
2. Implemented measurable health care standards are compared with implemented process, structure, and outcome criteria to identify quality of health care problems.
3. An appropriate representative sample of health care standards compared with structure, process, and outcome criteria is obtained to identify quality of health care problems.
4. Problem identification information is documented on a Continuous Quality Improvement Activity Form (see Exhibit 1010-1).
5. Problem identification information is communicated to individuals, as appropriate, according to Policy and Procedure 1010: Confidentiality of Quality Improvement Information, and Policy and Procedure 1001: Administrative Control.

Source: Adapted from J.M. Bulau, *Quality Assurance Policies and Procedures for Ambulatory Health Care,* p. 106, © 1990, Aspen Publishers, Inc.

Exhibit 20–19 Problem Identification Form

AMBULATORY HEALTH CARE ORGANIZATION
PROBLEM IDENTIFICATION FORM

Following Section To Be Completed by Individual Reporting the Problem

Name of Individual(s) Involved in Incident   Place of Incident

Date of Incident	Time of incident A.M. P.M.	Date This Form Completed	Time This Form Completed A.M. P.M.

Objective Narrative Description of Incident

Narrative Description of Identified Problems Resulting from Incident

Criteria Used for Problem Identification, e.g., from Standard, Policy and Procedure, Patient Bill of Rights, Code of Ethics

Corrective Action Implemented?   Date Corrective Action Implemented
❑ Yes   ❑ No   (please explain) _____

Narrative Description of Implemented Corrective Action

Recommendations for Additional Corrective Action

Following Section To Be Completed by Manager Reviewing Identified Problem

Review Date of This Form _____ Review Time of This Form _____

Narrative Description of Incident Investigation

Additional Corrective Action Implemented?   Date Corrective Action Implemented
❑ Yes   ❑ No   (please explain) _____

Narrative Description of Additional Corrective Action

continues

Exhibit 20–19 continued

Description of Outcome(s) Resulting from Additional Corrective Action

_____

Description Regarding Potential Impact of Quality Improvement Activity on Patient Ambulatory Health Care and/or Clinical Practice

_____

Identified Problem Referred for Quality Improvement Activity?
❑ Yes   ❑ No   (please explain) _____

Signature of Manager	Date of Signature

Following Section To Be Completed by Administrator of Ambulatory Health Care

Identified Problem Referred for Quality Improvement Activity?
❑ Yes   ❑ No   (please explain) _____

Signature of Administrator of Ambulatory Health Care

_____

Source: Adapted from J.M. Bulau, _Quality Assurance Policies and Procedures for Ambulatory Health Care,_ pp. 108–109, © 1990, Aspen Publishers, Inc.

Exhibit 20–20 Example of an Evaluation Policy and Procedure Statement

**AMBULATORY HEALTH CARE ORGANIZATION
QUALITY IMPROVEMENT
POLICY AND PROCEDURE
1014**

Subject: <u>Evaluation of Quality Improvement Program</u>
Drafted by: _____   Date drafted: _____
Revised by: _____   Date revised: _____
Approved by: _____   Date approved: _____
Supersedes date: _____   Page #: _____
Date effective: _____   Page: _____ of _____

POLICY

The Ambulatory Health Care Quality Improvement (AHCQI) Committee evaluates ambulatory health care organization quality improvement activities.

PURPOSE

1. To assess extent to which ambulatory health care organization quality improvement activities are appropriate, adequate, effective, and efficient.
2. To assess extent to which ambulatory health care organization resources for quality improvement activities are appropriate, available, and adequate.
3. To identify unnecessary duplicate quality improvement activities.
4. To ensure coordination and integration of quality improvement activities.
5. To determine if quality improvement program objectives are being met.
6. To ensure that the quality improvement program is consistent with internal and external legal and third party payer requirements.

PROCEDURE

1. The AHCQI Committee evaluates annually the ambulatory health care organization's total quality improvement program.

2. The AHCQI Committee review evalutes at least the following:
   a. written quality improvement plan, which includes:
      (1) mission statement
      (2) philosophy
      (3) objectives
      (4) administrative control
      (5) scope of quality improvement activities
      (6) standards
      (7) continuous quality improvement activities: problem assessment, identification, selection, study, corrective action, monitoring, evaluation, and reassessment
      (8) special quality improvement studies: study topic selection; data collection, analysis, and interpretation; conclusions; and recommendations
      (9) communication of quality improvement results
      (10) education
      (11) quality improvement policies and procedures
   b. organization
   c. administration
   d. medical quality improvement activities
   e. nursing quality improvement activities

continues

Exhibit 20–20 continued

f. therapy quality improvement activities

g. ancillary support services quality improvement activities

h. other activities

i. coordination of quality improvement activities

3. The AHCQI Committee submits the following report to the Administrator of Ambulatory Health Care and to the ambulatory health care organization's Ambulatory Health Care Advisory Committee: written report of its total evaluation and its recommendations for appropriate corrective action based on the evaluation results that specifically addressed item 2 above.

4. The Administrator of Ambulatory Health Care and Ambulatory Health Care Advisory Committee respond with appropriate action to the AHCQI Committee.

5. The AHCQI Committee evaluation results are documented on an Evaluation of Ambulatory Health Care Organization's Quality Improvement Program Form (see Exhibit 1014-1).

6. The AHCQI Committee evaluation results are communicated to ambulatory health care staff members.

7. Continuing-education classes are offered to ambulatory health care staff members, as necessary, to address educational needs identified by the AHCQI Committee evaluation results.

8. Evaluation of Quality Improvement Program information is communicated to individuals, as appropriate, according to Policy and Procedure 1010: Confidentiality of Quality Improvement Information, and Policy and Procedure 1001: Administrative Control.

9. The completed Evaluation of Ambulatory Health Care Organization's Quality Improvement Program Form is filed in the ambulatory health care organization's Evaluation of Ambulatory Health Care Quality Improvement Activities administrative file.

Source: Adapted from J.M. Bulau, *Quality Assurance Policies and Procedures for Ambulatory Health Care*, pp. 69–70, © 1990, Aspen Publishers, Inc.

Exhibit 20–21 Form To Evaluate an Ambulatory Health Care Organization's Quality Improvement Program

EVALUATION OF AMBULATORY HEALTH CARE ORGANIZATION'S
QUALITY IMPROVEMENT PROGRAM
YEAR OF EVALUATION: _____

OBJECTIVE: To assess the extent to which the ambulatory health care organization's quality improvement program is appropriate, adequate, effective, and efficient.

Topic	Topic Criteria	Topic Criteria Met			Topic Criteria Demonstrate Improvements				Corrective Action Taken	Comments
		Yes	No	Comments	Yes	No	N/A	Comments		
I. Quality Improvement Program Purpose: To ensure quality of ambulatory health care to all patients.	1. There is a written Quality Improvement Plan that includes:									
	a. Mission statement									
	b. Philosophy									
	c. Objectives									
	d. Administrative control									
	e. Scope of quality improvement activities									
	f. Standards									
	g. Problem assessment, identification, selection, study, corrective action, monitoring, evaluation, and reassessment									
	h. Study topic selection; data collection, analysis, and interpretation; conclusions; and recommendations									
	i. Communication of quality improvement results									
	j. Education									
	k. Quality improvement policies									
	2. The written Quality Improvement Plan is implemented.									
II. Organization Purpose: To ensure maximum efficiency in informing individuals of the organizational structure and lines of authority and their responsibilities and accountability.	1. There is an organizational or written description of the organization's Quality Improvement Program structure.									
	2. The organization operates in accordance with the formal Quality Improvement Plan.									

continues

Exhibit 20–21 continued

Topic	Topic Criteria	Topic Criteria Met			Topic Criteria Demonstrate Improvements				Corrective Action Taken	Comments
		Yes	No	Comments	Yes	No	N/A	Comments		
	3. There are objectives that identify expected outcomes of the Quality Improvement Program.									
III. Administration Purpose: To ensure the provision, management, and support of the organization's Quality Improvement Program. A. Governing Body	1. There is a governing body.									
	2. There are identified duties and responsibilities for the governing body.									
	3. The governing body functions in accordance with written rules and regulations.									
	4. Minutes of meetings show that the members have taken action on all business for which they are responsible.									
B. Advisory Group	1. The advisory group is representative of the community served.									
	2. There are identified quality improvement functions for the advisory group.									
	3. The advisory group functions in accordance with written rules and regulations.									
	4. Minutes of meetings show that the members have considered problems, offered recommendations to the governing body, and carried out their functions.									
C. Administrative Personnel	1. There is an appointed administrator and an alternate administrator.									
	2. There is an appointed Nursing Manager and an alternate supervisor available during operating hours.									

continues

Exhibit 20–21 continued

Topic	Topic Criteria	Topic Criteria Met			Topic Criteria Demonstrate Improvements				Corrective Action Taken	Comments
		Yes	No	Comments	Yes	No	N/A	Comments		
	3. There are identified quality improvement functions for administrative personnel.									
	4. Administrative personnel function in accordance with written rules and regulations.									
	5. Minutes of meetings show that the members have considered problems, offered recommendations to the governing body, and carried out their functions.									
D. Personnel	1. There are written job descriptions that identify current quality improvement qualifications, duties, and functions.									
E. Reports and Records	1. Quality improvement records and reports are kept according to policy guidelines, providing for									
	a. maintenance and protection									
	b. retention									
	c. availability and confidentiality									
	2. Contracts relative to quality assurance									
	a. are current									
	b. identify expectations of contractee and contractor									
F. Fiscal	1. Quality improvement budgets, audits, accounting, and billing are carried out according to provider policy.									
	2. Funding sources are multiple and adequate to meet costs.									
G. Statistical Information	1. There is a description of Quality Improvement Program statistical record keeping.									
	2. An annual report of Quality Improvement statistics is provided.									

continues

Exhibit 20–21 continued

Topic	Topic Criteria	Topic Criteria Met			Topic Criteria Demonstrate Improvements				Corrective Action Taken	Comments
		Yes	No	Comments	Yes	No	N/A	Comments		
	3. There are guidelines that identify how the statistical data are to be used and by whom.									
	4. Review of gathered statistics and data assists in the evaluation of quality health care.									
IV. Medical Quality Improvement Activities Purpose: To ensure physician input and supervision of medical Quality Improvement Activities.	1. There are written Quality Improvement Philosophy, Objectives, and Policies.									
	2. There are written guidelines that describe expected medical staff quality improvement functions.									
	3. These guidelines are implemented in accordance with current medical practice.									
	4. Medical consultation is available and utilized.									
V. Nursing Quality Improvement Activities Purpose: To ensure nursing input and supervision of nursing Quality Improvement Activities.	1. There are written Quality Improvement philosophy, objectives, and policies.									
	2. The nursing process (assessment, goal setting, planning, implementing, evaluating) is incorporated in quality improvement activities.									
	3. There are written guidelines that describe expected nursing quality improvement functions.									
	4. These guidelines are implemented in accordance with current nursing practice.									
	5. The nursing staff keep current in quality improvement theory and application by attending inservice meetings and by participating in continuing education.									

continues

Exhibit 20–21 continued

Topic	Topic Criteria	Topic Criteria Met			Topic Criteria Demonstrate Improvements				Corrective Action Taken	Comments
		Yes	No	Comments	Yes	No	N/A	Comments		
VI. Therapy Quality Improvement Activities Purpose: To ensure therapist input and supervision of therapy Quality Improvement Activities.	1. There are written guidelines that describe the scope of physical therapy, speech therapy, and/or occupational therapy quality improvement functions.									
	2. These guidelines are implemented in accordance with current therapy practice.									
	3. Therapists keep current in quality improvement theory and application by attending appropriate inservice meetings and by participating in continuing education.									
VII. Ancillary Support Quality Improvement Activities Purpose: To ensure ancillary support input and supervision of ancillary support quality improvement activities.	1. There are written guidelines that describe the scope of ancillary support quality improvement functions.									
	2. These guidelines are implemented in accordance with current ancillary support standards.									
	3. Ancillary support services staff keep current in quality improvement theory and application by attending appropriate inservice meetings and by participating in continuing education.									
VIII. Other Quality Improvement Activities										

continues

Exhibit 20–21 continued

Topic	Topic Criteria	Topic Criteria Met			Topic Criteria Demonstrate Improvements				Corrective Action Taken	Comments
		Yes	No	Comments	Yes	No	N/A	Comments		
IX. Coordination of Quality Improvement Activities Purpose: To ensure coordination of quality improvement activities so that efforts effectively complement all staff and support the objectives outlined in the Quality Improvement Program.	1. There are guidelines for liaison between and among all staff involved in quality improvement activities.									
	2. Staff meetings, including discussion of quality improvement activities, are held regularly.									
	3. There is an established method by which information is exchanged with other health care providers to ensure continuity of quality improvement activities.									

_____   _____
Signature of Administrator of Ambulatory   Date of Signature
Health Care

_____   _____
Signature of Ambulatory Health Care Quality   Date of Signature
Improvement Committee Chairperson

Following Section To Be Completed by Ambulatory Health Care Advisory Committee

Date of Ambulatory Health Care Advisory Committee Review: _____

_____   _____
Ambulatory Health Care Advisory Committee   Date of Signature
Chairperson Signature

Ambulatory Health Care Advisory Committee Recommendations for Corrective Action:

CORRECTIVE ACTION RECOMMENDATIONS	DATE CORRECTIVE ACTION OUTCOME WILL BE ASSESSED	INDIVIDUAL RESPONSIBLE	DATE CORRECTIVE ACTION OUTCOME ASSESSED	CORRECTIVE ACTION EFFECTIVE YES NO IF NO, EXPLAIN

Following Section To Be Completed by Governing Body

Date of Governing Body Review: _____

_____   _____
Signature of President   Date of Signature

Source: Adapted from J.M. Bulau, _Quality Assurance Policies and Procedures for Ambulatory Health Care,_ pp. 71–74, © 1990, Aspen Publishers, Inc.

SUGGESTED READING

American Medical Asociation. (1958). *Principles of medical ethics.* Chicago: Author.

American Nurses Association. (1973). *Standards: Nursing practice.* Kansas City, MO: Author.

Batalden, P.B., & O'Connor, J. (1980). *Quality assurance in ambulatory care.* Gaithersburg, MD: Aspen.

Bulau, J. (1990). *Quality assurance policies and procedures for ambulatory health care.* Gaithersburg, MD: Aspen.

Gould, E.J., & Wargo, J. (1987). *Home health nursing care plans.* Gaithersburg, MD: Aspen.

Joint Commission on Accreditation of Healthcare Organizations. (1991). *Ambulatory health care standards manual.* Chicago: Author.

Meisenheimer, C. (1985). *Quality assurance: A complete guide to effective programs.* Gaithersburg, MD: Aspen.

Schroeder, P. (1987). Standards of practice. *Journal of Nursing Quality Assurance 1*(2).

Schroeder, P., & Maibusch, R. (1984). *Nursing quality assurance: A unit-based approach.* Gaithersburg, MD: Aspen.

Solberg, L., et al. (1982). *The Minnesota project: A focused approach to ambulatory care quality assurance.* Minneapolis: Group Health Plan, Inc., HMO Minnesota, and Share Health Plan.

CHAPTER 21

Improving Quality in Home Care

Claire G. Meisenheimer

CHAPTER OBJECTIVES

After completing this chapter, the reader will be able to

- describe major forces influencing the shift of care from the hospital to the patient's home
- explain the standards applicable to home care
- design a comprehensive QI plan
- evaluate a performance improvement project using the PDCA model

The home has been, is, and will continue to be the cornerstone of the health care system. The shift of care from hospital to community settings is predicted to continue, with the increasing transferral of primary, secondary, and tertiary care services to the home (Burbach, Conrad, Schumacher, & Lindsay, 1991; Davis, 1993).

Home care is the fastest growing segment of the health care industry. Over 17,000 providers are delivering a variety of services, including skilled and semiskilled nursing care, pharmacy services, infusion therapy, durable medical equipment, infusion therapy, respiratory therapy, rehabilitation/assisted technology, hospice care, adult day care, prosthetics and orthotics, transportation, and custodial care, to some 7 million individuals (National Association for Home Care, 1995).

The proliferation of home health agencies (HHAs) from 208 in 1961 to an estimated 17,500 in 1995 includes some 8,747 Medicare-certified HHAs, 1,795 Medicare-certified hospices, and 7,019 "other" HHAs, home care aide organizations, and hospices that do not participate in Medicare. Although national expenditures for personal health care totaled $1.069 trillion in 1995 (National Association for Home Care [NAHC], 1995), home care expenditures constituted only a small fraction of national health spending. The home health benefit for Medicare recipients represented only about 8% of total benefit payments in 1995 and only 6.5% of the $108 billion in Medicaid benefit payments (NAHC, 1995). Although an estimated 9 to 11 million Americans need home care services, most will continue to receive services from so-called informal caregivers—family, friends, and others who provide uncompensated care (U.S. Bipartisan Commission on Comprehensive Health Care, 1990).

The home has always been the place where families have cared for their members, but as a major component of the health care delivery system, it has historically received attention only from individuals directly involved in community and public health activities. The current concerns about access to and cost and quality of care, however, have shifted home care into a new place of prominence. Major forces contributing to this shift include

375

- enactment of Medicare in 1965 and, more recently, OBRA regulations in 1980, increasing service access and cost and opening the market to proprietary agencies
- demographics—the over-65 population is larger than ever (11.2% in 1970 compared to 14% in 1990) and continuing to live longer, so that more years of health resources are required; projections for the year 2020 indicate that one person in five will be of traditional retirement age or older
- a trend away from institutionalization on account of human and cost factors (diagnosis-related groups encourage shorter length of stay)
- competitive market forces
- managed care contracting
- a capitated payment system in which everyone is expected to be more productive—fewer patient visits and accomplishment of a specific set of measurable outcomes
- outcomes data to compare with current industry benchmarks
- an increased awareness of the benefits of prevention and wellness programs
- advances in medical care and portable technology
- consumer demands for information, including requests for "report cards"

Although studies conducted in the past several years have shown cost savings data for individuals who are recuperating from hospitalization or experiencing a functional or cognitive disability and are unable to care for themselves (Bach, Intinola, Alba, & Holland, 1992; Casiro et al., 1993; Fields, Rosenblatt, Pollack, & Kaufman, 1991; Hughes et al., 1992; Pigott & Trott, 1993), the best argument for home care may be that it is a humane and compassionate way to deliver health care and supportive services. It can reinforce and supplement the care provided by family members and others and maintain the recipient's dignity

and independence. It does, however, provide challenges for professionals, legislators, accreditors, payers, and consumers.

In particular, rigorous, uniform, and comprehensive standards and norms and appropriate and achievable risk-adjusted outcomes have not been established for the quality of care provided to home health care clients, who are essentially invisible in their private homes and beyond the easy reach of public or professional scrutiny. The opportunities and challenges associated with developing a quality system in home care include the unique arena of practice—that is, the client's home—and the myriad of variables—physiological, environmental, physical, technological, and psychosocial—that must be managed to provide appropriate, effective care in a cost-efficient manner. The *outcomes* actually achieved by a client are the end product of a complicated interplay of the application/integration of (a) relevant information and skills by the client, (b) individual professional and paraprofessional practitioners, and (c) guidelines of policies and procedures of health care organizations and of agencies that finance, regulate, and accredit health care.

Heightening the efforts of home care is the paradigm shift to total quality management (TQM)/continuous quality improvement (CQI), a managerial philosophy and method that demands continuous and rigorous improvement in the total process of providing care, using statistical process control (SPC) tools for data-based decision making. Multiple causation of less-than-optimal system performance is assumed; isolated behaviors of individual professionals are *not* the focus.

Concentrating on systems, CQI recognizes the humanity and complexity of health care organizations; customer–supplier relationships are central to success. CQI emphasizes *all* customers and the involvement of the "owners" of all components of the system in seeking a common understanding of the issues and subsequent solutions for improving client outcomes through the delivery process.

QUALITY STANDARDS

Quality is regulated in home care by the federal government, individual states, accrediting organizations, insurers, and managed-care providers.

In the federal domain, Medicare's Conditions of Participation (COPs) must be met by all agencies receiving Medicare reimbursement. Emphasis on structure began to shift early in 1987 when the Health Care Financing Administration (HCFA), which administers Medicare and Medicaid, developed an interest in "outcomes." In 1991, Medicare issued its first standards revision since the passage of Medicare, including the Functional Assessment Instrument (FAI). Recent developments with *Medicare's OASIS: Standardized Outcome and Assessment Information Set for Home Health Care* (Shaughnessy, Crisler, & Schlenker, 1995), developed at the University of Colorado Center for Health Policy Research and HCFA and distributed by NAHC, point to changes in the assessment and improvement of quality in Medicare home health care.

This CQI approach to evaluating home health care has become the central theme of voluntary accrediting bodies such as the Joint Commission on Accreditation of Healthcare Organizations (Joint Commission) and the National League for Nursing's (NLN's) Community Health Accreditation Program (CHAP). Both agencies have received "deemed status" by HCFA, meaning that Medicare will accept evidence of accreditation in lieu of government inspection; at a minimum, they must cover the Medicare COPs.

- The Joint Commission, begun in 1988, has seen an increase in accreditation of 35% to 40% since 1993 (American Health Consultants, 1996). Complete requirements for TQM emphasize the involvement of HHA leadership in the initiation, design, and direction of CQI activities. Providers are to move away from a limited focus on clinical care to the management, support, and clinical aspects; from quality assurance (QA) in various departments or services to multidisciplinary approaches; and from an individual focus to a focus on systems and processes and an integrated assessment of appropriateness, effectiveness, and efficiency. For home care, various aspects of care include high-risk procedures (infection control and drug administration), high-volume procedures (such as personal care and care of the dying), and problem-prone procedures (service coordination, documentation, and billing).

- NLN (CHAP) issued the self-evaluation software, *Benchmarks for Excellence in Home Care,* in 1996. CHAP was the first organization to receive deemed status in 1992. The program establishes standards of excellence and emphasizes consumer rights and financial and organizational viability. Twenty-four indicators are included in five "pulse points" (consumer, clinical, organizational, financial, and risk management) intended to measure the many dimensions of excellence in home care.

- National Committee for Quality Assurance (NCQA) has issued a *Health Plan Employer Data and Information Set* (HEDIS 3.0 version is due in Spring 1997). It provides a standardized performance measurement set moving beyond prevention to care of the acutely and chronically ill and providing these data for report cards for broad populations, including Medicare and Medicaid patients.

- A newly formed (May 1996) Council on Healthcare Provider Accreditation (CHPA) program is currently writing a core set of standards for home medical equipment, home infusion, and rehabilitative assistive technology, to be ready by mid-1997.

Private

- University of Colorado Center for Health Policy Research and HCFA collaborated to produce *Medicare's OASIS* (Shaughnessy et al., 1995) by conducting demonstration projects to develop outcome measures.

Public

- Agency for Health Care Policy and Research (AHCPR), created in 1989 (formerly the National Center for Health Services Research), has produced research-based clinical guidelines for usage in a variety of settings, including home care. These various guidelines and measurement sets are intended to measure like outcomes for aggregates of client populations. Making clients' self-reports of their health status part of the standard of care will allow purchasers to buy a package of services, knowing the cost and quality of care an organization can provide.

Although hospitals were the first to be pushed by the business community to adopt CQI principles, all health care organizations are now undergoing a transformation, and their quality programs must be designed to be practical, flexible, and comprehensive in order to achieve improvement in a timely and priority fashion.

QUALITY IMPROVEMENT PLAN

A well-designed, comprehensive CQI program, such as the one in Exhibit 21–1, does not replace QA activities. Rather, it complements these activities by providing a broader systemwide framework that allows individuals the opportunity to make informed, data-based decisions for improving the process of delivery service.

Exhibit 21–1 Quality Improvement Plan

PURPOSE

The Visiting Nurse Association of Wisconsin (VNA) and its affiliates are committed to providing personalized, high-quality, cost-effective home health care services to its patients regardless of national origin, race, religion, sex, handicap, or financial status. The VNA shall develop a customer-driven Continuous Quality Improvement (CQI) program resulting in an organizational culture that delivers service excellence, cost effectiveness, and pride in individual performance.

The governing body accepts its responsibility for requiring and supporting the Continuous Quality Improvement program. The staff accepts its responsibility for carrying out quality improvement activities and is committed to resolving identified problems. The VNA shall strive to adhere to the quality improvement standards as defined in this quality improvement plan.

Conceptually, the Continuous Quality Improvement Program encompasses four (4) phases:

1. **Project Definition and Organization**
   * Identify the project
   * Establish the project and team
2. **Diagnostic Journey**
   * Analyze the symptoms
   * Formulate theories of cause
   * Test theories
   * Identify root causes
3. **Remedial Journey**
   * Consider alternatives
   * Design solutions and controls
   * Address resistance to change
   * Implement solutions and controls
4. **Holding the Gains**
   * Check performance
   * Monitor control systems

These phases are repeated continuously to ensure continued improvement in the processes within the organization.

VISION

We envision the VNA to be the leading home health provider in eastern Wisconsin by consis-

continues

Exhibit 21–1 continued

tently meeting patient's/caretaker's individualized needs at reasonable cost using standards of excellence that are considered to be of value to our customer.

QUALITY GOALS

1. To continually improve the quality of patient/client care in a cost-effective manner.
2. To assure that the quality of care provided by the professional and paraprofessional staff conforms to clinical standards of practice.
3. To assure that new programs or processes are designed well.
4. To understand, maintain, and/or improve systems and processes within the organization that will have a direct or indirect effect on outcomes.
5. To comply with all external requirements, i.e., Joint Commission Standards, state certification requirements, Medicare/Medicaid regulations, and OSHA requirements.

QUALITY OBJECTIVES

The quality improvement plan shall consist of ongoing process improvement activities and may include a periodic sampling of activities not initiated solely in response to an identified problem. The quality improvement plan shall be planned and evaluated at least annually and revised as necessary to:

1. ensure that high-quality care is provided by all services (either directly or by contract) at minimal risk to the patients
2. identify, track, and resolve problems in patient care, services, and customer satisfaction to ensure improvement or resolution of problems identified
3. identify and pursue opportunities to improve all systems and processes that impact upon patient care, service, and customer satisfaction
4. objectively and systematically monitor and evaluate quality and appropriateness of care

5. meet, and exceed where possible, state and federal regulatory and accreditation standards for quality improvement

CONFIDENTIALITY

All staff participating in quality improvement activities will adhere to the VNA's confidentiality policies. Results of activities and reports will not contain any identifiable customer information. Information will be coded or reported in aggregate, and identifiable patient information will be destroyed once data are summarized.

SCOPE OF CARE AND SERVICES

The home health agency provides multidisciplinary services that have been prescribed by a physician for patients of all ages.

To ensure a comprehensive, customer-driven CQI Program, monitoring and evaluation activities will encompass all:

1. disciplines providing care
2. types of service
3. types of patients
4. important functions within the organization

TYPES OF SERVICES

1. Registered Nurse
2. Licensed Practical Nursing
3. Physical Therapy
4. Occupational Therapy
5. Speech Therapy
6. Medical Social Work
7. Nutrition Consultation
8. Home Health Aide
9. DME/Infusion Therapy
10. Respiratory

SPECIALIZED PROGRAMS

1. Intravenous Therapy
2. Hospice
3. AIDS Care
4. Rapid Recovery
5. Advanced Heart Failure
6. Pediatrics

continues

Exhibit 21–1 continued

7. Enterostomal Therapy
8. Mobile Meals
9. Bath Service
10. Immunotherapy

ANCILLARY/CONTRACT SERVICES

1. Intravenous Therapy Products
2. Durable Medical Equipment
3. Contract Therapy
4. Contract Home Health Aide
5. Contract Nursing

TYPES OF PATIENTS

1. Acutely ill
2. Chronically ill
3. Terminally ill
4. Rehabilitative

IMPORTANT FUNCTIONS WITHIN THE ORGANIZATION

1. Rights, responsibilities, and ethics
2. Assessment
3. Care, treatment, and service
4. Education
5. Continuum of care
6. Leadership
7. Management of the environment of care
8. Management of human resources
9. Management of information
10. Surveillance, prevention, and control of infections
11. Improving organizational performance

IMPORTANT ASPECTS OF CARE AND SERVICE

Ongoing monitoring and evaluation activities will focus on important functions of the organization. These may be key functions, procedures, treatments, processes, or other activities that impact patient care, outcomes, or customer satisfaction either directly or indirectly. Areas of focus will include those activities identified as high risk, high volume, or problem prone.

ACCOUNTABILITY FOR AND IMPLEMENTATION OF THE QUALITY IMPROVEMENT PROGRAM

1. The **Board of Directors** of the Visiting Nurse Association of Wisconsin is ultimately responsible for the quality of care provided to patients by the agency subsidiaries and affiliates and for implementation of the Continuous Quality Improvement Program. The Board of Directors shall receive reports at specified times from the Professional Advisory Committee and the Director of Education and Quality.
2. The **Professional Advisory Committee** shall receive reports of the CQI Program at specified times from the Director of Education and Quality.
3. The **President/CEO** is given the responsibility of ensuring that the CQI program is implemented. Quarterly reports on CQI are given to the President/CEO and members of the Quality Council.
4. The **Quality Council** is responsible for:
   1. formulating the Quality Improvement Plan
   2. prioritizing the CQI activities
   3. providing resources: training, time for working on projects, diagnostic support, and facilitator support
   4. establishing teams
   5. reviewing progress
   6. acting upon and giving direction and/or support for recommended action
   7. giving recognition
   8. evaluating the CQI Program and reports

The **Management Team** comprises the Quality Council. The positions include:

President/CEO, Chairperson
Vice President, Operations
Vice President, Finance
Vice President, Business Development
Vice President, Operations of Aurora Home Medical

continues

Exhibit 21–1 continued

Director, Human Resources
Director, Information Systems
Director, Development & Community Relations
Director, Quality & Education
Systems Improvement Analysts
Operations Manager of Aurora Home Medical

The **Director of Quality** is responsible for the facilitation of the CQI Program and for ensuring that appropriate opportunities for improvement are undertaken. Responsibilities include:

1. reviewing and amending the CQI Program based on Quality Council recommendations
2. assisting the Quality Council and staff in identifying, developing, planning, and/or evaluating important functions, processes, or systems that impact patient outcomes
3. assuring that responsibility for data collection, reporting of findings, implementation of actions for improvement, and reporting follow-up status for each study or process improvement team have been assigned and proceed as planned
4. assuring that information from monitoring and evaluation activities is reported as delineated in the written plan for the CQI Program
5. reviewing and forwarding CQI reports to the President/CEO and Quality Council
6. providing the Board of Directors and Professional Advisory Committee with pertinent CQI program information

SELECTION OF ACTIVITIES

The Quality Council screens monitoring and evaluation activities and quality improvement projects for the purpose of choosing the activities/projects to be done. Criteria for the selection of those activities/projects are:

1. is consistent with the VNA mission, strategic goals and objectives, and organizational culture
2. involves urgency related to a need to respond promptly to pressures associated with actual or potential life safety, customer service, litigation, and adverse public relations
3. involves a high-volume, high-risk, and/or problem-prone process
4. addresses significant consequences of poor quality, i.e., cost, loss of patient volume, decreased satisfaction
5. does not duplicate a completed or in-process project
6. will include data that may serve multiple purposes, such as reporting for OSHA, Joint Commission, marketing, etc.
7. provides opportunities for multidisciplinary team participation

Application to the Quality Council for quality improvement activities/projects can be made to the Council and must include the following elements:

1. Definition of the problem/opportunity for improvement
2. Overall objective/goal
3. Identification of impact on internal/external customer
4. Identification of departments that need to be represented on the team to identify causes and implement solutions

MONITORING AND EVALUATION ACTIVITIES

CQI monitoring and evaluation activities will be ongoing, planned, and systematic. For each audit/indicator or outcome study developed, the following information will be delineated in a written plan that will include:

1. Audit/indicator or outcome topic
2. Purpose of study
3. Key indicators (with definitions, if needed)
4. Threshold for evaluation
5. Source(s) of data collection
6. Method of data collection
7. Sample size
8. Time frame for study

continues

Exhibit 21–1 continued

9. Person responsible for data collection, analysis, and reporting
10. Frequency of study/reporting

INDICATOR SELECTION AND DEVELOPMENT

The quality improvement monitoring and evaluation of selected indicators shall address all home care services provided directly and by arrangement. Indicators will be identified to monitor the quality of the identified important functions of the organization.

At least one relevant indicator will be developed to monitor each major function of the organization. In addition, indicators addressing patient satisfaction will be monitored quarterly and physicians, discharge planners, payers/contract sources, and employee satisfaction will be done annually.

Indicators and mechanisms to trigger evaluation will be revised as indicated and reviewed at least annually.

MECHANISMS TO TRIGGER EVALUATION

For each indicator, mechanisms will be established to identify levels, patterns, or trends in the indicator that will trigger further evaluation of the function. These mechanisms may include, but are not limited to, the following:

1. Setting a threshold for further evaluation
2. Setting upper and lower control limits
3. Using statistical data such as means and standard deviation
4. Identifying patterns or trends

When the mechanism is triggered, evaluation is used to determine whether an opportunity exists to improve care or processes that impact patient outcomes.

COLLECTION AND ORGANIZATION OF DATA

Data will be collected for each indicator at a specified time or at regular intervals. Data collection tools will be varied and will be appropri-

ate for the important aspect of care or service being studied and the indicators chosen. Sources of information for collecting data include, but are not limited to:

1. Medical records
2. Customer surveys
3. Records and reports from ancillary and contract services
4. Committee and departmental reports
5. Log books
6. Standards of care
7. Policies, procedures, protocols
8. Quality Improvement team reports
9. Home visits
10. Recommendations from: Joint Commission, state surveys, and other regulatory agencies
11. Staff/patient infection control data
12. Incident reports

Methods of data collection can be one or a combination of the following:

1. Documentation-based reviews (retrospective or concurrent)
2. Customer surveys
3. Direct observation of care
4. Pre- and post-testing

Methods of problem identification and tools for analysis may include the following:

1. Flowcharts
2. Cause-and-effect diagrams
3. Pareto charts
4. Histograms
5. Stratification
6. Scatter diagrams
7. Run charts
8. Control charts

Sample size will be determined for each study to adequately represent the population being studied.

ANALYSIS AND ACTION

Collected data will be tabulated at specified times. The level of performance will be compared to the pre-established thresholds or previ-

continues

Exhibit 21–1 continued

ous performance to identify if further evaluation is required.

If the threshold is exceeded, the findings will be evaluated by a qualified, designated person or team to determine if a problem or opportunity for improvement exists. If evaluation reveals that a problem or opportunity for improvement exists, a written plan for improvement will be implemented. The plan will include:

1. Nature of the problem or opportunity for improvement and the date identified
2. Who is responsible for improvement
3. Actions to be implemented. Actions may include, but are not limited to:
   a. individual counseling
   b. staff education/in-service
   c. patient service change
   d. system/process change
   e. administrative change (i.e., policy/procedure, staffing)
4. Reporting of results: To whom and when
5. Date information is to be evaluated again
6. Effectiveness of action taken

The effectiveness of actions taken will be evaluated as planned. Usually the monitoring activities which identified the problem/opportunity for improvement will be continued and utilized to determine if

1. the actions have resolved the problems;
2. improvement is achieved and sustained; or
3. the problem reoccurs.

The frequency of data collection, reporting, and analysis will be appropriately adjusted should the scope and severity of the problem identified warrant it.

DOCUMENTATION

A CQI Manual will be maintained by the Quality Director and organized to document the CQI Plan and its implementation.

The Quality Director will write a quarterly and annual quality report summarizing all quality activities. This report will be submitted to the President/CEO and the Quality Council. Reports will be prepared for the Board of Directors and the Professional Advisory Committee on a regular basis and as requested. Copies of the report will be placed in the CQI Manual and will be posted for discussion with staff.

CQI PROGRAM EVALUATION

The CQI Program will be evaluated annually and shall include the following:

1. Were the objectives of the program met?
2. Was the monitoring and evaluation effective?
3. Is the scope of the program sufficient to ensure quality?
   a. Is the program customer focused?
4. Was CQI information communicated accurately and to appropriate
   a. persons?
   b. committees?
   c. other groups?
5. Is there evidence of resolution of identified problems or action taken on opportunities for improvement?
6. Was CQI information used for quality planning?
7. What impact on customers has the CQI program had?

Courtesy of Visiting Nurse Association of Wisconsin, 1996, Milwaukee, Wisconsin.

As noted in Exhibit 21–1, a quality improvement plan should include (a) a statement of purpose, (b) a conceptual framework, such as Juran's (1988), to guide everyone in the continuous quality journey, (c) a brief, succinct vision statement clarifying the agency's values and beliefs that *all* employees can articulate, (d) scope of care and services provided, (e) important functions within the organization (i.e., functions identified by the Joint Commission), (f) "accountabilities" reflecting the importance of monitoring clinical and non-

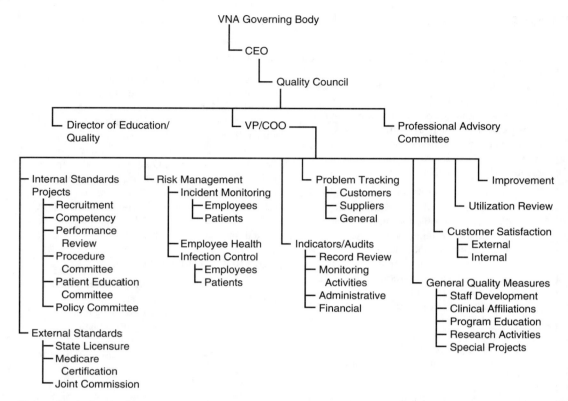

Figure 21–1 Composition of a CQI Quality Council. Courtesy of Visiting Nurse Association of Wisconsin, 1996, Milwaukee, Wisconsin.

clinical issues, including financial and human resource subsystems, for the purpose of improving client care, and (g) details describing data collection, analyses, and reporting mechanisms.

Figure 21–1 shows the composition of a Quality Council, with top leaders of each service/program and their communication patterns. It reflects the involvement and commitment of all disciplines and services to identify problems or issues of quality requiring data collection and management, corrective action, and continuing program assessment.

QUALITY OUTCOMES

Until the late 1980s, home care quality assurance was largely a reaction to the Medi-

care regulations, which focused primarily on structural standards (Kramer et al., 1990)—outcomes related to agency performance with limited reference to patient outcomes. Lalonde (1988) developed measures of seven key care elements, such as general symptom distress, medication adherence, and functional status, but these also found limited exposure and usefulness. In 1988, the Center for Health Policy Research and the Center for Health Services Research, located at the University of Colorado, initiated development of outcome-based quality improvement (OBQI) measures. HCFA adopted them in an effort to shift Medicare quality measurement from structure to outcomes and create a partnership between the home care industry and payers or regulators (Shaughnessy et al., 1995).

A patient care model is driven by the outcomes data that an agency and external customers deem appropriate for their patient populations. Although by Donabedian's (1980) quality model, structure, process, *and* outcome standards are all critical for a comprehensive QI program, the overriding reason for providing health care is to change a patient's health status over time by influencing positive patient outcomes through the use of appropriate human, technical, and financial resources.

Generating outcomes data that demonstrate high quality and low costs confirms value of care to providers and purchasers of health care and will win legislators and payers' approval, including managed care contracts, in this increasingly capitated home care industry. A major challenge in measuring outcomes is both to adjust for the natural progression of a condition or disability and to collect, reliably and comprehensively, the requisite data to analyze outcomes properly (Schlenker, Shaughnessy, & Crisler, 1995).

In addition to the Joint Commission, NLN, NCQA, and other performance measures, two sources that HHAs may find helpful to include in their assessment processes are (a) *Medicare's OASIS: Standardized Outcome and Assessment Information Set for Home Health Care*, developed for measuring outcomes for adult home care patients (National Association for Home Care, 1996); and (b) the AHCPR guidelines.

Medicare's OASIS: Standardized Outcome and Assessment Information Set for Home Health Care

The OASIS-A version, initially developed and released in 1995, was superseded by a new version, OASIS-B, in spring 1997. The OASIS-B is a comprehensive assessment instrument of approximately 85 items; most items are similar to those currently used by most HHAs, but with greater specificity to enhance continuity and consistency between assessors and to give them more opportunities to benchmark against each other and

against nationwide outcomes obtained from Medicare's outcome-based quality improvement national demonstration project.

As each revision undergoes further usage and review in over 50 demonstration agencies and other HHAs (American Health Consultants, 1996), updates will be provided to Medicare and individual agencies. Although some of the data items may change slightly prior to the final implementation of OASIS, it would be of value to agencies to fit the OASIS data items into their unique data set tailored to an individual agency's current assessment approach, including recertification and discharge procedures, so that they will be consistent with the Joint Commission and Medicare COP. The OASIS items have been arranged in a clinically meaningful sequence to facilitate incorporating them into current assessment instruments. For example, because "wounds" can present major problems for home care patients, assessing a patient's integumentary status at specific time points using Items 34 through 38 of OASIS-A, shown in Exhibit 21–2, can assist in measuring a patient's health status related to "wounds" and the effectiveness of subsequent treatment modalities to achieve desired outcomes.

AHCPR Guidelines: An HHA's Experience

AHCPR was established in 1989 by Congress to improve quality and effectiveness of health care and improve access to care. Guideline reports, quick reference guidelines for clinicians, and patient guides have been developed to address high-morbidity and high-mortality health problems. One set of guidelines is *Urinary Incontinence in Adults*.

Improving health status and quality of life for patients with urinary incontinence is a major quality and cost issue. Urinary incontinence affects 15 to 30% of noninstitutionalized elderly persons and exacts a high cost in publicly funded home health care services (Baker & Bice, 1995). The Visiting Nurse Association (VNA) of Eastern Montgomery County/

Exhibit 21–2 Medicare's Oasis-A: Standardized Outcome and Assessment Information Set for Home Health Care

INTEGUMENTARY STATUS

34. **Open Wound:**   Does this patient have an
open wound/lesion (e.g., surgical wound, stasis ulcer,
pressure ulcer, etc.)? This **excludes** "OSTOMIES."

☐ 0 – No [If No, go to Question 39]
☐ 1 – Yes

35. **Pressure Ulcers:** Use the table below to indicate the current number of pressure ulcers the patient has at each stage. (Circle one response for each stage.)

Ulcer Stages	Number of Pressure Ulcers				
	0 Zero	1	2	3	4 or or more
a) Stage 1: Nonblanchable erythema of intact skin: the heralding of skin ulceration. In darker-pigmented skin, warmth, edema, hardness, or discolored skin may be indicators.	0	1	2	3	4
b) Stage 2: Partial thickness skin loss involving epidermis and/or dermis. The ulcer is superficial and presents clinically as an abrasion, blister, or shallow crater.	0	1	2	3	4
c) Stage 3: Full-thickness skin loss involving damage or necrosis or subcutaneous tissue which may extend down to, but not through, underlying fascia. The ulcer presents clinically as a deep crater with or without undermining of adjacent tissue.	0	1	2	3	4
d) Stage 4: Full-thickness skin loss with extensive destruction, tissue necrosis, or damage to muscle, bone, or supporting structures (e.g., tendon, joint capsule, etc.)	0	1	2	3	4

36. **Most Problematic Ulcer:**   According to the preceding definitions, what is the stage of the most problematic pressure ulcer?

☐ 0 – No pressure ulcer
☐ 1 – Stage 1
☐ 2 – Stage 2
☐ 3 – Stage 3
☐ 4 – Stage 4

37. **Wounds Present:**   Indicate the numbers of each type of wound/lesion currently present on this patient. Note: If a wound (e.g., surgical) is partially closed but has more than one opening, consider each opening as a seperate open wound/lesion.

Type	Number of Wounds/Lesions				
	0 Zero	1	2	3	4 or or more
a) Stasis ulcer	0	1	2	3	4
b) Surgical wound	0	1	2	3	4

38. **Wound/Lesion Status:**   Indicate the status of each of the following types of open wounds/lesions. If the patient has more than one of a single type of wound/lesion, indicate the status of the one that is most problematic.

Type of Wound	No lesion of this type	Fully granulating	Early/Partial granulation	Not healing
a) Pressure ulcer	0	1	2	3
b) Stasis ulcer	0	1	2	3
c) Surgical wound	0	1	2	3

Source: Reprinted from the Center for Health Policy Research, 1995, Denver, Colorado.

Abington Memorial Hospital found that long-term Foley catheter use for incontinence was a significant source of urinary tract infections, sepsis, and mortality. Using the AHCPR guidelines, they examined their existing processes and alternative management techniques to improve quality of life for their incontinent patients. Various data sources such as long-standing anecdotal data of many nurses, phone calls from patients with indwelling catheters, requests to the education committee to develop a teaching tool for patients, and lack of consensus among nurses regarding the management of Foley catheters resulted in "monitoring of clients with an alteration in pattern of urinary elimination requiring instruction in Foley catheter care" being included in the 1993 Quality Assessment and Improvement (QAI) Plan as a quality initiative (Yuan, 1996).

Although various corrective actions were successfully employed, including education regarding catheter and continence management, nursing rounds, revision of the flowsheet, and documentation improvement, the reason the catheter was being used still needed to be investigated. A quality improvement clinical guidelines team was initiated to identify and evaluate the VNA's patient population with urinary incontinence and retention. Copies of AHCPR's clinical practice guideline, *Urinary Incontinence in Adults,* were distributed to all nurses.

To establish a baseline, the team (a) added questions to the Quarterly Record Review (Exhibit 21–3), (b) conducted a literature review, (c) flow charted the process currently carried out according to AHCPR's guidelines (Figure 21–2), (d) identified barriers to implementing AHCPR's clinical practice guideline for urinary incontinence, using a fishbone diagram (Figure 21–3), and developed a history-taking form (Exhibit 21–4) and an assessment tool (Exhibit 21–5) to identify specific types of incontinence.

Following the development of user-friendly patient education and documentation tools, education for medical and nursing staff, and the monitoring of instruction on care of the Foley catheter, Indicator 2A (Exhibit 21–6) was changed to "Within the limits of patient choice, Foley catheter use will comply with AHCPR guidelines" (Yuan, 1996). It was found that the number of patients with indwelling catheters on service was not significantly reduced, but the patient population was constantly changing due to the short-term use of Foley catheters following surgery and shortened hospital stays.

Outcomes related to important aspects of care are reported in the Performance Improvement Reports (Exhibits 21–6 and 21–7); they indicate significant improvements in nursing practice, and the (1996) revised AHCPR guideline, *Managing Acute and Chronic Urinary Incontinence,* will continue to provide opportunities for improvement in practice.

INTEGRATION OF PATIENT-FOCUSED AND ORGANIZATIONAL FUNCTIONS

The scope of the quality improvement program identifies the multidisciplinary approach to patient care and the types of services and programs including ancillary and contract services. One approach to organizing important functions within an organization is according to the Joint Commission's (1996) five patient-focused functions and six organizational functions. The Quality Assessment and Improvement Plan (Exhibit 21–8) indicates the frequency with which various indicators should be monitored. The Quality Assessment and Improvement calendar (Exhibit 21–9) reflects this integration of functions while recognizing the need for flexibility when assessments trigger defects or when opportunities for improvement and care processes need to be examined.

Linking Quality with Information Systems

Data sources and collection mechanisms are numerous. Manual systems have historically been cumbersome, time consuming, and questionable in terms of accuracy, timeliness, and

Exhibit 21–3 Quality Assurance Quarterly Record Review

I. AHCPR: Urinary Incontinence in Adults	YES	NO	N/A	COMMENTS
A. Was the genitourinary system assessed?				
B. Was a problem with incontinence/retention identified?				
C. Was a nursing diagnosis made related to incontinence/retention?				
D. What was the number of the nursing diagnosis (e.g., 72, 49)?				
E. Was referral to incontinence/retention specialist (e.g., Golden Horizons, urologist) offered?				
F. Was referral made to incontinence/retention specialist (e.g., Golden Horizons, urologist)?				
G. Is Foley present?				
H. If Foley present, does patient meet following guidelines for Foley catheter? 1. Severely impaired for whom bed and clothing changes are disruptive 2. Grade III or IV decubitus ulcer 3. Terminally ill				
I. If patient does not meet guidelines, was patient informed of increased risk of morbidity, e.g., UTI, urosepsis, and mortality?				

Courtesy of Visiting Nurse Association of Eastern Montgomery County/A Department of Abington Memorial Hospital, Willow Grove, Pennsylvania.

conclusiveness of data. Computerized systems are being marketed as the panacea to all the home care industry's woes. Integrated systems are being designed to allow all caregivers to use laptops or subnotebook computers in the "field" to complete, transmit, and receive clinical documentation from remote locations to ensure continuity of care. Some features to consider when selecting an integrated system are its ability to

- customize *all* segments of the system, including assessments and documentation

- facilitate patient care planning (the Joint Commission's "plan of treatment," HCFA's 485 and 487)
- provide medication data, including teaching materials
- quantify data collection and add user-defined indicators to evaluate existing care practices
- gather retrospective data related to risk management, such as incident tracking (falls, injuries, medication, patient/employee issues), infection control, and safety issues

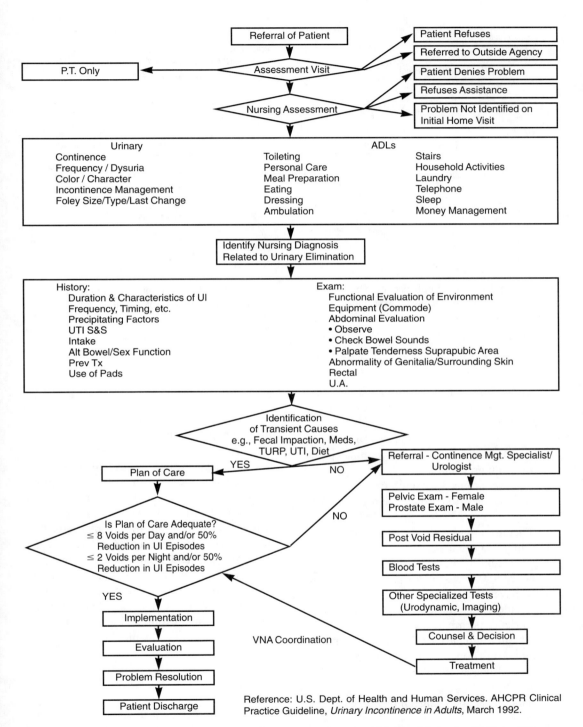

Figure 21–2 Clinical guidelines R/T urinary incontinence. Courtesy of Visiting Nurse Association of Eastern Montgomery County/A Department of Abington Memorial Hospital, Willow Grove, Pennsylvania.

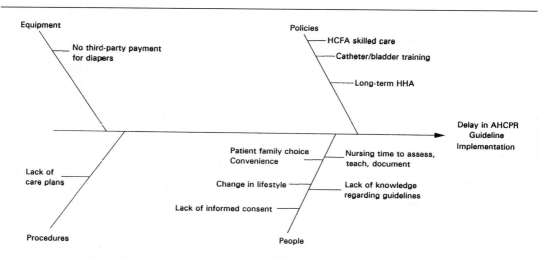

Figure 21–3 Barriers to implementation of AHCPR clinical practice guideline for urinary incontinence in adults. Courtesy of Visiting Nurse Association of Eastern Montgomery County/A Department of Abington Memorial Hospital, Willow Grove, Pennsylvania.

- capture unique criteria for evaluation on a patient level, care-provider level, and aggregate agency data
- provide clear, detailed metrics to quantify results of patient care and clinical pathways and procedures
- track variations and run variance reports on diagnoses, individuals, and geographic areas
- generate powerful reports, including graphical presentations
- provide online ICD-9 codes
- incorporate assessments predetermined by the payer source
- provide a flexible security system that can restrict or permit access
- link all segments of business, including home infusion therapy, hospice, private duty, Home Medical Equipment (HME), and physical therapy
- link clinical and financial outcomes

Please refer to Chapter 13 for greater detail regarding information systems.

Case Management

An internal case management system is a critical component to ensure program quality and acceptable outcomes for patients served in home care agencies. The case manager, frequently a nurse, monitors the patient's progress, coordinates the use of services/resources provided by an interdisciplinary team effectively to maximize functional improvement, ensures that care progresses within set time frames (i.e., uses caremaps), and serves as a liaison/advocate between the patient, the clinical team, the family, and, on occasion, the payer representative. Case management is facilitated through improved communication and ability to access resources. (Refer to Chapter 14 for greater detail.)

Customers

Quality improvement focuses on customer-provider-supplier relationships and requires the examination of who constitutes internal

Exhibit 21–4 Incontinence History

Assessment: Duration of incontinence _____

                    Prior treatment (medical/surgical/behavior modification) _____

                    Use of self-care items (pads/diapers) _____

Exam: Abnormality of genitalia _____

           Altered sexual function _____

Functional evaluation of environment: 1. Distance to bathroom/commode _____

                                        2. Barriers to bathroom access _____

                                        Clutter:　❑ Yes　　❑ No

                                        Stairs _____

Equipment: 1. Commode _____

                2. Adaptive equipment for toilet _____

                3. Other _____

UA Results	Date	Date	Date	Date	Date	Date
1. Leukocytes						
2. Nitrite						
3. PH						
4. PRO						
5. Glucose						
6. Ketones						
7. Urobilinogen						
8. Bilirubin						
9. Blood						

Note: Presence of leukocytes, nitrites, and blood indicate UTI.

Definitions:

61. **Stress Incontinence:** Involuntary loss of urine during coughing, sneezing, laughing, or other physical activity. Confirm diagnosis by observing urine loss during activities that increase abdominal pressure.

63. **Urge Incontinence:** Involuntary loss of urine associated with an abrupt and strong desire to void. Often associated with frequency, may be massive and sudden urine loss. (Mixed incontinence: may have components of urge or stress. Use diagnostic category that predominates.)

59. **Functional Incontinence:** Involuntary urine loss associated with altered environment, sensory, cognitive, and/or mobility deficits.

60. **Reflex Incontinence:** Involuntary loss of urine occurring at somewhat predictable times with a specific bladder volume. Often associated with neuro impairment.

62. **Total Incontinence:** Continuous unpredictable urine loss associated with neuro impairment, including neuropathy, dysfunction, or trauma.

Reference: Gordon, M. (1994). *Manual of nursing diagnosis.* St. Louis: Mosby. Courtesy of Visiting Nurse Association of Eastern Montgomery County/A Department of Abington Memorial Hospital, Willow Grove, Pennsylvania.

Exhibit 21–5 Assessment: Types of Incontinence

61–Stress Incontinence; 63–Urge Incontinence; 59–Functional Incontinence; 60–Reflex Incontinence; 62–Total Incontinence

PT. # _____ NAME _____ PG. _____

PARAMETERS/INTERVENTIONS GOAL:	DATE	DATE	DATE	DATE	DATE
By discharge ◄ 8 vpd ◄ 2 vpn and/or 50% reduction in incontinence episodes					
ASSESSMENT					
Char. continent voids/UI:					
Frequency					
Time of day					
Amount (cc/pads)					
Precipitating factors (ETOH, meds, caffeine)					
UTI S & S					
Intake: _____ ounces/day					
Bowel pattern					
Cognitive/mental state					
Exam: Abdominal shape					
Bowel sounds					
Palp suprapubic tenderness					
Perineal skin					
Rectal exam					
INSTRUCTION					
Kegel exercises					
Bladder/habit training					
Diet/fluid intake					
Skin care					
Reportable signs & symptoms					
INTERVENTION					
Evaluate effectiveness of treatment					
Coordination with UI spec.					
Note: See reverse for definitions of incontinence types, incontinence history, and UA. Complete reverse side and choose appropriate diagnosis.	RN SIG				

C - Care; D - Disc; E - Eval; N - Narrative; DNA - Does Not Apply; NA - Not assessed. Courtesy of Visiting Nurse Association of Eastern Montgomery County/A Department of Abington Memorial Hospital, Willow Grove, Pennsylvania.

Exhibit 21–6 Performance Improvement Report

Important Aspect #2: Clients with an Alteration in Pattern of Urinary Elimination with an Indwelling Foley Catheter

Department: VNA of EMC—Home Care & Hospice

INDICATOR/CRITERIA	STANDARD	FEB	MAR	APR	MAY	JUNE	JULY	AUG	SEPT	OCT	NOV	DEC	JAN
2A. Within the limits of patient choice, Foley catheter use will comply with AHCPR guidelines.	95%	98%	98%	100%	100%	98%	100%	100%	100%	100%	100%	100%	100%
2A1. Criteria for use of indwelling Foley catheter include:													
a. Patient has urinary retention and is:													
(1) severely impaired for whom bed and clothing changes are disruptive.													
(2) Grade III or IV decubitus ulcer													
(3) Terminally ill													
b. Surgical/medical intervention necessitates short-term use													
c. Patient refuses other intervention for continence													
d. No other treatment options available													
Meets criteria/informed Number of patients with Foley catheter		52	56	66	63	67	66	59	64	65	$\frac{59}{59}$	$\frac{57}{57}$	$\frac{49}{49}$

Courtesy of Visiting Nurse Association of Eastern Montgomery County/A Department of Abington Memorial Hospital, Willow Grove, Pennsylvania.

Exhibit 21–7 Performance Improvement Report

Important Aspect #2:   Clients with an Alteration in Pattern of Urinary Elimination Requiring Instruction in Foley Catheter Care

Department: VNA of EMC—Home Care & Hospice

INDICATOR/CRITERIA	STANDARD	MAY	JUNE	JULY	AUG	SEPT	OCT	NOV	DEC	JAN	FEB	MAR	APR	MAY	JUNE	JULY
2A. The patient/caregiver will be instructed in care of the Foley catheter.																
2A1. The patient/caregiver instructions will include:	95%															
a. cleansing around catheter with soap & water at least once daily		100%	100%	98%	100%	100%	100%	100%	100%	100%	100%	100%	100%	100%	100%	100%
b. fluid intake—1.5L min. (if no fluid restrictions)		100%	100%	100%	100%	100%	100%	100%	100%	100%	100%	100%	100%	100%	100%	100%
c. securing catheter		100%	100%	100%	100%	100%	100%	100%	100%	100%	100%	100%	100%	100%	100%	100%
d. positioning of drainage bag		100%	100%	100%	100%	100%	100%	100%	100%	100%	100%	100%	100%	100%	100%	100%
e. emergency removal		100%	100%	100%	100%	100%	100%	100%	100%	100%	100%	100%	100%	100%	100%	100%
f. emptying drainage bag every 8 hours		100%	100%	100%	100%	100%	100%	100%	100%	100%	100%	100%	100%	100%	100%	100%
g. maintenance of closed system		0%	0%	13%	56%	84%	88%	100%	100%	100%	93%	93%	94%	100%	100%	100%
Number of patients with Foley catheter.								46	56	57	42	57	51	50	58	58

Courtesy of Visiting Nurse Association of Eastern Montgomery County/A Department of Abington Memorial Hospital, Willow Grove, Pennsylvania.

Exhibit 21–8 Quality Assessment and Improvement Plan: Frequency of Indicator Monitoring

Department: VNA of EMC—Home Care & Hospice

IMPORTANT ASPECT/INDICATORS	JAN	FEB	MAR	APR	MAY	JUN	JUL	AUG	SEPT	OCT	NOV	DEC
1. Assessment and evaluation of satisfaction with services provided.												
1A. Patients/families will indicate satisfaction with professional services provided on the discharge patient questionnaire.	X	X	X	X	X	X	X	X	X	X	X	X
1B. Patients/families express satisfaction with professional care through written letters.	X	X	X	X	X	X	X	X	X	X	X	X
1C. Families will indicate satisfaction with hospice services provided.	X	X	X	X	X	X	X	X	X	X	X	X
1D. Physicians will indicate satisfaction with services provided to their patients.	X											
1E. Patients/families will indicate satisfaction with home health aide (HHA) services provided.	X	X	X	X	X	X	X	X	X	X	X	X
1F. Patients/families express satisfaction with personal care through written letters.	X	X	X	X	X	X	X	X	X	X	X	X
1G. Patients/families will indicate satisfaction with infusion therapy services provided.	X	X	X	X	X	X	X	X	X	X	X	X
1H. Patients/families will not express dissatisfaction with infusion therapy services through written letters.	X	X	X	X	X	X	X	X	X	X	X	X

continues

Exhibit 21–8 continued

IMPORTANT ASPECT/INDICATORS	JAN	FEB	MAR	APR	MAY	JUN	JUL	AUG	SEPT	OCT	NOV	DEC
2. Clients with an alteration in pattern of urinary elimination with an indwelling Foley catheter.	X	X	X	X	X	X	X	X	X	X	X	X
2A. Within the limits of patient choice, Foley catheter use will comply with AHCPR guidelines.												
3. 24-hour on-call system is available and responsible.	X	X	X	X	X	X	X	X	X	X	X	X
3A. RN responds to patients'/families' concerns after office hours.												
4. Precipitous discharge	X	X	X	X	X	X	X	X	X	X	X	X
4A. Prior to discharge from VNA service, patients for whom 3rd party reimbursement has been denied will be offered care options.												
5. Monitoring of care provided by contract agency and intervention as indicated.	X											
5A. Contract agency adheres to a quality assessment and improvement program periodically reviewed by home care director.			X			X			X			
6. Hospice care												
6A. Identification of hospice services includes the management of discomfort and symptom relief.												X

IMPORTANT ASPECT/INDICATORS	JAN	FEB	MAR	APR	MAY	JUN	JUL	AUG	SEPT	OCT	NOV	DEC
7. Infection control			X			X			X			X
7A. The RN demonstrates techniques to limit the spread of infection.												
7B. The RN follows the universal precautions approach to infection control.			X			X			X			X
7C. The HHA demonstrates techniques to limit the spread of infection.			X			X			X			X
7D. The HHA follows the universal precautions approach to infection control.			X			X			X			X
7E. Prevention and surveillance of infection related to infusion therapy via peripheral lines.			X			X			X			X
7F. Prevention and surveillance of infection related to infusion therapy via central lines.			X			X			X			X
8. Home health aide (HHA) services provided to patients with personal care needs.	X			X			X			X		
8A. The frequency of HHA visits is provided according to the plan to meet patients' personal care needs.		X	X		X	X		X	X		X	X
9. Interdisciplinary care												
9A. Assessment of the patient includes referral to all necessary resources (nurse specialist, PT, OT, ST, MSS, Hospice).						X		X	X			
10. Outcome of patient care for Nsg, HHA, PT, OT, SP, MSS												

continues

Exhibit 21–8 continued

IMPORTANT ASPECT/INDICATORS	JAN	FEB	MAR	APR	MAY	JUN	JUL	AUG	SEPT	OCT	NOV	DEC
10A. Patients discharged from services in Rehab groups 1–3 with a discharge reason of 1 (died) will have no quality-of-care concerns identified.	X	X	X	X	X	X	X	X	X	X	X	X
10B. Evaluation by KePRO of care provided results in no quality-of-care concern being identified on final determination.	X	X	X	X	X	X	X	X	X	X	X	X
11. Intravenous (IV) Therapy												
11A. The RN administering IV medication (e.g., antibiotics, Lasix) maintains an accurate record of the therapy provided.	X	X	X	X	X	X	X	X	X	X	X	X
11B. Surveillance of unscheduled inpatient admissions for patients receiving home IV therapy.	X	X	X	X	X	X	X	X	X	X	X	X
12. Competency												
12A. RN demonstrates technical skills needed to meet patient care needs as set forth in the physician plan of treatment and in accordance with standards of nursing practice.			X			X			X			X
13. Instructions to patients identified.												
13A. Patient/family will report that instructions provided by VNA personnel related to health care needs were clear.			X			X			X			X

Courtesy of Visiting Nurse Association of Eastern Montgomery County/A Department of Abington Memorial Hospital, Willow Grove, Pennsylvania.

Exhibit 21–9 Quality Assessment and Improvement Calendar

Department: VNA of EMC—Home Care & Hospice

	JAN	FEB	MAR	APR	MAY	JUN	JUL	AUG	SEPT	OCT	NOV	DEC
Utilization review and record review	X	X	X	X	X	X	X	X	X	X	X	X
Record review summary			X			X			X			X
Annual record review summary						X						
Patient questionnaires mailed	X	X	X	X	X	X	X	X	X	X	X	
Patient questionnaires follow-up	X	X	X	X	X	X	X	X	X	X	X	X
Analysis of unsolicited letters	X	X	X	X	X	X	X	X	X	X	X	X
Physicians' questionnaires mailed	X											
Assessment of important aspects of care	X	X	X	X	X	X	X	X	X	X	X	X
Evaluation of clinical competence	X	X	X	X	X	X	X	X	X	X	X	X
Monitoring and review of patient outcomes	X	X	X	X	X	X	X	X	X	X	X	X
Incident report follow-up	X	X	X	X	X	X	X	X	X	X	X	X
Annual agency evaluation									X			
Fiscal year												

Courtesy of Visiting Nurse Association of Eastern Montgomery County/A Department of Abington Memorial Hospital, Willow Grove, Pennsylvania.

and external customers. Individuals and groups may be both customers and suppliers, depending on the role they play at a given time. Traditionally, clients, physicians, suppliers, individuals providing contracted services, and third-party payers are considered external customers; internal customers are all employees who work together as teammates, communicate effectively, and constantly innovate and advance their capabilities. To improve quality, agencies must adopt a fundamental attitude of caring about the customer by assessing their satisfaction with patient-focused and organizational functions that are essential for achieving good outcomes. The shift to development of strong, caring relationships with internal and external customers has resulted in numerous forms and techniques to gather quantitative and qualitative data. Some examples include the Discharged Patient Questionnaire in Exhibit 21–10, the IV Discharged Patient Questionnaire in Exhibit 21–11, the Physician Satisfaction Survey in Exhibit 21–12, and a customer annual program evaluation (Exhibit 21–13). (Refer to Chapter 8 for more detailed discussion regarding the customer.)

Human Resources

Human resources are an agency's greatest asset. Structural outcomes such as an appropriate number of staff with relevant knowledge and skills form the foundation for quality patient care. Agencies must ensure that staff are uniformly oriented, competencies are assessed, and support is provided for self-development and continuous learning. Evaluating productivity behaviors ensures critical job skills for cost-effective quality of care (Benefield, 1996; Dansky & Brannon, 1996).

Home health aides constitute the largest segment of paraprofessional staff and provide the greatest amount of direct patient care. The sample Home Health Aide's Supervision and Competency Checklist (Exhibit 21–14) and Quarterly Record Review Form (Exhibit 21–15) track the competency of this critical worker.

Annual Evaluation Plan

To complete the quality improvement cycle, provide a new benchmark using current performance data, and recommend areas for performance improvement for the coming year, an agency must conduct an annual evaluation of processes. Relating to the Joint Commission's patient-focused functions and the organizational functions, the evaluation form in Exhibit 21–16 typifies the process in which all home care staff engage: seeking to understand what is working well and why and what is not working well and why.

The data are summarized; the managers evaluate the summary for patterns and trends and identify/recommend performance improvement projects, which are then forwarded to the quality improvement committee. Using the performance improvement selection criteria—high risk, problem prone, high volume, high cost—to identify critical CQI projects that support the agency's mission, vision, and values (patient-centered care, needs/expectations of staff, integrated system, and customer needs/satisfaction for the coming year), the committee members prioritize recommended projects, identify work team members, and implement projects, using the plan-do-check-act (PDCA) process shown in Exhibit 21–17.

Radical changes are taking place within the home health care industry. The opportunity and challenge for providers to contribute to the design and use of data to measure clinical and administrative outcomes, customer satisfaction, and adjustment factors for caseloads of varying severity (case mix) clearly represent a major philosophical and fundamental change from an adversarial relationship between providers, state and federal regulators, and the business industry to a collegial relationship. With the ability to demonstrate continuous improvement of cost-effective, quality care, an agency will strengthen its financial status and marketability in the community.

Exhibit 21–10 Discharged Patient Questionnaire

DISCHARGED PATIENT QUESTIONNAIRE # _____

1. What services were provided?
   ❑ Nursing   ❑ Speech therapy
   ❑ Home health aide (personal care)   ❑ Physical therapy
   ❑ Social worker   ❑ Dietitian
   ❑ Occupational therapy

2. Was the service what you expected it to be?

3. VNA personnel considered my family's special needs.

Poor	Fair	Satisfactory	Very Good	Excellent
1	2	3	4	5

4. I was satisfied with the personnel.

Poor	Fair	Satisfactory	Very Good	Excellent
1	2	3	4	5

5. Were there other services you would have liked us to provide? _____

6. Instructions provided by VNA personnel related to my health care needs were clear.

Poor	Fair	Satisfactory	Very Good	Excellent
1	2	3	4	5

7. Questions were answered adequately.

Poor	Fair	Satisfactory	Very Good	Excellent
1	2	3	4	5

8. This service helped me achieve my health care goals.

Poor	Fair	Satisfactory	Very Good	Excellent
1	2	3	4	5

9. Would you use this service again? _____

10. Would you recommend this service to others? _____

11. What suggestions would you make to improve the service? _____

_____

_____

12. Additional comments: _____

_____

_____

_____

_____

continues

Exhibit 21–10 continued

PLEASE COMPLETE FOR THOSE SERVICES RECEIVED

1. The nurse understood what my main health problem was.

Poor	Fair	Satisfactory	Very Good	Excellent
1	2	3	4	5

2. The nurse appeared skillful in carrying out procedures.

Poor	Fair	Satisfactory	Very Good	Excellent
1	2	3	4	5

3. The home health aide considered my individual needs.

Poor	Fair	Satisfactory	Very Good	Excellent
1	2	3	4	5

4. The home health aide provided personal care to my satisfaction.

Poor	Fair	Satisfactory	Very Good	Excellent
1	2	3	4	5

5. The physical therapist explained things in language that I could understand.

Poor	Fair	Satisfactory	Very Good	Excellent
1	2	3	4	5

6. The exercise program that the physical therapist gave me helped me to achieve my goals.

Poor	Fair	Satisfactory	Very Good	Excellent
1	2	3	4	5

7. The social worker acted in a supportive manner.

Poor	Fair	Satisfactory	Very Good	Excellent
1	2	3	4	5

8. The social worker gave me information about available resources.

Poor	Fair	Satisfactory	Very Good	Excellent
1	2	3	4	5

9. The speech therapist visited according to plan.

Poor	Fair	Satisfactory	Very Good	Excellent
1	2	3	4	5

10. The speech therapist helped me to communicate.

Poor	Fair	Satisfactory	Very Good	Excellent
1	2	3	4	5

11. The occupational therapist enabled me to improve my activities of daily living.

Poor	Fair	Satisfactory	Very Good	Excellent
1	2	3	4	5

12. The occupational therapist visit schedule met my needs.

Poor	Fair	Satisfactory	Very Good	Excellent
1	2	3	4	5

13. The dietitian provided a nutrition therapy plan that I could understand.

Poor	Fair	Satisfactory	Very Good	Excellent
1	2	3	4	5

Signature: _____ Date: _____

Courtesy of Visiting Nurse Association of Eastern Montgomery County/A Department of Abington Memorial Hospital, Willow Grove, Pennsylvania.

Exhibit 21–11 IV Discharged Patient Questionnaire

IV DISCHARGED PATIENT QUESTIONNAIRE # _____

1. What services were provided?
   ❑ Nursing   ❑ Intravenous therapy   ❑ Physical therapy
   ❑ Home health aide   ❑ Occupational therapy   ❑ Social worker
     (personal care)   ❑ Speech therapy

2. Was the service what you expected it to be?   ❑ Yes   ❑ No

3. Medication delivery was timely.
Poor	Fair	Satisfactory	Very Good	Excellent
1	2	3	4	5

4. Supplies were delivered in sufficient quantity to meet my needs.
Poor	Fair	Satisfactory	Very Good	Excellent
1	2	3	4	5

5. I was satisfied with the personnel.
Poor	Fair	Satisfactory	Very Good	Excellent
1	2	3	4	5

6. Were there other services you would have liked us to provide? _____
   _____

7. Instructions provided by VNA personnel related to my health care needs were clear.
Poor	Fair	Satisfactory	Very Good	Excellent
1	2	3	4	5

8. The evening/weekend on-call response was effective.
Poor	Fair	Satisfactory	Very Good	Excellent
1	2	3	4	5

9. This service helped me achieve my health care goals.
Poor	Fair	Satisfactory	Very Good	Excellent
1	2	3	4	5

10. Would you use this service again? _____
    _____

11. Would you recommend this service to others? _____
    _____

12. What suggestions would you make to improve the service? _____
    _____

13. Additional comments: _____
    _____

continues

Exhibit 21–11 continued

PLEASE COMPLETE FOR THOSE SERVICES RECEIVED

1. The nurse understood what my main health problem was.

Poor	Fair	Satisfactory	Very Good	Excellent
1	2	3	4	5

2. The nurse appeared skillful in carrying out procedures.

Poor	Fair	Satisfactory	Very Good	Excellent
1	2	3	4	5

3. The home health aide considered my individual needs.

Poor	Fair	Satisfactory	Very Good	Excellent
1	2	3	4	5

4. The home health aide provided personal care to my satisfaction.

Poor	Fair	Satisfactory	Very Good	Excellent
1	2	3	4	5

5. The physical therapist explained things in language that I could understand.

Poor	Fair	Satisfactory	Very Good	Excellent
1	2	3	4	5

6. The exercise program that the physical therapist gave me helped me to achieve my goals.

Poor	Fair	Satisfactory	Very Good	Excellent
1	2	3	4	5

7. The social worker acted in a supportive manner.

Poor	Fair	Satisfactory	Very Good	Excellent
1	2	3	4	5

8. The social worker gave me information about available resources.

Poor	Fair	Satisfactory	Very Good	Excellent
1	2	3	4	5

9. The speech therapist visited according to plan.

Poor	Fair	Satisfactory	Very Good	Excellent
1	2	3	4	5

10. The speech therapist helped me to communicate.

Poor	Fair	Satisfactory	Very Good	Excellent
1	2	3	4	5

11. The occupational therapist enabled me to improve my activities of daily living.

Poor	Fair	Satisfactory	Very Good	Excellent
1	2	3	4	5

12. The occupational therapist visit schedule met my needs.

Poor	Fair	Satisfactory	Very Good	Excellent
1	2	3	4	5

13. The dietitian provided a nutrition therapy plan that I could understand.

Poor	Fair	Satisfactory	Very Good	Excellent
1	2	3	4	5

Signature: _____   Date: _____

Courtesy of Visiting Nurse Association of Eastern Montgomery County/A Department of Abington Memorial Hospital, Willow Grove, Pennsylvania.

Exhibit 21–12 Physician Satisfaction Survey

VISITING NURSE ASSOCIATION OF EASTERN MONTGOMERY COUNTY

A Department of
Abington Memorial Hospital

PHYSICIAN SATISFACTION SURVEY

Your patients have used one or more of the services available through the Visiting Nurse Association of Eastern Montgomery County/A Department of Abington Memorial Hospital. Would you please take the time to complete and return this questionnaire in the enclosed self-addressed envelope? Please comment and make suggestions for improvements you believe would be helpful in making this association more effective in the community. Thank you for your cooperation in this evaluation process.

Marilyn D. Harris, RN, MSN

Marilyn D. Harris, RN, MSN
Executive Director

Services are provided to more than 1100 patients by more than 150 health care personnel each month, for a total of over 10,000 visits per month. These services could have included:

Skilled Nursing	Speech Therapy	Enterostomal Therapy	Home Health Aide
Medical Social Service	Psychiatric Nursing	Occupational Therapy	Maternal Child Health
Hospice	Physical Therapy	Continence Management	Hi-Tech Services

1. How satisfied are you with the quality of care given by this agency's personnel?

0	1	2	3	4
Not applicable	Very Satisfied	Satisfied	Dissatisfied	Very Dissatisfied

Comments: _____

_____

2. Communication is crucial to the coordination of patient care. Please indicate your level of satisfaction with access to patient-specific/agency information.

0	1	2	3	4
Not applicable	Very Satisfied	Satisfied	Dissatisfied	Very Dissatisfied

Comments: _____

_____

3. In this era of shortened hospital stays, are there any other programs or services that you would want this department to provide for your patients?

Comments: _____

_____

Signature: _____

Abington Memorial Health Center, 2510 Maryland Rd., Suite 250, Willow Grove, PA 19090-0520

Accredited with Commendation by the Joint Commission on Accreditation of Healthcare Organizations

Courtesy of Visiting Nurse Association of Eastern Montgomery County/A Department of Abington Memorial Hospital, Willow Grove, Pennsylvania.

Exhibit 21–13 Customer Annual Program Evaluation

VISITING NURSE ASSOCIATION OF EASTERN MONTGOMERY COUNTY

A Department of
Abington Memorial Hospital

This department is conducting its annual program evaluation. Your feedback would be most appreciated. A stamped return envelope has been included for your convenience.

Thank you for your participation in this evaluation process.

Marilyn D. Harris, RN

Marilyn D. Harris, RN, MSN
Executive Director

1. Why did you select this organization for the provision of service? _____

   _____

2. Was the service what you expected it to be? Yes _____ No _____ Why or Why not?

   _____

3. Level of satisfaction with the service provided.

poor	fair	satisfactory	very good	excellent
1	2	3	4	5

4. Were there other services you would have liked us to provide? _____

   _____

5. Would you recommend this organization to others? Yes _____ No _____

6. What suggestions would you make to improve the service provided by this organization?

   _____

7. The 1995 Joint Commission on Accreditation of Home Care standards requires that internal and external sources be surveyed to solicit expectations regarding the home care agency's dimensions of performance such as availability, timeliness, continuity, safety, respect and caring. Please comment.

   _____

   _____

   _____

   _____

   Signature

Abington Memorial Health Center, 2510 Maryland Rd., Suite 250, Willow Grove, PA 19090-0520

Accredited with Commendation by the Joint Commission on Accreditation of Healthcare Organizations

---

Courtesy of Visiting Nurse Association of Eastern Montgomery County/A Department of Abington Memorial Hospital, Willow Grove, Pennsylvania.

Exhibit 21–14 Home Health Aide Supervision and Competency Checklist

NAME _____

PROCEDURE _____

	Date	Outstanding	Satisfactory	Unsatisfactory	COMMENTS
Physical Personal Care Needs					
Mouth care					
Bath—tub bath/shower/bed/partial					
Skin care—back rub					
Foot care/nail care					
Hair care—shampoo—bed/sink/tub					
Transfers (body mechanics)					
Toileting					
Ambulation					
Positioning					
Homemaking Chores					
Care of client's room					
Bed linen					
Care of BR after bath or shower					
Care of kitchen after meal prep.					
Care of client's clothing					
Infection Control					
Appropriate use of universal precautions					
Hand washing techniques					
Emotional Support					
(Explains procedures)					
Provides for client privacy					
Appropriate relationship with client/family					
Confidentiality and ethics					
Other Special Procedures					
Temp, pulse, resp.					
Range of motion					
_____					
_____					
Personal Habits					
Appearance—neat and clean					
Approved uniform					
Record Keeping					
Accurately completes time logs/activity sheets					
Adheres to assigned schedule					
Attendance					

Courtesy of Visiting Nurse Association of Eastern Montgomery County/A Department of Abington Memorial Hospital, Willow Grove, Pennsylvania.

Exhibit 21–15 Home Health Aide's Quarterly Record Review Form

NURSING (HOME HEALTH AIDE)

CLIENT NAME: _____   DATE OF REVIEW: _____

CLIENT CASE NO: _____   PRESENT QUARTER: _____

PRIMARY NURSE NAME: _____   MONTHS INCLUDED: _____

STATUS OF RECORD: ACTIVE _____   _____
                                                SIGNATURE OF REVIEWER
              DISCHARGED ___

SERVICES INVOLVED:

	Yes	No	N/A	Comments
I. Assessment A. Does the clinical record include assessment of physical, psychosocial, and environmental needs of patient/family?				
B. Was the nursing assessment form updated upon each new plan of treatment or past each hospitalization?				
C. Were nursing diagnoses based on assessment factors?				
D. Did the primary nurse select the correct patient group on admission?				
E. If the patient's status changed, was the patient group changed accordingly?				
II. Planning A. Were client goals stated?				
B. Were the nursing parameters specific to the identified nursing diagnoses/problems?				
C. Was the plan of treatment (orders) current and signed by physician?				
D. Was the POT completed in accordance with agency policy?				
E. Were signed verbal orders obtained to cover any change in the plan of treatment?				
III. Implementation A. Was the frequency of nursing visits based on the assessment of the client's needs?				
B. Was the service provided consistent with the care plan?				

continues

Exhibit 21–15 continued

	Yes	No	N/A	Comments
C. Does the record contain evidence that the applicable subobjectives in the patient classification/objectives system were being acted upon?				
D. Did the nurse request consultative services of other disciplines when needed?				
E. Did the nurse regularly supervise the performance of the HHA/LPN?				
F. HHA consistent with client's needs?				
G. Did the nurse demonstrate evidence of his/her coordination of all services?				
H. Did the nurse hold conferences/joint visits with other services when appropriate?				
I. Did the nurse notify the physician/other team members of any significant changes in the client's status?				
J. Were service reports legible, dated, and signed?				
K. Did service reports include:				
1. Adequate information regarding the client's current condition?				
2. Specific treatments/instructions given?				
3. The date of the next visit?				
L. Were the following forms present and updated according to agency protocol:				
1. Authorization and release form?				
2. Medicare termination letter?				
3. HHA plan of care?				
4. Family information sheet?				
M. Does the record contain evidence that medications were checked for significant side effects and indications?				

continues

Exhibit 21–15 continued

	Yes	No	N/A	Comments
N. In the opinion of the reviewer, were services:				
Appropriately utilized?				
Over-utilized?				
Under-utilized?				
IV. Evaluation				
A. Were patient/family responses to nursing intervention documented?				
B. Were necessary modifications in the care plan made based on the nurse's evaluation?				
C. If discharged from nursing service:				
1. Was discharge a logical development of the care plan and client goals?				
2. Does the record contain a description of the patient/family change in knowledge, understanding and/or behavior as the result of the nurse's intervention?				
3. Was there evidence of the client's goals having been met?				
4. Was the discharge summary present and accurately completed?				
5. Were the nursing diagnoses on the discharge computer summary consistent with those on the problem list?				
6. Were the service codes (group # and goal attainment) listed on the discharge computer summary consistent with the evidence found in the record?				
7. Was the physician notified of client's discharge?				
V. Joint Commission Medication Management Patient/significant other was instructed in all new medications within 4 weeks A. Indication				
B. Dosage				
C. Frequency				
D. Route				
E. Adverse reactions				
F. Drug interactions				

Courtesy of Visiting Nurse Association of Eastern Montgomery County/A Department of Abington Memorial Hospital, Willow Grove, Pennsylvania.

Exhibit 21–16 HomeCare Southwest Agency Evaluation Tool

Evaluation of Southwest Washington Medical Center HomeCare's Total Program

OBJECTIVE: To assess the extent to which Southwest Washington Medical Center HomeCare's program is appropriate, adequate, effective, and efficient.

TOPIC	TOPIC CRITERIA	AREAS WORKING WELL	SUGGESTIONS FOR IMPROVEMENT
Rights and responsibilities	How well does the process for addressing & reporting patient rights work?		
	Do you believe our patients understand their rights and responsibilities?		
	How effective is our process on: 1. Rights and responsibilities 2. Advance directives 3. DNR 4. Confidentiality 5. Patient complaints 6. Resolution of ethical issues 7. Staff rights not to participate in aspects of care that are in conflict with cultural values or religious beliefs		
Assessment	Do we determine care and service for our patients based upon our: 1. Assessment admission/reassessment 2. Evaluation of that assessment 3. Development of a care plan based upon the evaluation 4. Do you understand your responsibilities relative to communicating payer source information throughout the agency?		

continues

Exhibit 21–16 continued

TOPIC	TOPIC CRITERIA	AREAS WORKING WELL	SUGGESTIONS FOR IMPROVEMENT
	5. Does documentation reflect the assessment process?		
	6. Does the documentation process support the assessment process?		
Human Resources	1. Orientation		
	2. Competency assessment		
	3. Performance evaluation		
Infection Control	1. How well does the infection control program meet your needs?		
Care, Treatment, and Service	1. Do we effectively develop, implement, monitor, and document patient-specific care plans?		
	2. Do we effectively modify patient-specific care plans based upon changes and reassessments?		
	3. How effective is the process for prescriptions or ordering of medications?		
	4. How effective is the process for preparation and dispensing of drugs?		
	5. How effective is the process for medication management, administration, monitoring, and reporting of adverse drug reactions?		
	6. Does the payer source impact care, treatment, and service?		

TOPIC	TOPIC CRITERIA	AREAS WORKING WELL	SUGGESTIONS FOR IMPROVEMENT
Education	1. Are patient education resources and activities effective?		
	2. Are staff education resources and activities effective?		
Continuum of Care	1. Does our referral or transfer process support sufficient information to allow meeting the patient needs with the appropriate level and type of care and service?		
	2. Do our systems support an optimum level of coordination and communication of patient care needs (i.e., inter/intradisciplinary, inter/intra-agency and external organization)?		
Performance Improvement	1. Has HomeCare Southwest's QI process made an impact on your job?		
	2. Do you have adequate understanding of the process? Explain it with examples of the process this past year.		
	3. What QI indicators, processes, or clinical outcomes do you believe should be studied further?		
Leadership	1. Is leadership effective in providing a working environment that supports Southwest Washington Medical Center/HCSW MVV?		

continues

Exhibit 21–16 continued

TOPIC	TOPIC CRITERIA	AREAS WORKING WELL	SUGGESTIONS FOR IMPROVEMENT
	2. Do you have adequate access to leadership?		
Management of the Environment of Care	1. How do you evaluate our patients' environment for safety?		
	2. How does HomeCare Southwest provide sufficient information to its patients for their safety, environment, and preparedness for emergency?		
	3. Do you know what the emergency preparedness and environmental safety plan is?		
	4. What should be reported as incidents and accidents?		
	5. How do you report incidents, accidents of patients, and employees?		
Management of Information	1. How well does the information system support your work?		
	2. What areas, if any, of the information system could be improved for the work you do?		
	3. What information do you need to do your job that you currently do not have?		
Accounting Department Evaluation	How well do the following processes work: 1. Admits		

TOPIC	TOPIC CRITERIA	AREAS WORKING WELL	SUGGESTIONS FOR IMPROVEMENT
	2. Pay source verification		
	3. Itinerary input		
	4. Claims processing		
	5. Month-end close		
	6. Billing chart set-up		
	7. DDE/EMC		
	8. Deposits/cash handling/petty cash		
	9. Posting/working EOBs		
	10. Aging		
	11. Write-offs		
	12. Payables		
	13. Computer system		
Support Services	1. Answering of telephones and relaying messages		
	2. Greeting people		
	3. Voice mail		
	4. Pagers		
	5. Patient satisfaction survey		
	6. Word processing		
	7. Mail distribution		
	8. Paycheck and mileage check distribution		
	9. Distributing keys, papers, and security code to new employees		

continues

Exhibit 21–16 continued

TOPIC	TOPIC CRITERIA	AREAS WORKING WELL	SUGGESTIONS FOR IMPROVEMENT
	10. Employee licensure file maintenance		
	11. Adding/omitting employees from our security list to Sonitrol		
	12. Office equipment (copy and fax machines) maintenance		
	13. Forms system management		
	14. Ordering, stocking, and distributing medical supplies		
	15. Office supply maintenance		
	16. Coordination of admit packets for disciplines		
	17. Supply input (billing)		
	18. Ordering and stocking kitchen supplies		
Medical Records	1. Doctor licensure verification process		
	2. Chart review process		
	3. Teamwork within medical records		
	4. Teamwork with other staff		
	5. Meetings/MR meetings/staff meetings		
	6. Supplies/equipment management process		
	7. Communication process		
	8. Corrections process		
	9. Patient satisfaction questionnaire mailing (once a month) process		

TOPIC	TOPIC CRITERIA	AREAS WORKING WELL	SUGGESTIONS FOR IMPROVEMENT
	10. Paperwork flow process		
	11. Training of medical records staff		
	12. Orientation for field staff		
	13. Coding (ICDA) process		
	14. Admits/secondary process		
	15. Recertification process		
	16. Note input process		
	17. Tracking process		
	18. Filing process		
	19. Itineraries process		
	20. Doctor changes/change of status process		
Intake (Processing of Incoming/Outgoing Calls, Referrals)	1. Physician communication process		
	2. Insurance/Medicaid authorization process		
	3. Access to intake coordinators (telephone or direct)		
	4. Relaying of incoming information (patient reports, verbal orders, etc.)		
	5. End-of-day referral process (referral log, distribution of referrals, etc.)		
	6. Night/weekend call information		

continues

Exhibit 21–16 continued

TOPIC	TOPIC CRITERIA	AREAS WORKING WELL	SUGGESTIONS FOR IMPROVEMENT
CarePlus (Private Duty Program)	How well do the following processes work:		
	1. Orientation		
	2. Scheduling		
	3. Documentation/charting		
	4. Care plans		
	5. Special instructions regarding patients		
	6. Staff meetings		
	7. Coordination of services with other programs such as home care/hospice		
	8. On call		
	9. Voice mail		
	10. Communication of pertinent information		
	11. Availability/support of office staff for issues/concerns/problems (i.e., Paul, Nancy, Phyllis)		

Courtesy of HomeCare Southwest, Southwest Washington Medical Center, Vancouver, Washington.

Exhibit 21–17 Performance Improvement Process

STEP 1   **Project Definition & Organization**

Project

To identify who will be the project team members and facilitator.
Define the project purpose and scope clearly.
Why is it important that this be addressed?
Define the measures of success.
What is the basis for this project?
How will progress be measured?

▲ Identify who will be the project team members and facilitator.
▲ Define the project purpose and scope clearly.
▲ Why is it important that this be addressed?
▲ Define the measures of success.
▲ What is the basis for this project?
▲ How will progress be measured?

STEP 2   **Diagnostic Journey**

Current Situation

To future focus the improvement effort by gathering data about the current situation

Cause Analysis

To identify and verify deep causes to pave the way for implementation of solutions

▲ What is the history?
▲ Can the problem or situation be depicted in a sketch or flow chart?
▲ What happens now when the problem appears?
▲ What are the symptoms?
▲ Where do symptoms appear?
▲ Where don't they?
▲ Who is involved?

▲ What solutions could address the verified deep causes?
▲ What criteria are useful for comparing solutions?
▲ What are the pros and cons of each solution? How do they relate to the causes?
▲ Which solutions seem most feasible and worth testing?
▲ How can feasible solutions be tested and evaluated on a small scale?
▲ What data will you collect?
▲ Which solution is most effective?
▲▲ What are the plans for implementing it full scale?

STEP 3   **Remedial Journey**

Solutions

To develop, pilot, and implement solutions that address deep causes.

Results

To evaluate both the solutions and the plans used to implement the methods.

▲ What solutions could address the verified deep cause?
▲ What criteria are useful for comparing potential solutions?
▲ What are the pros and cons of each solution? How do they relate to the causes?
▲ Which solutions seem most feasible and worth testing?
▲ How can feasible solutions be tested and evaluated on a small scale? What data will you collect?
▲ Which solution is most effective?
▲ What are the plans for implementing it full scale?

▲ How well do results meet the targets?
▲ How well was the plan executed?
▲ What can this tell you about planning for improvement?

STEP 4   **Holding the Gains**

Standardization

To maintain the gains from the solutions by standardizing work from this effort.

▲ What is the new standard method or process?
▲ Document the new method in graphic form.
▲ How will all employees who do this work be trained?
▲ What is in place to assure the gains are maintained? To prevent back-sliding?
▲ How will methods, processes, and results be monitored?
▲ What measures are in place to foster ongoing improvement of this standard method?

STEP 5   **Future Gains**

Future Plans

To anticipate future improvement and preserve the lessons from this effort.

▲ What remaining needs were not addressed by this project?
▲ What recommendations would you make for investing in these remaining needs?
▲ What did you learn from this project?
▲ How will the documentation be completed?
▲ What happens to it when it is finished?
▲ How will this project be brought to a close?

Courtesy of HomeCare Southwest, Southwest Washington Medical Center, Vancouver, Washington.

REFERENCES

American Health Consultants. (1996). Want an option to Joint Commission accreditations? *Homecare Quality Management, 2*(8), 99–100.

Bach, J., Intinola, P., Alba, A., & Holland, I. (1992). The ventilator-assisted individual: Cost analysis of institutionalization vs. rehabilitation and in-home management. *Chest, 101*(1), 26–30.

Baker, D., & Bice, B. (1995). The influence of urinary incontinence on publicly financed home care services to low-income elderly people. *Gerontologist, 35*(3), 360–369.

Benefield, L. (1996). Productivity in home healthcare: Assessing nurse effectiveness and efficiency. *Home Healthcare Nurse, 14*(9), 698–706.

Burbach, C., Conrad, M., Schumacher, K., & Lindsay, L. (1991). Issues in home health nursing education. *Home Healthcare Nurse, 9*(4), 22–28.

Casiro, O., McKenzie, M., McFayden, L., Shapiro, C., Seshia, M., MacDonald, N., Moffat, M., & Cheang, M. (1993). Earlier discharge with community-based intervention for low birth rate infants: A randomized trial. *Pediatrics, 92*(1), 128–134.

CHAP and Joint Commission Announce Cooperative Agreement. (1996). *N & HC: Perspectives on Community, 17*(6), 325.

Dansky, K., & Brannon, D. (1996). Using TQM to improve management of home health aides. *Journal of Nursing Administration, 26*(12), 43–49.

Davis, J. (1993). Evaluation of novice-home visitor preparation strategies. *Journal of Community Health Nursing, 10*(4), 249–258.

Donabedian, A. (1980). *Explorations in quality assessment and monitoring. Volume 1: The definition of quality and approaches to its assessment.* Ann Arbor, MI: Health Administration Press.

Fields, A., Rosenblatt, A., Pollack, M., & Kaufman, J. (1991). Home care cost-effectiveness for respiratory technology-dependent children. *American Journal of Diseases of Children, 145*, 729–733.

Hughes, S., Cummings, J., Waver, F., Manheim, L., Braun, B., & Conrad, K. (1992). A randomized trial of the cost effectiveness of VA hospital-based home care for the terminally ill. *Health Services Research, 26*(6), 801–817.

Joint Commission on Accreditation of Healthcare Organizations. (1996). *1997–1998 Comprehensive Accreditation Manual for Home Care.* Oakbrook Terrace, IL: Author.

Juran, H. (1988). *Juran on planning for quality.* New York: Free Press.

Kramer, A., et al. (1990). Assessing and Assuring the Quality of Home Healthcare. *Generations,* 51–53.

Lalonde, B. (1988). *Quality Assurance Manual of the Home Care Association of Washington.* Edmonds, WA: Home Care Association of Washington.

Medicare's OASIS: Standardized Outcome and Assessment Information Set for Home Health Care. (1996). National Association for Home Care: 1.

National Association for Home Care. (1995). *Basic statistics about home care 1995.* Washington, DC: Author.

Pigott, H., & Trott, L. (1993). Translating research into practice, the implementation of an in-home crisis intervention triage and treatment service in the private sector. *American Journal of Medical Quality, 8*(3), 138–144.

Schlenker, R., Shaughnessy, P., & Crisler, K. (1995). Outcome-based continuous quality improvement as a financial strategy for home health care agencies. *Journal of Home Health Care Practice, 7*(4), 1–15.

Shaughnessy, P., Crisler, K., & Schlenker, R. (1995). *Medicare's OASIS: Standardized outcome and assessment information set for home health care.* (Distributed by the National Association for Home Care.) Denver, CO: Center for Health Policy Research.

U.S. Bipartisan Commission on Comprehensive Health Care. (1990). *The Pepper commission final report: A call for action.* Washington, DC: U.S. Government Printing Office: S. Prt. 101–114.

Yuan, J. (1996). The evolution of an incontinence management program. Unpublished document, Visiting Nurse Association of Eastern Montgomery County/A Department of Abington Memorial Hospital, Abington, PA.

APPENDIX 21–A
Home Care Resources

Agency for Health Care Policy and Research
2101 East Jefferson Street
Rockville, MD 20852
(301) 594-1364
Fax: (301) 594-1364

National Association for Home Care
519 C Street, NE
Washington, DC 20002-5809
(202) 547-7424
Fax: (202) 547-3540

NAHC's Affiliates:

- Hospice Association of America: Founded 1985
- Forum of State Associations: Founded 1985
- National Association for Physicians in Home Care: Founded 1986
- Center for Health Care Law: Founded 1987
- Home Care Aide Association: Founded 1990
- World Organization for Care in the Home and Hospice: Founded 1992
- National Home Care and Hospice Congressional Network: Founded 1994
- Hospital Home Care Association of America: Founded 1994

National Committee for Quality Assurance (NCQA)
2000 L Street, NW, Suite 500
Washington, DC 20036
(202) 955-3500
Fax: (202) 955-3599

National League for Nursing
Community Health Accreditation Program (CHAP); Benchmarks for Excellence in Home Care
359 Hudson Street
New York, NY 10014
(212) 989-9393
Fax: (212) 989-9256

## CHAPTER 22

Home Medical Equipment: Home Oxygen and Durable Medical Equipment

Marsha Magnusen Hughes and Angella D. Mattheis

CHAPTER OBJECTIVES

After completing this chapter, the reader will be able to

- describe an organization's response to improving quality using the Joint Commission's framework, categorized by 11 functions
- identify performance standards and competencies required by staff to perform job responsibilities using measurable outcomes
- discuss various aspects of admission assessment and reassessment processes including safety measures

There has been a tremendous growth of home-delivered services due to the increasing numbers of older adults and the fact that inpatient stays are decreasing. The technology and portability of durable medical equipment (DME) and oxygen supplies have made more services available at home. Hundreds of millions of dollars were spent on home respiratory services and equipment in 1996, and those numbers will continue to rise in the future.

Patients, doctors, and payers need to be assured that ill individuals will receive the highest quality of care. The Joint Commission on Accreditation of Healthcare Organizations (Joint Commission) sets quality standards and applies the same standards to hospice, home care, and home medical equipment (HME)

companies. These standards emphasize continuous improvement of patient care. To become accredited in the future, organizations will not only need to demonstrate that they have the capacity to provide high quality care but also that they are actually delivering such care (Joint Commission 1993, p. 6). These standards are categorized according to 11 functions that intertwine with each other. An overview of the standards with examples and tools follows.

MANAGEMENT OF HUMAN RESOURCES

Walt Disney once said, "An organization is only as good as the people working there." The key to the success of the organization and the quality of service is the people who provide the service. The reputation of a company is directly tied to its employees—from the billing clerk to the delivery person. All represent the company. Therefore individuals need to have a clear understanding of their roles and what is expected in their role. The job description and performance standards need to be specific. Qualifications must be commensurate with job responsibilities. Personnel files must be maintained. Employees must be assessed periodically as to how they are performing their job duties.

An organization must have a process for determining competence. Competency must be assessed prior to going out into the field.

Competencies are the technical skills, subject matter, and judgment that must be mastered to ensure safe and optimum patient care or care of equipment. *Orientation* is the time period during which essential competencies are taught, and there must be measurable outcomes to verify that the employee is competent. Exhibit 22–1 gives an example of a home oxygen/DME competency tool, containing general categories in which the individual must be deemed competent by the preceptor.

Ongoing education is a good investment. A needs assessment should be done annually with staff and an educational calendar (Exhibit 22–2) developed.

RIGHTS, RESPONSIBILITIES, AND ETHICS

The Patient Self-Determination Act (1991) requires that upon entry into the health care system, a person be informed about advance directives. In HME companies, CPR status must be determined and a physician's order obtained if the patient wishes no resuscitation. This should be done by the highest trained

---

Exhibit 22–1 Home Oxygen/DME Competency Tool

The oxygen technician upon completion of orientation will have:

[ ] 1. Articulated the mission of the department and will have discussed rights, responsibilities, and ethics.
[ ] 2. Demonstrated an understanding of the physical layout and mechanics of the site.
[ ] 3. Read and discussed key personnel issues.
[ ] 4. Discussed and have an understanding of the chain of command and organizational structure.
[ ] 5. Acquired knowledge of basic billing and oxygen requirements.
[ ] 6. Demonstrated understanding of basic universal precautions.
[ ] 7. Reviewed documentation and guidelines and role played an admission visit.
[ ] 8. Reviewed components and techniques of assessment skills, proper reporting of situations, and use of resource personnel.
[ ] 9. Written a Plan of Care for 2 patients from chart reviews.
[ ]10. Articulated how to access community resources.
[ ]11. Discussed and can articulate philosophy/concepts of care of hospice and home care patients, and will have participated in an observational experience at an interdisciplinary conference.
[ ]12. Completed Manufacturers Oxygen Concentration School(s) within 6 months of hire.
[ ]13. Demonstrated proper setup and use of equipment and satisfactorily completed a return demonstration on patient education for each piece.
[ ]14. Discussed "on call" procedures and issues and participated with 2 nights of "on call" with an experienced employee.
[ ]15. Demonstrated correct maintenance technique and cleaning for each piece of equipment.
[ ]16. Demonstrated understanding of the special needs of tracheotomy and pulmonary aid patients by passing an exam with 90% accuracy.
[ ]17. Reviewed a self-learning module on teamwork.
[ ]18. Participated in a discussion on safety issues.

Instructor: _____   Oxygen Technician: _____
Date: _____

Courtesy of St. Agnes Hospital, HME Department, Fond du Lac, Wisconsin.

Exhibit 22–2 Educational Calendar for Home-Delivered Services Durable Medical Equipment

Month	Topic	Presenters
December 1995	Assessment/Communicating and Reporting	Kris ———, RN
January 1996	Plan of Care	Angie ———, RN
February 1996	Community Resources	Carol ———, MSW
	Trach and Pulmo Aid—Use of Respiratory Therapist	Larry ———, RT
March 1996		
3–5	Infection Control/Hand Washing	Gayle ———, RN
3–8	Care Planning	Angie ———, RN
3–18	Assessment Review	Kris ———, RN
3–25	Devilbiss Concentrator Demo	Comp Rep.
	Competency Book Completed	Kris ———, RN
April 1996	Personal Safety	FDL PD
	Concentrator School (2 Persons)	Devilbiss Co.
May 1996		
5–22	Hospice Retreat	Marsha ———, RN
	TB Mask Inservice—Fitting	Kris ———, RN
June 1996	Body Mechanics	PT and DME Instructor
July 1996	The Dying Patient—Respect, Comfort Dignity	Hospice (RN)
August 1996	Customer Relations	Debbie ———, RN
September 1996	Documentation Regulations	Marsha ———, RN
October 1996	Risk Management QI	Angie ———, RN
November 1996	POC Assessment/Review	DME Educator
December 1996	Time Management	Karla ———, RN

Courtesy of St. Agnes Hospital, HME Department, Fond du Lac, Wisconsin.

member in the field in your organization. If you have a nurse or a respiratory therapist, they could discuss this with the patient with more expertise than the delivery technician.

Patients and families need to have clear expectations about their rights and responsibilities. They need to read, have explained to them, sign, and receive copies of written documents on these topics (examples are shown in Exhibits 22–3 and 22–4).

Respect for the patient and family is key to providing a quality service. The organization should have a complaint system. There must also be a process for receiving, investigating, and following up on patient complaints.

Exhibit 22–5 is a sample written notification of how a patient can file a complaint.

Ethical issues may occur during the delivery of service. The organization needs to have a process to resolve patient conflict. All team members need to have a basic understanding of what an ethical conflict is and what they would do in such a situation. The resolution may be as simple as to notify the supervisor, the home oxygen nurse, or respiratory therapist. Unresolved, serious conflicts may ultimately need to go to the ethics committee.

One way to teach ethics is to incorporate it into a general competency statement. The com-

Exhibit 22–3 Patient Bill of Rights

We at St. Agnes Hospital Home Oxygen/DME feel that all our patients should be informed of their rights while we serve them.

1. While you are being cared for by St. Agnes Home Oxygen/DME, the patient and any member of their family will be treated with dignity, courtesy and respect by all employees.

2. If we are unable to meet any of your needs for any special service, every effort will be made to secure this equipment or service. If we are still unable to meet your needs, we will assist you in finding another home care company that can meet those needs.

3. The patient will receive equipment and supplies in a timely manner.

4. You will be informed of our policies, procedures and charges for services and equipment. This will include telling you of third party eligibility payment and an explanation of any forms that you may need to sign.

5. St. Agnes Hospital Home Oxygen/DME staff will identify themselves and explain what services they are providing.

6. Employees of St. Agnes Hospital Home Oxygen/DME will not discriminate against the patient in the receiving of equipment or services due to race, religion, sex, social standing, sexual preference, age or handicap.

7. The patient has the right to participate in all decisions concerning needs, and the right to refuse any of the services offered by St. Agnes Hospital Home Oxygen/DME.

8. All patient records and communications, either oral or written, will be treated with the strictest confidence.

9. The patient is allowed access to any of their records through St. Agnes Hospital's Medical Record Department.

10. The patient will be allowed to make any suggestions in the change of services they need or **to register any complaints to St. Agnes Hospital Home Oxygen/DME employee or the Director of Hospice/Home Oxygen at 414-924-4661** without any fear of discrimination or reprisal by any employee of St. Agnes Home Oxygen/DME.

11. The patient will be informed of the procedure for registering complaints and they have a right to have each complaint reviewed and resolved in a timely manner. The patient will receive an answer to the complaint from the Director of Hospice/Home Oxygen.

12. The patient understands grounds for discharge of services which include:
    a. The physician discontinues the therapy.
    b. The patient expires.
    c. The patient is non-compliant with therapy (the physician's orders). The physician will be notified and may discontinue the order.
    d. The patient alters the equipment and the equipment does not meet the safety standards or the patient abuses the equipment. The physician will be notified.

13. The patient will be informed and shown their responsibilities in the care of the equipment or services they acquire from St. Agnes Hospital Home Oxygen/DME.

SAH HOME OXYGEN/DME SIGNATURE _____   DATE _____

PATIENT SIGNATURE _____   DATE _____

Courtesy of St. Agnes Hospital, HME Department, Fond du Lac, Wisconsin.

Exhibit 22–4 Patient/Family Responsibilities Statement

1. The patient/family agrees to use the equipment for the purpose that it was intended. The patient will not alter or modify the equipment in any way. The equipment will be returned in good working condition with the exception of normal wear.

2. The patient/family agrees to report any problems with the equipment promptly so that replacement or repair can be made as soon as possible.

3. The patient/family agrees to allow St. Agnes Hospital Home Oxygen/DME staff access to equipment for any needed maintenance, repair, replacement or pick-up of equipment if it is no longer needed.

4. The patient/family agrees to use the equipment as the doctor has prescribed. Employees of St. Agnes Hospital Home Oxygen/DME are not authorized to make any changes to your prescription unless there is a direct order from the physician.

5. The patient/family agrees to keep the equipment in their possession at the address it was delivered. If you wish to move the equipment to another location, please call to see if this is possible.

6. The patient/family agrees to notify St. Agnes Hospital Home Oxygen/DME of any hospitalizations, change in insurance information, address, telephone, doctor, change in prescription or if the equipment is no longer needed.

7. The patient/family agrees to all financial responsibility of any equipment furnished by St. Agnes Hospital Home Oxygen/DME.

8. The patient/family will furnish a copy of all advance directives if requested.

9. The patient/family will be reasonably considerate of all agency staff.

The above has been discussed with the patient and the patient and/or family member accepts these responsibilities.

SAH HOME OXYGEN/DME SIGNATURE _____ DATE _____

PATIENT SIGNATURE _____ DATE _____

Courtesy of St. Agnes Hospital, HME Department, Fond du Lac, Wisconsin.

Exhibit 22–5 Sample Notification of System for Handling Patient Complaints

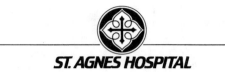

ST. AGNES HOSPITAL

PATIENT COMPLAINT SYSTEM
St. Agnes Hospital Home Oxygen/DME

The employees of St. Agnes Hospital Home Oxygen/DME take great pride in the service that they provide. Our primary goal is to satisfy the needs of each patient. If your needs are not being met, then our goal is not being met. Therefore, in the event of any problem, such as empty oxygen cylinders being delivered, rude employees, violation of your rights, late deliveries or any other problem, please contact us.

You may call us with any complaint or problem. Please call (414) 923-7950 and ask for the Director of Hospice/Home Oxygen. Your complaint/problem will be handled in a very confidential manner and an answer to this will be expedited as soon as possible.

We appreciate your support and confidence. This complaint system will help us to continue to deliver the highest quality care in an efficient manner.

Thank you,

The Staff of St. Agnes Hospital Home Oxygen/DME

Courtesy of St. Agnes Hospital, HME Department, Fond du Lac, Wisconsin.

petency tool can be divided into three major categories under each general statement: (1) subject, (2) content, and (3) evaluation mechanism, or measurable outcome.

Exhibit 22–6 is a sample breakdown for oxygen technician competency requirements on rights, responsibilities, and ethics.

Exhibit 22–7 is a sample quiz that is a measurable outcome for the competency on rights, responsibilities, and ethics.

The staff also has a right not to participate in aspects of care that are in conflict with cultural values or religious beliefs. This should be defined in policy (Exhibit 22–8).

Exhibit 22–6 Sample Competency Requirements for Oxygen Technicians on Rights, Responsibilities, and Ethics

The oxygen technician upon completion of orientation will have:
1. Articulated the mission of the department and passed an exam with 90% accuracy on rights, responsibilities, and ethics.

Subject	Content/Learning Options	Objective/Evaluation Mechanisms	Notes
Mission statement	Mission statement Policies: 1. Patient/family rights, responsibilities 2. Patient bill of rights 3. Patient complaints 4. Advance directives 5. Code of ethics 6. Conflict of care 7. Resolution of ethical conflicts Handouts 1. Patient Bill of Rights 2. Patient/Family Responsibilities 3. Patient complaint handout 4. Advance directive brochure Discussion: 1. Case study of ethical conflict 2. Case study regarding confidentiality Role-play or observation of orientee explaining rights and responsibilities to patient	Will score 90% on written exam	

Courtesy of St. Agnes Hospital, HME Department, Fond du Lac, Wisconsin.

Exhibit 22–7 Exam on Rights, Responsibilities, and Ethics

1. Write your mission statement.
   _____
   _____

2. Name one thing your hospital code of ethics states.
   _____
   _____

3. Must you participate in aspects of care that are in conflict with your cultural values or beliefs?
   Yes _____   No _____

4. How are ethical issues resolved in your agency?
   _____
   _____

5. How are complaints handled?
   _____
   _____

6. How do you address advance directives?
   _____
   _____

7. 8. Name two family rights.
   _____
   _____

9. 10. Name two family responsibilities.
   _____
   _____

Courtesy of St. Agnes Hospital, HME Department, Fond du Lac, Wisconsin.

ASSESSMENT

Assessment is the process of data gathering. How the data are analyzed depends on the education and training level of the staff involved. For example, oxygen technicians can only gather the data. They then depend on the rest of the team members, such as the respiratory therapist or nurses, to analyze the data. Assessment needs to be a continuous process that integrates information from other disciplines. Any member of the interdisciplinary team can perform an assessment as long as he or she passes a competency exam on that assessment. If the patient is involved in several areas of your agency, such as hospice and home oxygen, the assessments can be shared through interdisciplinary communication. Exhibit 22–9 is an example of an initial assessment form.

During the admission visit, the areas of assessment must include

- pertinent physical findings
- signs of neglect or abuse
- age-specific and gender-specific findings
- the problems, needs, and strengths of the patient
- the patient's psychosocial status
- the education needs of the patient and caregiver

Exhibit 22–8 Policy and Procedure Statement on Conflicts of Care

St. Agnes Hospital Policy and Procedure

Department:	Human Resources	Policy No.	43
SUBJECT:	Conflict of Care	Page	1 of 2
EFFECTIVE DATE:	April 1, 1995	Approved	

Vice President Human Resources

President & CEO

1.0   OBJECTIVE

To provide a mechanism to address any request by an employee not to participate in an aspect of patient care, including treatment due to the employee's cultural, ethical or spiritual beliefs. In no instance will the mission of the organization be compromised. Treatment and care will be provided to all persons in need without regard to disability, race, creed, color, gender, national origin, lifestyle, or ability to pay.

2.0   PROCEDURE

2.1   It is understood that situations may arise in which the prescribed course of treatment or care for a patient may be in conflict with the personal values or spiritual beliefs of a staff member.

2.2   If an employee has an objection to providing an aspect of care to a patient based on cultural, ethical or spiritual beliefs, he/she is to notify his/her supervisor and department director immediately of his/her concerns.

2.3   The department director will then evaluate the verbal request and respond to the employee appropriately while ensuring the continuity of patient care.

Every effort will be made to make reasonable accommodations for all justified employee requests for exclusion from patient care or treatment resulting from a conflict with the employee's personal values or beliefs. However, it must be realized that for reasons of staffing limitations, it may not be possible to grant a request.

2.4   If the request is granted, the department director is responsible for reassigning the care of the patient to ensure patient care will not be negatively affected. In no circumstances will a request be granted if it is felt that doing so would negatively affect the care of the patient.

2.5   If the request is denied, the employee will be expected to honor the decision of the department director and resume care of the patient. Failure to resume care will result in corrective action in accordance with Human Resources Policy #14.

2.6   If the employee wishes to have the request be given further consideration, they must make that request in writing and submit a copy to their Area Vice President and the Human Resources Department.

2.7   This request will be addressed by the Director of Human Resources and the Area Vice President within two working days of date of receipt of the request.

2.8   Employees will not be censured or penalized for filing such a request. If an employee feels that they are being treated in such a manner, he/she should contact the Human Resources Department.

2.9   A quarterly written report of requests not to participate in aspects of patient care will be sent to both the Executive Staff and the Ethics Committee for review.

Courtesy of St. Agnes Hospital, HME Department, Fond du Lac, Wisconsin.

Exhibit 22–9 Sample Form for Initial Assessment of Patient and Safety Inspection

PATIENT NAME: _____

DATE: _____

CAREGIVER: _____

TELEPHONE #: _____

ADMISSION ASSESSMENT
and SAFETY CHECKLIST
Home Oxygen/DME
St. Agnes Hospital, Fond du Lac, WI

ADMISSION ASSESSMENT: *Check box if it applies.*

FUNCTIONAL ASSESSMENT   ❑ no problem observed
- ❑ Mobility difficulties r/t weakness/paralysis
- ❑ Use of aids (list in plan of care)

NUTRITIONAL ASSESSMENT   ❑ no problem observed
- ❑ Open wounds
- ❑ States unable to prepare meals
- ❑ States unable to obtain food from store
- ❑ Appears malnourished

BATHROOM ASSESSMENT   ❑ no problem observed
- ❑ Unable to toilet self
- ❑ Unable to provide self hygiene

ENVIRONMENTAL ASSESSMENT   ❑ no problem observed
- ❑ Throw rugs present (instruct to remove)
- ❑ Needs to use stairs to access BR or to enter or leave building
- ❑ Running water not present
- ❑ Sharp objects present
- ❑ Living corridors present
- ❑ Poor lighting
- ❑ Lack of refrigeration
- ❑ No access to telephone
- ❑ Rodents/insects present
- ❑ Unkempt house (not clean)
- ❑ Lack of home temp control

PSYCHOSOCIAL ASSESSMENT   ❑ no problem observed
(if checked, elaborate in comment section)
- ❑ Limited support
- ❑ Handicaps present
- ❑ Presence of child in home
- ❑ Obvious use of drugs/alcohol
- ❑ Obvious lack of coping
- ❑ Obvious signs of anger
- ❑ Expresses discomfort with situation
- ❑ Family problems identified
- ❑ Caregiver needs not being met

Any checked box above must be addressed on plan of care.

COMMENTS: _____

_____

_____

_____

_____

_____

_____

_____

_____

_____

NS-4662-9 NIS (REV. 10/95)

SAFETY INSPECTION LIST: *A check signifies the area is okay.*

ELECTRICAL PLUGS
- ❑ are grounded
- ❑ are not overloaded

FIRE SAFETY
- ❑ received fire safety sheet
- ❑ smoke detectors in home and working
- ❑ fire extinguisher
- ❑ exits are accessible

EQUIPMENT
- ❑ location is good
- ❑ concentrator not near thermostat
- ❑ concentrator not near heating ducts
- ❑ cylinders stored safely
- ❑ no flammable or open flames near cylinders
- ❑ easy access to equipment

TEACHING HANDOUTS GIVEN TO PATIENT/FAMILY
- ❑ Disaster Instruction Sheet
- ❑ Fire Safety Sheet
- ❑ Patient Rights
- ❑ Patient/Family responsibilities
- ❑ Oxygen Teaching Checklist
- ❑ Cylinder and Regulator Checklist
- ❑ Advance Directives
- ❑ Patient Complaint System
- ❑ Specific Equipment Instruction sheet (see plan of care)
- ❑ Other: _____
- ❑ Other: _____

NOTES: _____

_____

_____

_____

_____

_____

_____

_____

_____

_____

_____

_____

_____

SIGNATURE: _____   DATE: _____

Courtesy of St. Agnes Hospital, HME Department, Fond du Lac, Wisconsin.

- the home environment
- the ability of the patient to use and maintain the equipment
- the caregiver's ability and willingness to provide support
- functional limitations
- nutritional assessment

When performing a functional assessment, some of the key elements to include are

- patient's mobility status
- patient's ability to operate and maintain the equipment
- patient's communication skills
- patient's memory
- patient's cognitive level
- orientation of the patient

A nutritional assessment is necessary to determine if the patient is at moderate to high risk for poor nutrition. The following are the key elements to assess:

- Are the patient's needs or problems nutritionally related?
- Does the patient have open wounds?
- Is the patient able to prepare his or her own meals?
- Is the patient able to obtain food?
- Has the patient experienced a significant weight loss or gain in a short period of time?

Assessment does not stop at admission. The patient needs to be reassessed for all the above areas, including

- patient's response to care
- changes in patient's condition
- changes in patient's diagnosis
- changes in patient's environment
- changes in patient's support system
- operation of the equipment
- storage and use of supplies
- risk of an infection or actual acquiring of an infection
- compliance with physician's orders
- maintenance and cleaning of the equipment

Communication is another important element of the assessment process. It can be accomplished through voice mail, written case communication, or face-to-face interaction. Effective communication can occur through the establishment of a morning report. At morning report, the interdisciplinary team will analyze the gathered data to identify and prioritize patient problems, needs, and level of services needed.

The actual information that is gathered by the interdisciplinary team needs to be defined by the organization's policies. The policies should include stipulations for, when, and by whom the assessments are to be completed. The assessment process is one of the most important functions in the delivery of care. Patients must be accurately assessed, and the assessment must be communicated to appropriate resource persons so that patients receive the care they need. Exhibits 22–10 and 22–11 are examples of helpful checklists for assessment and reassessment that technicians can use. Exhibit 22–12 shows a visit form.

CARE, TREATMENT, AND SERVICES

This function focuses on the means to provide individualized, planned, and appropriate care to meet patients' needs. To provide the highest quality of care, the care planning process must include four steps:

1. Planning—the process of gathering all the patient information and developing the necessary plan of action to meet the patient goals
2. Implementation—the process of actually carrying out the plan that was developed in the planning step
3. Monitoring—This is the process of reassessing the patient to determine if the initial plan developed is assisting the patient toward meeting his or her goals
4. Modification—the process of making any necessary changes to the patient's plan of care after discovering, by monitoring, that the initial plan of care is not meeting the patient's goals

Exhibit 22–10 Guidelines for Assessment

1. Any age- or gender-specific issues
   - Hearing
   - Vision
   - Memory
2. Problems and needs
   - Physical
   - Emotional
   - Financial
     - Give information on community care
     - Report to supervisor
3. Family and support system
   - Note if none or limited
   - Note significant comments regarding
4. Environment and safety
   - Safety checklist
5. Learning/education needs
   - Ability to communicate, language used
6. Ability of patient to use equipment
   - Admission assessment checklist
7. Change in MD orders or obvious changes in condition
8. Compliance with MD order
9. Compliance with use of equipment and cleaning
   - Change cannula every Monday
   - Change extension tubing first day of each month
   - Change water bottle monthly
   - Clean filter of concentrator daily
   - Clean filter of Pulmo Aid 1x month
10. Compliance with storage
    - Well-vented area
    - *Not* in car trunk or closet
    - M tank in stand
11. Patient and family know how to contact agency
12. Nutrition
    - Visible weight loss
    - States can't prepare meals
    - States can't obtain food
    - Open wounds
13. Any infections or falls
14. Any suspicion of abuse (elder, child, or chemical)
    - Notify supervisor
15. Need for other services
    - Home care
    - Hospice
    - Meals on Wheels
    - Community care
    - Pediatric clinical nurse specialist
16. Discharge planning needs
17. *Initial assessment must be completed within 48 hours of admission; all remaining documentation must be completed within 24 hours.*

Source: Data from *1995 Accreditation Handbook*, pp. 23–48, Joint Commission on Accreditation of Healthcare Organizations.

Exhibit 22–11 Guidelines for Reassessment

1. Response to care
   - Has the oxygen helped?
   - Is the walker height OK?
2. Problems and needs
   - Utilize information on care plan
3. Family and support system
   - Any changes or new observations
4. Environment and safety
   - Any change
   - No-smoking signs in place
5. Learning/education needs
   - Does the patient/family have any questions?
6. Ability of patient to use equipment
   - Request a return demonstration
7. Change in MD orders or changes in condition
   - Ask patient or family
8. Compliance with MD order
   - Observe and ask
9. Compliance with use of equipment and cleaning
   - Change cannula every Monday
   - Change extension tubing first day of each month
   - Change water bottle monthly
   - Clean filter of concentrator daily
   - Clean filter of Pulmo Aid 1x month
10. Compliance with storage
    - Well-vented area
    - *Not* in car trunk or closet
    - M tank in stand
11. Patient and family know how to contact agency
12. Nutrition
    - Visible weight loss
    - States can't prepare meals
    - States can't obtain food
    - Open wounds
13. Any infections or falls
14. Any suspicion of abuse (elder, child, or chemical)
    - Notify supervisor
15. Need for other services
    - Home care
    - Hospice
    - Meals on Wheels
    - Pediatric clinical nurse specialist
16. Understanding of backup system
    - What would you do if the electricity went off?
17. Discharge planning needs when appropriate
18. *All documentation must be completed within 24 hours.*

Source: Data from *1995 Accreditation Handbook*, pp. 23–48, Joint Commission on Accreditation of Healthcare Organizations.

Exhibit 22–12 Sample Visit Form

PATIENT NAME: _____	**VISIT FORM**
DATE: _____	Home Oxygen/DME
	St. Agnes Hospital, Fond du Lac, WI

CHECK IF APPLIES:	
Nutritional Assessment	Comments: _____
❑ visible weight loss	
❑ states can't prepare meals	
❑ states can't obtain food	
❑ open wounds	
Safety Inspection	
❑ properly using	
Goals of service met:	
❑ patient demo correct equip use	
❑ patient complies with MD orders	
❑ equip serviced (list)	
_____	
_____	Other agency involved:
Any problem with fam/support	
_____	
_____	Reported to:
SIGNATURE:	

NS-4661-9 NIS (REV. 1/96) OROGINAL - CHART • COPY - OTHER PROVIDER AS NEEDED

Courtesy of St. Agnes Hospital, HME Department, Fond du Lac, Wisconsin.

The plan of care provides a crucial piece of information. It should reflect all important facts involving the patient and his or her care. According to the Joint Commission (1993), every organization needs to have policies and procedures regarding (1) who develops the plan of care, (2) in what time frame it is to be completed, (3) when the plan of care needs to be reviewed, and (4) what makes up the plan of care.

The plan of care consists of the patient's problems and needs and must have corresponding goals for each of those problems or needs. After the goals have been established, actions need to be developed on how to meet these goals. Some important areas to address on the plan of care include

- home environment and safety
- knowledge deficit
- functional limitations
- any new problems
- the physician order
- services that are being provided
- any maintenance schedules

It is imperative that the plan of care be up to date and reviewed on a regular basis. The problems should be prioritized as the patient's needs change. The framework for the plan of care is developed by the ordering physician and then needs to be shared and evaluated with the patient. Exhibit 22–13 is an example of a plan of care used by the staff at St. Agnes Hospital Home Oxygen/DME Department.

Exhibit 22–13 Sample Plan of Care

PLAN OF CARE/SERVICE
Home Oxygen/DME
St. Agnes Hospital, Fond du Lac, WI

PATIENT NAME: _____

DATE: _____

CPR STATUS: _____

OTHER AGENCY INVOLVED: _____

ALLERGIES: _____

NO.	DATE	INI	PROBLEM/NEEDS	GOALS	SERVICES/ACTIONS
1.			Initial Problem	Patient will receive ordered DME & O2 on	Home O2 Tech will deliver ordered DME and
			Dx:	admit and subsequent visits.	O2. Patient will be scheduled.
					Telephone Call Q.
				O2 & DME will be maintained per manufac-	
			Order:	turer guidelines.	
			Need:		
					Tech will maintain equipment as outlined in
					manufacturer's guidelines.
					Concentrator check Q 90 days
					Due:
					DME maintenance check Q 6 months
					Due:
2.			Safety/Environment	Patient will demonstrate safe use of DME	Patient/caregiver will receive DME and O2
				and O2 as outlined in equipment orientation	instruction on safe use and safe home
				checklist and Home O2 precaution sheet.	environment as outlined in the equipment
					orientation checklist, Home O2 precaution
				Patient will comply with MD order.	sheet and admission assessment and safety
					checklist.
				Patient will maintain a safe home environ-	
				ment as outlined in Admission Assessment	
				and safety checklist and equipment	
				orientation checklist.	

SIGNED BY: _____

DATE: _____

NS-4663-9 NIS (REV. 4/96)

continues

Exhibit 22–13 continued

PATIENT NAME: _____

Page 2

PLAN OF CARE/SERVICE
Home Oxygen/DME
St. Agnes Hospital, Fond du Lac, WI

NO.	DATE	INI	PROBLEM/NEEDS	GOALS	SERVICES/ACTIONS
3.			Knowledge deficit		
4.			Functional limitations		
5.			New problems		

SIGNED BY: _____ _____ _____ _____

DATE: _____ _____ _____ _____

Courtesy of St. Agnes Hospital, HME Department, Fond du Lac, Wisconsin.

EDUCATION

Education is a key component of quality care. Patient education should be clearly defined in a policy such as that shown in Exhibit 22–14.

Education of the patient and family facilitates better patient outcomes through involvement of the patient and family. For an HME company, this means printed instructions regarding each piece of equipment delivered and a return demonstration done by the patient or caregiver.

Exhibit 22–15 is an example of a patient education form for a pulmoaide. These forms were developed using the manufacturer's guidelines. Risks and cleaning instructions should always be included.

The patient should receive education specific to his or her needs, abilities, and readiness. At the follow-up visit, another return demonstration should be done by the patient or caregiver to the agency employee.

Because oxygen accelerates combustion, it is essential that safety precautions be explained and left in writing. Exhibit 22–16 is an example of an equipment orientation checklist for oxygen.

Timely planning for discharge or transfer is essential in a patient-centered quality organization. That means that personnel must be well informed about other options in the community.

The organization must have staff with adequate credentials and training to instruct families when equipment is invasive or supports life functions, as in the case of suction machines or ventilators.

Because compliance with physician oxygen orders is a frequent problem, communication among staff members providing education to the patient must be consistent.

CONTINUUM OF CARE

In a responsible, quality HME organization, admission should include only those patients who can have their identified needs met by the staff.

Communication and coordination are essential to the patient receiving multiple services. Exhibit 22–17 is an example of a case communication that is used to communicate concerns to others. The original is placed in the chart, and the copy goes to the primary nurse of the hospice or home care agency. With respect to confidentiality, the patient signs a release of information if the information is going to a different organization.

Patients want consistency in staff and coordination of care. To improve continuity, patients can be assigned in geographical areas with a primary technician who then becomes familiar with them and their plan of care.

The organization must have a policy in place that determines what will occur if payment is denied and/or the patient is unable to pay. Exhibit 22–18 contains an example of such a policy.

IMPROVING ORGANIZATIONAL PERFORMANCE

To ensure quality, the organization needs to have a written continuous quality improvement (CQI) plan. It must be a planned, systematic, and organization-wide approach to designing, measuring, assessing, and improving performance. This plan does not have to follow a specific model; however, it must be in a written format. The CQI plan, in order to meet the Joint Commission's requirements, must address all 11 functions in regard to:

- high-risk indicators
- high-volume indicators
- problem-prone indicators

The plan needs to measure both the process and the outcome of the subject being studied. Indicators are measures that can be used to monitor care or service. The indicator should specify if a process or an outcome of a process is being measured. For example, an indicator stating that "all technicians will teach the patients on home safety issues" would be a *process* indicator. An indicator stating that "the

Exhibit 22–14 Policy Statement on Patient Education To Be Delivered by Home Oxygen Technicians and Nurses

---

Department: Home Oxygen/DME   **Policy: PF 19**

Subject: Patient Education

Objective: To define patient/family education.

1. Each home oxygen technician and the home oxygen nurse will demonstrate through competency #13 the proper setup of equipment and complete a return demonstration on patient education for each piece of equipment they instruct on.

2. The department has printed instruction sheets and provides the appropriate sheet to each patient/family when equipment is delivered.

3. Instruction components should include:
   a. Basic purpose and description, basic operating instructions, troubleshooting, correct use of supplies
   b. Safety precautions and warnings
   c. For equipment with known safety hazards, such as suction machines and oxygen modalities, equipment information and safety checks incorporating the manufacturer guidelines should be given to the patient or caregiver.
   d. When applicable, backup equipment and accessories and emergency plans
   e. Demonstration of correct equipment and observation of a return demonstration
   f. Any maintenance to be performed by the patient
   g. Any cleaning or disinfecting to be performed and infection control precautions
   h. Appropriate storage and transport of equipment

4. Admission Assessment and Safety Check List is completed at each admission (policy #PF 13). Basic home safety is addressed at this time, including fire, electrical, environmental, mobility and bathroom safety. The Patient Disaster Instruction sheet is given to the patient/family and explained at this time.

5. Knowledge deficient, functional limitations, and new problems are assessed for the POC initially and ongoing (Policy #9).

6. Reassessment of patient/family's abilities to operate and understand equipment is assessed verbally and through return demonstration by primary nurses and the oxygen technicians and oxygen nurse.

7. Problems and concerns regarding patient/family learning or compliance are brought to the nurse, supervisor or director by the field staff. Morning report is an opportunity for this to occur.

8. Education regarding other community resources is given throughout service and at the time of discharge.

Courtesy of St. Agnes Hospital, HME Department, Fond du Lac, Wisconsin.

Exhibit 22–15 Patient Education Checklist for a Pulmoaide

PULMOAIDE • EQUIPMENT CHECKLIST
St. Agnes Home Oxygen/DME, Fond du Lac, WI

EXPLAIN the following:

TO REDUCE THE RISK OF ELECTROCUTION:
- ❏ ALWAYS unplug this product IMMEDIATELY after using.
- ❏ DO NOT use while bathing.
- ❏ DO NOT place or store product where it can fall or be pulled into a tub or sink.
- ❏ DO NOT reach for product that has fallen into water. UNPLUG IMMEDIATELY.
- ❏ DO NOT place in or drop into water or other liquid.

TO REDUCE THE RISK OF BURNS, ELECTROCUTION, FIRE OR INJURY TO PERSONS:
- ❏ Product should NEVER be left unattended when plugged in.
- ❏ Close supervision is necessary when this product is used by, on or near CHILDREN AND PHYSICALLY CHALLENGED INDIVIDUALS.
- ❏ Use this product only for its intended use. Use the product only under physician's direction. Do not use attachments not recommended by the manufacturer.
- ❏ Never operate if it has a damaged cord or plug, if it is not working properly, if it has been dropped or damaged, or dropped into water; call qualified service personnel for examination and repair.
- ❏ Keep the cord away from HEATED or HOT surfaces.
- ❏ NEVER drop or insert any object into any opening.
- ❏ NEVER use while sleeping or drowsy.
- ❏ NEVER block the air openings of the product or place it on a soft surface, such as a bed or couch, where the air openings may be blocked. Keep the air openings free from lint, hair and the like. Blocked openings may cause the unit to shut down. Contact dealer immediately.
- ❏ DO NOT use outdoors or operate where aerosol (spray) products are being used or where oxygen is being administered in a closed environment such as an oxygen tent.
- ❏ This unit is oil-less. DO NOT lubricate.
- ❏ Risk of electric shock. Do not disassemble. Refer servicing to qualified service personnel.

CLEANING THE NEBULIZER – Your physician and/or equipment provider may specify certain cleaning procedures. If so, follow their recommendations. If not, clean according to the following instructions:
- ❏ Depending on usage and cleaning procedures, the life of your nebulizer may be extended for at least 15 days. Since the nebulizer is disposable, it is recommended that an extra nebulizer be kept at all times.
- ❏ Clean the nebulizer after every use and at least once a day.
- ❏ Remove the nebulizer and mouthpiece or pediatric face mask from the tubing.
- ❏ Disassemble nebulizer chamber by turning counterclockwise and separating.
- ❏ Fill two (2) plastic containers or bowls.
  Washing: hot water/detergent solution
  Soaking: hot water/vinegar solution (one (1) part vinegar to three (3) parts water).
- ❏ Thoroughly clean the nebulizer, mouthpiece or pediatric face mask in hot water/detergent solution.
- ❏ Remove the water/detergent solution and rinse with clear hot tap water.
- ❏ Soak in hot water/vinegar solution for 30 minutes.
- ❏ Rinse with hot tap water again and air dry thoroughly.
- ❏ If using medical disinfectant cleaners, follow manufacturer's instructions carefully.
- ❏ Keep the outer surface of the tubing dust-free by wiping regularly.
- ❏ The nebulizer air tubing does not have to be washed internally because only filtered air passes through the tubing.

NS-4260-9 NIS   ORIGINAL - CHART • COPY - PATIENT

continues

Exhibit 22–15 continued

PULMOAIDE · EQUIPMENT CHECKLIST
St. Agnes Home Oxygen/DME, Fond du Lac, WI

EXPLAIN the following:

CLEANING OR REPLACING THE FOAM INTAKE FILTER:
- ☐ Clean the filter once a month or sooner if filter discolors.
- ☐ Open cover of storage compartment to gain access to filter.
- ☐ Remove filter and clean with soap and water. Let dry thoroughly before use.
- ☐ Replace filter if it becomes clogged, torn or has a worn appearance.
- ☐ Regular filter cleaning/replacing is necessary to help ensure proper compressor performance.
- ☐ DO NOT RUN UNIT WITHOUT FILTER.

I understand how to operate my equipment and have been given an opportunity to ask questions.

HANDLER SIGNATURE _____ DATE _____

PATIENT SIGNATURE _____ DATE _____

Courtesy of St. Agnes Hospital, HME Department, Fond du Lac, Wisconsin.

---

patient will be able to verbalize three safety issues related to home safety" would be an *outcome* indicator.

The plan will need to address monthly tracking of specific adverse patient/employee occurrences. This can be accomplished by using an incident-reporting form that is uniform for all employees. Exhibit 22–19 is an example of a patient occurrence worksheet.

The following are important areas that need to be tracked and trended:

- patient complaint
- missed visit
- patient fall/injury
- employee fall/injury
- medication error
- medication reaction
- employee infection
- patient infection

The calendar in Exhibit 22–20 illustrates how an agency could map out how it meets the Joint Commission standards and addresses the important elements.

When using the Joint Commission standards as a basis for a CQI plan, you will need to focus on two areas of performance, *what* is done and *how well* it is done.

The dimensions are the characteristics of performance. The characteristics of what is done should include

- *Efficacy* (Is the oxygen that we supply to the patient giving the desired saturation level?)
- *Appropriateness* (Do we provide a walker to a patient who really needs a wheelchair?)

The characteristics that are included in *how well* it is done include

- *Availability* (Do we have a patient who requires a ventilator when we do not have ventilators?)

Exhibit 22–16 Equipment Orientation Checklist

PATIENT'S NAME: _____

EQUIPMENT: _____

_____

GENERAL INFORMATION

_____ Patient and others who will be operating equipment are present during instructions.

_____ Patient has operating instructions and ask all present to read thoroughly.

_____ Review doctor's prescription and explain should not turn up or down.

_____ Patient has name, address and phone number for routine and emergency problems.

_____ Do not make adjustments or attempt to repair machine.

_____ Explain how concentrator works.

_____ Explain E cylinder or D cylinder system and when it should be used.

_____ Tell them the electrical company knows they are on this type of equipment in case of power failure.

SAFETY INFORMATION

_____ Explain that oxygen accelerates combustion but as a substance is nonflammable.

_____ Explain fire hazards of combustible materials.

_____ Explain need for ventilation to prevent accumulation of oxygen.

_____ Explain warnings in operating instructions.

_____ Do not allow persons who have not read instructions to operate equipment.

_____ Explain the importance of no smoking in the same area that oxygen is being used and the use of no-smoking sign.

_____ Explain the importance of grounding all electrical equipment.

_____ Explain the importance of following cleaning procedure.

_____ Explain the audible alarm (if applicable).

_____ Explain the importance of proper positioning of the machine within any given room.

_____ Explain proper procedure for dealing with power failure.

_____ Explain proper use of the backup oxygen cylinder (if applicable).

DEMONSTRATE THE FOLLOWING

_____ How to turn power switch on

_____ Demonstrate how to attach the humidifier to the machine and fill with distilled water to proper level (if applicable).

_____ How to attach cannula and inspect for leaks.

_____ How to adjust the flow control to the prescribed flow rate.

_____ How to clean and disinfect humidifier (if applicable).

_____ Explain flow lock purpose (if applicable).

_____ Demonstrate how to dial in the proper flow rate.

_____ Explain when the filter should be cleaned.

_____ Have patient demonstrate the operation of the concentrator back to you.

_____ Use of Oxygen Concentrator Indicator (OCI) and when to call Home Oxygen (when red or yellow light on).

I understand how to operate my equipment and have been given an opportunity to ask questions.

HANDLER SIGNATURE _____   DATE _____

PATIENT SIGNATURE _____   DATE _____

Courtesy of St. Agnes Hospital, HME Department, Fond du Lac, Wisconsin.

Exhibit 22–17 Sample Case Communication

COMMUNICATION
St. Agnes Home Oxygen - Fond du Lac, WI
NS-5080-9 NIS • WHITE-CHART • CANARY-PRIMARY NURSE/THERAPIST

PATIENT: _____

TIME: _____

SIGNATURE/TITLE   DATE

Courtesy of St. Agnes Hospital, HME Department, Fond du Lac, Wisconsin.

- *Timeliness* (Do we deliver oxygen tanks before the patient's supply is empty?)
- *Effectiveness* (Is the walker we delivered adjusted to the right height?)
- *Continuity* (Are all disciplines involved always informed of the patient changes?)
- *Safety* (Are the patients educated on the proper use of their concentrator?)
- *Efficiency* (Do we supply the patient with tanks when a concentrator would be more appropriate?)
- *Respect and caring* (Do we deliver oxygen at 8:00 A.M. when the patient has asked to have it delivered at 12:00 P.M.?)

Organizations need to identify their own areas of concern and prioritize them. It is imperative to use a systems approach in CQI. Getting rid of the bad apples and keeping a poor system will not result in an improved system. People function at a high level because the process or system is operating at a high level.

One way to know how a system is functioning is to follow these steps: (1) plan the improvement, (2) do data collection, (3) check and study the results, and (4) act to hold the gain and improve the process. In a problem-solving situation, try to include representatives of all significant areas to plan a change. The involved persons investigating a specific problem compose a CQI task force. The responsibilities of the task force include

- developing the team mission
- gathering and analyzing data
- developing a plan for change
- making recommendations for the change

The members of the task force are usually involved in making a presentation on the recommendation.

The work of the task force is not done after implementation of the recommendations. The task force also needs to evaluate whether the recommendations are improving the process. Many recommendations may require further study to achieve a desired result. *The final results will show the importance of the time well spent.*

Exhibit 22–21 is an example of a tool that St. Agnes Hospital Home Oxygen Department uses to track and monitor equipment malfunction.

Exhibit 22–18 Sample Policy on Patient Transfer, Referral, and Discharge, Including Cases of Nonpayment

---

DEPARTMENT: Home Oxygen/DME   POLICY NO. PF5

SUBJECT: Patient transfer, referral or discharge

OBJECTIVE: To establish criteria for the discharge, transfer, or referral of a patient/client from or to St. Agnes Hospital Home Oxygen/DME.

PROCEDURE:

1. Patients will be transferred to another company for the following reasons:
   a. The patient is moving to another area that is outside the St. Agnes Hospital Home Oxygen/DME service area.
   b. The clinical equipment is beyond the scope of St. Agnes Hospital Home Oxygen/DME Services.
   c. The patient is dissatisfied with the services being provided to them by St. Agnes Hospital Home Oxygen/DME.

2. When the service is to be supplied via another provider, contact will be made with that provider either by telephone, written or both as to meet the patient needs and to prevent disruption of service. (See transfer letter.)

3. Patients will be discharged from the services of St. Agnes Hospital Home Oxygen/DME for the following reasons:
   a. The physician discontinues the therapy.
   b. The patient expires.
   c. The patient is noncompliant with the physician's orders. The physician will be notified and may choose to discontinue the orders.
   d. The patient destroys or alters the equipment safety. The physician will be notified.
   e. The patient refuses therapy.
   f. Patients who have not had any activity through St. Agnes Hospital Home Oxygen/DME for more than one year.

4. Patients discharged from Home Oxygen/DME will have a discharge form completed (NS-4660-9 NIS).

5. In the case of nonpayment, the physician will be notified. Attempts will be made to find an alternate funding source. The patient may then be referred to St. Agnes Hospital Community Care where ability to pay will be reviewed as well as need.

6. Referrals will be accepted from other companies to St. Agnes Hospital Home Oxygen/DME if:
   a. The patient is able to meet the admission criteria (Refer to Policy No. AD 8).
   b. St. Agnes Hospital Home Oxygen/DME is able to provide the services required by the patient.

Reviewed/Revised: 7/93, 7/94, 6/95

Courtesy of St. Agnes Hospital, HME Department, Fond du Lac, Wisconsin.

Exhibit 22–19 Worksheet for Reporting Adverse Patient Occurrence

DEPT. WHERE OCCURRENCE HAPPENED _____

DATE _____ TIME _____

NAME OF PHYSICIAN NOTIFIED _____

DATE _____ TIME _____

Addressograph or write patient's name, address and phone number

TYPE OF INCIDENT/OCCURRENCE (Identify the type of incident/occurrence using code number)

SECTION ONE: STATEMENT BY PERSON REPORTING INCIDENT/OCCURRENCE

_____
_____
_____

INTERVENTIONS TAKEN _____

PATIENT STATUS AFTER THE OCCURRENCE _____

☐ NO INJURY/MINOR INJURY   ☐ REQUIRES PHYSICIAN INTERVENTION   ☐ POSSIBLE HIGH RISK (NOTIFY RISK MANAGER IMMEDIATELY)

DID THE SITUATION INVOLVE MEDICAL SUPPLY OR EQUIPMENT?   ☐ YES   ☐ NO   IF "YES", SEE SAFE MEDICAL DEVICES POLICY

SIGNED _____ DATE _____

SECTION TWO: DIRECTOR'S ANALYSIS (TO BE COMPLETED BY DEPT. MOST CLOSELY INVOLVED IN OCCURRENCE)

PROBLEM IDENTIFIED:	CORRECTIVE ACTION:		
☐ LACK OF KNOWLEDGE	☐ NO FURTHER ACTION NECESSARY	☐ EDUCATION PROVIDED	☐ GROUP AWARENESS
☐ PERFORMANCE	☐ POLICY/PROCEDURE CHANGE	☐ STAFFING CHANGE	☐ SYSTEM CHANGE
☐ ADMINISTRATIVE	☐ OTHER (EXPLAIN) _____		
☐ COMMUNICATION			

ADDITIONAL COMMENTS _____
_____
_____

SIGNED _____ DATE _____

IF REPORT NEEDS TO BE SENT TO ANOTHER DEPT.
DATE CONTACT MADE, AND PERSON CONTACTED _____

SECTION THREE: PHYSICIAN/OTHER DEPT.

COMMENTS _____
_____

SIGNED _____ DATE _____

SECTION FOUR: QA DEPT.

COMMENTS _____

SIGNED _____ DATE _____

SECTION FIVE: RISK MANAGER INVESTIGATION/CORRECTIVE ACTION

SIGNED _____ DATE _____ PART TWO

Courtesy of St. Agnes Hospital, HME Department, Fond du Lac, Wisconsin.

Exhibit 22–20 St. Agnes Home Oxygen Quality Improvement Calendar

Indicator	Function	Process or Outcome	High Risk	High Volume	Problem Prone	Report Dates '96
Patient family satisfaction survey	PE LD Tx	0		X	X	March, June Sept., Dec.
Chart audit	Tx CC LD MI RRE A PE	0	X	X	X	March, June Sept., Dec.
Equipment malfunction	Tx EC	0	X	X		March, June Sept., Dec.
On call visits/TC issues	Tx CC PE	0		X	X	March, June Sept., Dec.
Tracking of: 1) Pt satisfaction	LD Tx	0		X		March, June Sept., Dec.
2) Pt/staff infection	IC HR	P	X	X		March, June Sept., Dec.
3) Pt/staff injury	HR	P	X			March, June Sept., Dec.
Missed visits	Tx CC	P/O	X	X		March, June Sept., Dec.

Note: Tx = Care, Treatment, Service   CC = Continuum of Care   HR = Human Resources
MI = Management of Information   PE = Patient Education   LD = Leadership
IC = Surveillance, Prevention, and Control of Infection   RRE = Rights, Responsibilities, and Ethics   EC = Management of Environment of Care   A = Assessment

Courtesy of St. Agnes Hospital, HME Department, Fond du Lac, Wisconsin.

Exhibit 22–21 Home Oxygen Equipment Malfunction Tracking Tool

PATIENT	DATE	PRIMARY TECH	EQUIPMENT #	PROBLEM	SOLUTION

Courtesy of St. Agnes Hospital, HME Department, Fond du Lac, Wisconsin.

LEADERSHIP

If the organization is part of an integrated system, the strategic plan of the integrated system will provide the framework for planning, directing, coordinating, providing, and improving health care services. The organization needs a clear organizational chart that defines reporting mechanisms. The governing body must have ultimate responsibility and legal authority and must have an orientation process.

Patient satisfaction surveys are a proven method of obtaining feedback regarding care and services. Exhibit 22–22 is an example of a patient survey.

An organization should have an emergency preparedness plan, and the staff should be able to articulate and understand this plan. The plan will be dependent on the type of staff, service provided, and service area. Exhibit 22–23 is an example of an emergency preparedness policy.

The Joint Commission will examine operational plans, capital expenditure plans, the budget process, staffing plans, risk management, and any measurements used to determine patient care and service needs. These plans and the process for developing priorities are all important ingredients for providing quality care.

Mechanisms should be in place to ensure uniformity of care to all patients and families. Care should be provided according to patients' needs rather than their insurance. For example, a Medicaid patient should receive the same service as a private-pay patient.

The day-to-day operations require good leadership. The person in charge of patient care must have authority to match the responsibility. He or she must also have the qualifications, clinical experience, and orientation to provide the scope of care and services required.

Policies and procedures must be developed and reviewed annually. For agencies desiring Joint Commission accreditation, the policy book can be organized under the 11 functions identified by the Joint Commission. Two indexes are developed: one lists the functions as chapters with the policies in each chapter, and the other index lists each policy alphabetically with the page number.

MANAGEMENT OF ENVIRONMENT OF CARE

The *environment of care* refers to the place where the patient receives care as well as sites in the organization itself. For an HME company, those environments would be the office, the home, the warehouse, and the delivery vehicles. Risks and hazards need to be minimized in all settings. Safety is a high priority. Exhibit 22–24 is an example of a home safety instruction sheet.

Every quality program needs to have a process for routine and preventative maintenance. Exhibit 22–25 is an example of a 6-month wheelchair maintenance checklist. A policy (such as that in Exhibit 22–26) should spell out the specifics of the maintenance check, and the competency of the technician should be determined by a return demonstration.

MANAGEMENT OF INFORMATION

The goal of the management of information is to develop a standard way to gather, store, and utilize information to improve organizational performance in patient care. Some of the sources for this information are

- policies and procedures
- patient charts
- meeting minutes
- annual governing reports
- planning documents

The Joint Commission requires an organization to have a policy on the security and confidentiality of records. An effective plan would include

- who has access to the charts
- what information is made accessible
- release of information
- removal, retention, and storage of the charts

Exhibit 22–22 Home Oxygen Patient Survey

Dear Patient:

St. Agnes Home Oxygen needs your feedback. Please offer your opinions so we may continue to provide quality care.

As a patient with our hospital's Home Oxygen department, we're interested in your candid responses to the short questionnaire printed below. This survey is anonymous and strictly confidential.

Enclosed is a postage-paid envelope for returning the questionnaire to our Quality Assurance staff, who help departments like Home Oxygen evaluate their services. Thank you for your help — your feedback is extremely valuable to us.

How would you grade the following qualities of St. Agnes Hospital's Home Oxygen staff?
Evaluate each one as you would grade a report card. Space has been provided after each question for any additional comments or suggestions you may have regarding your Home Care experience.

1. **Did Home Oxygen staff show up on time for their visits with you?** [ ] yes   [ ] no

    _____
    _____

2. **Our staff's ability to explain your oxygen equipment and supplies to you in an easy to understand manner:**
    [ ] A   [ ] B   [ ] C   [ ] D   [ ] F

    _____
    _____

3. **The friendliness of Home Oxygen staff:** .... [ ] A   [ ] B   [ ] C   [ ] D   [ ] F

    _____
    _____

4. **The appearance of Home Oxygen staff ....**   [ ] A   [ ] B   [ ] C   [ ] D   [ ] F

    _____
    _____

5. **Please grade our different Home Oxygen staff on how competent and helpful they were to you. Only grade those you came in contact with:**
    Office Personnel .... [ ] A   [ ] B   [ ] C   [ ] D   [ ] F
    Oxygen Technician .... [ ] A   [ ] B   [ ] C   [ ] D   [ ] F

    _____
    _____
    _____
    _____
    _____

6. **The working order and cleanliness of Home Oxygen equipment:**
    [ ] A   [ ] B   [ ] C   [ ] D   [ ] F

continues

Exhibit 22–22 continued

7. **The Home Oxygen staff's ability to answer your phone calls in a timely and proper fashion:**
   [ ] A   [ ] B   [ ] C   [ ] D   [ ] F

_____

_____

8. **Did you feel that Home Oxygen staff met with you frequently enough to meet your needs?**
   [ ] A   [ ] B   [ ] C   [ ] D   [ ] F

_____

_____

9. **Did you feel your needs were met when you had to call after hours?**
   [ ] A   [ ] B   [ ] C   [ ] D   [ ] F

_____

_____

10. **How did you learn about St. Agnes Hospital Home Oxygen:**
   [ ] Hospital Discharge/Social Worker   [ ] Advertisement
   [ ] Family/Friend/Word of Mouth   [ ] Other (please specify) _____
   [ ] Physician

   _____

Signature (optional): _____

Courtesy of St. Agnes Hospital, HME Department, Fond du Lac, Wisconsin.

• confidentiality of the information in the charts
• protection of the charts from damage or loss

Information that is gathered needs to have a check system in place to ensure accurate, complete, timely, and reliable information. One possibility is an audit system. The audit can be done by any competent individual in the organization. The results need to be shared with all staff members for educational purposes. During these educational sessions, the importance of data collection will be demonstrated. The process of data collection will improve by having an extensive orientation in which documentation is included in the competency tool.

The Joint Commission is clear as to what needs to be included in a chart:

• patient identification, such as
  1. name
  2. address
  3. sex
  4. phone number
  5. date of birth
  6. emergency contact numbers
  7. height and weight
• the initial assessment
• reassessments of the patient
• evidence of suitability of the home environment
  1. availability of telephone, water, electricity, running water

Exhibit 22–23 Sample Emergency Preparedness Plan

DEPARTMENT: Home Oxygen/DME   **POLICY NO.** EM 3

SUBJECT: Emergency Preparedness Plan

OBJECTIVE: To have a plan designed to provide continuing care/service in the event of a weather emergency or disaster that would result in interruption of patient services.

PROCEDURE:

1. Staff members will gather at the Home Care/Hospice building if the emergency occurs during regular scheduled work hours.

2. If the emergency occurs during off hours, the employee should report to work at the next scheduled work time unless called to come in earlier.

3. If phones are down, car phones are used.

4. The individual on call for the day will be responsible to triage and make a list with patients requiring priority needs and will check the schedule for continuous use oxygen and those due for delivery.

5. Wisconsin Power and Light will be called to identify what areas are affected by power outage if necessary.

6. Emergency visits will be done as soon as possible.

7. Telephone usage will be limited to emergency use only.

8. Staff will document attempts to communicate and see patients on the communication form.

9. Normal documentation will be completed.

10. Patients should call after the emergency, especially if they relocated.

11. Within 24 hours after emergency, the director or designee will review how plan was followed and make recommendations for improvement.

Reviewed/Revised: 6/95, 10/95

Courtesy of St. Agnes Hospital, HME Department, Fond du Lac, Wisconsin.

Exhibit 22–24 Patient Disaster Instruction Sheet

In the event of SEVERE WEATHER or TORNADO WARNINGS:

1. Move to basement if possible.

2. If no basement is available, move to a room with no windows or to a room with as few windows as possible in the center of the home—away from glass.

3. If other shelter is available (such as in a trailer court), take cover in shelter.

4. If you are unable to move to a shelter, protect yourself by throwing a blanket over your body to prevent possible injury.

In the event of a FIRE:

1. As soon as a fire is seen, dial 911. Report if oxygen in home.

2. Do not attempt to extinguish fire.

3. Leave home if you are able from available exits.

4. If unable to exit safely, close door to block out fire.

5. Wet towels and put around door.

6. Lie on the floor until help arrives.

7. Turn oxygen off if able.

In the event of an EARTHQUAKE:

1. If tremors are felt, go to a doorway in your home.

2. The procedure set up by the County Sheriff will be followed for appropriate evacuation.

In the event of a POWER OUTAGE:

1. Use candles or a flashlight as an alternative light source. (Only use candles if no flashlight is available. Use extreme caution with candles to prevent fire.)

2. Listen if possible for updated reports on weather. If severe warnings develop, act accordingly to ensure your safety.

3. If you are on oxygen, hook up to portable oxygen until power resumes. Do not use candles near oxygen.

Courtesy of St. Agnes Hospital, HME Department, Fond du Lac, Wisconsin.

Exhibit 22–25 Wheelchair Safety Inspection Checklist

❑ Wheelchair opens and closes with ease.

❑ Wheelchair rolls straight (no excessive drag or pull to one side).

❑ Wheel locks do not interfere with tires when rolling.

❑ Wheel locks easy to engage.

❑ Wheel locks pivot points free of wear or looseness.

❑ Crossbraces inspected for wear or bending.

❑ Crossbraces pivot bolt secure but loose enough to keep all four wheels on ground when crossing uneven surfaces.

❑ Clothing guards — inspect for bent or protruding metal and ensure all fasteners are secure.

❑ Arms — secure but easy to release; adjustment levers engage properly.

❑ Adjustable height arms operate and lock securely.

❑ Arm rests — inspect for rips in upholstery.

❑ Base of arm rest sits flush against arm tube.

❑ Seat and back upholstery — inspect for rips or sagging.

❑ Wheels — axle nut and sealed bearings tension correct.

❑ No excessive side movement or binding when wheel lifted from ground and spun.

❑ Handrims — inspect for signs of rough edges or peeling chrome.

❑ Inspect for bent or broken spokes.

❑ All spokes uniformly tight.

❑ Inspect axle for proper tension by spinning caster; caster should come to a gradual stop.

❑ Adjust bearing system if wheel wobbles noticeably or binds to a stop.

❑ Tires — inspect for flat spots and wear.

❑ If pneumatic tires, check for proper inflation.

❑ Clean and wax all chrome-plated parts.

❑ Clean upholstery and armrests.

HANDLER SIGNATURE _____   DATE _____

Courtesy of St. Agnes Hospital, HME Department, Fond du Lac, Wisconsin.

Exhibit 22–26 Sample DME Maintenance Competencies

The oxygen technician upon completion of orientation will have:
15. Demonstrates correct maintenance technique and cleaning for each piece of equipment.

Subject	Content/Learning Options	Objective Evaluation Mechanisms	Notes
Maintenance and Cleaning	1. Receive and review Guidelines for Maintenance and Cleaning all DME (focusing on how to perform correct cleaning and maintenance and frequency to be done): 　a. Electric and Manual Beds 　b. Wheel Chairs 　c. Lifts 　d. Oxygen Concentrator 　e. Trapeze 　f. Pulmonaide 　g. Walker 　h. Shower Chair and Commode 　i. Overbed Table 　j. Suction Machine 　k. Canes 2. Receive a demonstration on cleaning each of the above pieces of equipment. 3. Review how to correctly complete a cleaning/maintenance log for a piece of DME equipment, and receive a sample log.	1. Correctly performs a return demonstration on maintenance and cleaning of each piece of equipment. 2. Correctly completes a log for each piece of equipment cleaned.	
Recall of Equipment	1. Receive and review EM 1—Recall of Device, Supply, Equipment or Product.		
Medical Device Reporting	1. Receive and review IC 8—DME Medical Device Reporting.		
Equipment Safety	1. Receive and review IC 9—Initial Electrical Checks. 　a. All equipment must be checked through Materials Management. 2. Receive and review IC 10—Use of Adaptor Plugs.		

Courtesy of St. Agnes Hospital, HME Department, Fond du Lac, Wisconsin.

2. appropriate storage
3. accessibility
4. presence of infestation or pests
- safety measures to protect the patient
- a visit note for each home contact, which includes
  1. what care was provided
  2. date
  3. who provided the care
- functional limitations
- instructions for discharge
- activity restrictions
- changes in patient's condition
- plan of care
- patient education
- physician orders
- other agencies involved
- patient diagnosis
- allergies and sensitivities
- laboratory results
- rights and responsibilities
- financial agreements
- communication with patient and other care providers

Having a planned, systematic approach to gathering, storing, and utilizing data can prove to benefit both patient care and organizational improvement. Having all members involved in the approach can save time and money.

SURVEILLANCE, PREVENTION, AND CONTROL OF INFECTION

To supply DME in the home environment, the supplier must have in place a systematic approach to infection prevention and surveillance. The Joint Commission is clear on activities that must be included in your infection control plan: (1) surveillance, (2) identification, (3) reporting, (4) prevention, and (5) control of infection.

The goal of the infection control plan is to improve patient outcomes by identifying and

reducing the risk of infections. The plan must include policies and procedures that address the following areas:

- care that is provided
- education of involved persons on the prevention of infection
- a system for tracking infections that occur
- compliance with local, state, and federal regulations
- Centers for Disease Control guidelines

It needs to be clear to anyone who enters the system what procedures are in place to prevent the potential or spread of infections. The procedures need to include the following areas:

- personal hygiene
- precautions to be taken to protect the staff, patients, and caregivers
- aseptic procedures
- appropriate cleaning, disinfecting, or sterilization of the equipment
- supplies intended for single use

The organization needs to have in place a consistent orientation process to train all team members on the surveillance, prevention, and control of infections. This process needs to be reviewed on an annual basis by a competent person. The information that is gathered needs to be reviewed and analyzed on a quarterly basis to implement any needed improvements in patient care. Exhibit 22–27 is an example of an infection-reporting form.

Figure 22–1 is an example of a graph tracking infection incidence. Exhibit 22–28 is an example of an infection tracking log.

Quality care takes time, energy, and dedication from all members of the organization. The definition of quality is an evolving process. Time spent in monitoring and improving quality will improve patient outcomes as well as staff performance.

Exhibit 22–27 Infection Report Form

Patient's first name and last initial: _____ Office: _____

Diagnosis: _____

Primary nurse: _____

Date of onset of infection: _____ Medical record #: _____

Last hospitalization: Admission date: _____ Discharge date: _____

Name of hospital: _____

Infection site and symptoms associated with infection:

Skin/wound: _____

_____

Upper/lower respiratory: _____

_____

Urinary tract infection: foley present ❏ yes ❏ no _____

_____

Sepsis: _____

_____

IV: _____

_____

Other: _____

_____

_____

Interventions (include test and treatments, state if no treatment sought and why):

_____

_____

_____

_____

Causative organism if known: _____

Outcome: _____

_____

RN completing form: _____

Courtesy of St. Agnes Hospital, HME Department, Fond du Lac, Wisconsin.

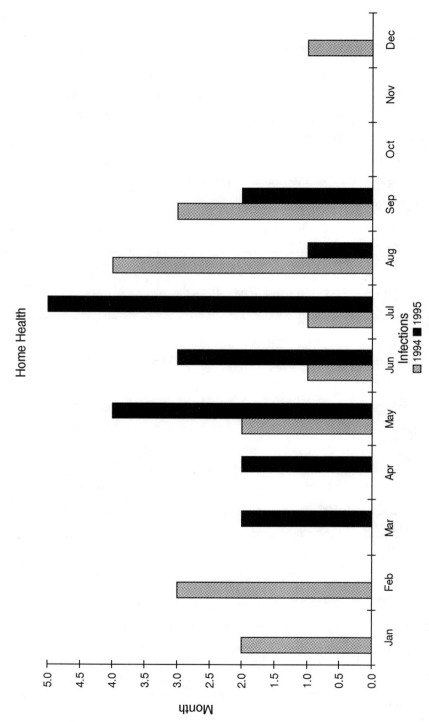

Figure 22–1 Sample graph tracking infection incidence. Courtesy of St. Agnes Hospital, HME Department, Fond du Lac, Wisconsin.

Exhibit 22–28 Infection Tracking Log

☐ Hospice
☐ Home Care

| Date | Medical Record # | Infection Site | | | | | Interventions | Causative Organisms | Outcome | Branch |
		Skin-Wound	URI/LRI	UTI	Sepsis	IV	Other			

Courtesy of St. Agnes Hospital, HME Department, Fond du Lac, Wisconsin.

REFERENCES

Health Care Financing Administration. (1985). *Manual for federally qualified health maintenance organizations.* Author.

Health Care Financing Administration. (1989). *Manual for federally qualified health maintenance organizations.* Author.

Joint Commission on Accreditation of Healthcare Organizations. (1993). *Quality improvement in health care.* Oakbrook Terrace, IL: Author.

National Commission for Quality Assurance. (1996). *Standards for the accreditation of managed care organizations* (3rd ed.). Washington, DC: Author.

Wisconsin Department of Health and Social Services, Contract for Medicaid HMO Services between HMO and WI Department of Health and Family Services, July 1996–December 1997.

Chapter 23

Quality Improvement in Hospice Care

Katrina Sargent-Deziel

CHAPTER OBJECTIVES

After completing this chapter, the reader will be able to

- describe various sources of standards applicable to hospice care
- detail elements necessary to design a comprehensive quality improvement plan
- conduct a chart audit
- draft satisfaction surveys for family members and physicians
- discuss an interdisciplinary team "closure summary" following the death of a patient

Hospice care began in the United States in the early 1960s when Dame Cicily Saunders, founder of St. Christopher's Hospice in London, England, visited and introduced her philosophy of care for people with terminal illnesses to health care workers in America. Her mission was to manage pain and symptoms, while maximizing the patient's comfort and dignity of the end of life, that is, palliative care (NHO, 1994). This philosophy was built on the belief that terminally ill patients often received unnecessary treatments that only prolonged their suffering. Many felt that patients were receiving surgery, radiation, or chemotherapy even though there was no hope of a cure. Patients were being aggressively treated, but their spiritual, social, and psychological needs were being left unmet. Saunders enthusiastically sought to empower patients and their families with a more "holis-

tic" view of care. She encouraged health professionals to address not only their patients' physical needs but also their spiritual, social, emotional, and economic needs.

Saunders' lectures inspired many people in America who were working with the terminally ill. They began to implement the hospice concept of care and to discuss ways to ensure that patients with terminal illnesses received quality care. Because hospice staff responsible for providing the care have also been the people most dedicated to the quality of care their patients receive, quality improvement has always been central to the hospice movement. Quality improvement is a formal organization of activities designed to identify problems in the quality of care, determine possible solutions to alter situations in the next similar case, implement those solutions, and then evaluate their effectiveness. In an organization with a continuous quality improvement (CQI) program, quality is not merely the province of a few specialists who respond to errors and complaints; rather it is the province of all staff, who are encouraged to work continuously toward the best possible care for all. Some quality improvement activities in hospice care include

- Chart audits: clinical, bereavement, and inpatient charts
- Surveys and questionnaires: family evaluation forms; physician assessment forms; be-

461

reavement follow-up; evaluations by hospice volunteers, clergy, and funeral directors

• Meetings: monthly quality improvement meetings, weekly interdisciplinary group meetings, committee meetings such as medical advisory and utilization review

Quality improvement programs in hospice care seek to ensure that a high standard of patient and family care is provided. Unlike traditional health care, hospice programs see both the dying patient and family as a unit of care because both are affected by the terminal illness. The interdisciplinary team will respond to the needs of both the patient and the caregiver.

Hospice refers to a philosophy of care more than to a place in which care is provided. Among the many hospices in the United States, there are hospital-based programs, programs housed in independent, free-standing facilities, hospice programs that provide services to residents in nursing homes, and programs designed to provide care to patients who choose to die at home. Though all hospice programs recognize the physical, social, psychological, and spiritual needs of patients and their families, how the interdisciplinary team responds to the unique problems may vary. This is, in part, related to the communities that hospices serve, the facilities with which they are affiliated, and the state standards or the standards they set themselves.

If a hospice is affiliated with a hospital accredited by the Joint Commission on Accreditation of Healthcare Organizations (Joint Commission), the hospice must meet the Joint Commission's standards for home care. Independent hospices must follow state regulations and Medicare/Medicaid regulations if they are Medicare/Medicaid certified. The Health Care Financing Administration (HCFA) is the federal agency that is responsible for the medical review of hospice claims except for third-party claims.

STANDARDS

The recognized stamp of quality care is the Joint Commission's accreditation. The

1997–1998   Comprehensive   Accreditation Manual for Home Care, applicable to hospices and home medical equipment, includes functionally organized performance-based standards, and programs applying for accreditation must meet the intent of the standards. The standards are divided into the following 11 functions:

• Rights, Responsibilities, and Ethics
• Assessment
• Care, Treatment, and Services
• Education
• Continuum of Care
• Improving Organizational Performance
• Leadership
• Management of the Environment of Care
• Management of Human Resources
• Management of Information
• Surveillance, Prevention, and Control of Infection

Individual states also set standards through interpretation of their individual state hospice licensure laws. Fifty-eight percent of all hospices in the United States are currently licensed. An example of the way a state might address quality assurance can be found in the Wisconsin Department of Health and Social Services, under HSS 131.37, "Quality Assurance":

> 1. GENERAL REQUIREMENT. The hospice shall develop and maintain a quality assurance program that evaluates the quality and effectiveness of the program and its services in all patient and family care settings.
> 2. MEETINGS. The individual responsible for the quality assurance program may draw on selected members of the interdisciplinary group to conduct studies, and shall convene meetings of hospice staff at least annually to review progress and findings and to produce recommendations for improvements in policies and practices.

3. ANNUAL REPORT. The quality assurance program findings shall be developed into an annual report for the governing body along with appropriate recommendations for changes to current policies and procedures based on those findings.

Standards vary from state to state. Generally, they all demand that a quality improvement plan be in place. Many require retrospective chart audits on at least 10% of the charts to assess the effectiveness of programs and determine if services are meeting patients' needs. Additionally, they usually require that licensed hospices report to the board of directors on a quarterly basis on the quality of their programs.

The majority of hospices (75%) are also Medicare and/or Medicaid certified. Medicare/Medicaid regulations are more detailed than the state regulations and are what drives those hospices in the practical day-to-day business of quality improvement. Exhibit 23–1 shows these regulations as of 1996.

Exhibit 23–1 Medicare/Medicaid Regulations

Tag Number	Regulation	Guidance to Surveyors
L141	*418.66 Condition of Participation—Quality Assurance*	*418.66 Guidelines:* This self-assessment should include all services that were provided and the patients' and caregivers' response to those services. It should also include those services that might have been provided but were omitted. Special attention should be given to the ability of the hospice to deal with symptom management, pain control, stress management, continuity of care, and inpatient care. Suggestions for improving care and any problems identified in providing hospice care should receive the appropriate consideration from the hospice management or governing body.
L142	A hospice must conduct an ongoing, comprehensive, integrated self-assessment of the quality and appropriateness of care provided, including inpatient care, home care, and care provided under arrangements. The findings are used by the hospice to correct identified problems and to revise hospice policies if necessary.	
		418.66 Probes: What type of system does the hospice use to monitor and evaluate the care and services it provides to its patients and their caregivers/families? How does the hospice receive, record, investigate, and resolve patient grievances or complaints? Who has the overall responsibility for the development and implementation of the quality assurance program?
	Those responsible for the quality assurance program must:	How do the medical director and interdisciplinary group (IDG) implement procedures to monitor quality that include at least the following:

continues

Exhibit 23–1 continued

Tag Number	Regulation	Guidance to Surveyors
L143	(a) Implement and report on activities and mechanisms for monitoring the quality of patient care;	• Problem implementation evaluations and monitoring of staff performance; • Recommendations to the administrator and governing body for improving patient care; • Implementation of recommendations resulting from evaluation and studies?
L144	(b) Identify and resolve problems; and	
L145	(c) Make suggestions for improving patient care.	
L146	*418.68 Condition of Participation-Interdisciplinary Group*	*418.68 Guidelines:* Members of the IDG must be hospice employees of the agency or organization of which the hospice is a sub-division (e.g., a hospital) who are appropriately trained and assigned to a hospice unit. All IDG members have the same responsibilities regardless of whether they are employed directly, assigned, or volunteer employees of the hospice. An employee is one who meets the common law definition of *employee* as found in title II of the Social Security Act or one who is a volunteer under the control of the hospice.
L147	The hospice must designate an interdisciplinary group or groups composed of individuals who provide or supervise the care and services offered by the hospice.	
		The hospice may involve other members of the care team in the IDG's activities. A hospice with more than one IDG must designate a specific group to establish policies governing care and services.
		The IDG should conduct an ongoing assessment of each patient's and caregiver's or family's needs.
		"Supervision" of care may be accomplished by conferences, evaluations, discussions, and general oversight, as well as by direct over-the-shoulder observations.
		418.68 Probe: How does the hospice ensure that all individuals on the IDG have been trained and are competent to perform in the area(s) assigned?

Source: Reprinted from Wisconsin State Hospice Licensure, Chapter 50, 4SS131.

The National Hospice Organization (NHO), a national, not-for-profit professional organization, sets quality assessment and improvement standards for patient care (Exhibit 23–2). They are set forth as professional guidelines by the NHO and are only guidelines; they are not regulatory.

Exhibit 23–3 is an example of a quality improvement plan based on Kansas's state regula-

Exhibit 23–2 National Hospice Organization's Quality Assessment and Improvement Standards for Hospice Programs

Quality Assessment and Improvement

Principle:

Hospice is committed to continuous assessment and improvement of the quality and efficiency of its services.

Standard:

The governing body authorizes and supports a quality assessment and improvement program to assess and improve the quality and efficiency of the governance, management, clinical, and support processes.

Outcome:

1. Hospice follows a written plan for continually assessing and improving all aspects of operations which include:
   • goals and objectives
   • the identity of the person responsible for the program
   • a system to ensure systematic, objective, regular reports are prepared and distributed to appropriate areas
   • the method for evaluating the quality and appropriateness of care
   • a method for resolving identified problems
   • application to improving the quality of patient care
2. The plan is reviewed at least annually and revised as appropriate.
3. The governing body and administration strive to create a work environment where problems can be openly addressed and service improvement ideas are encouraged.
4. Quality assessment and improvement activities are based on the systematic collection, review, and evaluation of data which, at a minimum, include:
   • services provided by professional and volunteer staff
   • outcome audits of patient charts
   • reports from staff, volunteers, and clients about services
   • concerns or suggestions for improvement in services
   • organizational review of the hospice program
   • patient/family evaluations of care
   • high-risk, high-volume, and problem-prone activities
5. When problems are identified in the provision of hospice services, there is evidence of corrective actions, including ongoing monitoring, revisions of policies and procedures, educational intervention, and changes in the provisions of services.
6. The effectiveness of actions taken to improve services or correct identified problems is evaluated.

Source: National Hospice Organization, Arlington, Virginia.

tions, Medicare/Medicaid regulations, and the NHO's standards.

An approach to evaluating quality within the framework of the Joint Commission's 11 functions is shown in Exhibit 23–4 (CQI plan) and 23–5 (QI Calendar). In accordance with CQI principles, the plan in Exhibit 23–4 singles out for scrutiny indicators that are high risk, high volume, or problem-prone.

Exhibit 23–3 Sample Quality Improvement Plan

STANDARDS AND INDICATORS

The following standards are presented for inclusion in the 1996 Quality Improvement Plan:

Standard 1:   Hospice will strive for customer satisfaction.

NHO Principle(s):

- Hospice is committed to continuous assessment and improvement of the quality and efficiency of its services.

- The hospice interdisciplinary team collaborates continuously with the patient's attending physician to develop and maintain a patient-directed, individualized plan of care.

A. *Indicator:* Hospice Satisfaction Survey will show satisfaction with services.

Methodology: All families will receive a survey during the 4th month of their bereavement. Areas of concern will be reported quarterly with a comprehensive analysis/summary completed by an outside consultant annually.

B. *Indicator:* Physicians will indicate satisfaction with services.

Methodology: To be developed.

C. *Indicator:* Patients discharged alive or transferred will express satisfaction with the continuity of care.

Methodology: To be developed.

Standard 2:   A comprehensive interdisciplinary program is available to assist patients/families to maintain the highest level of comfort in all aspects of care.

NHO Principle(s):

- Hospice offers palliative care to all terminally ill people and their families regardless of age, gender, nationality, race, creed, sexual orientation, disability, diagnosis, availability of a primary caregiver, or ability to pay.

- The unit of care in hospice is the patient/family.

- The hospice interdisciplinary team collaborates continuously with the patient's attending physician to develop and maintain a patient-directed, individualized plan of care.

- Hospice provides a safe, coordinated program of palliative and supportive care, in a variety of appropriate settings, from the time of admission through bereavement, with the focus on keeping terminally ill patients in their own homes as long as possible.

A. *Indicator:* Hospice, Inc. will evaluate the quality of pain management throughout the patient's disease process and in all settings.

Methodology: To be developed.

continues

Exhibit 23–3 continued

B. *Indicator:* Patients and their caregivers will have no more than 2 HCAide substitutes in a 30-day period.

Methodology: The monthly aide schedules will be reviewed for a minimum of 10% of patients receiving HCA services and 100% of patients receiving Senior Care Act services. Reviews will be conducted by the Health Care Aide Coordinator. The Vice President of Medical/Nursing Services will monitor for compliance.

C. *Indicator:* Patient's primary caregiver will maintain or increase coping ability with grief and loss issues after two social work visits.

Methodology: Each quarter the Director of Bereavement and Clinical Social Work, or designee, will audit 10% of new admission charts from each team to determine if the score on the Beck Hopelessness Scale remained the same or decreased by the third social work visit.

D. *Indicator:* Patients experience physical, psycho-social, and spiritual coping as evidenced by no attempted suicide.

Methodology: All attempted suicides will be reported to the Risk Management Committee. The committee will report to Quality Council quarterly.

E. *Indicator:* Patient's spiritual comfort is adequately addressed as evidenced by a decrease on the Spiritual Distress Scale for any concerns ranked "5" or higher after two pastoral care counseling visits.

Methodology: The Director of Pastoral Care will monitor 10% of patient charts quarterly. These charts will include only those patients with identified spiritual distress as defined in the indicator. Progress reports will be reviewed to ensure the distress identified via the Spiritual Distress Scale is addressed by the chaplain.

Standard 3: A comprehensive and diverse bereavement program is available to assist the bereaved to integrate the experience of loss in their life.

NHO Principle(s):

• Hospice provides a safe, coordinated program of palliative and supportive care, in a variety of appropriate settings, from the time of admission through bereavement, with the focus on keeping terminally ill patients in their own homes as long as possible.

A. *Indicator:* Bereaved will experience physical, psycho-social, and spiritual coping as evidenced by no attempted suicide.

Methodology: Attempted suicides will be reported to the Risk Management Committee. The committee will report to Quality Council quarterly.

B. *Indicator:* Bereaved adolescents and adults will identify increased coping ability with grief and loss issues after participating in time-limited groups.

continues

Exhibit 23–3 continued

Methodology: The Director of Bereavement and Clinical Social Work will review the charts of those attending time-limited groups to determine if the Beck Hopelessness Scale score has decreased after participation in the time-limited group.

C. *Indicator:* Respondents to the Bereavement Self-Assessment tool will show maintenance or improvement in their physical, spiritual, and psychological health.

Methodology: Being developed.

Standard 4: The patient medical record will be complete and accurate to ensure continuity of care, effective interdisciplinary communication, and maximized financial reimbursement.

NHO Principle(s):

• Hospice maintains a comprehensive and accurate record of services provided in all care settings for each patient/family.

A. *Indicator:* Documentation for the care being provided in the home by the Health Care Aide is consistent with the assignment, reflected in the Assignment Request, Plan of Care, Nursing Notes, and HCA Notes.

Methodology: Nursing Support Services Coordinator will conduct monthly chart audits on 10% of charts of patients receiving HCA services completing the appropriate screen.

B. *Indicator:* The patient record reflects continuity between the Plan of Care and the services being rendered.

Methodology: A minimum of 10% of the active charts and 10% of the closed charts of patients served during the quarter will be reviewed by the Quality Council quarterly. The Vice President of Medical Services will monitor for ongoing compliance.

C. *Indicator:* The patient record reflects continuity between the Plan of Care and treatments being rendered.

Methodology: A retrospective study will be conducted. 100% of patients who received radiation therapy during the 1st quarter will be reviewed by the nursing QI committee in the 3rd quarter. 100% of patients who received chemotherapy in the 2nd quarter will be reviewed by the Nursing QI committee in the 4th quarter.

Standard 5: The agency will ensure resources are maximized and safeguarded.

NHO Principle(s):

• Hospice is accountable for the appropriate allocation and utilization of its resources in order to provide optimal care consistent with patient/family needs.

continues

Exhibit 23–3 continued

- Hospice maintains a comprehensive and accurate record of services provided in all care settings for each patient family.

A. *Indicator:* Cash flow will be maximized as evidenced by billings for applicable services being sent within 30 days of the end of the month in which the service(s) occurred.

   Methodology: The Controller will audit quarterly 10% of monthly billings for timeliness.

B. *Indicator:* Patients admitted and cared for by Hospice, Inc. are appropriate as evidenced by the Utilization Review Admission and Continued Stay Screens, including the NHO Clinical Parameters when indicated.

   Methodology: All admissions during the month of January will be screened. 10% of active charts will be screened by Health Information for appropriate Continued Stay during the second quarter.

C. *Indicator:* Hospice patients are discharged appropriately as evidenced by the UR Hospice Discharge Screen and Discharge Summary.

   Methodology: All dismissals during the month of December will be screened by Health Information.

D. *Indicator:* Changes in level of care to Acute Inpatient are appropriate as evidenced by the UR Hospital Admission Screen.

   Methodology: 100% of acute admissions will be screened by Health Information during the 1st and 3rd quarters.

E. *Indicator:* Changes in level of care from Acute Inpatient are appropriate as evidenced by the UR Hospital Discharge Screen.

   Methodology: 100% of discharges from acute care will be screened by Health Information during the 1st and 3rd quarters.

F. *Indicator:* The financial resources of the agency are managed appropriately as evidenced by the annual report of the external auditing agency.

   Methodology: An independent Certified Public Accounting firm will conduct a complete audit of the financial statements and practices of Hospice, Inc. yearly.

G. *Indicator:* Develop indicator regarding Risk Management.

Standard 6:   The agency will ensure its human resources are developed and safeguarded.

NHO Principle(s):

- A highly qualified, specially trained team of hospice professionals and volunteers work together to meet the physiological, psychological, social, spiritual, and economic needs of hospice patient/families facing terminal illness and bereavement.

continues

Exhibit 23–3 continued

A. *Indicator:* Hospice volunteers are adequately prepared to meet patient/family needs as evidenced by increased comfort/knowledge as identified on the assessment tool.

> *Methodology:* Using the Volunteer Skill-Based Inventory, the Volunteer Department will survey 100% of each volunteer orientation class. One month after their first assignments, the volunteers will be asked to complete another inventory. The Volunteer Department will compare the results of both surveys.

B. *Indicator:* Hospice staff are prepared and adequately perform their job duties.

> *Methodology:* Employees will evaluate the effectiveness of their orientation at the end of their first six months of employment. Supervisors will complete the six-month evaluation of the employee. The HR Director will compile the responses and report to QC during the 3rd quarter.

C. Develop indicator regarding diversity.

Standard 7:   The agency will continue to meet its mission with the highest quality programs possible.

NHO Principle(s):

- Hospice has an organized governing body that has complete and ultimate responsibility for the organization.

- The hospice governing body entrusts the hospice administrator with overall management responsibility for operating the hospice, including planning, organizing, staffing, and evaluating the organization and its services.

- Hospice is committed to continuous assessment and improvement of the quality and efficiency of its services.

A. *Indicator:* The agency will meet or exceed the NHO Standards as evidenced by a score of 2.5 or more on all areas of the evaluation tool.

> *Methodology:* The Standards Committee will evaluate the Hospice, Inc. programs based on the NHO Standards of a Hospice Program of Care. This evaluation will be conducted yearly and reported during the 4th quarter.

B. *Indicator:* The agency will pass the Medicare survey with no Conditions of Participation out of compliance and minimal deficiencies.

*Indicators also required by another governing body such as Medicare, Senior Act Grant, etc.

continues

Exhibit 23–3 continued

QI PLAN 1996

POLICY/PROCEDURE REVIEW CALENDAR
1996

POLICY REVIEW	JAN	FEB	MAR	APR	MAY	JUN	JUL	AUG	SEP	OCT	NOV	DEC
ADMIN										X	X	X
COMMUNITY RELATIONS							X	X	X			
COUNSELING/ SUPPORT SER	X	X	X									
FINANCE	X	X	X									
MED/NSG SER				X	X	X						

UTILIZATION REVIEW
1996

POLICY REVIEW	JAN	FEB	MAR	APR	MAY	JUN	JUL	AUG	SEP	OCT	NOV	DEC
HOSPICE ADMISSION	X											
CONTINUED STAY				X	X	X						
HOSPICE DISCHARGE												X
ACUTE ADMISSION	X	X	X			X	X	X				
ACUTE DISCHARGE	X	X	X			X	X	X				

QUALITY COUNCIL
POLICY/PROCEDURE REVIEW
1996

MED/NSG PROC	JAN	FEB	MAR	APR	MAY	JUN	JUL	AUG	SEP	OCT	NOV	DEC
GENERAL 800-860				X	X	X						
MEDICATION 860-900							X	X	X			
SYSTEMS 900-950										X	X	X
LAB/ DIABETES 950-975	X	X	X									

continues

Exhibit 23–3 continued

QUALITY COUNCIL
INDICATOR REVIEW/1996

INDICATORS	1	2	3	4	5	6	7	8	9	10	11	12
STANDARD 1												
FAMILY SATISFACTION			X									
PHYSICIAN SATISFACTION											X	
DISCHARGED PT/SATISFACTION						X				X		
STANDARD 2												
PAIN MGMT BASELINE	X											
PAIN MGMT				X								
HCA SUBS							X					
CAREGIVER COPING			X			X			X			X
PT SUICIDE ATTEMPTS			X			X			X			X
SPIRITUAL COMFORT				X								
STANDARD 3												
BEREAVED COPING			X			X			X			X
BEREAVED ADOLESCENTS			X			X			X			X
BEREAVED SELF-ASSESS			X			X			X			X
STANDARD 4												
CONSISTENT HCA DOCUMENT			X			X			X			X
POC/SERVICES CONTINUITY			X			X			X			X
POC/TREATMENT CONTINUITY e.g., RAD TX			X			X			X			X

continues

Exhibit 23–3 continued

INDICATOR REVIEW/1996

INDICATORS	1	2	3	4	5	6	7	8	9	10	11	12
STANDARD 5												
TIMELY BILLINGS			X			X			X			X
ADMIT UR	X											
DISCHARGE UR												X
ACUTE DISCH LEVEL OF CARE			X						X			
FINANCE AUDIT									X			
RISK MGMT		X										
STANDARD 6												
VOLUNTEERS PREPARED					X							
STAFF PREPARED									X			
DIVERSITY			X			X			X			X
STANDARD 7												
NHO STANDARDS									X			
MEDICARE SURVEY									X			

Note: POC = Plan of Care; RAD TX = radiation treatment; UR = utilization review.

Courtesy of Hospice, Incorporated, 1996, Wichita, Kansas.

Exhibit 23–4 Continuous Quality Improvement Hospice Plan

Indicator	Function	Process or Outcome Measure	High Risk	High Volume	Prone	Problem Report Dates '96
Patient Satisfaction	PE, LD, Tx	O	X	X		Jan, March, June, Sept, Dec
Infection Control	IC	P/O	X	X		Jan, March, June, Sept, Dec
Inpatient Respite	Tx, CC	P	X		X	June, Dec
Nursing Home Survey	CC, LD, Tx, PE	O			X	Sept
Tracking of Pt Complaints	LD, Tx	O	X			Jan, March, June, Sept, Dec
Missed Visits	Tx, CC	P/O	X			Jan, March, June, Sept, Dec
Employee Injury	HR	P	X			Jan, March, June, Sept, Dec
Pt Falls Injury	A, PE, EC, HR	P	X	X	X	Jan, March, June, Sept, Dec
Med Error	Tx	O	X			Jan, March, June, Sept, Dec
Med Reaction	A, Tx, IM	O	X			Jan, March, June, Sept, Dec
Patient/Employee Infection	IC, HR	P/O	X	X	X	Jan, March, June, Sept, Dec

Note: Tx = Care, Treatment, Service   CC = Continuum of Care   LD = Leadership
MI = Management of Information   PE = Patient Education   EC = Management of Environment of Care
IC = Surveillance, Prevention, and Control of Infection   RRE = Rights, Responsibilities, and Ethics
HR = Human Resources   A = Assessment

Courtesy of St. Agnes Hospital Hospice, Fond du Lac, Wisconsin.

Exhibit 23–5 QI Calendar for Hospice

Survey Criteria	March 95	April 95	May 95	June 95	July 95	Aug 95	Sept 95	Oct 95	Nov 95	Dec 95	Jan 96	Feb 96	March 96	April 96	May 96	June 96
Patient Satisfaction PE, LD, Tx	R	C	C	C	C	C	R/C	C	C	R/C	C	C	R/C	C	C	R/C
Infection Control IC	C	C	C	R/C	C	C	R/C	C	C	R/C	C	C	R/C	C	C	R/C
Inpatient/Respite Tx, CC	C	C	C	R	C	C	C	C	C	C	C	C	C	C	C	R
Nx Home Survey CC, LD, Tx, PE			C				R									
Monthly Tracking of:																
1. Pt Satisfaction Complaints LD, Tx	R	C	C	R/C	C	C	R/C	C	C	R/C	C	C	R/C	C	C	R/C
2. Missed Visits Tx, CC	R	C	C	R/C	C	C	R/C	C	C	R/C	C	C	R/C	C	C	R/C
3. Employee Survey Hr	R	C	C	R/C	C	C	R/C	C	C	R/C	C	C	R/C	C	C	R/C
4. Pt Falls/Injury A, PE, EC, HR	R	C	C	R/C	C	C	R/C	C	C	R/C	C	C	R/C	C	C	R/C
5. Med Error Tx	R	C	C	R/C	C	C	R/C	C	C	R/C	C	C	R/C	C	C	R/C
6. Med Reaction A, Tx, IM	R	C	C	R/C	C	C	R/C	C	C	R/C	C	C	R/C	C	C	R/C
7. Employee Infection IC, HR	R	C	C	R/C	C	C	R/C	C	C	R/C	C	C	R/C	C	C	R/C

Note: C = Collect data; R = report data.
Courtesy of St. Agnes Hospital Hospice, Fond du Lac, Wisconsin.

TOOLS

Exhibit 23–6 is one example of a chart audit form used by Hospice of Portage County. Twenty percent of charts are reviewed each year using this tool. The responsibility is divided between the interdisciplinary team members. The executive director and nursing care coordinator decide what charts will be reviewed on the basis of the complexity of each case. If a number of challenges have been faced by the hospice team in caring for a particular patient/family and if problems are more likely to surface in auditing the chart, it is likely that the chart will be reviewed.

Exhibit 23–7 is another example of a chart audit form. It represents minimum standards that one quality improvement team felt should be met for all patients and is completed on two charts every quarter.

For a variety of reasons, a hospice patient's caregivers may need a respite from daily caregiving, and a patient may take advantage of an inpatient/respite program. The checklist shown in Exhibit 23–8 has proven helpful in evaluating the inpatient/respite experience.

Hospice staff meet regularly to discuss patients and evaluate their care. Weekly meetings are one effective way to ensure that a high quality of care is being provided. Family surveys, such as that shown in Exhibit 23–9, are another.

Exhibit 23–10 (Family Evaluation Form) is an example of a questionnaire that is mailed to families following the death of their loved one. The completed survey is reviewed and provided to the patient's primary physician on a quarterly basis to measure the effectiveness of the patient's care.

The Hospice Hope Evaluation Survey (Exhibit 23–11) is another approach to gathering patient and family satisfaction data.

The Physician Assessment Form (Exhibit 23–12) is an example of a physician evaluation form that is sent to doctors following the death of one of their patients. Once completed, it is circulated at the weekly interdisciplinary team meeting for all of the staff to review.

The closure summary tool (Exhibit 23–13) is another example of a tool that hospice staff may use to meet Medicare/Medicaid guidelines for monitoring care and assessing the quality of care provided to their patients. This tool is completed by the interdisciplinary team for every patient following his or her death. Possible solutions are discussed, and recommendations are referred to the Quality Assurance Committee, who meet quarterly to review these recommendations. This process allows staff to discuss their personal feelings about the case and bring closure to it. Ultimately, it helps to improve quality of care for future patients.

Exhibit 23–6 Care Documentation/Quality Improvement

Patient # _____ _____ Active _____ Closed

Review done by _____ Date reviewed _____ Quarter _____

Diagnosis _____ Length of stay in program _____

Medicare/Medicaid Appropriateness	Yes	No	N/A

If non-cancer diagnosis

1. Documentation on admission of medical
   guidelines appropriateness

	Yes	No	N/A
Meets criteria	_____	_____	_____
Karnophsky scale completed	_____	_____	_____
Activities of Daily Living completed	_____	_____	_____
MD agrees to guidelines	_____	_____	_____

2. Ongoing (at benefit) discussion, reevaluation
   and documentation of progressive
   symptoms

	Yes	No
1st benefit	_____	_____
2nd benefit	_____	_____
3rd benefit	_____	_____
4th benefit	_____	_____

Patient/Family Care	Yes	No

1. Asterisk aspects of teaching/counseling
   plan have documentation   _____ _____

   What areas:

2. Does it include date, whom, and initials?   _____ _____
3. Education protocol on Death and Dying.
   Did documentation include patient/family
   readiness to learn?   _____ _____

Pain Management	Yes	No	N/A

1. Pain opened as problem?   Date _____
2. Initial pain assessment completed? Date _____
3. If pain unopened, was pain assessed
   by staff (how many visits)_____
   and documented?   _____ _____ _____
4. Was pain medication ordered?   _____ _____ _____
5. If pain opened, was patient/family
   informed of pain management interventions
   other than medicines?   _____ _____ _____
      If yes, what:

   _____

   _____

continues

Exhibit 23–6 continued

Stress Management	Yes	No	N/A
1. Family conference considered and documented, include date, whom, etc.			

Date

Continuity of Care

Patient was transferred to _____ on _____

	Yes	No
1. If planned, was transfer/discharge problem opened prior to: Date:_____		

	Yes	No
2. Did staff person accompany or visit patient within two hours?		
3. Was care plan available and reviewed with new facility staff when transferred?		
4. Was family instructed regarding differences of facilities?		

In-Patient Care	Yes	No
1. Pages documented in hospice chart (compare with hospital chart)		
2. Hospice plan of care identifies the admission unmanaged symptom as a need in first 24 hours		

Nursing Home	Yes	No	N/A
1. Collaboration of Nursing Home/Hospice on charts (both)			
2. Pre MDS/RAP review on charts (both)			
3. Post MDS/RAP review on chart (both)			
4. Hospice attended quarterly review and documented			
5. Quarterly MDS/RAP review on charts (both)			

(MDS/RAP = Minimum Data Set/Resident Assessment Protocol)

Bereavement Services	Yes	No	
Date of death_____ (day of week and date)			
1. IDT care conference update on bereavement after two weeks following death for two months			If no, why?____

IDT = Interdisciplinary Team

Courtesy of Hospice of Portage County, Inc., Stevens Point, Wisconsin.

Exhibit 23–7 Quality Care Review

Patient Number _____	Active _____ Closed _____ Case No. _____
Diagnosis _____	
Period reviewed _____	Date reviewed _____
Review done by _____	Length of stay _____

I. Physician's Orders	Yes	No	N/A
1. Medical plan reflects current health history	____	____	____
2. Orders signed and carried out on a timely basis	____	____	____
3. IDT order reflected palliative care measures and anticipated outcomes	____	____	____

II. Observation of Symptoms and Reactions	Yes	No	N/A
4. Related observations to course of disease	____	____	____
5. Related observations to complications due to therapy (medications or procedures)	____	____	____
6. Made continuing observations regarding patient's condition, notification of physician when necessary	____	____	____

III. Patient/Family Care	Yes	No
Date admitted _____		
7. Patient/family rights reviewed	____	____
8. Care plan completed date _____		
9. Safety and security of patient discussed	____	____
10. Current medication profile in record with evidence of patient/family instructions	____	____
11. Supported patient/family in reaction/adaptation to condition and care	____	____
12. Care plans revised in accordance with assessment	____	____
13. Interaction/relationship with patient/family documented	____	____
14. Patient and family informed as to plan of care	____	____
15. Patient and family informed of plan for medical emergency	____	____
16. Evidence of continuing monitoring of patient's primary problems and appropriate action taken	____	____
17. Evidence of patient/family teaching regarding expected disease and dying process	____	____

continues

Exhibit 23–7 continued

IV. Inter-Disciplinary Team	Yes	No
18. Coordination of services:		
a. IDT conferences are documented and found in chart	_____	_____
b. Evaluation of the need for other services with referral documented	_____	_____
c. Evidence of evaluation closure	_____	_____
d. Medical record entries by all caregivers	_____	_____

V. Death Date of Death _____	Yes	No
19. Documentation regarding death date, time, place, and circumstances	_____	_____
20. Discharge summary is recorded and dated	_____	_____

VI. Bereavement	Yes	No
21. Documentation of bereavement services offered	_____	_____
22. Bereavement care plan initiated	_____	_____

Courtesy of Hospice of Portage County, Inc., Stevens Point, Wisconsin.

Exhibit 23–8 Inpatient/Respite Admission Checklist

Patient Name: _____   Date of Admission: _____

Date of Discharge: _____

Criteria To Be Checked	Performed at Time of Admission (Initial and Date)	Performed at Time of Discharge (Initial and Date)
1. Rationale for inpatient/respite documented in nurse's notes.		N.A.
2. Physician order obtained for inpatient/respite status (should be written on telephone order form).		N.A.
3. Documented in nurse's notes that Hospice RN called report to floor and that code status was relayed.		N.A.
4. Call inpatient admitting and inform them that a hospice patient is coming, either inpatient or respite.		N.A.
5. Call DME, Volunteers, Pastors, and HHA if necessary to inform them of inpatient status.		N.A.
6. Update patient's POC at time of admission and photocopy for admitting facility. Also photocopy current medication list, admission assessment, and last nursing visit. (These should be received by admitting facility within 8 hours of admission—either in person or faxed.)		N.A.
7. Primary RN or designee will visit patient daily and document on inpatient progress notes. RN will also check POC daily to ensure its completeness and that only one POC exists.	N.A.	
8. RN will monitor any test, medication changes, or procedures and document knowledge and concurrence of these changes.	N.A.	
9. For sites other than St. Agnes, a copy will be made of the inpatient/respite sites chart, and this will become part of the hospice record.	N.A.	
10. Assistant director reviews chart, writes and notes noncompliance, reviews with primary nurse, and documents. Assistant Director Evaluating:	Comments:	

Note: POC = Plan of Care.

Courtesy of St. Agnes Hospital Hospice, Fond du Lac, Wisconsin.

Exhibit 23–9 Family Satisfaction Survey

Family Satisfaction Survey

Please indicate the response which best represents your satisfaction with the hospice services you and your family received. Please add any comments on the back of this page. Thank you.

Based on the care your family received, would you recommend hospice services to others?	Yes	No
Were you given a clear explanation of what services were available through hospice and how to access them?	Yes	No
Did your hospice provide you with adequate information about "advance directives" like the living will?	Yes	No

1. How satisfied were you with the patient's pain control after admission to hospice?

Very dissatisfied	Dissatisfied	Neutral	Satisfied	Very satisfied
1	2	3	4	5

2. How satisfied were you with control of the patient's other symptoms after admission to hospice?

Very dissatisfied	Dissatisfied	Neutral	Satisfied	Very satisfied
1	2	3	4	5

3. How satisfied were you with the education and training you received on caring for your family member?

Very dissatisfied	Dissatisfied	Neutral	Satisfied	Very satisfied
1	2	3	4	5

4. If you contacted the evening or week-end on-call service, how satisfied were you with the response?

Very dissatisfied	Dissatisfied	Neutral	Satisfied	Very satisfied
1	2	3	4	5

5. How satisfied were you with hospice's efforts to help manage your stress and anxiety during the illness of your family member?

Very dissatisfied	Dissatisfied	Neutral	Satisfied	Very satisfied
1	2	3	4	5

6. How satisfied were you with hospice's efforts to assist you with spiritual concerns?

Very dissatisfied	Dissatisfied	Neutral	Satisfied	Very satisfied
1	2	3	4	5

7. Were you satisfied that the patient was referred to hospice at the appropriate time during the course of the terminal illness?

Very dissatisfied	Dissatisfied	Neutral	Satisfied	Very satisfied
1	2	3	4	5

continues

Exhibit 23–9 continued

8. How satisfied were you with the hospice's efforts to support the patient's quality of life?				
Very dissatisfied	Dissatisfied	Neutral	Satisfied	Very satisfied
1	2	3	4	5

If there was one thing hospice could do better, what would it be?

Comments

Patient Information

How long received hospice services (circle one):	<1 month	1 to 3 months	3 to 6 months	6 to 9 months	9 to 12 months	> 1 year

Diagnosis (circle one):
Cancer   AIDS   Alzheimer's   Heart Disease Lung   Other:

Age: **Sex: M   F**

Race (Circle one):
African-American   Hispanic   Asian   Native American   Caucasian   Other:

Courtesy of Hospice of Portage County, Inc., Stevens Point, Wisconsin.

Exhibit 23–10 Family Evaluation Form

Family Evaluation Form		
1. The philosophy of Hospice is to promote comfort to the extent possible for the dying person and family. Was this accomplished in the following areas:		
Pain management	Yes	No
Physical	Yes	No
Emotional issues	Yes	No
Spiritual dimension	Yes	No
If no, what symptom or concern do you feel was not addressed?		
2. Hospice staff and volunteers believe that care given should respect your wishes, beliefs, and values. Do you feel these needs were respected?	**Yes**	**No**
If no, please explain		
3. Effective communication between you and the Hospice staff is essential to providing Hospice care. Do you feel there was good communication?	**Yes**	**No**
If no, please explain		
Please identify any other areas for improvement that would assist us in the provision of Hospice care.		
Signature:		
Relationship:	Date:	

Courtesy of Hospice of Portage County, Inc., Stevens Point, Wisconsin.

Exhibit 23–11 Hospice Hope Survey

We would like to learn what you think about Hospice services and how you think they could be improved. Please answer the following questions, writing detailed comments or suggestions wherever you want. If you do not write your name on the questionnaire, your answers will remain anonymous.

Please circle the letter that best expresses your evaluation of the care provided by our staff. The grades you choose from are based on the same principle as grading systems used in school. "A" is the best grade and "C" is the worst mark. Your comments and suggestions will enable us to improve the quality of care we provide in the coming years. Mail your completed questionnaire in the enclosed, stamped, self-addressed envelope. Thank you for your time interest in completing this promptly and returning it to our office.

1. Physical care — comfort measures; skin, bowel, and bladder care.   A   B   C   NA
   Comments: _____
   _____

2. Pain and symptom control — use of appropriate medications; response to input   A   B   C   NA
   from the patient and family members; interventions with physicians; general
   comfort of the patient.
   Comments: _____
   _____

3. Emotional support — listening to concerns of patient and family members; taking   A   B   C   NA
   necessary action when possible; assisting family unit with variety of emotions
   expressed.
   Comments: _____
   _____

4. Spiritual care — a willingness to discuss questions regarding the meaning and   A   B   C   NA
   purpose of life, if desired, or assistance in coordinating visits by church leader or
   chaplain.
   Comments: _____
   _____

5. Financial issues — adequate direction given when requested regarding insurance   A   B   C   NA
   coverage, financial concerns, SSI, legal issues.
   Comments: _____
   _____

6. Volunteer assistance — volunteers, when provided, give adequate support and   A   B   C   NA
   assistance.
   Comments: _____
   _____

7. Involvement at the time of death — visits or telephone calls to family members;   A   B   C   NA
   presence at wake or funeral.
   Comments: _____
   _____

continues

Exhibit 23–11 continued

8. Contact after death — bereavement care.   A   B   C   NA
   Comments: _____

   _____

9. Suggestions for improvement: _____

   _____

Sign only if you wish: _____

Courtesy of St. Agnes Hospital Hospice, Fond du Lac, Wisconsin.

Exhibit 23–12 Physician Assessment Form

Physician Assessment Form

Patient:

1. Was the initial referral handled smoothly?	Yes	No	Unknown
Comments:			

2. Did the Hospice Nurse Coordinator keep you informed of the patient's condition on a regular basis?	Yes	No	Unknown
Comments:			

3. How was the care in the following areas?	Good	Satisfactory	Poor
Pain control			
Technical nursing care			
Emotional support			
Patient/family education			
Use of community resources			

4. Please comment on the following:

Positive aspects of the program

Suggestions for program change

Physician:

Date:

Courtesy of Hospice of Portage County, Inc., Stevens Point, Wisconsin.

Exhibit 23–13 A Closure Summary

CLOSURE SUMMARY

Date: _____   Record Number _____

[Three RNs, a social worker, a home health aide, a bereavement coordinator, a volunteer coordinator, and a volunteer]

Overall assessment or impression of care from friends, family, staff:

Daughter expressed appreciation of the care her father received to different team members. Memorials were donated to hospice.

2. IDT Evaluation of:

Assessment

It was appropriate.

Implementation

No problems with care plan implementation as far as primary caregiver (PCG) and hospice staff concerned. It was difficult dealing with opposing family members. PCG was unable to trust that brothers or sister would come when they said they would and give her a break.

Dimensions of Care:

Physical symptoms

Antihistamine helped relieve itching and made it easier for patient to sleep at night. Lift chair helped to keep feet elevated, decrease edema, and increase comfort. Pain was managed with a low dose of long acting morphine.

Psycho-social

Social worker provided ongoing counseling to family who had difficulty resolving conflict. Problems were complicated by son's alcohol problem.

Spiritual

Hospice chaplain provided spiritual support appropriate to patient and primary caregiver's wishes.

Staffing

Home health aide helped with bath three days a week. A volunteer visited twice a week and provided respite to primary caregiver.

Communication

Family had functional problems that were exacerbated when father became ill. Social worker helped to keep focus on patient's needs and wishes.

Continuity of Care

Good.

Documentation

Complete.

In-Patient Care

Not appropriate. Patient remained at home.

3. Stress management for staff and ideas/solutions to alter situation in next similar case:

Have two staff respond to call at time of death in situations where staff safety may be a concern.

4. Recommendations to QA for changes:

Establish crisis protocol for situations where there is a great deal of family discord. Write care plan for death event when family issues are more complicated and increased tension likely to cause problems.

Courtesy of Hospice of Portage County, Inc., Stevens Point, Wisconsin.

CONCLUSION

As the elderly population increases, we can expect a growing interest in the use of hospice services to provide more control for patients and improve the end-of-life experience for the patient and family. The National Hospice Origination (1996) reported that nationwide, nearly 15% of the 1.5 million Americans who died form illness or disease received hospice services; 45% of these in Florida, reflecting the high concentration of elderly there.

Lash and Dunn (1996) stated that hospice cost savings come from changing the service model from intermittent delivery of need for high-cost inpatient and home care services to a lower-acuity care plan by avoiding unnecessary medical costs. By providing interdisciplinary clinical, social, and mental health services such as in-home personal care; pain management, including pharmacy services; education and counseling; crisis management, including 24-hour access to the hospice team; and bereavement counseling, integrating hospice services into the health care continuum will help patients and families achieve quality of life benefits during the last 6 months of life.

REFERENCES

Joint Commission on Accreditation of Healthcare Organizations. (1996). *1997–1998 Comprehensive accreditation manual for home care.* Oakbrook Terrace, IL: Author.

Lash, B., & Dunn, S. (1996). The growth of hospice services in a managed care environment. *The Remington Report, 4*(4), 28–32.

National Hospice Organization. (1994). *The basics of hospice.* Arlington, VA: Author.

National Hospice Organization Annual Report DATA 1994–1995. (1996). Arlington, VA: Author.

Wisconsin Department of Health and Social Services. *Quality assurance.* HSS 131.37. Author.

SUGGESTED READING

Siebold, C. (1992). *The hospice movement: Easing death's pains.* New York: Twayne.

## CHAPTER 24

Improving Quality in Integrated Health Care Systems

Kathryn L. Clark and Allen Nottingham

CHAPTER OBJECTIVES

After completing this chapter, the reader will be able to

- define the concept of integrated delivery systems (IDSs)
- describe the differences between a vertically integrated system and a horizontally integrated system
- identify challenges for developing a quality improvement program in IDSs
- draft a performance improvement plan for an IDS

Integrating the concept of quality into health care systems presents an exciting and challenging opportunity for health care leaders of today and tomorrow. With the rapid changes occurring in health care today, leaders are challenged to make certain that quality of care is of utmost importance during the redesign of institutions, models of care delivery, and contracted relationships of various service vendors and systems. Although integrated systems are able to achieve higher levels of patient care with lowered costs, they must be cautious in responding to change too quickly because of the risk of losing the element of quality in the process (Coddington, Moore, & Fischer, 1994).

The purpose of this chapter is to describe how quality may be incorporated into the strategic planning of health care institutions striving to become integrated with other providers of care. Maintenance of quality within the developing integrated system will also be discussed. Through a review of the literature, personal communications with experts and practitioners, and our own experiences in the fields of quality and health care systems, strategies for planning and implementation of quality within integrated health care systems will be presented.

Jargon related to quality in health care is varied and often confusing. The terms *quality improvement, total quality management*, and *continuous quality improvement* may be used to reflect clinical and management efforts to assess and improve current patient care delivery practices and performance of services. For the purposes of this chapter, quality improvement (QI) will refer to selected techniques, strategies, tools, and methods used in an organization to monitor and improve the spectrum of quality processes.

QUALITY IMPROVEMENT

Institutions may invest in QI for a variety of reasons, including accreditation requirements, cost control, improving/maintaining community reputation, pressure from payers, and belief in a QI philosophy. Rationale for and commitment to QI will vary by institution and will be influenced by the institution's mission and vision statements.

As a management philosophy and management method, QI has distinguishing characteristics and functions, which include

1. empowering clinicians and managers to analyze and improve current quality processes
2. adopting a philosophy that customer preferences determine quality of services and processes
3. incorporating a multidisciplinary approach
4. motivating individuals for a cooperative approach based upon data and rationale (McLaughlin & Kaluzny, 1994)

With the implementation of quality processes within an organization to improve services, personnel become motivated and more involved in identifying current practices and services and providing solutions. Problems, or areas of needed improvement, are not owned by an individual or a single department but rather by multiple players within the organization. Thus a multidisciplinary approach removes the "blame" and focuses the QI team upon the identified problem, not specific personnel involved. Several teams may be involved in the process, especially when multiple departments or institutions are integrated.

INTEGRATED DELIVERY SYSTEMS

Integrated delivery systems (IDSs), or integrated health care systems, are partnerships between hospitals, physicians, and health plans to provide the complete spectrum of medical services for customers (Beckham, 1993). The challenge is to do so while managing the cost, quality, and accessibility of care. Capitation, direct contracting, and risk assumption will be the groundwork for such systems or alliances.

IDSs may or may not be multihospital systems. Some will own their facilities or employ physicians or physician groups; others will form a cooperative partnership or network driven by a shared vision and collaboration for

improvement of current methods of providing care for customers (Coile, 1994). Health care will be streamlined, organized, and "seamless."

Integration may be vertical or horizontal. Concise definitions of vertical and horizontal integration may vary greatly depending upon the players involved and the philosophies and functioning of each IDS.

Vertical integration within a unit, department, or health care institution or region realigns resources and services upstream or downstream. Duplication, costs, and personnel may be reduced in an effort to provide more efficient services and management. Vertical integration implies efforts among organizations or institutions to improve access to health care. For example, several institutions or health clinics providing similar services may integrate to reduce duplication of services and begin "sharing" resources, while maintaining autonomy of practice.

Horizontal integration involves partnerships across similar institutions and services. The relationship stresses partnership, not ownership. Hospitals, physicians, and health plans operate under common management and financial incentives to coordinate needs of payers and patients with available resources. Organizations that are considered to be horizontally integrated are interested primarily in reducing costs. Hospitals associated with Volunteer Hospitals of America (VHA) have been able to reduce costs through contracting with specific vendors. Massive sales translate into reduced costs of doing business while maintaining operations and services.

HISTORICAL PERSPECTIVE

Although integration in health care has only recently gained recognition as a model for the future, the organizational concept began in the business sector. DuPont Chandler, the historian of business at the Harvard Business School, wrote in 1962 how successful retail and manufacturing firms dominated their respective industries through realignment of the organization and integration of suppliers and distributors.

Large integrated firms, like General Motors, Standard Oil, and General Electric, acquired competing firms and integrated suppliers and distributors into the organization. Middlemen and their profits were incorporated, providing transport systems and raw materials at reduced costs. Integrated firms had the advantage over their less-integrated competition through coordination of production and marketing and domination of their respective industries (Goldsmith, 1994).

An early example of an integrated system in a health care system existed in Oklahoma in 1971. Columbia Presbyterian Hospital in Oklahoma City began a remote cardiac monitoring (RCM) network of rural hospitals throughout Oklahoma linked to Columbia Presbyterian through dedicated telephone lines (see Figure 24–1). RCM allows the transmission of rural patients' cardiac rhythms to the central monitoring unit (CMU) of Presbyterian for continuous interpretation and analysis. Data and voice can be transmitted simultaneously, thus allowing observation of rhythms and communication between the CMU and RCM personnel (Nottingham & Camp, 1987). The network grew primarily through word of mouth as rural hospitals recognized the need for improved cardiac care and were financially able to adopt the service.

In the late 1970s, vertically integrated systems evolved in health care. Kaiser and other group health cooperatives experienced rapid growth due to the integration of finances and delivery services. Large, investor-owned hospital systems purchased smaller, independent hospitals. Rush-Presbyterian-St. Luke's Health System in Chicago served as an example of a vertically integrated health system with an academic health center, a network of regional hospitals, a prepaid health plan, an inner-city community health center system, and private practitioners (Beckham, 1993).

Currently, multiple IDSs are growing through the influence of managed-care principles and practices. Successful systems are visionary risk takers that provide the opportunity and incentives for participation, peer communication, and education (Brown & Mayer, 1996; Durbin, Haglund, & Dowling, 1993).

The vertically integrated system of Columbia/HCA Healthcare Corporation has developed nationwide with careful consideration of unique services and areas of expertise within each Columbia organization. Currently, the Columbia network includes 343 hospitals and related service centers, 135 ambulatory surgery centers, and 200 home health agencies (Columbia/HCA Healthcare Corporation, 1995). Centers of Excellence have been recognized that allow the patient to move within the Columbia network in a more "seamless" fashion. Patients requiring heart or bone marrow transplantation, for example, may be transferred to a Columbia hospital with recognized expertise in those treatment modalities, along with all data information. Transportation and lodging costs for family members are recognized and financially supported. Duplication of processes is reduced while maintaining continuity of care.

The Oklahoma Division of Columbia/HCA Healthcare Corporation includes urban, suburban, and rural hospitals, specialty hospitals, surgicare centers, urgent care centers, senior health centers, and a physician practice management group (see Figure 24–2). Providing quality throughout such a diverse group of members requires a thorough understanding of each institution's operational definition of quality and its preferred monitoring practices for evaluation and improvements of services provided.

With the rapidly growing challenges in health care, attention to quality is critical for the success of the system and the provision of appropriate patient care. Values of the organizational philosophy will help attain efficiency and quality in the integrated system. Organizational quality may be enhanced through double-loop

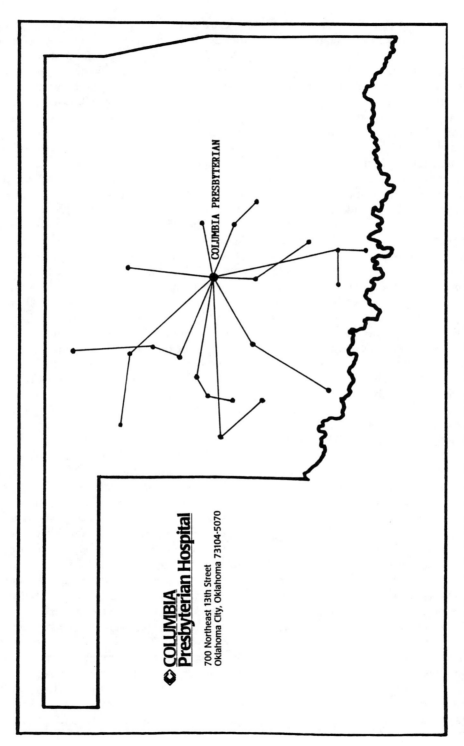

Figure 24–1 Presbyterian's Remote Cardiac Monitoring Network in the late 1980s. Courtesy of Columbia Presbyterian Hospital, Remote Cardiac Monitoring Department, Oklahoma City, Oklahoma.

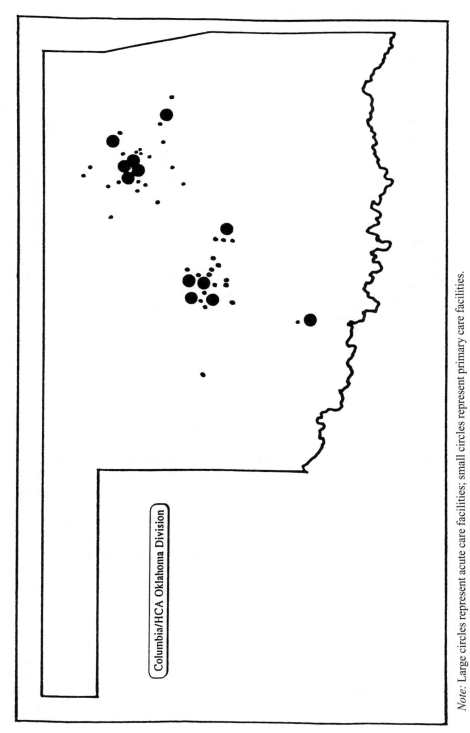

Note: Large circles represent acute care facilities; small circles represent primary care facilities.

Figure 24-2 Integrated Delivery System of the Oklahoma Division of Columbia/HCA Healthcare Corporation, 1996. Courtesy of Columbia/HCA Healthcare Corp., Oklahoma Division, 1996.

learning, the examination of the quality of QI (Elliott, 1996).

QUALITY IMPROVEMENT IN IDSs

Hospitals, physicians, and health care plans are working diligently to provide appropriate care with limited resources and to do so with the quality that Americans have come to expect of health care providers. Beckham (1993) argued that quality defined from the customer's perspective must be actively and accurately determined, not assumed.

No matter what type of integration is used, long-term success will be determined by the QI programs throughout the system. In fact, increasing numbers of payers are awarding contracts to providers that focus upon clinical quality. Both concepts must be based upon a vision statement that is understood and supported by all members of the system. The characteristics of both integration and QI include a customer focus upon service and access, empowerment of the provider, a multidisciplinary approach, and cooperation of facilities and staff (see Exhibit 24–1).

Although organizations may be able to define their mission and vision statements for marketing purposes, operational definitions provide supportive data of the organization's true belief in what is seen as the purpose and vision for the future of the organization, employees, and customers. Thus QI is not merely

---

Exhibit 24–1 Characteristics Shared by Integrated Delivery Systems and the Quality Improvement Philosophy

Characteristics Shared by IDSs and QI:
• Customer Focus
• Empowerment of Staff
• Multidisciplinary Approach
• Cooperation and Collaboration

displayed in brochures, manuals, and readily visible framings but rather is seen in the operation of the organization and its success.

Developing the Environment

IDSs function as organizations with supportive goals and strategic planning. To direct energies of the organizations and employees toward innovation and success, cultures of the various institutions must be analyzed for unique and comparable beliefs, values, and assumptions.

Organizational cultures are grounded in history and tradition and reflect what is truly important to the organization, as well as individual employees. Organizations considering integration must recognize the cultures that are to be "combined" and determine if sufficient compatibilities exist to foster success. Integration will not flourish if the environment of the delivery system does not facilitate collaboration and teamwork in developing QI programs system-wide.

Communication across the system promotes cooperation and an open environment supportive of needed change. Leaders at all levels of the organization remain a strong driving force of system communication. Input from employees, especially regarding quality issues, must be encouraged and valued.

Successful integration systems believe in participation at all levels of the organization and a team-based approach to management. Energies of cross-functional and cross-divisional teams may be quite successful in solving organizational problems. But team members must be empowered to make necessary decisions and recommendations for problem resolution and improvement in the system.

Challenges for Implementation

Challenges for developing QI in an integrated system are often due to lack of established standards or protocols for each respective organizational component of the system. A functional QI program within the IDS requires standards or protocols that are appropriate for every member organization. Cross-functional and cross-divisional work teams are excellent resources for developing and implementing standards or protocols.

Accreditation standards have been developed by the Joint Commission on Accreditation of Healthcare Organizations (Joint Commission),

the National Committee for Quality Assurance (NCQA), and the Accreditation Association for Ambulatory Health Care (AAAHC) (Kedrowski, 1995). Yet these standards may be service specific, not IDS specific, and may need to be adapted by each IDS for better utilization. See Exhibit 24–2 for an example of a medical quality plan based upon Joint Commission standards.

Exhibit 24–2 Medical Quality Plan Based upon Joint Commission Standards

---

COLUMBIA PRESBYTERIAN HOSPITAL - OKC
PERFORMANCE IMPROVEMENT PLAN
Primary Care Providers, Family Practice Clinics

1.0 PURPOSE

The primary purpose of the Performance Improvement Plan is to study and improve patient outcomes. The performance of patient care is evaluated for patients in specific age groups who are diagnosed and treated by the primary care providers in the family practice facilities. This evaluation will be accomplished by:

1.1 Organizing performance improvement activities of the primary care providers around specific patient care groups who are high risk, high volume, and problem prone.

1.2 Evaluating individual performance regarding medical diagnosis, treatment planning, and patient outcomes.

1.3 Coordinating and integrating efforts to improve patient outcomes with other individuals involved in the process of providing patient care.

2.0 RESPONSIBILITY FOR QUALITY CARE

The Medical Director of the employed family practice providers is accountable for directing the Quality Plan activities for the department in accordance with regulatory and accrediting standards, and acts as the Quality Plan Coordinator. The Medical Director or a designee is responsible for identifying indicators, collecting data, evaluating data, and assisting in the development of actions to address identified problems or concerns.

The ultimate responsibility for the quality of patient care rests with the Board of Trustees who receives reports from the hospital's Vice President of Medical Staff Services.

3.0 SCOPE OF CARE AND SERVICES

Primary care services are provided in an ambulatory setting by licensed family practice physicians, physician assistants, and nurse practitioners employed by Columbia Presbyterian. Patients include newborn through adult, and services include assessment, diagnostic testing, treatment planning, medical intervention, and patient education. Minor procedures which may be performed in the ambulatory setting include circumcisions, flexible sigmoidoscopies, repair of lacerations, and vasectomies.

4.0 APPROACH

4.1 An assessment is conducted of the accrediting and regulatory standards, and of the high risk/high volume/problem prone patients. From that assessment, identification is made of processes needing improvement.

continues

Exhibit 24–2 continued

        4.1.1 Selecting appropriate medications, based on diagnosis and cost.

        4.1.2 Providing continuing education for the employed family practice provider, augmented when possible by the results of performance improvement activities.

        4.1.3 Assessing and diagnosing patients.

        4.1.4 Providing appropriate medical interventions.

        4.1.5 Planning medical care.

        4.1.6 Coordinating follow-up care/making indicated referrals.

        4.1.7 Educating patients and significant others.

        4.1.8 Dating/timing entries in the medical record.

        4.1.9 Managing high risk/high volume/problem prone patients such as:

                4.1.9.1 Pediatric patients with otitis media.

                4.1.9.2 Chest pain patients.

                4.1.9.3 Patients admitted to an acute care facility within one week of being seen in the family practice facility.

                4.1.9.4 Diabetics on insulin.

4.2 Dimensions of performance will be identified for each of the processes (4.1.1 through 4.1.8). Those dimensions will include at least one of the following: efficacy, appropriateness, availability, timeliness, effectiveness, continuity, safety, efficiency, and respect/caring.

For each of the patient groups (4.1.9), concurrent and/or retrospective chart review will be performed by a reviewer to evaluate:

        4.2.1 Appropriate diagnosis based on the assessment.

        4.2.2 Appropriateness of the treatment plan based on the diagnosis.

        4.2.3 Continuity of care when referrals are part of the treatment plan.

        4.2.4 Other more specific criteria to be identified.

4.3 Data collection plan: Approaches to collect data are being evaluated. Currently a contracted reviewer gathers physician specific data that are then evaluated by the Medical Director. This will need to be expanded upon in order to trend data according to patient groups. Under consideration is an automated data collection plan.

4.4 Assessment: The collected data on processes will be interpreted using Quality Improvement statistical methods. An understanding of variation will be incorporated into the data assessment. The collected data on the patient group will be interpreted by the family practice provider group and utilized to improve care.

4.5 Actions to Improve: If the evaluation of the data identified an opportunity for improvement, actions will be recommended and taken. Attempts to improve the process with the PCDA cycle will be implemented. The findings from the concurrent and retrospective chart reviews will be incorporated into peer review and into continuing education opportunities for the providers.

4.6 Assess the actions and maintain the gain: Whether the actions actually improve care or services will be determined, and further evaluation and action will be initiated.

4.7 Communicate results to relevant individuals and groups: In the periodic meetings of the family practice provider group, findings will be discussed. In addition, quarterly status reports regarding findings will be forwarded to the Vice President of Medical Staff Services, who will report appropriate findings to the Board of Trustees.

5.0 FOCUS OF PLAN

An emphasis is placed upon the improvement of processes that affect the care of patients. Judgments about quality from patients will be incorporated into improvement efforts. Collab-

continues

Exhibit 24–2 continued

oration and interdisciplinary work will be accomplished by working with other staff involved in the care of patients.

6.0 ANNUAL PROGRAM APPRAISAL

The objectives, scope, organization, and effectiveness of the Performance Improvement Plan will be evaluated annually and revised as necessary. Emphasis will be placed on areas monitored and evaluated, problems/opportunities for improvement that are identified, success of actions taken, and improvement made in patient care. This will be written and retained with the department's quality records.

7.0 SIGNATURES

_____   _____
V.P. Medical Staff Services /Date   Medical Director, Family Practice

---

COLUMBIA PRESBYTERIAN - OKC
Family Practice Medical Quality

Action Plan

The following diagram demonstrates the reporting relationship of the Family Practice Medical Quality Improvement Committee to the Board of Trustees of the hospital and demonstrates how the quality findings are used to improve care:

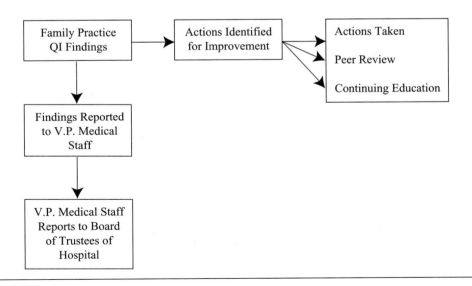

continues

Exhibit 24–2 continued

COLUMBIA PRESBYTERIAN - OKC

Quality Improvement Effort Status Report

Department/Clinic Reporting: _____

Process Improving: _____

Instructions: Enter activities, referring to FOCUS-PDCA stages; attach relevant data, flowcharts, plans
since last report. Sign after last entry.

Month/Year	Narrative

continues

Exhibit 24–2 continued

COLUMBIA PRESBYTERIAN - OKC

Quality Report

Process: _____   Department/Clinic: _____
_____   Signature: _____

Dimension of Performance: _____   Month/Year: _____

Indicator	Threshold Act./Exp	Evaluation of Findings	Actions Taken	Follow-up Plan

Courtesy of Columbia Presbyterian Hospital, Columbia Practice Management Department, Oklahoma City, Oklahoma.

Normative and summative evaluations may be helpful in determining appropriateness of used quality monitoring tools and use of outcomes data. Use of comparable monitoring tools by each component member of the health care system will provide accurate collection of data and subsequent relevance as a means of improving quality. Input from involved institutions, units, and/or services will support a more functional monitoring tool and encourage individual involvement in the QI process.

Vision, operational definitions of quality, current practices, and multidisciplinary involvement will foster the development of QI programs designed to advance clinical practices and the health care system as a whole. Timely feedback from the evaluation process demonstrates usefulness of the program and the critical importance of the clinical practitioner in providing continuously monitored, quality patient care and services (Elliott, 1996). Rapid reporting mechanisms enhance the opportunity to incorporate needed change. Outcomes data supported with current research further provide the incentives for change and improvement considerations.

Henry Ford Health System (HFHS) in Detroit is an excellent example of an integrated health system that has used QI as a business strategy. HFHS has evolved into a system that includes a tertiary hospital, four community hospitals, two medical groups with a total of 920 physicians, 35 ambulatory care satellites, a health maintenance organization (HMO), and nursing homes and home health care agencies. On the basis of the Deming/Shewhart cycle for continuous improvement, HFHS uses customer feedback in each cycle of its strategic planning and has developed a process of raising and resolving systemwide issues at the system level and at the operating level. Thus its strategic plan for QI facilitates communication system-wide and fosters innovation, teamwork, and evaluation throughout the process (Sahney & Warden, 1993; Young, Ward, & McCarthy, 1994).

Columbia Presbyterian Hospital in Oklahoma City incorporated QI in the initial development of RCM. Ongoing education through team conferences has provided opportunities for nurses and physicians from the rural hospitals and Presbyterian to identify problems or concerns regarding the system and to propose methods for improvement. Service, education, and equipment are adapted to meet the changing needs of the rural hospital (see Exhibit 24–3). Chart audits are used to determine accuracy of cardiac rhythm interpretation, to determine appropriateness of clinical consultations, and to identify actual/potential problems in communication (see Exhibit 24–4). Education, communication, feedback, and vision promote QI and continued success of the program.

CHALLENGES FOR INTEGRATION

QI is a critical element of success for IDSs, and everything that QI offers is a requirement for success. Vision statements must be clearly articulated. Organizational cultures require thorough assessments and incorporation into the mission of the IDS. Team work groups must be empowered to make necessary decisions and to do so with urgency and optimism (Griffith, 1995).

Quality is an attitude, a philosophy that must be pervasive throughout the IDS. Innovative, flexible IDSs will succeed in their ability to meet the demands for quality mandated by the customer while improving processes throughout the organization. The real challenge lies in the ability to do so in a cost-effective, streamlined, and "seamless" system designed to meet the demands of managed care and health care reform while providing the quality of care expected by the consumer. Leaders must be risk takers, motivators, and visionaries, for QI is not a means to an end but a continuous journey toward improving processes, reducing variation, and increasing performance.

Exhibit 24–3 Tool Used for Documentation of Education Resulting from QI Findings.

◆ COLUMBIA
Presbyterian Hospital

700 Northeast 13th Street
Oklahoma City, Oklahoma 73104-5070

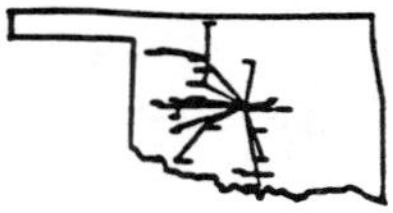

EDUCATION ACTIVITY REPORT

ACTIVITY INFORMATION: **PARTICIPATION:**

Location _____   Nursing _____

Date _____   Physician _____

Type _____   Other _____

  I. Topic Presented:

 II. Speaker:

III. Purpose:

 IV. Objectives:

 V. Methodology:

VI. Evaluation:

VII. Comments:

Courtesy of Columbia Presbyterian Hospital, Remote Cardiac Monitoring Department, Oklahoma City, Oklahoma.

Exhibit 24–4 Tool Used To Gather QI Data Regarding Cardiac Rhythm Interpretation and Recommendations for Follow-up.

```
                    REMOTE CARDIAC SERVICES
                      Chart Audit Tool


    Remote Monitoring Units ═══════════════════════════════

    Date     _____


    Number of Charts Audited     _____

    Number of Rhythm Strips Audited    _____

    Number of Correct Interpretations    _____

    Misinterpreted Rhythms    _____

              _____

              _____




    In-House ═══════════════════════════════════════════════

    Date     _____


    Number of Charts Audited     _____

    Number of Rhythm Strips Audited    _____

    Number of Correct Interpretations    _____

    Misinterpreted Rhythms    _____

              _____

              _____



    Recommendations    _____

              _____

              _____
```

Courtesy of Columbia Presbyterian Hospital, Remote Cardiac Monitoring Department, Oklahoma City, Oklahoma.

REFERENCES

Beckham, J.D. (1993). The architecture of integration. *Healthcare Forum Journal, 36*(5), 56–63.

Brown, H.P., & Mayer, T. (1996, May/June). Physicians and hospitals: New partnerships. *Health Systems Review,* 35–37.

Chandler, D. (1962). *Strategy and structure: Chapters in the history of the American industrial enterprise.* Boston: MIT Press.

Coddington, D.C., Moore, K.D., & Fischer, E.A. (1994). In pursuit of integration. *Healthcare Forum Journal, 37*(2), 53–56.

Coile, R.C. (1994). Guiding the integrated delivery network. *Healthcare Forum Journal, 37*(6), 16–23.

Columbia/HCA Healthcare Corporation. (1995). *1995 annual report.* Nashville, TN: Author.

Durbin, S., Haglund, C., & Dowling, W. (1993). Integrating strategic planning and quality management in a multi-institutional system. *Quality Management in Health Care, 1*(4), 24–34.

Elliott, R.L. (1996). Double loop learning and the quality of quality improvement. *Journal on Quality Improvement, 22*(1), 59–66.

Goldsmith, J.C. (1994). The illusive logic of integration. *Healthcare Forum Journal, 37*(5), 26–31.

Griffith, J.R. (1995, May/June). The infrastructure of integrated delivery systems. *Healthcare Executive,* 12–17.

Kedrowski, S.M. (1995). Quality improvement: Is there common ground in accreditation programs? *AAACN Viewpoint, 17*(6), 6.

McLaughlin, C.P., & Kaluzny, A.R. (1994). Defining total quality management/continuous quality improvement. *Continuous quality improvement in health care: Theory, implementation, and applications.* Gaithersburg, MD: Aspen.

Nottingham, A., & Camp, V. (1987). Remote cardiac monitoring: Nursing collaboration is the key. *Dimensions of Critical Care Nursing, 6*(3), 176–180.

Sahney, V.K., & Warden, G.L. (1993). The role of CQI in the strategic planning process. *Quality Management in Health Care, 1*(4), 1–11.

Young, M.J., Ward, R., & McCarthy, B. (1994). Continuously improving primary care. *Joint Commission Journal on Quality Improvement, 20*(3), 120–126.

## CHAPTER 25

Improving Quality in Long-Term Care

Mary E. Cohan and Sandra M. Mareno

CHAPTER OBJECTIVES

After completing this chapter, the reader will be able to

- identify the essential components for developing a quality improvement program
- design a quality improvement plan for a long-term care facility
- define key clinical and administrative indicators
- describe a quality improvement team's use of continuous quality improvement tools (flowchart, fishbone diagram, and force field analysis of various products) to improve the quality of wound and skin care.

Comprehensive quality improvement (QI) programs in health care were first developed for acute care hospitals. As nursing home regulation has moved away from minimal standards toward a more comprehensive and proactive view of QI, many of the methods developed in the acute care setting have been successfully applied to long-term care. The differences in philosophy and patient population need to be kept in mind when developing a QI program. In the acute care setting, the emphasis is on quality of health care and on an episode of care. In the long-term care setting, quality of life and residents' rights compound the quality of health care issues. Any given nursing home may serve both long-stay residents and short-stay residents with either restorative or termi-

nal care goals. Long-term care facilities provide both medical care and personal care. The typical resident is a frail elderly person who has a number of chronic medical conditions with periodic superimposed acute illnesses. Thus the focus of QI is shifted from a defined episode of care and toward ongoing monitoring and evaluation of physical, functional, and psychosocial indicators.

Nursing homes must abide by both state and federal standards. The Omnibus Budget Reconciliation Act (OBRA) of 1987 required formal QI programs to be a part of nursing home care as of October 1990 (Department of Health and Human Services, 1989). A QI committee must meet at least quarterly. The OBRA standards are also a source for key indicators to be monitored. More long-term care facilities, particularly those with subacute care units, are seeking additional accreditation from the Joint Commission on Accreditation of Healthcare Organizations (Joint Commission). The Joint Commission (1996) specifically addressed management's responsibility to provide leadership, support, and resources for an ongoing QI program. They require that processes most important to resident outcomes be continuously and systematically assessed and improved. Demonstration of an effective QI program is an important piece of the survey process. Much of the shift from traditional quality assurance to QI in the long-term care industry has occurred since 1990.

QUALITY PLAN

Development of a QI program begins with support and leadership from the governing body. In small long-term care facilities that do not have a board of directors, this initiating role may be fulfilled by the chief executive officer (CEO) or administrator. Some of the initial steps involved in developing a quality plan are listed below.

1. Define the mission statement and goals of the organization. The mission statement of the organization forms the basis for the QI program. The goals of long-term care are (1) to restore and maintain function, (2) to maximize quality of life, (3) to support residents' rights and autonomy, and (4) to provide comfort and dignity to the dying.

2. Define quality service. Quality can be defined as the provision of service that consistently meets or exceeds the sponsoring group's mission, professional standards, and customer expectations. Each facility needs its own working definition of quality based on its mission statement.

3. Educate management and staff about the QI process. Education cannot be overemphasized. A quality advisor should be appointed to coordinate the QI program and educational efforts. In many long-term care facilities, the infection control nurse or education coordinator will take on this role part time. Larger organizations with more than one facility or multiple levels of care may need a full-time quality advisor. Initially, all managers should receive training in the QI process, and a standard language and format should be adopted for team use. Generally, this training will be done by an outside consultant or at an off-campus seminar. These managers may then assist in training other employees, and eventually the training will become a part of employee orientation and continuing education. Each time a cross-functional team is chartered, more intense training is required.

4. Identify products and services. In general, long-term care provides medical and personal care for frail elderly persons. The list of products and services provided by a given facility will be more inclusive. For example, a long-term care facility may provide therapeutic services such as physical, occupational, and speech therapy; housing; an accessible environment; education; and support services. Each department also needs to identify the products and/or services that it provides.

5. Identify customers. The direct customers for the long-term care facility may be the residents, family members, and significant others, but the more indirect customers may include the local community, attending physicians, employees, and payer sources.

6. Identify the core processes involved in providing long-term care. Defining the core processes allows one to cross department lines and to view care provision as multidisciplinary. The core processes involved in long-term care are

- Admitting Process
- Assessment Process
- Care Planning Process
- Care Provider Process
- Evaluation Process
- Discharge Process

7. Develop ways to identify areas for improvement. Surveys of internal and external customers can provide valuable information. Most long-term care facilities have a formal venue for voicing and responding to concerns from external customers. State ombudsmen act as resident advocates and follow up on complaints. In addition, suggestion boards, hot lines, and formal complaint policies for employees can be valuable sources of information. OBRA, state, and Joint Commission standards can help target key areas to monitor.

8. Outline the structure of a QI program in your particular facility. An organizational chart for quality assessment and improvement is shown in Figure 25–1. Details of the following description of the QI structure are facility specific but can be applied in similar situations.

The corporation has funded and developed a position for a part-time quality advisor to coordinate the QI program. This person chairs the Quality Steering and Quality Core Committees, trains and advises the cross-functional teams,

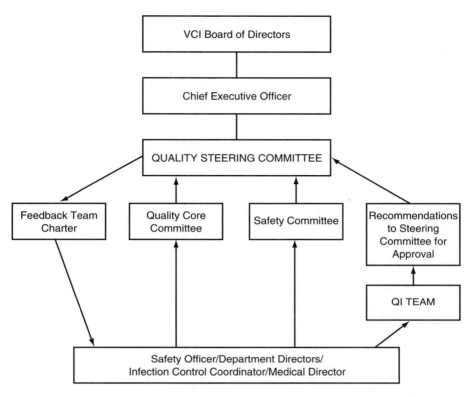

Figure 25–1 Organizational chart for sample QI program. Courtesy of Villa Clement, Inc., Milwaukee, Wisconsin.

and reports to the board of directors. Corporations with multiple facilities may use a full-time quality advisor.

The Quality Steering Committee monitors the overall quality direction of the corporation. The committee consists of the president/CEO, medical director, mission development director, administrators, vice presidents of finance, director of human resources, directors of nursing, retirement community directors, and the quality advisor. Members meet monthly to identify and review corporate critical indicators, charter cross-functional teams and evaluate their recommendations, recommend ongoing educational needs and opportunities, and approve quality policies. Ongoing QI is reported to the Quality Steering Committee through the Quality Core Committee.

Much of the work of developing and monitoring written indicators and thresholds for

evaluation and discussion of problems and appropriate actions occurs at the Quality Core Committee meetings. The department directors are grouped to facilitate meaningful feedback and discussion (Exhibit 25–1). Each group of department directors attends quarterly meetings. In addition, all meetings are attended by the administrators, the mission development director, the vice president of finance, and the quality advisor.

In this example, the Safety Committee is separated from the Quality Core Committee and reports directly to the Quality Steering Committee. This was done because the safety issues in long-term care are very technical and highly regulated. In addition to state, federal, and Joint Commission guidelines, there are strict Occupational Safety and Health Administration (OSHA) and local fire codes. The committee has members from all departments and

Exhibit 25–1 Quality Core Committee Reporting Groups

<u>Group 1</u> Medical Services Nursing Medical Records Infection Control Pharmacy Dietitian Risk Management	<u>Group 2</u> Rehabilitation Services Activities Social Services Volunteers Pastoral Care Beauty Shop
<u>Group 3</u> Environmental Services Laundry Maintenance Dietary Services Employee Inservice/Orientation Safety Orientation/Education	<u>Group 4</u> Business Office Human Resources Employee Health Materials Management Admissions Apartments/Adult Day Care

Courtesy of Villa Clement, Inc., Milwaukee, Wisconsin.

all levels of management and meets monthly to monitor (1) general safety, (2) life safety, (3) equipment management, (4) utilities management, (5) security, and (6) hazardous materials.

Cross-functional teams are chartered by the Quality Steering Committee. Team membership and frequency and number of meetings are determined by the issues to be addressed. The QI teams report their recommendations back to the Quality Steering Committee for approval.

KEY INDICATORS

Some of the key clinical and management indicators that are monitored on an ongoing basis are listed in Exhibits 25–2 and 25–3. Many of these are from state, federal, and Joint Commission guidelines. The Minimum Data Set (MDS), which is required by OBRA for each long-term care resident, is another source for clinical indicators. Thresholds are set from these standards and from published studies. Because QI stresses continuous improvement and trending, indicators may be monitored with control charts that set facility-specific thresholds two standard deviations above and below the mean.

QI TEAM STUDIES

Clinical and administrative team studies are critical to the QI process. This section provides examples of studies performed at two long-term care facilities sponsored by the same organization. In-depth descriptions of the team studies on wound and skin care and wandering provide details of the team process and QI tools and techniques used.

The following are some of the department-specific projects that have been conducted:

1. Human resources has revamped the orientation process on the basis of satisfaction surveys.
2. A nurse-physician communication study was conducted to develop the most efficient method of communicating with physicians.
3. Pastoral care addressed congestion and inadequate seating at religious services.
4. Nursing developed an interdisciplinary behavior management team to monitor the key clinical indicators related to behavior assessments and the use of physical and chemical restraints.

Exhibit 25–2 Key Clinical Indicators

1. Facility Infection Rates
   Number of infections per 1,000 resident days
   Number of residents with urinary tract infection with foley catheter
   Total number of residents with foley catheters
2. Serious Occurrences/Incidents
   Number of falls
   Number of falls with serious injury
3. Nutrition Indicators
   Number of residents with 5% or greater weight loss triggering a new Minimum Data Set
4. Medication Utilization
   Number of medication errors
   Number of significant medication errors
   Number of residents receiving:
      psychotropics
      antipsychotics
      antidepressants
      antianxiety/hypnotics
   Number of residents for which alternatives to psychotropics have been tried
5. Restraints
   Number of residents with physical restraints
   Number of residents for which alternatives have been tried
6. Change in Activity of Daily Living (ADL) Condition
   Change in two or more ADLs triggering a new Minimum Data Set
   Number with improvement
   Number with decline
7. Skin Management
   Total number of pressure ulcers
   Number of pressure ulcers per stage
   Number of facility-acquired ulcers
8. Minimum Data Set Completion within 14 Days

Courtesy of Villa Clement, Inc., Milwaukee, Wisconsin.

Wound Care Team

Pressure sore development is considered a critical outcome measure in the long-term care industry. Prevention and treatment are both important in the care of high-risk nursing home residents. A comprehensive skin care protocol is required by state, federal, and Joint Commission guidelines.

A QI team formed to address wound and skin care was charged with the task of auditing the effectiveness of current wound care treatments, using resources to determine and evaluate alternatives, and establishing diagnosis-specific care protocols, care standards, and expected outcomes.

The team identified direct customers of the wound care process as residents, nurses, pharmacy, physicians, and material management. Indirect customers were listed as family, admissions, and adjunctive therapies.

To determine variation in the current procedure, a flowchart of the wound care process was developed (Figure 25–2), and pharmacy audits were conducted of the products used to treat pressure sores. Discrepancies in the deci-

Exhibit 25–3 Key Administrative Indicators

1. Sponsorship
   Community benefit plan
2. Quality of service provided
   State/federal/Joint Commission compliance
   Percent Joint Commission compliance
      State survey compliance
      Number of self reports substantiated
   Resident satisfaction
      Post admission survey
      Resident focus group survey
3. Human Resources
   Turnover %/Retention rate
   Employee satisfaction
   Exit Interviews
4. Meeting Community Needs
   Utilization
      Percent occupancy
      Number of admissions
   Community Needs
      Reasons for denied admissions
      Referral source
      Reason for refusal from client
   Safety
      Safety management
      Life safety
      Equipment management
      Utilities management

Courtesy of Villa Clement, Inc., Milwaukee, Wisconsin.

sion-making process and in the steps required to treat and document wounds in a consistent and appropriate manner were identified.

A fishbone diagram was completed (Figure 25–3). The following root causes for inconsistent wound care were identified and ranked:

1. no standardized protocols
2. lack of knowledge of wound care
3. lack of experience
4. specific treatments requested by physicians
5. limited staff time
6. unavailability of product/cost
7. noncompliance from residents

8. nonstandardized assessment forms and terminology

As a first step, the team focused on educating themselves. Team members attended several local seminars and reviewed the literature for additional information. Major manufacturers of wound care products were identified, and their representatives were asked to complete a product specification questionnaire for all categories of wound products. Representatives from certain companies were then interviewed to review new products and techniques for wound healing. From these sources, a standardized definition for each wound stage was

Wound Care Process

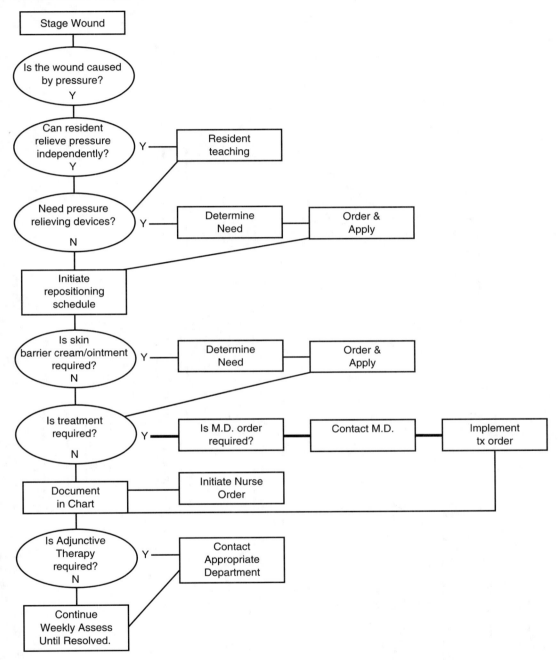

Figure 25–2 Wound care team: Flowchart. Courtesy of Villa Clement Inc., Milwaukee, Wisconsin.

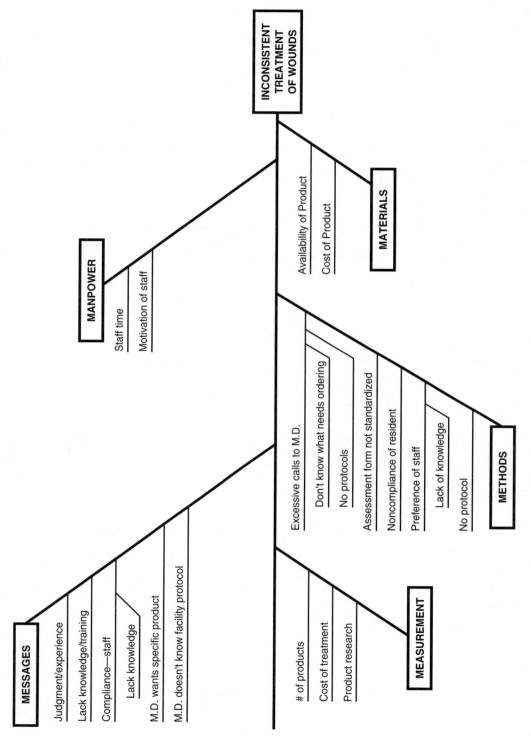

Figure 25–3 Wound care team fishbone diagram. Courtesy of Villa Clement Inc., Milwaukee, Wisconsin.

formulated. Body pressure points at risk for pressure ulcers were listed and grouped. Protocols for assessment were developed.

A *force-field analysis* was completed for various products by category for each stage of wound care. On the basis of these results, several products were selected for trial and evaluation with current residents. Clinical effectiveness, cost, and ease of use were considered in the selection process. From these studies, a list of products to be used was developed.

A force-field analysis was completed to compare various types of beds, mattresses, and support services. The pressure-relieving properties of various mattress replacements and specialty beds and their reimbursement guidelines were considered. Various wound cleansing and irrigation solutions were evaluated for toxicity levels, effectiveness, and cost.

Final recommendations by the team addressed the areas identified as root causes of inconsistent wound and skin care:

- *No standardized protocols.* The team developed corporate pressure-wound care protocols that included the following sections: skin care philosophy, assessment, education, wound care procedures, adjunctive therapies, products, infection control, and monitoring.
- *Lack of knowledge of wound care.* The team recommended that all licensed nursing staff receive a two-part, in-depth education in-service consisting of the anatomy and physiology of wound care and healing and that there be ongoing in-servicing of the *Wound and Skin Care Protocol Manual.*
- *Lack of experience.* The team recommended that a facility wound care coordinator be appointed. This person would coordinate wound rounds and in-services; maintain the manual by updating policies, procedures, and wound products; be a resource to the product evaluation committee when wound care products were discussed; and update the list of physicians who approved of the wound and skin protocols. In addition, the team recommended that weekly wound rounds be conducted on each unit with an outside wound care nurse specialist, the facility wound care coordinator, the charge nurse, and a physical therapist when appropriate. During these rounds, all identified wounds would be assessed for appropriate treatment, measured and documented on the skin assessment flowsheet, and assessed for progress in healing.

- *Specific treatment requested by physicians.* The team recommended that all physicians receive a copy of the Wound Care Protocol, accompanied by a letter of explanation from the medical director.
- *Limited staff time.* The team identified areas where implementation of protocols would reduce nursing time:

1. The wound kit would decrease nursing time in ordering supplies and calls to Central Supply for initial setup.
2. Central Supply would have only one charge instead of charges for separate items.
3. There would be a decreased number of calls to physicians for orders.
4. Protocols would decrease the time spent in decision making for treatment selection.
5. A well-defined product list would decrease the time spent by nursing and Central Supply on specialty orders.
6. New forms would decrease duplication of wound documentation.

- *Unavailability of products and cost.* The team recommended that a contract be developed with one primary wound care product provider. Product-specific protocols would limit the number of treatment choices, and approved products would be readily available for use. Distribution and storage of wound care products varied at the two facilities. The recommended protocol included use of a wound kit containing common items. These kits would aid in storage organization, save time in the or-dering process, ensure the charge of all items, and provide a clean field for wound treatment.

- *Noncompliance of residents.* Noncompli-ance of residents regarding treatments and positioning is an ongoing problem and should be dealt with on an individual basis by Nursing and Social Services.
- *Nonstandardized assessment forms and terminology.* The team recommended the implementation of the newly standardized assessment forms as found in the Wound Protocols.

Wandering Team

Wandering can be defined as moving about without a fixed course, aim, or goal and with-out regard for safety. This is a common prob-lem with cognitively impaired nursing home residents. Maintaining the safety of the cogni-tively impaired wanderer is a challenge in long-term care that requires extra staff time and environmental modifications.

The staff's frustrations regarding their diffi-culty in providing a safe and secure environ-ment for wandering residents prompted the creation of a cross-functional team. The team was charged to study the current wandering management system and to develop a system to ensure resident safety and quality of life. Using the brainstorming method, the team identified the customers affected by wander-ing as residents, staff, and family members/significant others. These customers were sur-veyed regarding effectiveness of the current wandering system, potentially hazardous areas, and freedom of access for identified wanderers throughout common areas. Survey results revealed that all concerned customers valued the freedom of access for all residents. The team goal was to provide an environment for all residents to move throughout the build-ing and remain safe.

Potentially hazardous areas identified by the surveys were organized into a Pareto chart (Figure 25–4). Using the Pareto principle, the team focused on the three greatest areas of concern: exits, lower level, and stairwells.

To help determine trends in wandering activ-ity, nursing staff documented the alarms trig-gered at the existing equipment. These data were organized by date and time of incident in a scatter diagram (Figure 25–5).

The team flowcharted the process for identi-fying residents who exhibit wandering behav-ior and the documentation and communication process for monitoring wandering. A cause-and-effect fishbone diagram was completed that identified the following root causes:

1. There is an unwillingness to diminish freedom of the residents.
2. Information about wanderers is not dis-seminated to all staff.
3. Staff education is lacking.
4. Identified wanderers refuse to wear bracelets.
5. There is inconsistent location of infor-mation related to resident appointments and activities.

Staff involvement and education were ad-dressed and corrected by implementation of a "quick fix." The quick fix included develop-ment of a policy and procedure statement for redirecting an identified wanderer and for re-sponse to a code to locate a resident, develop-ment of a binder for each department contain-ing photographs of all identified wanderers, and staff in-servicing. The refusal of wanderers to wear an alarm bracelet was also addressed in a quick fix by using alternate placement and the addition of a neon bracelet.

Final recommendations to address all areas of the building included keypad locks on stair-well doors, an upgraded alarm system to in-clude all exits, and an elevator lock-out system to deter residents from accessing the lower level after 6:00 P.M. An outside fenced court-yard was built to provide an opportunity for

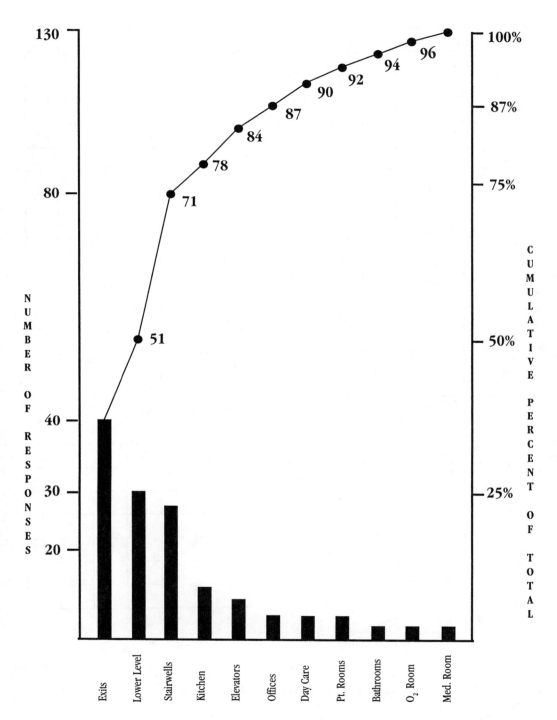

Figure 25–4 Wandering team employee survey of potentially unsafe areas: Pareto chart. Courtesy of Villa Clement Inc., Milwaukee, Wisconsin.

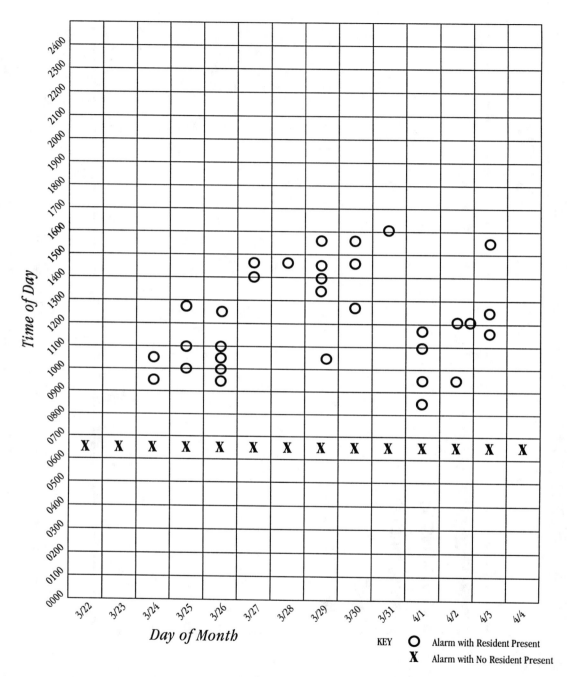

Figure 25–5 Wandering team: Scatter diagram of alarm activation. Courtesy of Villa Clement Inc., Milwaukee, Wisconsin.

residents to go outside in a safe, controlled environment. Documentation was simplified, and a standardized format for communication of residents' activities was developed.

Recommendations, including a detailed schedule of financial impacts, were presented to the Quality Steering Committee for approval. An implementation team was appointed to develop an action plan, including time frames to ensure completion of recommendations.

CONCLUSION

As new information management systems for the MDS become available, the whole database for long-term care QI will be enhanced. Computer databases of clinical information for single facilities and groups of facilities will aid in the identification and monitoring of key clinical indicators. This should streamline the process of identifying opportunities for improvement.

REFERENCES

Joint Commission on Accreditation of Healthcare Organizations. (1996). *1996 comprehensive accreditation manual for long-term care.* Oakbrook Terrace, IL: Author.

U.S. Department of Health and Human Services. (1989). *Medicare and Medicaid: Requirements for long-term care facilities: Final rule and request for comments.* Washington, DC: Government Printing Office.

CHAPTER 26

Improving Quality in a Managed Care Environment: An HMO Example

Linda Gonia

CHAPTER OBJECTIVES

After completing this chapter, the reader will be able to

- describe the standards mandated by the state and federal governments as well as standards of voluntary accrediting agencies (Joint Commission, NCQA, AAAHC) governing the managed care environment
- identify components of a request for proposal or request for bid required by employer groups contracting with managed care organizations, including evidence of a quality improvement program
- design various satisfaction surveys for patients, including Medicaid members, to assess their satisfaction with the performance of various departments
- discuss the policies and procedures for credentialing or recredentialing employed and contracted physicians
- identify key clinical and administrative indicators to measure organizational performance

The quality management (QM) program of a health care delivery system is shaped by many forces. The internal forces that shape a QM program begin with the organization's mission statement. Mission statements can vary in length and scope. Some mission statements are vague with regard to QM; others are

very detailed. The QM program that will be described is based on the following mission statement:

The **Mission** of Family Health Plan Cooperative (FHPC) is to develop and operate quality, cost-effective health care programs that achieve the following goals:

- to pursue high standards of quality in the delivery of health care;
- to operate health care programs in a manner that achieves cost-effectiveness to the benefit of the consumer;
- to foster innovation in the development of health care programs;
- to give the health consumer choice as to the type of health care system they wish to use;
- to develop an organized system of health care offering a comprehensive set of benefits with maximum accessibility;
- to give the health consumer a voice and some control in the operations of the health care delivery system; and
- to encourage members to participate in the practice of preventive health maintenance as an alternative to crisis-oriented care.

521

The goal of the FHPC QM program is to support FHPC's mission. The FHPC QM program defines *quality* as meeting or exceeding the needs of members and employers, based on measurable standards and guidelines. It is important to note that the QM program exists within an organization's culture and the organization's hierarchical structure. Building a program that does not recognize these facts will result in the failure of the program.

EXTERNAL FORCES

Three main types of external forces shape an organization's QM program: state and federal requirements, voluntary accrediting bodies, and employer groups.

State and Federal Requirements

Any organization that provides services for patients receiving medical assistance must have a QM program that satisfies the requirements of the Department of Health and Human Services (or the equivalent) of the state in which services are provided. Although the particular requirements will differ from state to state, each will include some variations on the same theme. For example, the requirements for the state of Wisconsin include the following:

1. an annual plan and evaluation of the quality improvement (QI) program
2. specified representatives on QI committees (e.g., from obstetrics/gynecology, pediatrics, and mental health)
3. regular QI meetings (at least quarterly), complete with documentation (minutes and reports)
4. integration of utilization management, risk management, and complaint handling into the QM program
5. monitoring and evaluation of clinical care and service provided in institutional settings, noninstitutional settings, and specialty areas (including subcontracted care and service)

6. measurement regarding access (wait time for an appointment and distance to provider)
7. a credentialing and recredentialing program
8. a health promotion/preventive services program
9. satisfaction surveys or other forms of communication (Wisconsin Department of Health and Social Services [1996–1997])

Any organization that provides services for patients receiving Medicare must have a QM program that satisfies the requirements of the Health Care Financing Administration (HCFA). The five basic requirements expected of health maintenance organizations (HMOs) are

1. *Ongoing QI program*—Have an ongoing QI program for the health services furnished.
2. *QI methodology*—Stress health outcomes to the extent consistent with the state of the art.
3. *Peer review*—Provide review by physicians and other health professionals of the process followed in providing health services.
4. *Systematic data collection*—Use systematic data collection of performance and patient results, provide interpretation of these data to the HMO's practitioners, and institute needed changes.
5. *Remedial action*—Include written procedures for taking appropriate remedial actions whenever inappropriate or substandard services were furnished or services that should have been furnished were not.

Voluntary Accrediting Bodies

An organization may attempt to gain endorsement by an outside accrediting body, such as the National Committee for Quality Assurance (NCQA) or the Accreditation Association for Ambulatory Health Care, Inc. (AAAHC).

NCQA

The NCQA is an independent, nonprofit institution, established in 1979, that reviews and accredits managed-care organizations. NCQA has worked with a broad group of contributors to develop a set of standards that reviewers use to evaluate a managed-care organization. Compliance with the NCQA *Standards for Accreditation of Managed Care Organizations* (1996) indicates that a managed-care organization is committed to quality. Standards are in the following six categories:

1. *Quality management and improvement*—Does the plan fully examine the quality of care given to its members? How well does the plan coordinate all parts of its delivery system? What steps does it take to make sure members have access to care in a reasonable amount of time? What improvements in care and service can the plan demonstrate?
2. *Utilization management*—Does the plan use a reasonable and consistent process when deciding what health services are appropriate for individuals' needs? When the plan denies payment for services, does it respond to member and physician appeals? Does the plan protect against underutilization? Are decisions made by individuals with sufficient expertise to make them?
3. *Physician credentials*—Does the plan meet specific NCQA requirements for investigating the training and experience of all physicians in the network? Does the plan look for any history of malpractice and fraud? Does the plan keep track of all physicians' performance and use that information for their periodic evaluation?
4. *Members' rights and responsibilities*— How clearly does the plan inform members about how to access health services, how to choose a physician or change physicians, and how to make a complaint? How responsive is the plan to

members' satisfaction ratings and complaints?

5. *Preventive health services*—Does the plan encourage members to have preventive tests and immunizations? Does the plan support physician efforts to deliver preventive services? Is there evidence of monitoring of the success of preventive care? Is there evidence of improvement where monitoring suggests an opportunity?
6. *Medical records*—How consistently do the medical records kept by the plan's physicians meet NCQA standards for quality care? For instance, do the records show that physicians follow up on patients' abnormal test findings?

Managed-care organizations receive a score of *full compliance, significant compliance, partial compliance, minimal compliance, noncompliance*, or *not applicable* for each standard in a category and the category overall. Compliance is assessed by

1. review of written documentation and records provided by the organization
2. on-site observations by surveyors
3. information gained by surveyors during relevant interviews with members of the organization
4. review of medical records
5. assessment of member service teams, including systems such as complaint and grievance, member education, and member survey

An accreditation decision is made based on compliance with standards. The decision rendered is either for full accreditation, accreditation with recommendations, 1-year accreditation, provisional accreditation, or denial/revocation of accreditation status.

The Health Plan Employer Data and Information Set (HEDIS) is a set of performance measures developed by NCQA for the purpose of accreditation and producing "Report Cards." HEDIS 3.0 is the third version of HEDIS to be distributed by NCQA and was released in Spring 1997. HEDIS 3.0 differs from prior HEDIS documents in that it

- is "outcomes," or results, oriented
- addresses the full spectrum of health care
- brings private-sector and public-sector measurement together
- includes standardized measurement across the full range of issues
- includes a process for ongoing improvement

HEDIS 3.0 integrates and expands HEDIS 2.5 for commercial members, Medicaid HEDIS for Medicaid members, and new measures for Medicare-risk members into a single, nonduplicative set of measures. HEDIS 3.0 integrates public and private reporting requirements in health care. The HEDIS 3.0 measures cover eight broad categories of health plan performance that are important to purchasers and consumers:

- *Effectiveness of care*—These measures assess how well the care delivered by a managed-care plan is achieving the clinical results it should.
- *Accessibility/availability of care*—These measures assess whether care is available to members when they need it, in a timely and convenient manner.
- *Satisfaction with the experience of care*—These measures are intended to provide information about whether a health plan is able to satisfy the diverse needs of its members.
- *Cost of care*—These measures help consumers to estimate the stability of the health plan.
- *Stability of the health plan*—These measures help consumers to estimate the stability of the health plan.
- *Informed health care choices*—These measures help consumers to assess how their health plan has equipped them to make health care decisions.
- *Use of services*—These measures permit users to understand patterns of service use across different health plans.

- *Health plan descriptive information*—This section is a narrative of the attributes and operating characteristics of the health plan itself. (HEDIS 3.0: NCQA, July 1996, pp. 1–5)

Accreditation Association for Ambulatory Health Care

The AAAHC is a voluntary accrediting organization that was founded in 1979. AAAHC standards provide a peer-based survey process by which ambulatory care providers can be publicly recognized for complying with standards of quality. The following types of organizations may apply for an accreditation survey:

1. ambulatory health care clinics
2. ambulatory surgery centers
3. birthing centers
4. college and university health services
5. community health centers
6. dental group practices
7. diagnostic imaging centers
8. endoscopy centers
9. HMOs
10. hospital-sponsored ambulatory care clinics and surgery centers
11. multispecialty group practices
12. occupational health services
13. office surgery centers and practices
14. oral and maxillofacial surgeons' offices
15. radiation oncology centers
16. single-specialty group practices
17. surgical recovery centers
18. urgent and immediate care centers (Accreditation Handbook for Ambulatory Health Care, 1994–1995, pp. 4–7)

The AAAHC has a series of standards in the following 22 areas:

1. *Rights of Patients*—recognizes the basic human rights of patients.
2. *Governance*—has a governing body that sets policy and is responsible for the organization.
3. *Administration*—is administered in a manner that ensures the provision of

high-quality services and that fulfills the organization's mission, goals, and objectives.

4. *Quality of Care Provided*—provides high-quality health care services in accordance with the principles of professional practice and ethical conduct and with concern for the costs of care.

5. *Quality Assurance Program*—maintains an active, organized, peer-based, quality assurance program as an integral part of professional and administrative practice.

6. *Clinical Records*—maintains a clinical record system from which information can be retrieved promptly. Clinical records are legible, documented accurately in a timely manner, and readily accessible to health care practitioners.

7. *Professional Improvement*—strives to improve the professional competence and skill, as well as the quality of performance, of the health care practitioners and other professional personnel it employs.

8. *Facilities and Environment*—provides a functionally safe and sanitary environment for its patients, personnel, and visitors.

9. *Anesthesia Services*—are provided in a safe and sanitary environment by qualified health care practitioners who have been granted privileges to provide those services by the governing body.

10. *Surgical Services*—are performed in a safe and sanitary environment by qualified practitioners who have been granted privileges to perform those procedures by the governing body.

11. *Overnight Care and Services*—provides overnight care and related services; such care and services meet the needs of the patients served and are provided in accordance with ethical and professional practices and legal requirements.

12. *Dental Services*—are provided or made available by an accreditable organization to meet the need of the patients and are provided in accordance with ethical and professional practices and legal requirements.

13. *Emergency Services*—implies by its activities, advertising, or practice that it provides emergency services on a regular basis to meet life-, limb-, or function-threatening conditions; such services meet the needs of the patients and are provided in accordance with ethical and professional practices and legal requirements.

14. *Immediate/Urgent Care Services*—implies by its activities, advertising, or practice that it provides medical care of an urgent or immediate nature on a routine or regular basis; such care meets the needs of the patients and is provided in accordance with ethical and professional practices and legal requirements.

15. *Pharmaceutical Services*—meet the needs of the patients and are provided in accordance with ethical and professional practices and legal requirements.

16. *Pathology and Medical Laboratory Services*—meet the needs of the patients and are provided in accordance with ethical and professional practices and legal requirements.

17. *Diagnostic Imaging Services*—meet the needs of the patients and are provided in accordance with ethical and professional practices and legal requirements.

18. *Radiation Oncology Treatment Services*—meet the needs of the patients and are provided in accordance with ethical and professional practices and legal requirements.

19. *Occupational Health Services*—are organized to ensure a safe and healthy workplace for employees through the recognition, evaluation, and control of illness and injury in or from the workplace and to meet the needs of the employees served, and are provided in accordance with ethical and professional practices and legal requirements.

20. *Other Professional and Technical Services*—even though not specifically mentioned in the *Handbook,* meet the needs of the patients and are provided in accordance with ethical and professional practices and legal requirements.
21. *Teaching and Publication Activities*—has policies governing those activities that are consistent with its mission, goals, and objectives.
22. *Research Activities*—establishes and implements policies governing research that are consistent with its mission, goals, objectives, and clinical capabilities. (Accreditation Handbook for Ambulatory Health Care, 1994–1995)

HMOs receive a score of *substantial compliance, partial compliance, noncompliance, unsure,* or *not applicable* for each standard in a category and the category overall. An accreditation decision is made based on compliance with standards. The decision rendered is for accreditation, deferral, or nonaccreditation. Granting accreditation reflects AAAHC's confidence that, on the basis of its survey, an organization demonstrates the attributes of an accreditable organization as outlined by the standards.

Employer Groups

An organization's QM/QI program is also shaped by information required by current employer groups, prospective employer groups, and brokers. As health care has become more competitive, the information requirements from these groups has become more sophisticated. Contracts are offered to a health plan based on the responses gathered in the Request for Proposal (RFP) or Request for Bid (RFB) process. If the QM program of your organization does not address their concerns as specified in the RFP/RFB, you risk losing a contract or not being offered one. The following is a list of the topics contained in a typical RFP/RFB pertaining to QM:

- wait time for appointments
  1. primary care provider
  2. specialists
  3. mental health/substance abuse
- phone access
- referral process
- HMO medical and QM committees
  1. structure
  2. reporting
  3. frequency of meetings
  4. chairperson
  5. function
  6. rotation of members
- review criteria
  1. inpatient criteria
     - medical/surgical
     - obstetrical
     - psychiatric
     - outpatient criteria
- utilization
  1. ICD-9 diagnoses
  2. DRG
  3. drug
- HEDIS
- clinical studies
- disease-specific clinical guidelines/protocols
- preventive service guidelines for adult and pediatric care
- procedures for follow-up/intervention to health screening and other diagnostic tests
- credentialing/recredentialing
- provider performance monitoring
- peer review
- member satisfaction surveys
- complaint handling/resolution

QUALITY MANAGEMENT PROGRAM

The QM program of an organization must be sufficiently comprehensive to address the needs of all the internal and external audiences. Many of these needs may overlap, but some are very distinct for a particular audience. The initial step in building a committee structure requires the organization's membership to review its continuum of care. The various providers and services included in that continuum must be represented in the committee structure to ensure oversight activities related to each aspect of care; an example is shown in Figure 26–1.

Developing reporting relationships is critical. Because health care delivery is such a dynamic process, very few activities are so compartmentalized that they do not have an impact on another segment of the organization. In recognizing this fact, the leaders of the organization must support and facilitate communication vertically and horizontally throughout the organization. As shown in Figure 26–1, all committees, task forces, and work groups are connected through the Quality Coordinating Team. The Quality Coordinating Team is made up of the FHPC senior managers, committee chairs of the major standing committees, and the quality manager.

As shown in Exhibit 26–1, the scope of this team includes the full range of clinical care, clinical service, and administrative QI activities throughout the organization. Part of its mission is

> to evaluate the needs of our members, employers, various third party agencies, and trade organizations based on demographic traits, utilization characteristics, epidemiological status, provider changes, general re-enrollment, dis-enrollment, and other satisfaction survey results; assign quality improvement activities, and track improvement activities through completion and follow-up.

To paraphrase, the mission of this team is to evaluate needs on the basis of data.

Satisfaction Surveys

The primary source of data is the member, and one method of gathering these data is through satisfaction surveys. The HMO must have a process to maintain a relationship with its members that promotes two-way communication and contributes to quality of care and service. Some examples of surveys of satisfaction with services are those conducted by the FHPC Clinic Services Quality Committee, including pharmacy (Exhibit 26–2), radiology (Exhibit 26–3), medical records (Exhibit 26–4), and nursing department services (Exhibit 26–5). Figures 26–2 and 26–3 show 1995 survey results. These surveys are conducted to gain a snapshot rating of the department, to review member responses to open-ended questions, and to develop a customer service action plan for the coming year.

Medicaid member satisfaction surveys (Exhibit 26–6) specifically must be conducted by the FHPC public affairs department during a contract period per federal waiver requirements.

An HMO must also have a mechanism for considering the provider's performance by reviewing member complaints and member satisfaction surveys, quality studies that have rated the provider, and the provider's record of utilization management. The FHPC Affiliated Providers Quality Committee conducts and reviews the member surveys regarding satisfaction with specialists' care (Exhibit 26–7); data are displayed in Figures 26–4 and 26–5. Satisfaction with care provided by the primary care physicians is displayed in Figure 26–6 (Spider Diagram). These versions of "report cards" are being viewed by payers, providers, and consumers as mechanisms for accountability: controlling health care costs while maintaining and improving quality health care is the goal.

Credentialing/Recredentialing Employed and Contracted Physicians

An HMO must have written policies and procedures (Appendix 26–A) for provider selection and qualifications (see credentialing review form in Exhibit 26–8). The HMO must periodically monitor (no less than every 2 years) the provider's documented qualifications to ensure that the provider still meets the HMO's specific professional requirements (see the recredentialing review form in Exhibit

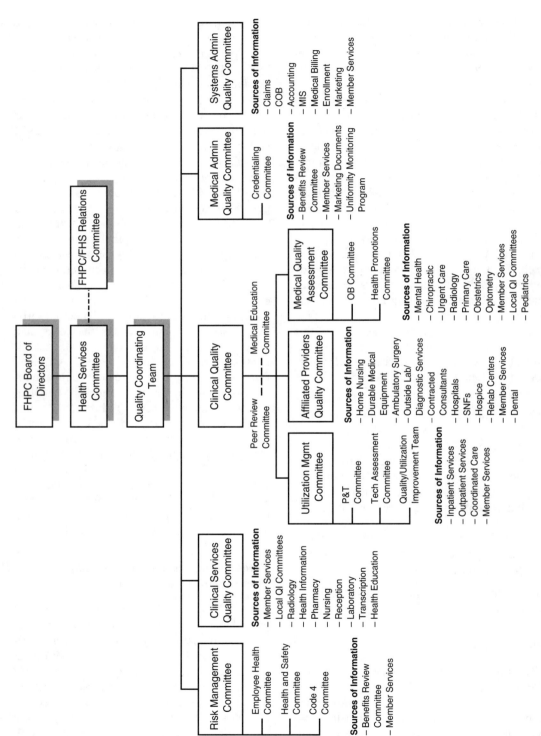

Figure 26–1 Family Health Plan Cooperative's organizational structure, March 31, 1996. Courtesy of Family Health Plan Cooperative, Milwaukee, Wisconsin.

Exhibit 26–1 Scope of Quality Coordinating Team Activities at FHPC across Continuum of Care

	Our Practitioner Offices/Support Services	Hospitals	Skilled Nursing Facilities	Nursing Homes	Specialist's Offices	FHPC Labs/Other Diagnostic Services	Outside Labs/Other Diagnostic Services	Ambulatory Surgery Facilities	Durable Medical Equipment Vendors	Home Nursing Vendors	Administration
Quality of Care –Structure –Process –Outcomes	CQC (MQAC)	CQC (APQC)	CQC (APQC)	CQC (APQC)	CQC (APQC)	CQC (MQAC)	CQC (APQC)	CQC (APQC)	CQC (APQC)	CQC (APQC)	
Services	CSQC MAQC	CQC (APQC)	CQC (APQC)	CQC (APQC)	CQC (APQC)	CSQC MAQC	CQC (APQC)	CQC (APQC)	CQC (APQC)	CQC (APQC)	MAQC SAQC
Utilization	UMC (MQAC)	UMC (APQC)	UMC (APQC)	UMC (APQC)	UMC (APQC)	UMC (MQAC)	UMC (APQC)	UMC (APQC)	UMC (APQC)	UMC (APQC)	

File: Scope
Date: 03/30/95

Key:
MAQC = Medical Administration Quality Committee
CQC = Clinical Quality Committee
RMC = Risk Management Committee
APQC = Affiliated Providers Quality Committee

SAQC = Systems Administration Quality Committee
UMC = Utilization Management Committee
CSQC = Clinical Services Quality Committee
MQAC = Medical Quality Assessment Committee

Courtesy of Family Health Plan Cooperative, Milwaukee, Wisconsin.

Exhibit 26–2 Member Survey on Satisfaction with **Pharmacy** Department Services

Please rate the *Family Health Plan Cooperative* (FHPC) Pharmacy based on your experiences. Mark the best response to each statement.

	Poor	Fair	Good	Very Good	Excellent	Not Applicable
1. Friendliness and courtesy of the pharmacy staff	1	2	3	4	5	N/A
2. The time spent waiting in the lobby for a new prescription to be filled	1	2	3	4	5	N/A
3. Information on new prescriptions is explained in an understandable manner	1	2	3	4	5	N/A
4. The thoroughness and completeness of answers I received to questions I asked	1	2	3	4	5	N/A
5. Privacy provided to me during my prescription consultation	1	2	3	4	5	N/A
6. Refills are available when I was told they would be	1	2	3	4	5	N/A
7. The amount of time the Pharmacist spends with me	1	2	3	4	5	N/A
8. The overall usefulness of the telephone system for ordering refills	1	2	3	4	5	N/A
9. The overall usefulness of the telephone system for obtaining pharmacy or prescription information	1	2	3	4	5	N/A
10. The time I wait on the telephone before I am helped when I call during regular pharmacy hours	1	2	3	4	5	N/A
11. Response of pharmacy staff to my special needs ("Staff goes the extra mile")	1	2	3	4	5	N/A
12. Overall, how would you evaluate pharmacy serivces at *FHPC?*	1	2	3	4	5	N/A

13. If you could improve one thing about the *FHPC* Pharmacy, what would it be? _____

_____

14. What do you like best about the *FHPC* Pharmacy? _____

_____

_____

continues

Exhibit 26–2 continued

We would like you to think about another aspect of pharmacy services. We would like to know how important each of the following services is to you. For each of these services, please check the response that best describes how important that pharmacy service is to you.

15. I can order refills using the phone system.
_____ 1. Absolutely essential
_____ 2. Very important
_____ 3. A little important
_____ 4. Not too important
_____ 5. Not important at all

16. I can obtain information regarding my prescription using the phone system.
_____ 1. Absolutely essential
_____ 2. Very important
_____ 3. A little important
_____ 4. Not too important
_____ 5. Not important at all

17. Refills are available within 24 hours.
_____ 1. Absolutely essential
_____ 2. Very important
_____ 3. A little important
_____ 4. Not too important
_____ 5. Not important at all

18. Refills are available within 48 hours.
_____ 1. Absolutely essential
_____ 2. Very important
_____ 3. A little important
_____ 4. Not too important
_____ 5. Not important at all

19. Waiting time in lobby is less than 15 minutes for a new prescription.
_____ 1. Absolutely essential
_____ 2. Very important
_____ 3. A little important
_____ 4. Not too important
_____ 5. Not important at all

20. I am given privacy during my consultation.
_____ 1. Absolutely essential
_____ 2. Very important
_____ 3. A little important
_____ 4. Not too important
_____ 5. Not important at all

21. I feel free to ask questions or raise concerns about new or refill prescriptions.
_____ 1. Absolutely essential
_____ 2. Very important
_____ 3. A little important
_____ 4. Not too important
_____ 5. Not important at all

22. Take-home information on my prescriptions is available.
_____ 1. Absolutely essential
_____ 2. Very important
_____ 3. A little important
_____ 4. Not too important
_____ 5. Not important at all

Courtesy of Family Health Plan Cooperative, Milwaukee, Wisconsin.

Exhibit 26–3   Member Survey on Satisfaction with **Radiology** Department Services

Please rate the *Family Health Plan Cooperative* (FHPC) Radiology (X-ray) Department based on your experiences. Mark the best response to each statement.

	Poor	Fair	Good	Very Good	Excellent	Not Applicable
1. Was the Radiology staff friendly and courteous? (Were you greeted in a professional manner?)	1	2	3	4	5	N/A
2. Was the appearance of the Radiology staff appropriate?	1	2	3	4	5	N/A
3. Was the Radiology staff professional before, during, and after your exam?	1	2	3	4	5	N/A
4. Was the waiting area comfortable and attractive?	1	2	3	4	5	N/A
5. Was the X-ray room comfortable and private?	1	2	3	4	5	N/A
6. Were instructions given by the Radiology staff clear and specific?	1	2	3	4	5	N/A
7. Was the Radiology staff responsive to your questions and concerns?	1	2	3	4	5	N/A
8. Were you satisfied with the hours of appointment availability?	1	2	3	4	5	N/A
9. Were you satisfied with your ability to get in for an appointment?	1	2	3	4	5	N/A
10. Overall, how do you rate FHPC Radiology?	1	2	3	4	5	N/A

11. What did you like best about FHPC Radiology? _____

12. Where do you feel that we could improve? _____

13. What type of X-ray exam was performed?

    Plain X-ray _____ Fluoroscopy _____ EKG _____ CT _____ Ultrasound _____ Mammography _____

14. Additional comments: _____

_____

_____

continues

Exhibit 26–3 continued

We would like to get your opinions about another part of Radiology services. Please rate the following services in order of importance to you. Your preferences will be important in planning how to provide these services in the future. Thank you.

15. Ability to get in for a fluoroscopic exam within one week.
  _____ 1. Absolutely essential
  _____ 2. Very important
  _____ 3. A little important
  _____ 4. Not too important
  _____ 5. Not important at all
  _____ 6. Not applicable

16. Ability to get in for an ultrasound exam within one week
  _____ 1. Absolutely essential
  _____ 2. Very important
  _____ 3. A little important
  _____ 4. Not too important
  _____ 5. Not important at all
  _____ 6. Not applicable

17. Ability to get in for a CT scan within one week.
  _____ 1. Absolutely essential
  _____ 2. Very important
  _____ 3. A little important
  _____ 4. Not too important
  _____ 5. Not important at all
  _____ 6. Not applicable

18. Ability to get in for a mammogram within one week.
  _____ 1. Absolutely essential
  _____ 2. Very important
  _____ 3. A little important
  _____ 4. Not too important
  _____ 5. Not important at all
  _____ 6. Not applicable

19. Waiting less than 15 minutes for your Radiology appointment.
  _____ 1. Absolutely essential
  _____ 2. Very important
  _____ 3. A little important
  _____ 4. Not too important
  _____ 5. Not important at all
  _____ 6. Not applicable

20. Ability to have all scheduled Radiology exams done at the same location (i.e., CT ultrasound, etc.).
  _____ 1. Absolutely essential
  _____ 2. Very important
  _____ 3. A little important
  _____ 4. Not too important
  _____ 5. Not important at all
  _____ 6. Not applicable

21. Importance of being notified of all Radiology test results.
  _____ 1. Absolutely essential
  _____ 2. Very important
  _____ 3. A little important
  _____ 4. Not too important
  _____ 5. Not important at all
  _____ 6. Not applicable

Courtesy of Family Health Plan Cooperative, Milwaukee, Wisconsin.

Exhibit 26–4 Member Survey on Satisfaction with **Medical Records** Department Services

Please rate the *Family Health Plan Cooperative* (FHPC) Health Information (Medical Records) Department based on your experiences. Mark the best response to each statement.

	Poor	Fair	Good	Very Good	Excellent	Not Applicable
1. Friendliness of the Health Information staff (Were you greeted by your proper name/salutation?)	1	2	3	4	5	N/A
2. Appearance of the Health Information staff	1	2	3	4	5	N/A
3. Professionalism of the Health Information staff	1	2	3	4	5	N/A
4. Overall appearance and cleanliness of the window area and/or Health Information Dept	1	2	3	4	5	N/A
5. Understandability of the instructions given to you by Health Information to complete forms	1	2	3	4	5	N/A
6. Timeliness in which you were waited upon (within 5 minutes)	1	2	3	4	5	N/A
7. Response of the Health Information staff to your special needs ("Staff goes the extra mile")	1	2	3	4	5	N/A
8. The thoroughness or completeness of answers you received to questions you asked	1	2	3	4	5	N/A
9. The way your visit with Health Information staff was concluded (with a friendly, sincere comment)	1	2	3	4	5	N/A
10. How well you were directed to your next stop within the clinic	1	2	3	4	5	N/A
11. The hours that the Health Information Department is open for business	1	2	3	4	5	N/A
12. Your overall sense of confidentiality while visiting the health center	1	2	3	4	5	N/A
13. Ability to get your forms completed within one week of your request	1	2	3	4	5	N/A
14. Overall, how would you evaluate the Health Information services at FHPC?	1	2	3	4	5	N/A

15. What do you like best about the FHPC Health Information Department?

_____

16. If you could improve one thing about the FHPC Health Information Department, what would it be?

_____

_____

continues

Exhibit 26–4 continued

We would like you to think about another aspect of the Health Information Services. We would like to know how important each of the following services is to you. For each of these services, please check the responses that best describe how important the Health Information Services are to you.

17. Ability to get a form completed within one week.
    _____ 1. Absolutely essential
    _____ 2. Very important
    _____ 3. A little important
    _____ 4. Not too important
    _____ 5. Not important at all
    _____ 6. Not applicable

18. Importance of getting a form completed the same day.
    _____ 1. Absolutely essential
    _____ 2. Very important
    _____ 3. A little important
    _____ 4. Not too important
    _____ 5. Not important at all
    _____ 6. Not applicable

19. Waiting less than 5 minutes for assistance at the Health Information window.
    _____ 1. Absolutely essential
    _____ 2. Very important
    _____ 3. A little important
    _____ 4. Not too important
    _____ 5. Not important at all
    _____ 6. Not applicable

20. Ability to go to a consultant's office and have your FHPC information and X-rays there waiting for you, rather than hand-carrying it.
    _____ 1. Absolutely essential
    _____ 2. Very important
    _____ 3. A little important
    _____ 4. Not too important
    _____ 5. Not important at all
    _____ 6. Not applicable

Courtesy of Family Health Plan Cooperative, Milwaukee, Wisconsin.

Exhibit 26–5 Member Survey on Satisfaction with **Nursing Department** Services

Please rate the *Family Health Plan Cooperative* (FHPC) Nursing Department based on your experiences. Mark the best response to each statement.

	Poor	Fair	Good	Very Good	Excellent	Not Applicable
1. Friendliness and courtesy of the nursing staff	1	2	3	4	5	N/A
2. Appearance of the nursing staff	1	2	3	4	5	N/A
3. Professionalism of the nursing staff	1	2	3	4	5	N/A
4. Nurses' personal interest in you and your medical problems	1	2	3	4	5	N/A
5. Response of the nursing staff to your special needs ("Staff goes the extra mile")	1	2	3	4	5	N/A
6. The way your visit with nursing staff was concluded (with friendly, sincere comment)	1	2	3	4	5	N/A
7. Callbacks from nursing staff are made when you were told they would be	1	2	3	4	5	N/A
8. The overall usefulness of the telephone system for obtaining advice from a nurse	1	2	3	4	5	N/A
9. The usefulness of the phone advice you received from the nurse	1	2	3	4	5	N/A
10. You were informed if your appointment was going to be delayed more than 15 minutes	1	2	3	4	5	N/A
11. The thoroughness and completeness of answers you received to questions you asked	1	2	3	4	5	N/A
12. The usefulness of teaching visits (for prenatal care, diabetes, allergy, etc.) conducted by the nurse	1	2	3	4	5	N/A
13. The difference between types of nurses is made apparent to you (either verbally or by a name tag)	1	2	3	4	5	N/A
14. Overall, how would you evaluate the nursing services at *FHPC?*	1	2	3	4	5	N/A

15. What do you like the best about the *FHPC* Nursing Department? _____

16. If you could improve one thing about the *FHPC* Nursing Department, what would it be? _____

_____

_____

continues

Exhibit 26–5 continued

We would like you to think about another aspect of nursing services. We would like to know how important each of the following services is to you. For each of these services, please check the response that best describes how important that nursing service is to you.

17. Ability to get advice from a nurse.
    _____ 1. Absolutely essential
    _____ 2. Very important
    _____ 3. A little important
    _____ 4. Not too important
    _____ 5. Not important at all
    _____ 6. Not applicable

18. Being informed if your appointment is going to be delayed more than 15 minutes.
    _____ 1. Absolutely essential
    _____ 2. Very important
    _____ 3. A little important
    _____ 4. Not too important
    _____ 5. Not important at all
    _____ 6. Not applicable

19. Ability to schedule teaching visits with a nurse.
    _____ 1. Absolutely essential
    _____ 2. Very important
    _____ 3. A little important
    _____ 4. Not too important
    _____ 5. Not important at all
    _____ 6. Not applicable

20. Ability to tell the difference between different types of nursing staff by their uniforms.
    _____ 1. Absolutely essential
    _____ 2. Very important
    _____ 3. A little important
    _____ 4. Not too important
    _____ 5. Not important at all
    _____ 6. Not applicable

Courtesy of Family Health Plan Cooperative, Milwaukee, Wisconsin.

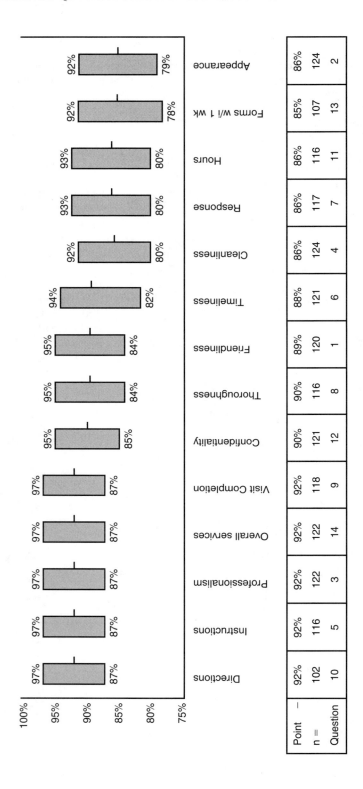

Point	–	92%	92%	92%	92%	92%	90%	90%	89%	88%	86%	86%	86%	86%	85%	86%
n =		102	116	122	122	118	121	116	120	121	124	117	116	124	107	124
Question		10	5	3	14	9	12	8	1	6	4	7	11	13	2

Date: 03/12/96
*Confidence Interval = 95%

Figure 26–2 Health Information Department 1995 Member Satisfaction Survey Results, Questions 1–4 (Percentage Responding *Excellent* and *Very Good**). Courtesy of Family Health Plan Cooperative, Milwaukee, Wisconsin.

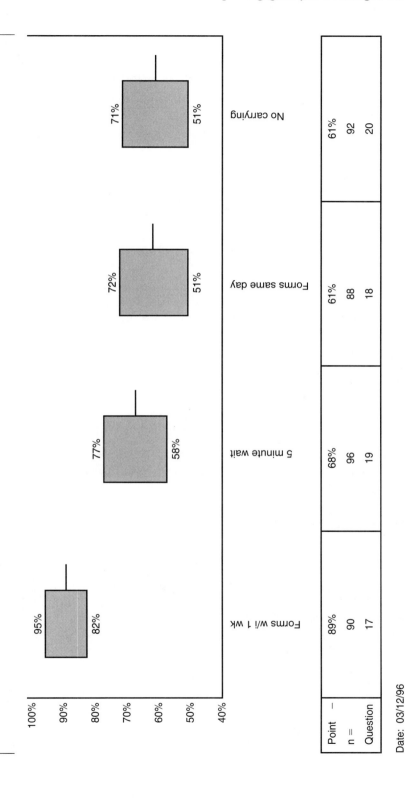

Point	—			
n =	90	96	88	92
Question	17	19	18	20

	Forms w/i 1 wk	5 minute wait	Forms same day	No carrying
Point	89%	68%	61%	61%
n =	90	96	88	92
Question	17	19	18	20

Date: 03/12/96
*Confidence Interval = 95%

Figure 26–3 Health Information Department 1995 Member Satisfaction Survey Results, Questions 17–20 (Percentage Responding *Absolutely Essential* and *Very Important**). Courtesy of Family Health Plan Cooperative, Milwaukee, Wisconsin.

Exhibit 26–6 Medicaid Member Satisfaction Survey

1. In the past 12 months, have you or your children had visits to any of the following places? Please circle all of the answers that are true.

   a. Doctor's clinic or office
   b. Emergency room
   c. Hospital bed, one night or more
   d. Have not had any visits

2. At any time in the past 12 months, were you or your children unable to get an appointment to see your regular doctor when you needed to? YES _____   NO _____
   If you checked YES, circle all the reasons why you were unable to get an appointment.

   a. Don't know how to make an appointment
   b. Doctor's office canceled visit
   c. I couldn't get in soon enough
   d. Waited too long in doctor's clinic or office
   e. Other reason (write in): _____
   _____

3. When do you or your children go to the doctor? Please circle all true answers.

   a. When sick or hurt
   b. For regular checkups and shots, even if not sick
   c. When pregnant
   d. When I need to talk to someone
   e. After I try home medicine and it doesn't work
   f. Don't go to or don't believe in doctors. Why? _____
   _____
   g. Other reason (write in): _____
   _____

4. When your family goes to the doctor, what types of transportation do you use? Please circle each type that you use to get to the doctor.

   a. Drive own car
   b. Family member or friend drives
   c. Bus
   d. Taxi
   e. Other (write in):

5. In the past 12 months, did you or your children ever miss an appointment to see your regular doctor? Please check YES or NO: YES _____   NO _____
   If you checked YES, please circle all the reasons why:

   a. Forgot
   b. Hard to get a ride
   c. No money for ride
   d. Couldn't get time off from work or school
   e. Babysitter problems
   f. Doctor's office too far

continues

Exhibit 26–6 continued

g. Doctor's visit costs too much
h. Don't speak English well
i. Other reason (write in):

_____

6. How would you say the health care that you get is? Check the best answer:
GOOD _____   FAIR _____   POOR _____

If you are not happy with the health care you get, please tell us why:

_____
_____
_____

7. What would make it easier for your family to get health care? Circle the 3 best reasons:

a. Help with a ride
b. Doctor closer to my home
c. Shorter wait to get appointment
d. Help with babysitting
e. Shorter wait in doctor's waiting room
f. Evening appointments
g. Weekend appointments
h. Help with speaking or understanding English
i. Better directions from the doctor about when to come in
j. Other (write in):

_____

8. Please tell us your year of birth: _____

Please return this survey in the enclosed envelope. No stamp is needed.

THANK YOU!

Courtesy of Family Health Plan Cooperative, Milwaukee, Wisconsin.

26–9). Credentialing and recredentialing are conducted by the FHPC Medical Administration Quality Committee in accordance with the current NCQA standards. As with Medicaid requirements, physicians, optometrists, dentists, and chiropractors must be initially credentialed at the time of hire and recredentialed every 2 years subsequently.

As indicated in Exhibit 26–10, key indicators are reviewed on a monthly basis. A variance report is prepared to explain deviations from standard. On the basis of review of the key indicators over time, action plans may be developed in response to changes in performance. Chart reviews are also conducted in ac-

cordance with current NCQA standards in conjunction with recredentialing.

The success of a managed-care organization is based on meeting the needs of individual members and employer groups while satisfying the needs of the medical staff and the requirements of regulatory bodies as well as voluntary accreditating agencies. Although the managed-care revolution is still in a relatively rudimentary stage of development with "report cards" and other mechanisms for measuring outcomes, the potential is great for health care quality performance to assist in lowering costs and to demonstrate value to all stakeholders.

Exhibit 26–7 FHPC Member Survey: Satisfaction with Specialist Care

At Family Health Plan Cooperative (*FHPC*), quality health care is our standard. We continually assess the performance of our plan and it is important to know what *you* think about the care you received. Please take a few minutes to complete this survey about the specialist you or your family member visited. Please mark the best response to each statement.

Specialist's Name: _____

	Poor	Fair	Good	Very Good	Excellent	Not Applicable
1. Your access to specialty care	1	2	3	4	5	N/A
2. The process of scheduling an appointment with the specialist	1	2	3	4	5	N/A
3. The specialist's thoroughness of examinations and accuracy of diagnoses	1	2	3	4	5	N/A
4. The specialist's attention to what you have to say	1	2	3	4	5	N/A
5. The specialist's thoroughness of treatment including how well the doctor and staff follow through on your care	1	2	3	4	5	N/A
6. The friendliness and courtesy of the specialist's staff	1	2	3	4	5	N/A
7. Cleanliness and appearance of the specialist's office	1	2	3	4	5	N/A
8. The length of time you wait between making an appointment with the specialist and the day of your visit	1	2	3	4	5	N/A
9. How long you usually have to wait for the specialist when you arrive on time for a scheduled appointment	1	2	3	4	5	N/A
10. Location of the specialist's office	1	2	3	4	5	N/A
11. How well the whole system works together to coordinate your medical care, including how well different people and departments communicate with you and with each other about your care	1	2	3	4	5	N/A
12. Overall, how would you evaluate the specialist?	1	2	3	4	5	N/A

13. What did you like the best about the *FHPC* specialist? _____

14. If you could improve one thing about the *FHPC* specialist, what would it be? _____

Optional Information

15. Name: _____

16. Member Number: _____

17. May we contact you if we would like more information?
 — 1. No
 — 2. Yes

18. Phone Number: _____

Please complete the following background questions.

19. How long have you belonged to *FHPC?*
 1. Less than 1 year
 2. One to less than 3 years
 3. Three to less than 5 years
 4. Five to less than 10 years
 5. Ten years or more

20. Your age?

Courtesy of Family Health Plan Cooperative, Milwaukee, Wisconsin.

21. Your gender?
 — 1. Female
 — 2. Male

22. Type of membership?
 1. Through an employer group
 2. Medicare
 3. Medicaid
 4. Self pay

23. Your home site?
 1. Airport
 2. Bluemound
 3. Edgerton
 4. Parkway
 5. Port Road
 6. Silver Spring
 7. Waukesha

Fold and tape the completed survey, and drop it in a mailbox. We have paid for the postage. Thank you.

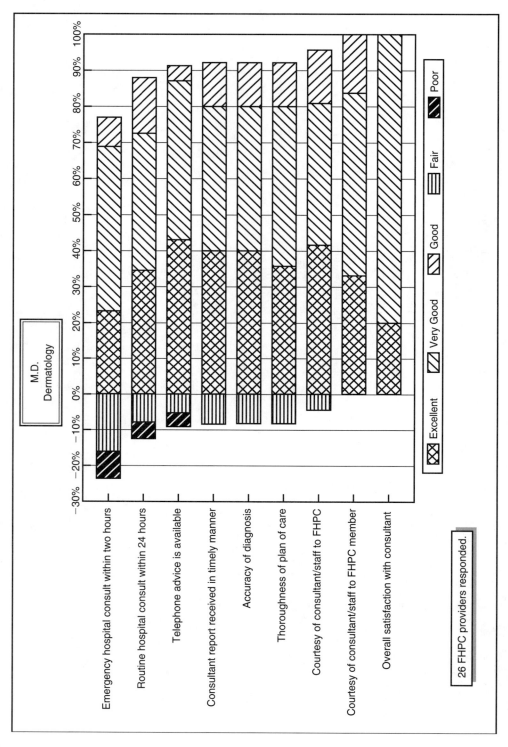

Figure 26–4 Data on FHPC providers' satisfaction with a specialist. Courtesy of Family Health Plan Cooperative, Milwaukee, Wisconsin.

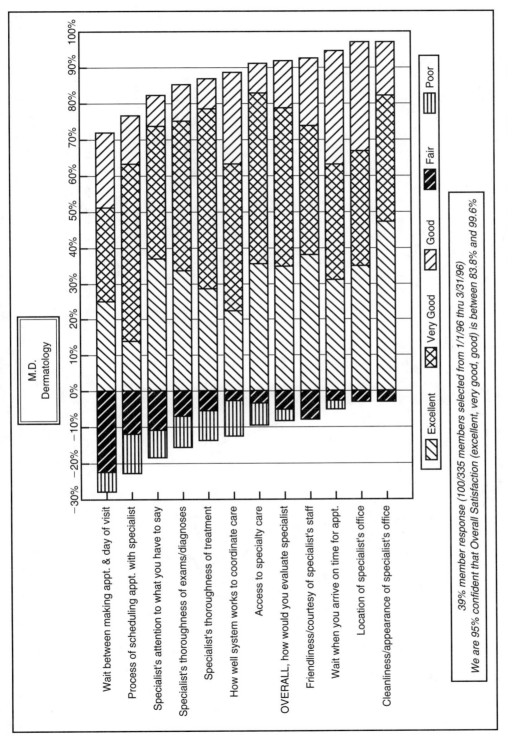

Figure 26–5 Data on FHPC members' perceptions of care provided by a specialist. Courtesy of Family Health Plan Cooperative, Milwaukee, Wisconsin.

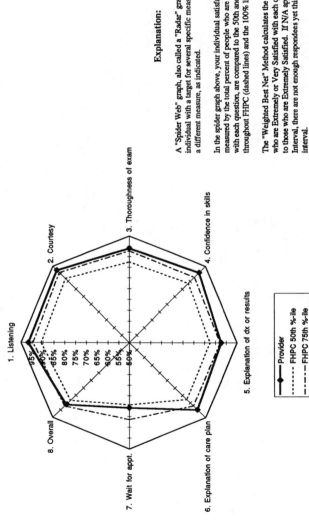

Member Satisfaction Survey
Surveys Completed From 1/96 through 7/25/96

"**Weighted Best Net**" Method
Number of respondees: 30
95% confidence interval: ± #N/A

Explanation:

A "Spider Web" graph, also called a "Radar" graph, is used to compare an individual with a target for several specific measures. Each "spoke" represents a different measure, as indicated.

In the spider graph above, your individual satisfaction levels (diamonds), as measured by the total percent of people who are Extremely or Very Satisfied with each question, are compared to the 50th and 75th %-ile for providers throughout FHPC (dashed lines) and the 100% line (fine line).

The "Weighted Best Net" Method calculates the percentage of all respondees who are Extremely or Very Satisfied with each question, giving higher weight to those who are Extremely Satisfied. If N/A appears in the Confidence Interval, there are not enough respondees yet this year to calculate a confidence interval.

Questions one through six are related to communication, and tend to have the highest importance to patients when they decide whether to maintain a relationship with a provider or a health plan.

Figure 26–6 Spider diagram of member survey data on satisfaction with primary care providers. Courtesy of Family Health Plan Cooperative, Milwaukee, Wisconsin.

Exhibit 26–8 Credentialing Review Form

Provider Name:		Date Initiated:	
Specialty:		Date Committee Reviewed:	
Group Name:		☐ Interim Review	

Provisional Approval by Medical Director (Initials) _____ Date: _____

VARIATION FROM POLICY (Check all that apply)

☐ Wisconsin License Limitation
☐ DEA Privilege Restriction
☐ Other Non-verifiable Information
☐ History of Substance Abuse
☐ History of Felony Conviction
☐ Hospital Practice Limitation
☐ No Privileges at Affiliated Hospital
☐ History of Malpractice Claims
☐ Site Visit Report
☐ Not Board Certified

FILE INCLUDES:

☐ Signed Application
☐ Wisconsin License
   ___ Verified with State
☐ Confirmation of Hospital Privileges
   ___ St. Michael
   ___ WAMH
   ___ SSMC   ___ SGM
   ___ St. Francis
   ___ Waukesha Memorial
   ___ Other _____

☐ DEA Certificate _____ Initials _____ Date
☐ Malpractice Coverage
                    _____ Initials _____ Date
☐ National Practitioner Data Bank
☐ Medicare Sanction Report (10/95)
   Not listed: _____ Initials _____ Date

EDUCATION	PER ABMS DIRECTORY	LETTER
Medical School		
Internship		
Residency		
Fellowship		
Board Certified		

Initials _____ Date: _____

COMMITTEE RECOMMENDATIONS

☐ Acceptance, 2 years, No restrictions
☐ Acceptance, 2 years, List restrictions:
_____

☐ Provisional Acceptance
       ___ 1 Year, Review Board Status
       ___ 1 Year, Reason _____
       ___ Other: _____
☐ Rejected. Reason: _____
   Report to NPDB

_____   _____
Chair of Credential Committee   Date of Action

Courtesy of Family Health Plan Cooperative, Milwaukee, Wisconsin.

Exhibit 26–9 Recredentialing Review Form

Provider Name: **Date Initiated:**

Specialty: **Date Committee Reviewed:**

Group Name: ☐ Interim Review

Provisional Approval by Medical Director (Initials) _____ Date: _____

VARIATION FROM POLICY (Check all that apply)

☐ Wisconsin License Limitation
☐ DEA Privilege Restriction
☐ Other Non-verifiable Information
☐ History of Substance Abuse
☐ History of Felony Conviction
☐ Hospital Practice Limitation
☐ No Privileges at Affiliated Hospital
☐ History of Malpractice Claims
☐ Site Visit Report
☐ Not Board Certified

FILE INCLUDES:

☐ Signed Application
☐ Wisconsin License
   __ Verified with State
☐ Confirmation of Hospital Privileges
   __ St. Michael
   __ WAMH
   __ SSMC   __ SGM
   __ St. Francis
   __ Waukesha Memorial
   __ Other _____
☐ DEA Certificate ____ Initials ____ Date
☐ Malpractice Coverage
       ____ Initials ____ Date
☐ National Practitioner Data Bank
☐ Medicare Sanction Report (10/95)
   Not listed: ____ Initials ____ Date
☐ Data from QA
   __ Meets Standards
   __ Does not Meet Standards

☐ CME Credits

CERTIFICATION	PER ABMS DIRECTORY	LETTER
Board Certified		

Initials _____ Date: _____

COMMITTEE RECOMMENDATIONS

☐ Acceptance, 2 years, No restrictions
☐ Acceptance, 2 years, List restrictions:
_____

☐ Provisional Acceptance
   ____ 1 Year, Review Board Status
   ____ 1 Year, Reason:_____
   ____ Other:_____
☐ Rejected. Reason:_____
   Report to NPDB

_____   _____
Chair of Credential Committee   Date of Action

Courtesy of Family Health Plan Cooperative, Milwaukee, Wisconsin.

Exhibit 26–10 Key Indicators Reviewed Monthly

1996 HEALTH CENTER KEY INDICATOR EXPLANATION		
DEPARTMENT	**INDICATOR**	**CALCULATION/SAMPLE SIZE**
ADMINISTRATION	PRIMARY CARE CAPACITY OF HEALTH CENTERS	Calculated by the monthly panel report at each health center
CROSS-FUNCTIONAL TRANSCRIPTION	TOTAL DICTATION CYCLE TIME PRIORITY This includes: dictation turnaround time: actual transcription; findings folder turnaround time; misc. filing turnaround time.	Adds all values of dictation turnaround time, actual transcription turnaround time, (priority separate from routine), findings folder turnaround time and misc filing turnaround time for each site. Reported monthly from each site to Parkway, and they report all findings to Center Point.
	ROUTINE This includes: dictation turnaround time; actual transcription; findings folder turnaround time; misc. filing turnaround time.	Same as above.
	AGGREGATE (Not reported to Board)	10 per week per site - Determine number of days between filing date and date patient seen
HEALTH INFORMATION	WORKERS COMP RELEASE OF INFORMATION TURNAROUND TIME (Report Weekly)	100% sample of all work completed within the period to determine if it was completed within 7 calendar days. If site is manually logging the work, the calculation is done in the log book. If the site has the computer program, the computer produces a list of all work completed that week and the TAT. The calculation is then done from this list.
	NON-WORKERS COMP RELEASE OF INFORMATION TURNAROUND TIME (Report Weekly)	Same as above.
	ACCURACY OF MISC. FILING (Information in the correct chart)	30 chart sample (per site) of charts ready for appointments. All charts reviewed on the same day for one particular site. Each chart is examined to determine if all paperwork belongs to the member listed on the outside of the folder. All errors from 1 year or less are counted.
	PLACEMENT OF REPORTS IN CHART (Information in the correct location in the chart)	Same method as above. Charts are examined to determine if the paperwork is in the correct location within the chart. All misplaced reports are evaluated by the Supervisor to determine if they were correctly placed at the time they were filled. All errors from 1 year or less are counted.
	MISCELLANEOUS FILING TURNAROUND TIME WEEKLY	100% sample. The number of days since the misc filing box was emptied is recorded. The total of these figures is divided by the number of storage boxes to be filed.
LABORATORY	LAB WEEKDAY ONLY LAG TIME First two available appts., not necessarily together, before 9 a.m.	Lag times are measured weekly on Fridays before Noon.
		The number of days until 2 or more openings are available before 9:00 am.
	COLLECTION/DISPATCH ERRORS SITE CONTROLLABLE Based on site total tests.	100% of errors times 5000 divided by the total number of tests drawn for the month
	COLLECTION/DISPATCH ERRORS NON-FHPC LABS (Roche and WAMH)	100% of errors times 500 divided by the number of WAMH/Roche tests drawn for

continues

Exhibit 26–10 continued

		Based on site send out tests.	the month
		LAB LOBBY WAIT TIMES	Selected sample of the first patient at the top of every hour - sticker time vs actual draw time
		STAT U/A TURNAROUND TIME	100% sample of STAT urines; time specimen received vs the time results reported out
NURSING		PEDIATRIC IMMUNIZATIONS	10 healthcheck or N.O. encounter forms:
		HEDIS data elements regarding pediatric immunization are consistent between encounter form and medical record. (Report Weekly)	Check for whether the chart is documented correctly and whether the encounter is bubbled correctly.
		VITAL SIGN DOCUMENTATION	Same 10 encounter forms as above. Check
		Height and weight plotted accurately for all well child check visits. (Report Weekly)	to determine that height and weight are plotted accurately on growth chart.
		CALL-BACK TIME	10 acute callbacks per week, randomly selected
		Nurse triage (nursing advice/same day appointments), callbacks/attempted callbacks, during routine clinic hours. (Report Weekly)	from miscellaneous filing. The time they called versus the time we called back. (These callbacks do not require a chart pull)
		PATIENT TEACHING LAG TIMES	Lag times are measured weekly on Fridays before Noon.
		Calendar days for first available nurse teaching appointments during dedicated nurse teaching sessions. (Report Weekly)	The number of days until the next available opening.
		AVOIDABLE ED VISITS	100% sample of all ER callbacks. Codes
		Review of all ED admissions during routine clinic hours (Reasons 8,9,10 avoidable).	1 through 10 are assigned by the RN. Codes 8,9, and 10 are considered avoidable.
NURSING (Cont'd)		SKIN TEST LAG TIME	Count all calendar days from date of referral
		Count all calendar days from date of referral to date of next available skin test appointment	to date of next available skin test appointment
		ALLERGIST LAG TIME	Count all calendar days from date skin test
		Count all calendar days from date skin test results submitted to allergist to date patient notified of recommendations.	results submitted to allergist to date patient notified of recommendations.
PHARMACY		REFILL TURNAROUND TIME FOR REFILLS THAT REQUIRE MD/NP/PA SIGNATURE	
		REFILL TURNAROUND TIME FOR REFILLS THAT WERE PREVIOUSLY AUTHORIZED	
		WAITING TIME IN LOBBY	Selected sample of the first patient at the top of
		Time a member spends waiting in lobby for a new prescription.	every hour - check in time vs actual time dispensed
		DISPENSING ERRORS	Number of dispensing errors times 10,000
		Rate per 10,000 Rxs.	and then divided by the number of scripts dispensed for the month
PHYSICIANS		% OF AVOIDABLE RESCHEDULED APPTS.	Number of appointments cancelled for vac, CME,
		Vacation/CME requests/Admin mtgs.	and admin mtgs divided by the total number of appointments for the month. Tracked by individual provider to examine problems.
		% OF UNAVOIDABLE RESCHEDULED APPTS.	Number of appointments cancelled for hosp, pers
		Hospital admits, personal, sick, OB.	sick and OB divided by the total number of appointments for the month.
		LAG TIMES	Lag times are measured weekly on Fridays
		ACUTE APPOINTMENTS	before Noon.
		(Report Weekly)	The number of days until there are 4 acute appointments available, measured individually for each provider. Average the results of all providers to determine the average for the site.

continues

Exhibit 26–10 continued

		LAG TIMES	Lag times are measured weekly on Fridays before Noon.
		ROUTINE APPOINTMENTS	
		(Report Weekly)	The number of days until there is 1 hr of routine appointments available, measured individually for each provider. Average the results of all providers to determine the average for the site.
		DATA BASE PHYSICALS	The number of days until there are 2 consecutive
		(Report Weekly)	days of at least 1 database available, measured individually for each provider. Average the results of all providers to determine the average for the site.
RADIOLOGY		TECHNOLOGY LAG TIMES - ROUTINE APPTS	All Lag times are measured weekly on Fridays before Noon.
		MAMMOGRAPHY	The number of days until the next routine
		(Report Weekly)	appointment opening.
		ULTRASOUND	The number of days until the next routine
		(Report Weekly)	appointment opening.
		FLUORO	The number of days until the next opening.
		(Report Weekly)	
		CT (Report Weekly)	The number of days until there are 2 openings.
		X-RAYS RETURNED TO DEPARTMENT	
		X-RAY DEPARTMENT WAITING TIME	
		The time between x-ray request (from one-ply) until time the patient is called into the dept.	
RECEPTION		TELEPHONE SERVICE FACTOR	Provided by Telephone software
		Percent of calls answered within the standard.	
		(Report Weekly)	
		PHONE ABANDONED RATE	Provided by Telephone software
		Calls abandoned	
		(Report Weekly)	
		AVERAGE HOLD TIME OF ALL CALLS	Provided by Telephone software
		Average speed of answer	
		(Report Weekly)	
		AVERAGE HOLD TIME OF ALL CALLS	Provided by Telephone software
		Average speed of answer	
		(Report Weekly)	
		POST-CALL PROCESSING TIME	Provided by Telephone software
		Time that phones are in "not ready".	
		(Report Weekly)	
		CALLS ANSWERED PER AVAILABLE	Provided by Telephone software
		AGENT PER HOUR (Peak Hours)	
		(Report Weekly)	
UCC/TRIAGE		TELEPHONE TURNAROUND TIME	
		Time between member's call and response from triage nurse.	
		CHART REVIEW	
		Completeness of documentation.	

Courtesy of Family Health Plan Cooperative, Milwaukee, Wisconsin.

REFERENCES

National Committee on Quality Assurance. (1996). *Standards for the accreditation of managed care organizations* (3rd ed.). Washington, DC: Author.

Wisconsin Department of Health and Social Services, Contract for Medicaid HMO Services between HMO and WI Department of Health and Family Services, July 1996–December 1997.

APPENDIX 26–A
Policy and Procedure for Provider Selection and Qualifications

POLICY:

In order to promote the highest quality of care for its members, it is the policy of Family Health Plan Cooperative to ensure that its employed and contracted physicians meet minimum standards relative to educational accomplishments, professional standing, and technical ability. The educational accomplishments, professional standing, and technical ability are verified by the collection of specific credentials on a routine basis. Credentials are reviewed by the Credentials Committee which is chaired by the Medical Director. The Credentials Committee reports its actions to the Health Services Committee of the Board of Directors through the Medical Administration Quality Committee. This policy shall be reviewed annually by the Credentials Committee.

SCOPE:

The Committee's scope is limited to all employed physicians and other independent practitioners of the organization and the contracted consulting physicians that provide the first level of consultation in the following fields:

> Allergy, Cardiology, Cardiovascular Surgery, Dermatology, Endocrinology, Gastroenterology, General and Vascular Surgery, Genetic Counseling, Infectious Diseases, Nephrology, Neurology, Neurosurgery, Obstetrics and Gynecology, Oncology/Hematology, Neurosurgery, Ophthalmology, Oral Surgery, Orthopedics, Otolaryngology, Pediatrics, Plastic Surgery, Podiatry, Psychiatry, Pulmonary Medicine, Radiation Oncology, Rheumatology, Thoracic Surgery, and Urology.

The Committee may, at its discretion, review the credentials of other contracted consultants to ensure they meet the standards of educational accomplishments, professional standing, and technical ability.

1. STANDARDS

    A. The physician holds a valid license to practice medicine in the State of Wisconsin.

       License limitations shall be considered in light of the impact of the limitation on the physician's contracted responsibility.

Courtesy of Family Health Plan Cooperative, Milwaukee, Wisconsin.

B. The physician has clinical privileges with relationship to their respective specialty in good standing at an affiliated hospital.

Consideration shall be given to physicians whose practice is non-hospital based.

FOR CONSULTANTS ONLY:

Scope of privileges shall be considered in light of the impact of the consultant's contracted responsibilities.

C. The physician has a valid DEA certificate. The absence of a valid DEA certificate or a restricted certificate shall be considered in light of the impact upon the physician's contracted responsibilities.

D. The physician shall be a graduate of a recognized medical school and shall have completed a residency accredited by ACGME in the area of service.

E. The physician shall be able to secure and maintain professional liability insurance that is adequate in the opinion of Family Health Plan and at least meets the requirements set forth in Section 655.23(4) Wisconsin Statutes.

F. The physician shall be board certified in the specialty for which he/she is contracted to provide service to Family members, from a board recognized by the appropriate certifying organizations listed below:

> American Board of Medical Specialists
> American Osteopathic Association
> American Podiatric Medical Association/Council on Podiatric Medical Education

A physician who has been employed by FHPC or contracted with FHPC prior to 1/1/95 who is not yet board certified shall be expected to obtain board certification within a designated period of time as determined by the Medical Director.

A physician who begins employment with FHPC or contracts with FHPC after 1/1/95 shall be expected to obtain board certification within two years of beginning with FHPC or within two years of becoming eligible to take the board exam.

The Medical Director has the discretion to take into consideration performance, experience, reputation, and needs of FHPC to make exceptions. This discretion will also apply to physicians who have achieved board certification in a specialty and are fellowship trained in their contracted specialty, but who have not achieved board certification in the contract specialty.

All physicians who achieve board certification shall be expected to maintain this certification.

G. The physician shall be in adequate health to provide contracted responsibility.

FOR HIGH VOLUME SPECIALISTS: High volume specialists are defined as those specialty services that account for 5 percent or more of the physician referrals. The following specialties are considered high volume: Orthopedics, Psychiatry, and Obstetrics/Gynecology.

H. The consultant shall provide services in an office that is functionally safe and sanitary.

I. The consultant shall maintain a clinical record system from which information can be readily accessible to the providers of health care.

2. RE-CREDENTIALING

After the initial credential review and approval, the physician's credentials are reviewed at least every two years to ensure continued compliance with the above standards.

3. HOSPITAL BASED PHYSICIANS (Not employed by FHPC)

This category includes but is not limited to radiologists, pathologists, emergency medicine physicians, and anesthesiologists who practice primarily at an affiliated hospital or ambulatory surgery center. Family Health Plan Cooperative shall rely upon the hospital to credential and privilege hospital-based consultants.

4. OTHER DELEGATION OF CREDENTIALING

From time to time, with the approval of the Credential Committee, credentialing of a selected group of providers may be delegated to another organization. The specific requirements of the organization accepting the credentialing responsibility shall be in a written agreement approved by the Credential Committee.

PROCEDURE

1. CREDENTIALING PROCESS

The following procedure is used for all physicians to Family Health Plan Cooperative. For all physicians, an application and credential information is required.

A. Credential Committee:

The Credential Committee as defined in the FHPC Quality Improvement Plan includes: The committee is composed of the Medical Director, the Chief of Primary Care, the Health Center Chiefs of Primary Care, the Manager of Affiliated Providers, and the Manager of Professional Staffing. The Committee meets monthly or more often if necessary to review and approve credentials. The Committee has the authority to request additional ad-hoc members as it deems necessary to provide adequate peer review.

B. The following data are requested.

1. License.
2. DEA Number.
3. Medical School and completion date.
4. ECFMG if applicable.
5. Internship.
6. Residency program and completion date.
7. Post residency training.
8. Board certification or eligibility.
9. Past and present hospital privileges and affiliations.
10. Past and present practice affiliations.
11. Professional liability coverage and history (NPDB).
12. Attestation as to history of substance abuse.

13. Attestation as to history of criminal/felony convictions.
14. Professional references.

C. The information provided is verified by telephone or by writing to the appropriate source or through the ABMS Compendium.

1. Medical examining board (Department of Regulation and Licensing).
2. Professional liability carrier.
3. Affiliated hospitals.
4. Medical college.
5. Residency program.
6. Fellowship program.
7. Specialty board.
8. ECFMG if foreign medical school graduate.
9. National Practitioner Data Bank.
10. Letters of recommendation.
11. DEA Certificate.

D. Additional information is gathered regarding provider status with Medicare and Medicaid.

E. Report of site visit if applicable. (For Consultants Only)

F. After verification of credentials, the prospective physician's application is presented to the Credential Committee for approval.

All reviews and actions of the Credential Committee shall be documented and retained in the physician's file.

G. The recommendations of the Credential Committee, including any limitations, reduction, suspension, or termination of privileges, along with a description of the appeal process described herein, will be communicated to the prospective physician and documented in the credential file. If any limitations, reductions, suspensions, or termination of privileges are set forth by the Credential Committee, proper individuals, including the NPDB as required by law, will be notified of the physician's limitations.

1. If the physician desires to appeal the recommendation of the Credential Committee, the physician must submit to the Credential Committee a written request for an appeal along with any information and documentation to support the physician's appeal position within thirty (30) days of the notice of the Credential Committee recommendation.

2. If the prospective physician does not respond in writing within thirty (30) days, the right for further appeals shall be considered to have been waived by the physician.

3. The Credential Committee shall reconsider the physician's application in light of any additional information and documentation provided at its next monthly meeting. The physician may request to appear at the Credential Committee meeting to present relevant information.

4. The Credential Committee shall notify the prospective physician of its decision within thirty (30) days of the Credential Committee meeting.

5. The prospective physician shall have thirty (30) days from the receipt of this decision by the Credential Committee to request an appeal via certified mail to the Medical Director of FHPC.

6. The Medical Director shall consider all the available information provided by the Credential Committee and the prospective physician. The Medical Director shall make a determination and notify the prospective physician within thirty (30) days of the receipt of the appeal request which is final.

H. After receipt and verification of credentials, current information is placed in the physician's file. Date of approval is noted.

2. RE-CREDENTIALING PROCESS

A. A completed re-credentialing application and the following information is obtained from each employed physician every two years:

1. Current active Wisconsin license. (Photostatic copy)
2. DEA number, active without restrictions. (Photostatic copy)
3. Evidence of professional liability coverage at the limits required by Wisconsin Statutes, Section 655.23(4).
4. Privileges at Family Health Plan affiliated hospitals sufficient to provide the required services to Family Health Plan patients.
5. Any change in board certification or eligibility or hospital privileges.
6. Professional liability history.

FOR EMPLOYED PHYSICIANS ONLY:

7. Record of accredited AMA or AOA CME credits sufficient for maintenance of Wisconsin licensure.

B. The information is verified every two years by a telephone call or by writing the appropriate source or the ABMS Compendium.

1. Medical examining board (Department of Regulation & Licensing).
2. National Practitioner Data Bank.
3. Affiliated hospitals.
4. Specialty board.
5. Professional liability carrier.

C. Additional information is gathered in regards to physician's status with the Medicare/Medicaid programs.

D. Data regarding member complaints, results of utilization or quality reviews, and member satisfaction surveys are collected from various sources in the organization and presented to the Credentials Committee for consideration along with the verified items in II A. and the renewal application.

E. Report of site visit, if applicable. (For Consultants Only)

F. After verification of credentials, the physician application is presented to the Credential Committee for approval.

All reviews and actions of the Credential Committee shall be documented and retained in the provider credential files.

G. The recommendations of the Credential Committee, including any limitations, reduction, suspension, or termination of privileges, along with a description of the appeal process described herein, will be communicated to the prospective physician and documented in the credential file. If any limitations, reductions, suspensions, or termination of privileges are set forth by the Credential Committee, proper individuals, including the NPDB as required by law, will be notified of the physician's limitations.

1. If the physician desires to appeal the recommendation of the Credential Committee, the physician must submit to the Credential Committee a written request for an appeal along with any information and documentation to support the physician's appeal position within thirty (30) days of the notice of the Credential Committee recommendation.

2. If the prospective physician does not respond in writing within thirty (30) days, the right for further appeals shall be considered to have been waived by the physician.

3. The Credential Committee shall reconsider the physician's application in light of any additional information and documentation provided at its next monthly meeting. The physician may request to appear at the Credential Committee meeting to present relevant information.

4. The Credential Committee shall notify the prospective physician of its decision within thirty (30) days of the Credential Committee meeting.

5. The prospective physician shall have thirty (30) days from the receipt of this decision by the Credential Committee to request an appeal via certified mail to the Medical Director of FHPC.

6. The Medical Director shall consider all the available information provided by the Credentials Committee and the prospective physician. The Medical Director shall make a determination and notify the prospective physician within thirty (30) days of the receipt of the appeal request.

H. Date of re-credential approval is noted in file.

CHAPTER 27

Improving Quality in Natural and Alternative Health Care Practice

Roxana Huebscher

CHAPTER OBJECTIVES

After completing this chapter, the reader will be able to

- consider some of the differences between conventional and nonconventional health practices
- describe various evaluative measures appropriate for NAHC practices
- evaluate quality of NAHC practices using foci of ethical, comfort, caring, confidential, and hygienic care

Natural/alternative health care (NAHC) refers to "those health care practices, outside the mainstream (conventional) nursing/medicine domain, including forms of care that we have not previously considered health care" (Huebscher, 1994, p. 67). A few of these nonconventional health care practices are listed in Exhibit 27–1.

To provide our clients with a truly comprehensive and holistic approach to care, health care providers (HCPs) must become knowledgeable about NAHC practices and must advocate for effective NAHC forms of care, especially if it is having a positive impact on the client. Criticizing the "unknown" prevents clients from receiving *all* beneficial care and discounts their ability to take charge of their own health. By gaining knowledge about various practices—conventional and nonconventional—HCPs can refer clients appropriately

and ensure a broader range of health care options. Evaluating the quality of the NAHC practices becomes an integral part of health care provision.

STANDARDS

NAHC options are usually less invasive than conventional therapies. However, there is a dearth of research for many of the NAHC practices (just as there is not a solid research base for many of the conventional forms of care we use). Thus assessing quality of NAHC services may require unconventional or unique criteria for the evaluative process. We can expect ethical, caring, competent, confidential, and hygienic care from NAHC practitioners. However, at this time, we cannot expect the same conventional theoretical orientation, rigorous research base, time frames for care, or legislative regulation. Nor should we, for often the whole purpose of NAHC is to provide broader and alternative approaches to treatment. NAHC treatments are often time intensive, and many of the NAHC methods do not lend themselves to double-blind, placebo-controlled studies.

There are educational, professional, and sometimes state criteria for chiropractors, naturopathic doctors (NDs), acupuncturists, and biofeedback therapists, to name a few. The American Holistic Nurses Association (AHNA) offers a Holistic Nurses Certification program

Exhibit 27–1 Systems and Techniques of Natural/Alternative Health Care

Acupressure	Feldenkrais	Reflexology
Acupuncture	Healing Touch	Reiki
Affirmations	Heller Work	Rolfing
Alexander	Herbals	Shamanism
Aromatherapy	Homeopathy	Shiatsu
Ayurveda	Hypnosis	Spiritual Practices
Bach Flower	Imagery	Support Groups
Bibliotherapy	Laying on of Hands	Tai Chi
Biofeedback	Macrobiotics	Therapeutic Touch
Bowen	Massage	Traditional Chinese Medicine
Chakra balancing	Meditation	Trager
Chiropractic	Naturopathy	Vitamins/Minerals
Colonics	Neuromuscular Work	Water Therapies
Craniosacral	Polarity	Yoga
Crystals	Prayer	

and cosponsors, with the Academy for Guided Imagery, a Nurses Certificate Program in Interactive Imagery. Not all practices have a form of certification or credentialing. Conversely, Healing Touch Practitioners may complete a certification program or simply take a workshop. AHNA, for example, has endorsed a Healing Touch Certification Program, although it is not offered through their organization. This course is a lengthy process and involves several levels of training and education. However, some persons may take a workshop or read one of several books on offering touch and then will practice Healing Touch. In addition, it is a common religious practice to offer laying on of hands, which is also considered healing touch.

Thus a different type of evaluation of the more uncommon/unusual practices is needed. This does entail more effort on the evaluator's part, but the NAHC provider can usually provide needed contacts. Thus, in appraising standards and quality of care for a particular NAHC practice, information gathering about what the NAHC practice is and about the education/training process, licensure/certification/credentialing (if applicable), professional organizations, and peer review becomes important. Appendix 27–A offers a sampling of some NAHC resources.

NAHC Practice Example: Massage/Bodywork

An overview of the prominent NAHC practice of massage or bodywork illustrates and provides insight into the variety and complexity of treatments available. Massage/bodywork therapy includes a wide array of modalities, ranging from Swedish massage to deep tissue, neuromuscular, and sports massage to Bowen, Feldenkrais, Heller Work, Rolfing, Polarity, Shiatsu, and TragerWork, to name several examples. Massage therapists may need a city, county, or state license to practice, or they may not. Twenty-two states, and Washington D.C., regulate massage (Mower, 1996); 20 states offer some type of credential ("State Massage Laws," 1996). Several states have State Massage Boards, including Arkansas, Delaware, Florida, Hawaii, Nebraska, New Hampshire, New York, North Dakota, Ohio, Oregon, Rhode Island, Texas, Utah, and Washington. Obviously, the state legislation varies. Thus state regulation may be part of quality criteria for some. However, if legislation is not available, other criteria are needed.

Several professional massage organizations have set standards, including the American Massage Therapy Association (AMTA), the

International Myomassethics Federation, and the National Association of Nurse Massage Therapists (NANMT). In addition, the AMTA has set standards for the National Sports Massage Team. The Associated Bodywork and Massage Professionals (ABMP) and the International Massage Association offer insurance to bodywork providers. Also, there are various specialty groups such as the American Polarity Therapy Association, the Jin Shin Do Foundation for Bodymind Acupressure, and the Shiatsu Practitioners Association. And as of May 1996, over 20,000 massage and bodywork practitioners had passed the National Certification Examination for Therapeutic Massage and Bodywork (Mower, 1996). Thus, even though there may not be state regulation of all bodyworkers, there are professional standards set and numerous organizations.

INSTITUTIONAL AND PEER EVALUATION

Along with city and state regulations and professional ongoing standards, institutional and peer evaluation become the major focus for measuring outcomes for alternative practices and are appropriate for all NAHC evaluations. Exhibit 27–2 (Natural/Alternative Health Care Practice Institutional Evaluation Form) and Exhibit 27–3 (Peer Evaluation of Provider/Practice) are examples of peer evaluations. Finding an experienced person in a like practice or someone who is familiar with the philosophy, technique, and uses for the form of care is essential when using a person as a peer. Any research base or existing outcomes for the practice, even if anecdotal, are worth studying.

Exhibit 27–2 Natural/Alternative Health Care Practice: Institutional Evaluation Form

NAHC Provider Name: NAHC Practice:

Type of Care:

Philosophical Basis (i.e., how it works):

NAHC Provider Name:

Educational Background of Provider:

Location of Educational Facility/Pertinent Background/Provider's Principal Instructors:

Provider Certification/Credentialing/Licensure:

Previous Experience (initial):

Continuing Education (ongoing):

Peer Evaluation:

Client Evaluations:

Additional Comments: _____

_____

_____

Exhibit 27–3 Peer Evaluation of Provider/Practice

Name of Provider:

Type of Practice:

Name of Peer (person evaluating):

Criteria for being named a peer:

Does the Provider meet the standard of care for (*practice*)? ☐ Yes ☐ No

Please describe why or why not.

How would you describe the level of care that the provider practices? (i.e., Novice, Advanced Beginner, Proficient, Expert, or some other term)

Are appropriate products used? (if applicable) ☐ Yes ☐ No

Are they of good quality? ☐ Yes ☐ No

Is the environment conducive to the type of practice/process? ☐ Yes ☐ No

Please explain.

Additional comments:

CLIENT SATISFACTION/OUTCOMES

Knowing what the client needs and expects is critical to the health of the client and the HCP's practice. All clients have experienced various forms of conventional care. Striving to achieve the best possible outcomes for every client means gathering data by using client satisfaction tools. Exhibit 27–4 (Client Satisfaction with NAHC Care), centering on comfort and healing, emphasizes important foci in NAHC practices.

Comfort is central to any health care provision. Many NAHC practices provide comfort and relaxation. Kolcaba (1991, 1992) provided a taxonomic structure for this important but difficult-to-define term by referring to relief, ease, and transcendence. *Relief* refers to having a need met; *ease* refers to a sense of well-being, calmness, and contentment; and *transcendence* "represents a comfort need that has

been met in such a way that the patient is energized or inspired to perform optimally" (Kolcaba, 1992, p. 6): that is, transcendence is rising above the concern. Kolcaba (1991, 1992) represented each of these three comfort needs as having physical, psychospiritual, environmental, and social dimensions. Achieving comfort hopefully will begin or lead to healing. Providers can ask questions in these areas to assess effectiveness of care.

Healing refers to the client's having a better sense of wholeness. NAHC practices often open the door to healing. Healing does not necessarily mean curing, meaning the elimination of the disease or pathology. Many persons do live with chronic disease or pathology. In contrast to curing, "We are healed when we can bring forth harmony out of the discordant strains of our life"—when we have "balance and equanimity in the midst of discomfort and agitation" (Levine, 1989, p. 196). Healing is a

Exhibit 27–4 Client Satisfaction with NAHC Care

---

1. For what reason did you see (provider's name/practice), i.e., what was your area of "need/
   expectation"?
   (Include physical, psychological, spiritual, social/environmental reasons.)

2. Were you *comfortable* with the *person* providing the care? Yes: ___ No: ___
   If not, please offer suggestions for improvement.

3. Were you *comfortable* with the *process/practice*? Yes: ___ No: ___
   If not, please tell us what you were not comfortable with.

4. Did you have the "need" met for which you sought care? Yes: ___ No: ___
   Please describe how it *was* or *was not* met:

5. Could you say that the *process/practice* increased your feeling of well-being?
   Yes: ___ No: ___? If yes, how?

6. Did you feel your *healing process* was assisted? Yes: ___ No: ___
   Please describe:

Any other comments you would like to make?

---

process that "facilitates health, and thus whole-ness" (Quinn, 1985, p. 116). "In fact, our basic wholeness may be rediscovered in the present moment if we lean into the pain and confusion of our lives" (Welwood, 1985, p. 165). Although healing and comfort are relatively subjective, elusive, and ethereal processes, they are outcomes of care and major aspects of quality.

CONCLUSION

HCPs need to understand that NAHC practices have a different, and not necessarily "wrong," theoretical orientation. They also need to recognize that there may not be a rigorous research base or standard legislative regulation for NAHC practices. NAHC practices often take more time, and this aspect of care must also be recognized as a given. With these issues in mind, clients can still expect the standards of ethical, caring, competent, confidential, and hygienic care from NAHC practitioners. Combined with peer review, educational, organizational, legal, and research documentation, and, most of all, client comfort and healing, quality evaluation of NAHC practices can become standard for conventional HCPs.

REFERENCES

Huebscher, R. (1994). What is natural/alternative health care? *Nurse Practitioner Forum, 5*(2), 66–71.

Kolcaba, K. (1991). A taxonomic structure for the concept of comfort. *Image, 23*(4), 237–240.

Kolcaba, K. (1992). Holistic comfort: Operationalizing the construct as a nurse-sensitive outcome. *Advances in Nursing Science, 15*(1), 1–10.

Levine, S. (1989). The healing for which we took birth. In R. Carlson and B. Shield, *Healers on healing,* 196–203. Los Angeles: Tarcher.

_____ (1996). State massage laws nationwide. *Massage, 62,* 124.

Mower, M. (1996). Certified touch: The impact of national certification. *Massage, 62,* 60–96.

Quinn, J. (1985). The healing arts in modern health. In D. Kunz (Ed.), *Spiritual aspects of the healing arts,* 116–124. Wheaton, IL: Theosophical Publishing House.

Welwood, J. (1985). Rediscovering basic wholeness. In D. Kunz (Ed.), *Spiritual aspects of the healing arts* 165–173. Wheaton, IL: Theosophical Publishing House.

SUGGESTED READING

French, M. (1996). The mind-body-spirit connection: An introduction to alternative therapies. *Advance for Nurse Practitioners, 4*(11), 38–40, 46.

Natural/Alternative Health Care. (1994). *Nurse Practitioner Forum, 5*(2).

Younghin, E., & Israel, D. (1996). *A Review and Critique of Common Herbal Alternative Therapies, 21*(10), 39–62.

JOURNALS

• Alternative Therapies in Health Medicine

• Alternative & Complimentary Therapies

APPENDIX 27–A

Selected Resources for Natural and Alternative Health Care

American Alliance of Aromatherapy
PO Box 309
Depoe Bay, OR 97341
800-809-9850

American Art Therapy Association, Inc.
1202 Allanson Rd.
Mundelein, IL 60060
708-949-6064

American Association of Acupuncture and
   Oriental Medicine
433 Front Street
Catasauqua, PA 18032
610-433-2448

American Association for Music Therapy
PO Box 80012
Valley Forge, PA 19484
610-265-4006

American Association of Naturopathic
   Physicians
2366 Eastlake Ave
Suite 322
Seattle, WA 98102
206-328-8510

American Association of Professional
   Hypnotherapists
PO Box 29
Boones Mill, VA 24065
703-334-3035

American Association for Therapeutic Humor
222 South Meramec, Suite 303
St. Louis, MO 63105
314-863-6232

American Botanical Council (Herbals)
PO Box 210660
Austin, TX 78720
800-373-7105

American Chiropractic Association
1701 Clarendon Blvd.
Arlington, VA 22209

American Herb Association
PO Box 1673
Nevada City, CA 95959
916-265-9552

American Herbalists Guild
PO Box 1683
Sequal, CA 95073
408-464-2441

American Holistic Medical Association
4101 Boone Trail
Suite 201
Raleigh, NC 27607
919-787-5146

American Holistic Nurses Association
4101 Lake Boone Trail
Suite 201
Raleigh, NC 27607
919-787-5181

American Institute of Homeopathy
1585 Glencoe
Denver, CO 80220
303-370-9164

American International Reiki Association, Inc.
2210 Wilshire Boulevard, #831
Santa Monica, CA 90403

American Massage Therapy Association
1130 W North Shore Ave
Chicago, IL 60626
312-761-2682

American Naturopathic Association
1413 K Street, First Floor
Washington, DC 20005
202-682-7352
202-289-2027

American Naturopathic Medical Association
PO Box 96273
Las Vegas, NV 89193
702-897-7053

American Oriental Bodywork Therapy
    Association
6801 Jericho Turnpike
Syosset, NY 11791
516-364-5533
Fax 516-364-5559

American Osteopathic Association
142 East Ontario Street
Chicago, IL 60611

American Polarity Therapy Association
2888 Bluff St
Suite 149
Boulder, CO 80301
303-545-2080

American Psychological Association,
    Division 30
Psychological Hypnosis
750 First Street, NE
Washington, DC 20002
202-336-5500

American Society of Clinical Hypnosis
2200 East Devon Ave, Suite 291
Des Plaines, IL 60018
708-297-3317

American Society for Phytotherapy &
    Aromatherapy International (ASPAI)
PO Box 3679
South Pasadena, CA 91031

Associated Bodywork and Massage
    Professionals
28677 Buffalo Park Road
Evergreen, CO 80439-7347
303-674-8478
800-458-2267 x626

Association for Applied Psychophysiology &
    Biofeedback
(formerly Biofeedback Society)
10200 West 44th Ave, #304
Wheat Ridge, CO 80033
303-422-8436

Body of Knowledge/Hellerwork
406 Berry Street
Mt. Shasta, CA 96067
916-926-2500
Fax 916-926-6839

The Feldenkrais Guild
706 Ellsworth St, SW
PO Box 489
Albany, OR 97321
800-775-2118
Fax 503-926-0572

The International Alliance of Healthcare
    Practitioners (Upledger Institute)
    (Includes craniosacral, St. John's, Aston
    Therapeutics, Zero Balancing,
    Visceral Manipulation)
11211 Prosperity Farms Road
Palm Beach Gardens, FL 33410
561-622-4334

International Association of Infant Massage
1720 Willow Creek Circle
Suite 510
Eugene, OR 97402
800-248-5432

International Association of Yoga Therapists
109 Hillside Avenue
Mill Valley, CA 94941
415-383-4587

International Chiropractors Association (ICA)
1110 N. Glebe Rd., Suite 1000
Arlington, VA 22201
703-528-5000
(800) 423-4690
Fax 703-528-5023

International Foundation for Homeopathy
2366 Eastlake Ave, E, #329
Seattle, WA 98102
206-324-8230

International Imagery Association
PO Box 1046
Bronx, NY 10471
Please write for information.

International Institute of Reflexology
PO Box 12642
St Petersburg, FL 33733
813-343-4811

International Medical and Dental
  Hypnotherapy Association
4110 Edgeland, Suite 800
Royal Oaks, MI 48073-2251
810-549-5594

International Myomassethics Federation
4227 N Olson Ave
Shorewood, WI 53211
800-433-4463

National Association of Massage Therapy
PO Box 1400
Westminster, CO 80030

National Association for Music Therapy
8455 Colesville Rd, Suite 930
Silver Spring, MD 20910
301-589-3300

National Association of Nurse Massage
  Therapists
PO Box 1150
Abita Springs, LA 70420
504-892-6990

National Center for Homeopathy
801 N Fairfax Street
Suite 306
Alexandria, VA 22314
703-548-7790

National Certification Board for Therapeutic
  Massage and Bodywork
1735 N Lyon St
Suite 950
Arlington, VA 22209

National Directory of Chiropractic
PO Box 10056
Olathe, KS 66501
800-888-7914
Fax 913-780-0658

National Iridology Research Association
PO Box 1278
Glenneyre #153
Laguna Beach, CA 92651

National Society for Clinical and Experimental
  Hypnosis
6728 Old McLean Village Drive
McLean, VA 22101-3906
703-556-9222

Natural Oils Research Association
BGB Plaza, Suite H
894 Route 52
Beacon, NY 12508

North American Society of Teachers of the
  Alexander Technique
PO Box 517
Urbana, IL 61801
217-367-6956

Nurse Healers-Professional Associates
1827 Haight St., Suite 157
San Francisco, CA 94117

The Rolf Institute of Structural Integration
205 Canyon Boulevard
Boulder, CO 80302
303-449-5903

Rosen Method Professional Association
2550 Shatttuck Ave
Berkeley, CA 94704

Society for Light Treatment and Biological
  Rhythms
10200 West 44th Avenue, Suite 304
Wheatridge, CO 80033
303-424-3697
Fax 303-422-8894

Trager Institute
21 Locust Ave
Mill Valley, CA 94941
415-388-2688

Worldwide Aquatic Bodywork Association
PO Box 889
Middletown, CA 95461

Note: Some of these references are business
organizations.

## CHAPTER 28

Improving Quality in Psychiatric and Mental Health Care

George Byron Smith and Cindy Parsons

CHAPTER OBJECTIVES

After completing this chapter, the reader will be able to

- explain various ANA, NCQA, Joint Commission, and other standards applicable to psychiatry/mental health
- design a comprehensive quality improvement plan for psychiatry/mental health
- describe the department-specific quality improvement plan and the interface with the organization-wide QI plan
- discuss a multidisciplinary team approach to improving quality that includes developing services, programs, and products (teaching protocols, critical paths)
- identify outcomes assessment tools that can be used in caring for psychiatric/mental health patients

The pursuit of quality in psychiatric-mental health care continues to evolve. Over the past 20 years, it has evolved from a quality assurance (QA) focus to a quality improvement (QI) focus. The current trend of quality in psychiatric-mental health services is to a performance improvement (PI) focus. PI is characterized by an organizational commitment to quality that concentrates on the consumer and continuously improves practices and systems.

STANDARDS

QI programs for psychiatric-mental health systems currently reflect standards of professional organizations, the Joint Commission on Accreditation of Healthcare Organizations (Joint Commission), the National Committee for Quality Assurance (NCQA), federal regulatory agencies, and state regulations when the facility is state supported. Exhibit 28–1 shows the standards of psychiatric care outlined by the American Nurses Association (ANA). The NCQA is an independent, not-for-profit organization dedicated to assessing and reporting on the quality of managed-care plans, including Managed Behavioral Healthcare Organizations (MBHOs). The committee is made up of quality experts, regulators, and representatives from employers, consumer and labor organizations, health plans, and organized medicine.

NCQA's mission is to provide information that will enable purchasers and consumers of managed health care to distinguish among health plans and to make informed choices based on quality and cost. NCQA accomplishes this mission through accreditation of managed-care plans and through performance measurement of published report cards on managed-care plans. NCQA measures performance using the Health Plan Employer Data

Exhibit 28–1 Standards of Psychiatric-Mental Health Clinical Nursing Practice

Standards of Care

Standard I. Assessment
The psychiatric-mental health nurse collects client health data.

Standard II. Diagnosis
The psychiatric-mental health nurse analyzes the assessment data in determining diagnosis.

Standard III. Outcomes Identification
The psychiatric-mental health nurse identifies expected outcomes individualized to the client.

Standard IV. Planning
The psychiatric-mental health nurse develops a plan of care that prescribes interventions to attain expected outcomes.

Standard V. Implementation
The psychiatric-mental health nurse implements the interventions identified in the plan of care.

Standard Va. Counseling
The psychiatric-mental health nurse uses counseling interventions to assist clients in improving or regaining their previous coping abilities, fostering mental health, and preventing mental illness and disability.

Standard Vb. Milieu Therapy
The psychiatric-mental health nurse provides, structures, and maintains a therapeutic environment in collaboration with the client and other health care providers.

Standard Vc. Self-Care Activities
The psychiatric-mental health nurse structures interventions around the client's activities of daily living to foster self-care and mental and physical well-being.

Standard Vd. Psychobiological Interventions
The psychiatric-mental health nurse uses knowledge of psychobiological interventions and applies clinical skills to restore the client's health and prevent further disability.

Standard Ve. Health Teaching
The psychiatric-mental health nurse, through health teaching, assists clients in achieving satisfying, productive, and healthy patterns of living.

Standard Vf. Case Management
The psychiatric-mental health nurse provides case management to coordinate comprehensive health services and ensure continuity of care.

Standard Vg. Health Promotion and Health Maintenance
The psychiatric-mental health nurse employs strategies and interventions to promote and maintain mental health and prevent mental illness.

Advanced Practice Interventions Vh–Vj

Standard Vh. Psychotherapy
The certified specialist in psychiatric-mental health nursing uses individual, group, and family psychotherapy, child psychotherapy, and other therapeutic treatments to assist clients in fostering mental

continues

Exhibit 28–1 continued

health, preventing mental illness and disability, and improving or regaining previous health status and functional abilities.

Standard Vi. Prescription of Pharmacologic Agents
The certified specialist uses prescription of pharmacologic agents, in accordance with the state nursing practice act, to treat symptoms of psychiatric illness and improve functional health status.

Standard Vj. Consultation
The certified specialist provides consultation to health care providers and others to influence the plans of care for clients, and to enhance the abilities of others to provide psychiatric and mental health care and effect change in systems.

Standard VI. Evaluation
The psychiatric-mental health nurse evaluates the client's progress in attaining expected outcomes.

Standards of Professional Performance

Standard I. Quality of Care
The psychiatric-mental health nurse systematically evaluates the quality of care and effectiveness of psychiatric-mental health nursing practice.

Standard II. Performance Appraisal
The psychiatric-mental health nurse evaluates own psychiatric-mental health nursing practice in relation to professional practice standards and relevant statutes and regulations.

Standard III. Education
The psychiatric-mental health nurse acquires and maintains current knowledge in nursing practice.

Standard IV. Collegiality
The psychiatric-mental health nurse contributes to the professional development of peers, colleagues, and others.

Standard V. Ethics
The psychiatric-mental health nurse's decisions and actions on behalf of clients are determined in an ethical manner.

Standard VI. Collaboration
The psychiatric-mental health nurse collaborates with the client, significant others, and health care providers in providing care.

Standard VII. Research
The psychiatric-mental health nurse contributes to nursing and mental health through the use of research.

Standard VIII. Resource Utilization
The psychiatric-mental health nurse considers factors related to safety, effectiveness, and cost in planning and delivering client care.

Source: Reprinted with permission from *A Statement on the Scope and Standards of Psychiatric-Mental Health Clinical Nursing Practice* by American Nurses' Association, pp. 25–40. © 1994 by the American Nurses Association.

and Information Set (HEDIS), a standardized set of approximately 60 performance measures for managed-care plans.

The original version of HEDIS did not include separate measures for MBHOs. During the 1980s, consumers and payers became increasingly concerned about the escalating cost of psychiatric-mental health care services. With over 300 MBHOs in operation today and over 100 million Americans covered by managed behavioral health care plans, there has been an increased demand for national standards to measure quality and accountability in psychiatric-mental health care (NCQA, 1996).

In 1995, NCQA convened a Behavioral Health Task Force to assist in developing standards that would reflect consensus on desired managed behavioral health care performance. Through the implementation of the Behavioral Health Accreditation Standards, NCQA intended to:

- provide consumers, employers, purchasers, and the MBHOs with a comprehensive set of accreditation standards to assess the quality of managed behavioral health care plans
- foster accountability among managed behavioral healthcare organizations for the quality of services their members receive
- encourage effectiveness in the provision of behavioral health care, through integration with general medical care, prevention, and early intervention (NCQA, 1996).

The Behavioral Health Task Force created the Behavioral Health Standards, which were released in 1997 with HEDIS 3.0. The standards are organized into seven categories:

1. *Quality Management and Improvement*—requires the MBHO to continuously assess and improve the quality of clinical care and services provided to members.
2. *Accessibility, Availability, Referral, and Triage*—focuses on the accessibility and availability of behavioral health care services, as well as network adequacy.
3. *Utilization Management*—focuses on the utilization and management of resources and services.
4. *Credentialing and Recredentialing*—requires that an MBHO's licensed behavioral health care practitioners have the necessary education, training, and clinical experience to provide care that meets quality standards.
5. *Members' Rights and Responsibilities*—outlines the expectation that MBHOs promote two-way communication for members and foster member contributions to the quality of clinical care.
6. *Preventive Behavioral Health Care Services*—addresses the prevention and early detection of behavioral problems, mental disorders, and substance abuse disorders in the member population.
7. *Clinical Evaluation and Treatment Records*—since treatment records are essential for documenting, integrating, guiding, and evaluating behavioral health care services delivery, this category of standards requires MBHOs to set standards, systematically review for conformity, and institute corrective actions when standards are not met (NCQA, 1996).

The Behavioral Health Standards from HEDIS 3.0 will be used primarily to review managed-care organizations (MCOs) that currently provide behavioral health services. MCOs will continue to be reviewed under NCQA's Managed Care Organization Standards, but also will be given the option to have their behavioral health programs accredited under the Behavioral Health Standards. However, NCQA anticipates that eventually all managed behavioral health programs will be assessed against the Behavioral Health Standards (NCQA, 1996).

QUALITY IMPROVEMENT PLANS

QI programs in psychiatric-mental health occur at two levels—organization-wide and department-specific. Exhibit 28–2 shows the organization-wide QI plan of Tampa General Healthcare (TGH); Figures 28–1 and 28–2 show the diagrams of the performance improvement reporting structure and the nursing shared governance structure to which that plan refers.

Exhibit 28–3 shows the QI plan specifically for TGH's psychiatric-mental health department. Studies conducted in psychiatric-mental health care are based on the American Nurses' Association Standards for Psychiatric-Mental Health Clinical Nursing Practice (shown in Exhibit 28–1). Responsibilities of the director

---

Exhibit 28–2 Organization-wide QI Plan for Tampa General Healthcare

Purpose
The purpose of this plan is to provide an overall framework for the Quality Improvement (QI) program at Tampa General Healthcare (TGH) by:
  1) delineating the medical staff, administrative staff and committee structure and responsibilities related to the program, and
  2) defining the process of Quality Improvement.

Part One: Philosophy/Structure
  I. Mission/Vision/Values
    A. Vision
       "Tampa General Healthcare is the Leader and Innovator in Quality healthcare, recognized as a resource of value in our communities."

    B. Mission Statement
       The Tampa General Healthcare System strives to improve the health status in our communities through partnerships, medical practice, advancements in education and research, and excellence in compassionate care and customer service.

    C. Organizational Values
       We, the employees, physicians, volunteers, foundation and board of Tampa General Healthcare believe in: patient family centered care; care provided through a team approach; clinical and service excellence; and leadership for community healthcare access.

    D. Strategic Plan Initiatives
       Maintain the ability of Tampa General Healthcare to: generate and sustain regional market leadership with active medical staffs; ensure financial viability and flexibility; strengthen partnerships within our communities; promote partnerships to advance the quality of medical practice, care research, and education; enhance partnerships with employees to create a work environment that fosters individual development, promotes team work, customer service, and our organization values.

  II. Mechanisms for Improvement
     The staff at TGH are highly involved in several mechanisms designed to improve organization performance. These include satisfaction surveys, patient population teams, the department-generated QI team program and the departmental quality monitoring activities.
     If an opportunity for individual performance improvement is identified through quality improvement efforts or sentinel events, the mechanism for improvement includes performance evaluations, individual coaching, counseling and peer review.

continues

Exhibit 28–2 continued

III. Scope of Plan

The Quality Performance Plan of Tampa General Healthcare encompasses the activities of all departments, services, and practitioners as their activities impact patient care and customer satisfaction.

A. Goal

To better achieve our mission, the overall goal of The Tampa General Healthcare quality improvement plan and process is to continuously improve the quality of care and the value of our service to our customers by:

1. Enhancing the satisfaction of our patients/families and all other customers
2. Improving clinical outcomes
3. Reducing consumption of resources and overall cost associated with provision of services.

This is accomplished through an ongoing analytic and educational approach that examines systems, processes, and data, and seeks organizational collaborative involvement with those who perform the services. All employees are required to be educated in the methodology and tools for ongoing quality improvement.

B. Structure and Responsibilities

The organizational structure of QI facilitates integration of the QI process with operational responsibilities. Data collection from monitoring activities and results from other Quality initiated activities is processed through hospital and/or medical staff channels with horizontal and vertical communications and problem-solving as indicated to facilitate continual improvement [see Figure 28–1].

1. Hospital Authority

The Hillsborough County Hospital Authority Board is ultimately responsible for the oversight of the quality of services that are provided at TGH. This responsibility is delegated to the Medical Executive Committee and Senior Management. Through their joint efforts, they are responsible for ensuring the implementation of a consistent program of quality improvement throughout the facility.

2. Quality Council

The Quality Council is composed of all members of the Senior Management Team and Senior Medical Staff. It is co-chaired by the Secretary-Treasurer of the Medical Staff and Senior Vice President of Nursing/Clinical Services. Responsibilities include the development and implementation of the QI program to meet the strategic plan initiatives, assessment and prioritization of the QI program, allocation of resources necessary for QI, and reporting to the Hospital Authority Board on the status of Quality Improvement Program activities. Data examined by this committee include patient, physician and staff satisfaction surveys, institutional indicators, Atlas data, Quality Improvement Committee Summary of activities reports and the Re-Engineering Task Force summary report.

3. Re-Engineering Task Force

The Re-Engineering Task Force is composed of members of the Senior Management Team and Medical Staff. The focus of this group is to improve both internal and external customer service and processes. Data examined by this task force include the results of patient satisfaction, physician satisfaction, and staff surveys. There is an emphasis on employee development.

continues

Exhibit 28–2 continued

4. Quality Improvement Committee

The Quality Improvement Committee membership consists of selected department Directors and Medical Staff representatives from major clinical departments/sections. The responsibilities are to assist and direct the Medical Staff and Hospital service areas in identification of QI opportunities; to review potential interdepartmental projects in a systematic manner; to assign interdepartmental QI teams; to monitor progress of QI teams and ensure follow-up; to review all monitors and studies; to manage flow of information to appropriate clinical/nonclinical teams; to analyze findings from review activities; to conduct focused reviews and studies on specific topics as issues are identified; to oversee the Atlas Program and findings and make recommendations on studies to the Multidisciplinary Teams as appropriate; to develop an annual institutional report; and to suggest modifications to the QI Plan. Data sources include Patient, Physician and Staff Satisfaction Surveys, Institutional Indicators, Multidisciplinary Team findings, Atlas data, department-initiated QI team activities, Blood and Drug Utilization findings, Invasive and Operative Procedures Review findings, report of regulatory or external agencies findings, and other related data sources for quality improvement. Physician specific quality issues are addressed by the physician membership through peer review.

5. Multidisciplinary Teams

There are currently five Multidisciplinary Teams (MDTs): Medicine, Surgery, OB/Gyn/Peds, Psychiatry and Ambulatory. Physician specific quality issues identified by multidisciplinary teams are to be discussed by the physician members and reported through routine clinical minutes. The focus of the activities of the multidisciplinary teams will be to assist in identification of best practices for specific patient populations and to provide a forum for addressing the needs of specific patient populations as well as meeting regulatory requirements. Improvement in the care of these specific patient populations will be monitored through the development of indicators which will include frequency, ALOS, charges/cost, morbidity and mortality at a minimum. Additional indicators will be developed specific to the patient population needs and tracked as part of outcomes management.

6. Hospital Organization

a) Senior Management Team

The Senior Management Team is accountable to the Hospital Authority Board for the overall quality of patient care provided to patients and families in the healthcare system. The functions of the Senior Management Team include: receiving reports of quality improvement monitoring and evaluation activities and department-initiated quality improvement teams and assessing the appropriateness of quality improvement activities in relationship to their importance to the strategic plan, patient care and their impact on patient care and reporting these activities to the Quality Improvement Council.

b) Hospital Departments

All hospital departments participate in the Quality Improvement Program. Each Vice President is responsible for overseeing the Quality Improvement Plans in their area of responsibility. Each department director is responsible for implementation of Quality Improvement process according to this plan. This responsibility includes: developing and maintaining a QI plan, maintaining the department/unit quality improvement man-

continues

Exhibit 28–2 continued

ual for each fiscal year, evaluating and implementing suggestions that affect the department that are communicated through the department-initiated QI teams, supporting the Quality Improvement Committee and Multidisciplinary Team (MDT) by communicating with staff and participating as appropriate. Department activities focus on enhancing value to customers through new or improved services, reducing errors, defects and waste, improving productivity and effectiveness in the use of all resources.

c) Risk Management

The Risk Management Department works in collaboration with the Quality Management Department in identification of opportunities for improvement. Information is shared between departments as appropriate. When Quality Management staff identify events that may require Risk Management intervention, this information is reported to Risk Management. When Risk Management staff identify incidents requiring physician review, an expedited peer review process is initiated in Quality Management. When incidents occur with multidisciplinary involvement, Risk/Quality teams are initiated to address the areas for improvement.

d) Nursing Staff Organization

The Senior Vice President of Nursing/Clinical Services is accountable to the Hospital Authority for the overall quality of nursing care rendered to patients and families in the healthcare system. The oversight functions include: final authority for overall nursing standards in all departments which have nursing staff, developing and implementing an effective and ongoing program to monitor, evaluate, and improve the quality of nursing care delivered to patients and families, receiving and acting on the information generated from nursing quality improvement activities and reviewing all patient council minutes. This is accomplished through the Nursing Shared Governance Structure [see Figure 28–2].

Shared Governance is an organization structure which promotes quality by creating a network structure for decision making. The structure is characterized by issue resolution by those most knowledgeable about and involved with a given issue. The structure builds peer relationships and encourages teamwork. The four shared governance councils are:

Nursing Practice Forum: composed of clinical caregivers (RNs and LPNs). Focus is on delivery of care, customer service for patients, families and employees. Components of direct care and systems to improve care as well as quality of work life issues, and the work environment are included in this structure.

Nursing Management Council: composed of nurse managers and assistant nurse managers. Focus is on care methodology and resource allocation. Responsible for systems that impact the nursing clinical areas as a whole.

Advanced Clinical Practice Council: composed of ARNP, CNS, CRNA, and certified nurse midwife level practitioners. Focus is on developing and overseeing credentialing, program/case management, and issues impacting nurses in advance practice.

Nursing Quality Council: composed of representatives from each clinical area plus representatives from Quality Management, Risk Management, and Center for Education, Development and Research (CEDAR). Focus is on monitoring care delivery and reviewing/revising nursing standards of care and practice.

continues

Exhibit 28–2 continued

The Councils are coordinated by the Shared Governance Coordinating Council, and report to the Nursing Leadership Council.

7. Medical Staff Organization

  a) Medical Staff Executive Committee

  The Executive Committee is accountable to the Hospital Authority for the overall quality of medical care rendered to patients and families in the healthcare system. The oversight functions of the Executive Committee include: receiving and acting upon recommendations of the Quality Council, assessing the compliance of the Medical Staff with Joint Commission standards, receiving and evaluating reports of the monitoring and evaluation of clinical departments/sections and monitoring committees, providing feedback to the Quality Improvement Council and the Medical Staff, and reporting the quality improvement activities of the Medical Staff to the Hospital Authority.

  b) Medical Staff Department/Section

  1) Clinical Chiefs—The Clinical Chief of each clinical department/section is responsible for implementing the QI process for monitoring and evaluating: The quality, appropriateness, care and treatment of patients served by the department, and the clinical performance of all individuals with clinical privileges in the department. It is the responsibility of the Clinical Chief to assure that opportunities to improve care are addressed and important problems of patient care are identified and resolved. The Clinical Chief will work cooperatively with the Quality Management Department staff, hospital staff and multidisciplinary teams.

  2) Clinical Department—must approve indicators for department specific aspects of care selected for monitoring and evaluation. Indicators for timely completion of medical records, clinical pertinence, blood usage, medication use, and operative and other invasive procedures performed by more than one department will be the same for all clinical departments. Indicators for quality and appropriateness of surgical and invasive procedures performed only by practitioners within a department will be approved by the practitioners within the department performing the procedure.

  3) Peer Review—the clinical chiefs of each department/section will appoint a physician who is responsible for performing peer review for the department's quality improvement program.

  4) Medical Staff Members—medical staff members are responsible for serving on the multidisciplinary teams, reviewing medical staff issues, participating in opportunities for improvement and reporting activities at the department/section meetings as appropriate.

IV. Communication/Reporting

  1. Interdepartmental

  As significant events or patterns/trends identify opportunities for improvement which involve more than one department, communication will be sent to the appropriate department by the department identifying the issue. The receiving department will be expected to respond to the communication within five days of receiving it.

continues

Exhibit 28–2 continued

2. Medical Staff Department to Medical Staff Department
   As opportunities for improvement are identified which involve other clinical departments, communications will be sent to the appropriate clinical chief by the clinical chief of the department identifying the events/issues. This process will be facilitated by the peer review process. The clinical chief of the department receiving the communication is expected to respond within one month except in the case of expedited reviews for Risk Management.

3. Hospital Staff to Medical Staff
   As opportunities for improvement are identified concerning Medical Staff, communication is sent to the Quality Management Department. The Quality Management staff will address the concerns with the appropriate Medical Staff and provide feedback as appropriate.

4. Medical Director/Medical Staff Leadership
   When the hospital department has a medical director, the findings of ongoing monitoring and department-initiated QI teams' activities will be reviewed with him/her a minimum of quarterly as outlined in the department QI Plan. The Medical Director will document review of information by signing the quarterly status report before it is shared with the Vice President.

5. Hospital Senior Management
   On a quarterly basis, the summary of the monitoring activities and department-generated QI team activities for each department will be reported to the appropriate Vice President. Reports to the Vice President will be documented on the quarterly report form. The Vice President will document their review of the information by signing on the appropriate signature line. The Vice President and Department Director will identify others with whom the information should be communicated and identify significant issues that should be brought to the attention of the Quality Council.

6. Medical Staff
   Results of monitoring and evaluation and peer review activity shall be communicated to the Executive Committee through submission of, at a minimum, quarterly clinical minutes.

7. Medical Staff Executive Committee
   The Medical Staff Executive Committee will give quarterly reports of medical staff quality improvement activities to the Hospital Authority.

8. Quality Improvement Council
   Significant issues and results of the Quality Improvement activities of each department are reported to the Council by the appropriate Vice President. The Institutional Indicator Report, results of external surveys, patient satisfaction survey results and other information as available will be submitted to the Hospital Authority on a quarterly basis.

9. Professional Credentials Committee
   Results of the Medical Staff monitoring and evaluation activities for each physician are reported to the Professional Credentials Committee through the Medical Staff Office for use in re-appointing or renewal or revision of privileges and appraisal of competence.

10. Human Resources
    When the results of the Quality Improvement activity identify an opportunity for improvement in individual employee performance, that information is incorporated into the performance evaluation of the employee.

continues

Exhibit 28–2 continued

V. Confidentiality
Confidentiality of Peer Review and Quality Improvement data is governed by the hospital's Confidentiality policy.

VI. Coordination with Mandated Review Activities
This Plan describes the minimum structure and operating characteristics of the healthcare system-wide Quality Improvement program. Specific review subjects and procedures mandated by external agents are recognized as an official part of this plan.

VII. Annual Review
The Quality Improvement plan and program will be evaluated annually and modified as necessary based upon the effectiveness of the program. This document may be amended by action of the Quality Council. Final approval remains with the Hospital Authority Board of Trustees.

VIII. Objectives and Goals for 1995/1996
Short-term Goals
- Implement the revised organizational structure to support QI by October 1995.
- Incorporate the following targets for improvement as identified.
  – Quality Council will define the priorities for improvement and establish mechanisms to address the top three priorities by November 1995.
  – Implement the use of Atlas (Medis) and target, at a minimum, three specific patient populations where opportunities exist by November 1995.
  – Establish Multidisciplinary Teams to address by January 1996.
- Develop Clinical Indicator Report ("Report Card")
- Prepare for 1996 on-site Joint Commission survey.
- Initiate and prepare TGH for competing for the Sterling Award in 1998.
- Establish Information Systems improvements which support quality improvement activities.

Part Two: Process of Quality Improvement
When the need for a new service or process is identified, the design is based on the following: The organizational mission and strategic plan, the needs and expectations of customers, current information about designing processes, and performance and outcomes in other organizations.

The department directors, managers, and staff members and the Medical Staff are responsible for the provision of high quality services to patients and families as well as participation in quality improvement activities. Responsibility for the coordination of hospital departments and Medical Staff quality improvement activities is delegated to the Director of Quality Management/Utilization Management.

I. Plan Development
Each hospital and medical staff department/section will develop a quality improvement plan which identifies: scope of care/services provided, responsibility for quality improvement efforts of the department/area and customers of the department. From the department scope of services, measures will be identified to assess how well the department is meeting its customers' requirements. Department activities should focus on enhancing value to customers through new or improved services, reducing errors, defects and waste, improving responsiveness and cycle time performance, and improving productivity and effectiveness in the use of all resources. These measurements, called quality indicators, are to be approved by the Vice President, Medical Director and/or Chief of Service and link to the mission statement or improvement of services,

continues

Exhibit 28–2 continued

outcomes, or costs. The plan should include those indicators directed by institutional initiatives and external requirements.

II. Required Activities
Processes that are selected to be measured include those that affect a large percentage of patients/families, are high risk or may be problem prone. Related processes as defined by the Joint Commission will be considered in the development of all indicators (e.g., blood usage, medication use, operative and invasive procedures).

A. Required aspects of Medical Staff quality improvement program
The Quality Improvement activities of the Medical Staff must include:
1. Medical Record review for clinical pertinence and timely completion
2. Blood and blood components usage
3. Medication use
4. Operative and other invasive procedures
5. Pharmacy and therapeutics
6. Infection control
7. Utilization management
8. Risk management
9. Consideration of the Joint Commission IMS indicators

Quality Improvement activities of the Medical Staff are integrated with hospital departments as appropriate. Other activities may be mandated by hospital-initiated quality improvement projects.

B. Required aspects of hospital quality improvements
All Joint Commission functional requirements must be measured over time. Patient, families, physician and staff satisfaction surveys will be performed. Department QI programs will address the components noted in I. Plan Development.
Quality control activities will be performed at a minimum in the Clinical Lab, Diagnostic Radiology and Nuclear Medicine, Nutrition Services and Radiation Oncology.

III. Indicators
Indicators development should be relevant to the key processes and outcomes identified as necessary to meet the scope of care or services of the department. The development of indicators is generally driven by three factors: 1) external regulatory requirements, e.g., Joint Commission, AHCA, CARF; 2) internal quality initiatives which may involve more than one department, e.g., institutional indicators, patient population specific processes and outcomes; 3) department specific, i.e., selected by the department to meet internal department improvement needs.

All indicators are to be characterized by the dimension of performance, key functions, and rationale for selection, using the forms provided by the Quality Management Department.

Goals should be set for each indicator, although the ultimate goal is continuous improvement. Benchmarks should be used when they are supported by literature and other research methodologies.

IV. Sources of Data
Decision-making requires access to information regarding hospital performance. This information is collected and reported from multiple sites internally. In addition, access to external com-

continues

Exhibit 28–2 continued

parative information is an important factor in identifying benchmarks. This allows TGH to identify best practices and seek to improve performance. Internal and external data bases include:

Internal
- Medical Records
- Information Systems
  – MDC Cost Reports
  – Other reports as required
- MedisGroups (Atlas) Patient Severity System
- MAXSYS quality/utilization tracking system
- Parsonnett Risk-Stratification System (open heart surgery)
- Patient Satisfaction Surveys
- Physician Satisfaction Surveys
- Staff Surveys
- Other internal/external customer surveys
- Other data sources as identified

External
- HCCB Data—severity adjusted by R-DRG—Florida
- HCCB Data—severity adjusted by APR-DRG (TBD)—Florida
- Atlas Comparative Data Base (total, teaching and Florida)
- Current national standards
- Practice parameters
- Current literature
- PRO-generated collaborative study results and other routine comparative reports
- Other comparative sources as identified

V. Priorities
Priorities are determined at all levels of the organization. Departments, each of the standing quality related committees, the Quality Council and the Multidisciplinary Teams (MDTs) will review opportunities for improvement by using a priority matrix.

VI. Collection and Organization of Data
To ensure that only relevant, useful, and necessary data are collected, the questions to be answered by the data are framed before data collection begins. After data are collected, they will be organized and compared to performance goals.

VII. Analysis and Evaluation of Data
The assessment of the data will include comparisons with: self (levels, patterns, and trends); others (reference databases, professional literature); standards (policies, practice guidelines); regulatory and legal requirements; and best practice (bringing performance up to leadership level, critical pathways). Statistical tools will be used as appropriate.

VIII. Action
Action is directed at improving processes. A systematic approach is employed. This includes:
- Testing the strategy for change.
- Assessing data following test pilot to determine improvement.
- System-wide implementation.

continues

Exhibit 28–2 continued

When deciding to improve a process, the improvement team will consider the importance of the function, the organization's ongoing data collection, the resources required to make the improvement, and the organization's mission and priorities. It is recommended that the solution matrix be used as appropriate. Actions may include one or more of the following: Policy and procedure change, redesigning of a process, education, and individual counseling.

IX. Assess and Document Improvement Process
Implementation of process improvements will be assessed by the organization's leadership to determine whether improvements occurred, to ensure that improvements are lasting, and to identify further opportunities for improvement.

X. Annual Evaluation
The Quality Improvement Program will be evaluated annually by hospital departments and clinical departments/sections using the annual evaluation tools. A list of specific improvements and outstanding concerns will be part of this evaluation.

Courtesy of Tampa General Healthcare, Tampa, Florida.

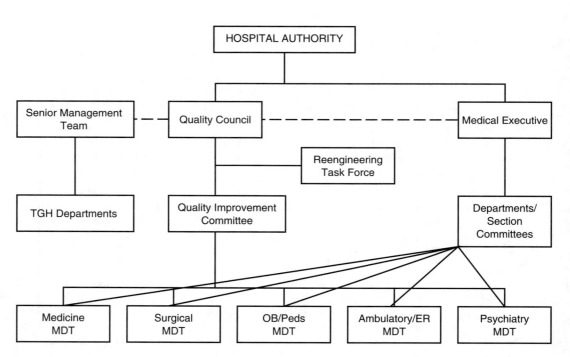

Figure 28–1 TGH performance improvement reporting structure. Courtesy of Tampa General Healthcare, Tampa, Florida.

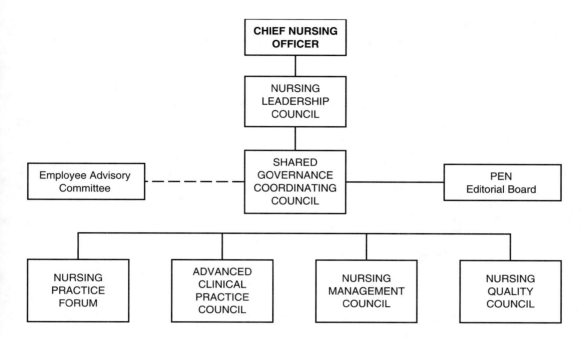

Figure 28–2 TGH nursing shared governance structure. Courtesy of Tampa General Healthcare, Tampa, Florida.

of patient care services, the case manager, the department staff, and the multidisciplinary team are clearly defined in the Quality Improvement Plan, as well as outlined in the Quality Improvement Structure and Responsibilities document (Exhibit 28–4).

QI planning at either level takes a multidisciplinary approach targeted primarily toward organizational priorities such as high-risk, problem-prone, or high-volume practices or procedures. *High-risk targets* are practices and procedures that place the population being served at risk for injury, complications, or potentially poor outcomes. Examples in psychiatric-mental health include electroconvulsive therapy (ECT), psychotropic management, seclusion and restraint, and use of safety devices. *Problem-prone targets* are practices or procedures that tend to be problematic for providers. Examples include practices that have high rates of error or patient or employee

injuries. *High-volume targets* are practices or procedures that a majority of the population being served would receive. Examples include admissions and discharges to programs, high-volume diagnoses, psychoeducational therapies, and medication administration.

As the psychiatric-mental health department plan in Exhibit 28–3 discusses, there are several "institutional indicators" of department volume and quality management/risk management on which data are routinely collected and reported quarterly (Exhibit 28–5). In addition, indicators for intensive QI study are selected annually using a Quality Management Matrix (Exhibit 28–6) that categorizes the indicators by rationale (high risk, high volume, and/or problem prone) and also classifies them according to the 11 functions of patient care established by the Joint Commission and eight dimensions of performance. The matrix selections are then discussed and agreed upon by

Exhibit 28–3 QI Plan for Tampa General Healthcare Psychiatric-Mental Health Department

1. Responsibility

   The department's Senior Leaders and members of the Psychiatric Multidisciplinary Team (MDT) set priorities for performance improvement activities designed to improve patient and family outcomes. Activities are coordinated and reported through department Quality Council.

2. Scope of Services

   Provision of psychiatric-mental health care to inpatient and ambulatory patients and families 24 hours a day, 7 days a week.

3. Key Processes

   Clinical Services (groups and individual therapies), Dietary (nutrition consults), Nursing (Standards of Care, Seclusion/Restraint, Fall Risk, Detoxification), Multidisciplinary (treatment planning and sentinel events, such as code blue, suicide gestures, sexual activity, medication management).

4. Customers (identify E—External and I—Internal)

__E/I__	Patients	__I__	Nursing Staff	__I__	Pharmacy
__E__	Families	__E__	Physical Therapy	__I__	Dietitian
__E/I__	Physicians	__I__	Social Services	__I__	Activities Therapy
__I__	Support Departments				

5. Indicators

   Quality improvement efforts include: 1) enhancing value to our customers through new and improved products and services; 2) reducing errors, defects and waste; 3) improving responsiveness and cycle time performance; and 4) improving productivity and effectiveness in the use of all resources. These efforts may be approached through the routine monitoring and evaluation activities or through the department generated improvement ideas. Data collection tools are used in evaluating documentation and/or performance [see Exhibit 28–8]. In addition, department volume and quality management/risk management indicators are collected and reported quarterly [see Exhibit 28–5].

   Indicators to be monitored this year are identified by the Psychiatric Multidisciplinary Team on the Quality Management Matrix [see Exhibit 28–6]. Using the key at the bottom of the page, the team indicates the function, dimension of quality, and rationale for selection of the indicator and a goal.

   I.   Patient Care Function: Seclusion and Restraint

      1. There is documentation that clinical justification exists for seclusion and/or restraint (Physician & Nursing)—100%

      2. Less restrictive measures were utilized prior to initiating seclusion and/or restraint (Physician, Nursing, Team)—100%

      3. A physician's order is requested within one hour of placing the patient in seclusion and restraint (Nursing)—100%

      4. The physician's order is time limited (Physician)—90%

continues

Exhibit 28–3 continued

5. The physician's order is co-signed by the physician (Physician)—100%

6. If seclusion and/or restraint is used for greater than 12 hours, the patient is re-evaluated by the physician as evidenced in the progress note within 24 hours of the seclusion and/or restraint episode (Physician)—100%

7. If seclusion and/or restraint is necessary three or more times in a seven-day period, the Master Treatment Plan is revised to reflect this and changes in treatment (Physician)—90%

II. Patient Care Function: Assessment/Treatment Team Planning

1. The Psychiatric Admission Assessment is completed in a timely manner as outlined in Policy and Procedure (Team Members)—90%

2. Problems identified in the assessments that are not treated are deferred to aftercare (Physician)—90%

3. A preliminary discharge plan is in place within 24–48 hours of admission or placement problem is noted when applicable (Case Management)—90%

4. All disciplines participate in multidisciplinary treatment plan and sign the attendance form, including their title (Team Members)—90%

5. The patient participated in treatment planning, signed acknowledgment of participating in developing the plan, and received a copy of master treatment plan within five days of admission (Nursing)—90%

6. The treatment plan is reviewed every five days while the patient is hospitalized (Team Members)—90%

III. Patient Care Function: Medication Usage/Laboratory

1. There is a progress note denoting rationale for introduction of new or changed medication (Physician)—90%

2. Progress notes indicate response to new/changed medication (Physician)—95%

3. All PRN medications administered are assessed for effectiveness (Nursing)—95%

4. Medication education is noted in progress notes (Nursing)—90%

5. Drug levels are ordered on patients receiving digoxin, theophylline, lithium, tegretol, or dilantin (Physician)—100%

6. Emergency treatment orders are written for each medication if authorization for treatment not signed and renewed every 24 hours (Physician)—100%

7. The patient is over 65 years old and creatine clearance has been ordered (Physician)—90%

8. The patient is not receiving more than one type of oral benzodiazepine simultaneously (Physician)—98%

9. Patients receiving greater than seven medications have a documented medication evaluation (Physician)—95%

continues

Exhibit 28–3 continued

10. Female patients have a negative urine pregnancy test prior to receiving benzodiazepines, nueroleptics, or lithium (Physician)—95%

IV. Patient Care Function: Electroconvulsive Therapy (ECT) Preparation

1. Diagnosis of major depression, mania, schizophrenia or atypical psychosis is documented in medical record (Physician)—100%

2. Medical assessment inclusive of effects of prior ECT, History & Physical, EKG prior to treatment, X-ray films, MSE, memory function and anesthetic evaluation (Physician)—100%

3. Informed consent inclusive of specified treatment course, right to withdraw consent, alternatives to treatment, risks/benefits of treatment, where, when, and by whom treatment is to be performed, description of treatment (Physician)—100%

4. Documentation that psychotropic medications are reviewed prior to treatment (Physician)—100%

5. Evidence of a documented second opinion is in the medical record (Physician)—100%

6. No more than three treatments performed in a week (Physician & Nursing)—100%

7. Prolonged and/or inadequate seizure duration is explained in the medical record (Physician)—100%

8. Post-ECT progress note included electrode placement, parameter settings at treatment, seizure duration, orientation and memory function and adverse effects or lack thereof are noted (Physician)—100%

9. Pretreatment work-up sheet complete (Nursing)—100%

10. "Authorization for Treatment" signed (Physician & Nursing)—100%

11. Vitals recorded on admission back to unit post-ECT (Nursing)—100%

12. Initial progress note on the unit post-ECT assesses mental status (Nursing)—100%

13. Fall precautions initiated for 24 hours after treatment (Nursing)—100%

V. Patient Care Function: Standard of Care for Patients Diagnosed with Schizophrenia

1. The psychiatric admission assessment addresses: a) psychotic symptoms (Physician & Nursing); b) suicide/violence potential (Physician & Nursing); c) behavior problems and/or bizarre behavior (Physician & Nursing); activities of daily living (Physician & Nursing); side effects from medications, especially movement disorders (Physician); baseline level of functioning (Case Management); and strengths/weaknesses (Physician)—95%

2. The patient is started on psychotropics within three days of admission unless otherwise indicated (Physician)—100%

3. The master treatment plan addresses alteration in thought process, i.e., delusions and/or hallucinations (Team Members)—100%

continues

Exhibit 28–3 continued

4. The master treatment plan addresses the potential for violence to self/others if patient has a history of violence and/or is violent at the time of admission (Team Members)—100%

5. The physician documents the presence of improvement in psychotic symptoms in the progress notes (Physician)—100%

6. Focus documentation indicates the assessments of psychotic symptoms (Nursing)—95%

7. Discharge plans address placement issues at the time of admission, i.e., does patient have a home or place to return to at discharge? If not, are alternatives noted in social history section of admission assessment (Case Management)—95%

8. Discharge plans identify referrals for support groups and follow-up care (Case Management)—90%

VI. Patient Care Function: Standard of Care for Patients Diagnosed with Major Depression

1. Signs/Symptoms in Psychiatric Admission Assessment support diagnosis as defined by DSM-IV (Physician)—95%

2. The patient's strengths and weaknesses are identified in the Psychiatric Admission Assessment (Physician)—95%

3. Patient is placed on safety checks if suicidal. Suicidal is defined as any patient expressing suicidal ideation who has a plan or past history of attempts (Physician)—95%

4. Patient is placed on antidepressant medications within three days of admission (Physician)—95%

5. Lab work is ordered prior to administration of medication—CBC, SMAC, UA (Physician)—95%

6. Goals of treatment are met upon transfer to a lesser level of care or an explanation as to why they are not is documented in progress notes, discharge summary or treatment plan (Team Members)—90%

VII. Patient Care Function: Standard of Care for Patients Diagnosed with Substance Abuse

1. Admission Assessment includes: a) history of physical abuse (Case Management); history of drug and/or alcohol abuse in the 7 days prior to admission (Physician & Nursing); race, gender and ethnic origin (Physician, Nursing, & Case Management); mental status exam includes immediate, recent and remote recall (Physician); and physical problems associated with dependence (Physician)—95%

2. Lab tests ordered on admission include CBC, SMAC, Urine Drug Screen, and UA. Results present within three days of admission (Physician & Nursing)—95%

3. Admission breathalizer result is recorded upon admission—if applicable (Crisis Assessment Center)—95%

4. Withdrawal score is documented on admission (Physician)—95%

continues

Exhibit 28–3 continued

5. Physician orders include: withdrawal checks (TADW), PRN medications for a positive score—if no, stop here (Physician)—95%

6. Symptoms of withdrawal are assessed until order is discontinued or results are negative—TADW times 48 hours, then discontinue if results are negative for 24 hours, seven days for benzodiazepines (Physician & Nursing)—95%

7. All withdrawal checks (TADW) scores are recorded three times daily—once each shift (Nursing)—95%

8. For every withdrawal check (TADW) score greater than 15, or specified range in order, a PRN medication is administered (Physician & Nursing)—100%

9. Abnormal findings (changes in vital signs, cognitive status or physical status or poor response to PRN medications) are reported to the physician within 30 minutes of RN assessment (Nursing)—100%

10. Problems, goals, interventions related to the risks of alcohol/drug detox are identified in master treatment plan (Team Members)—95%

11. Progress notes indicate the patient and/or family is involved in discharge planning (Team Members)—100%

12. Appointments for continued care are scheduled within one week of discharge or reason for delay noted (Case Management)—95%

VIII. Patient Care Function: Treatment and Consult Use

1. Consult request includes: a) date requested and b) rationale—100%

2. Consult completion includes: a) recommendations addressing original request, b) consultant name and signature, and c) date of completion—100%

IX. Patient Care Function: Management of Aggressive Behaviors

1. Psychiatric Emergency evaluations are maintained to process behavior management incidents. Incidents are reviewed on a case-by-case basis and referred to committee for review as needed (Team Members)—100%

2. Sentinel Events: a) death before or after transfer, b) occurrence of alleged sexual activity, c) suicide gesture/attempt, d) elopement of involuntary patients and e) medical emergencies (Team Members)—100%

6. Annual Evaluations
The department's Quality Improvement program will be evaluated annually and results will be submitted to the Quality Management Department by October 15.

7. Reports
A report will be submitted to the Quality Management Department quarterly and to the Director and Vice President as appropriate. Quarterly reports are due in the Quality Management Department on January 15 (Qtr 1: October–December); April 15 (Qtr 2: January–March); July 15 (Qtr 3: April–June); October 15 (Annual Evaluation, new QI Plan, and Qtr 4: July–September). Reports will include results of internal department team QI activities.

Exhibit 28–4 Quality Improvement Structure and Responsibilities

Quality Council

- Membership
    - Co-Chairs: Secretary/Treasury of Medical Staff
                       Senior Vice President, Patient Services

    - Chief Executive Officer
    - VP Financial Services
    - VP Support Services
    - VP Ancillary Services
    - VP Ambulatory Services
    - Medis Physician Advisor
    - Chief of Staff
    - Vice Chief of Staff
    - Medical Director
    - Medical Director, Psychiatry
    - Medical Director, Surgical
    - Board Representative
    - OB/Peds Multidisciplinary Team Representative
    - Medicine Multidisciplinary Team Representative
    - Ambulatory Multidisciplinary Team Representative
    - Director, Quality, Outcomes and Utilization Management

- Responsibilities
    1. Develop and implement QI program to meet strategic plan initiatives
    2. Assess and prioritize QI project
    3. Appoint teams as needed
    4. Operationalize improvement activities that are consistent with the Tampa General Healthcare Strategic Plan
    5. Evaluate the QI program
    6. Allocate resources necessary for QI projects
    7. Report to the Hospital Authority Board

- Data
    - Patient and Family, Physician, and Staff Satisfaction Surveys
    - Institutional Indicators
    - Medis Data
    - Quality Improvement Committee Summary
    - Re-Engineering Committee Summary

Quality Improvement Committee

- Membership
    - Co-Chairs: Secretary/Treasury of Medical Staff
                      Director, Quality, Outcomes and Utilization Management

    - Director, Risk Management
    - Medis Physician Advisor
    - Safety Officer
    - Director Pharmacy
    - Quality Leadership Process
    - Medical Director, Surgical
    - Medical Director, Ambulatory
    - Medical Director Blood Bank
    - Manager Infection Control

continues

Exhibit 28–4 continued

    – Department Directors
      – Laboratory
      – Radiology
      – Information Systems
      – Operations Consulting
    – Medical Staff Representatives from:
      – Medicine
      – Surgery
      – OB
      – Pediatric
      – Orthopedics
      – Pathology
      – Radiology
      – ENT
      – Psychiatry

• Responsibilities
1. Assist and direct the Medical Staff and hospital service areas in identification of QI opportunities
2. Physician Peer Review
3. Review potential interdepartmental projects in a systematic manner
4. Assign and coach interdepartmental QI teams
5. Monitor progress of QI teams and ensure follow-up
6. Review all monitors and studies
7. Manage the flow of information to appropriate clinical and nonclinical teams
8. Analyze findings from review activities
9. Conduct focused reviews and studies on specified topics as issues are identified
10. Make recommendations to the Quality Council for interdepartmental teams when appropriate
11. Oversee Medis program and findings. Make recommendations for study to Multidisciplinary Teams as appropriate
12. Develop clinical indicator report and monitor results
13. Suggest modification to the QI plan
14. Report to Quality Council

• Data
    – Patient and Family, Physician, and Staff Satisfaction Surveys
    – Institutional Indicators
    – Medis Data
    – Multidisciplinary Teams
    – Employee Improvement Suggestions (QLP)
    – Blood Utilization
    – Drug Utilization
    – Invasive operative and procedure review
    – Regulatory visits/external agencies reports
    – Re-Engineering summary data
    – Hospital Department Indicators
    – Medical Staff Department

continues

Exhibit 28–4 continued

- Section Monitors
- Peer Review
- Risk Management
- Utilization Management
- Infection Control
- Safety
- Outcomes Management
- Patient Complaints Management

Multidisciplinary Teams (MDT)
Psychiatry and Behavioral Medicine

- Membership
  - Co-Chairs: Physician
    Administrative Representative
  - Physician Representatives (4) Psychiatry
  - Medical Director
  - Nurse Manager, Adult Psychiatry
  - Director, Patient Services for Psychiatry
  - Quality Leadership Process
  - Representatives from:
    - Emergency Care Center
    - Community Mental Health System
    - Charge Nurse Representative
    - Staff Nurse Representative
    - Case Manager
    - Pharmacy
    - Activity Therapy
    - Quality Management/Utilization Management
    - Clinical Services
    - Risk Management
    - Safety Representative
    - Other ancillary departments as appropriate

- Responsibilities
  1. Have physician and other professional discipline Peer Review
  2. Assist in identification of "best practices" for specific patient populations utilizing critical paths, other tools, and variance reports, to document performance improvement
  3. Identify indicators for specific patient populations
  4. Focus on processes and activities that affect quality of care and services
  5. Place emphasis on functions such as assessment, reassessment, medication management, treatment, patient and family education, patient rights, and safety
  6. Ensure appropriate utilization of resources
  7. Evaluate care and take appropriate actions when patterns or trends in indicator data identify opportunities for improvement
  8. Evaluate effectiveness of actions

continues

Exhibit 28–4 continued

9. Participate in continuing education opportunities related to patient care process improvement and outcomes
10. Recommend interdepartmental teams on process related concerns
11. Report to Quality Improvement Committee

- Data
  - Patient and Family, Physician, and Staff Satisfaction Surveys
  - Drug Utilization
  - Medis data
  - Special Procedures
  - System Indicators
  - Risk Management/Patient Complaint
  - Infection Control
  - Outcomes Management
  - Psychiatric-Mental Health Services Indicators
  - Utilization Management
  - Surveyor Data
  - Quality Control/Quality Improvement Data

Courtesy of Tampa General Healthcare, Tampa, Florida.

the Psychiatric Multidisciplinary Team (MDT). The MDT also establishes frequency of monitoring, sample size (number of cases or percentage of all cases), and a QI calendar (Exhibit 28–7). Studies are performed by teams composed of multidisciplinary staff, case managers, managers, and directors. In QI activities, all levels of staff are expected to participate in the assessment, analysis, and PI process. Exhibit 28–8 shows a QI collection and evaluation tool used to record attainment (yes/no) of the improvement objective determined for each indicator.

QUALITY LEADERSHIP PROCESS

Although continuous quality improvement (CQI) has initiated new and exciting opportunities to improve practice and systems, it has also created the need for new skills in team building and team cohesion to produce quality psychiatric-mental health care services. The cornerstone of QI is to involve staff at all levels of the organization in the problem-solving

process. This QI process involves identifying, implementing, and evaluating system improvements. TGH promotes a team approach to problem solving using the Quality Leadership Process (QLP). QLP provides a structured method for all employees to

- Improve products and services
- Develop skills and positive attitudes
- Promote communication
- Enhance quality of work life
- Strengthen working relationships

The interdisciplinary team approach of QLP uses the storyboard technique for examining problems, processes, or systems to improve the quality (Figure 28–3). The storyboard is a technique used by teams to solve problems as well as to document and display improvement activities and results. It provides a structured way to

- Define problems/opportunities and narrow scope: Avoid working on problems that are too general, too large, or beyond the control or influence of team members.

Exhibit 28–5 Psychiatric-Mental Health Department Institutional Indicators

VOLUME INDICATORS
- Number of Patient Days
- Number of Patient Admissions
- Number of Patient Discharges
- Number of Psychiatric Emergency Codes (Code 44)
- Code 44 Rate
- Total Seclusion & Restraint Occurrences
- Seclusion & Restraint Rate
- Readmits 31 Days Post-Discharge
- Readmit Rate
- Transfers to Medical Services
- Transfer Rate
- Patient Length of Stay $<=$ 5 Days
- Rate
- ALOS
- Medication Errors
- Medication Error Rate

QUALITY MANAGEMENT/RISK MANAGEMENT INDICATORS
- Involuntary Patient Admissions
- Involuntary Admit Rate
- Court Ordered Treatment Patients
- Court Ordered Conversion Rate
- Against Medical Advice (AMA)
- AMA Rate
- Elopements
- Elopements Rate
- Patient Falls
- Fall Rate
- Unit-Specific Fall Rates
- Medical Emergency Codes (Code 12)
- Medical Emergencies
- Suicide Gesture/Attempt
- Seizures
- Alleged Sexual Activity
- Patient Injuries
- Patient Injury Rate
- Self-Inflicted Injuries
- Fall Related Injuries
- Recreational Related Injuries
- Medical Device Related Injuries
- "Other" Category of Injuries
- Patient Injury during Psychiatric Emergency Code
- AHCA Reportable Injuries
- Visitor Injuries
- Employee Injuries
- Mortality
- Mortality Rate

Courtesy of Tampa General Healthcare, Tampa, Florida.

- Analyze situations: Require thorough analysis of the situation and avoid jumping to unfounded conclusions.
- Collect data: Gather data and use factual information to understand the problem and justify the proposed solution.
- Obtain input from people involved: Obtain information and support for changes from the individuals performing the work, the customers, and the suppliers.
- Plan implementation and evaluate results: Ensure that the solution is adequately evaluated and implemented according to a well-thought-out plan that includes a pilot or trial implementation (Baxter Healthcare Corporation).

As shown in Figure 28–3, the storyboard process has nine steps.

1. Define requirements.
2. Collect and organize data.
3. List and prioritize improvement opportunities.
4. Define improvement objective.
5. Analyze and select most significant root cause.
6. Generate potential solutions.
7. Select best solution.
8. Implement solution.
9. Track effectiveness.

One psychiatric-mental health service specific example of the use of QLP is a multidisci-

Exhibit 28–6 Comprehensive Quality Measurement Matrix—Psychiatric-Mental Health Services Department Plan

Quality Measurement Indicators	Important Functions*											Dimensions of Performance••								Rationale***
INDICATORS	PE	TX	CC	PF	RI	LD	IM	HR	EC	IC	PI	Perf	Feat	Reli	Resp	Cred	Tang	Cour	Secu	
Treatment Plan		X					X					X	X	X		X	X			F, R, P, I, E
Medication Management	X			X							X	X	X	X	X	X				F, R, E
ECT Preparation		X					X					X		X	X	X				F, R, P
Psychiatric Emergency	X	X							X			X		X	X				X	R
Seclusion & Restraint		X							X		X									R, P, E
Fall Risk Program	X								X		X	X		X	X					R, P

Indicator	Rationale***
Consult Use	F, R
Standard of Care: Major Depression	P
Standard of Care: Schizophrenia	P
Sentinel Events: Medical Emergency	I, P
Documented Sexual Activity	I, P
Suicide Gesture Requiring Medical Intervention	I, P

*Important Functions Key:
PE: Patient Assessment
TX: Care of Patient
CC: Continuum of Care
PF: Patient/Family Education
RI: Patient Rights/Ethics
LD: Leadership
IM: Mgt. of Information
HR: Mgt. of Human Res.
EC: Environment of Care
IC: Infection Control
PI: Perf. Improvement

**Dimensions of Perf. Key:
Perf: Performance
Feat: Feature
Reli: Reliability
Resp: Responsiveness
Cred: Credibility
Tang: Tangibles
Cour: Courtesy
Secu: Security

***Rationale Key:
F: High Frequency
R: High Risk
P: Problem Prone
I: Institutional Indicator
E: Externally Required

Courtesy of Tampa General Healthcare, Tampa, Florida.

Exhibit 28–7 Psychiatric-Mental Health Services Quality Improvement Calendar

Aspect of Care	Jan	Feb	Mar	Apr	May	Jun	Jul	Aug	Sep	Oct	Nov	Dec
Seclusion & restraint			X	O					X	O		
Treatment plan			X	O						X	O	
Medication management	O					X	O					X
ECT prep					X						X	
Elopement				X	O					X	O	
Psychiatric emergency (Code Green)		X				O			X			O
Major depression		X	O					X	O			
Schizophrenia					X	O					X	O
Substance abuse			X	O					X	O		
Deaths*	X O	X O	X O	X O	X O	X O	X O	X O	X O	X O	X O	X O
Sexual activity*	X O	X O	X O	X O	X O	X O	X O	X O	X O	X O	X O	X O
Medical emergency (Code Blue)*	X O	X O	X O	X O	X O	X O	X O	X O	X O	X O	X O	X O
Suicide attempt	X O	X O	X O	X O	X O	X O	X O	X O	X O	X O	X O	X O

Note: X = Information collected; O = Data evaluated and reported.

*Each occurrence is evaluated and reported to MDT, then aggregated at the end of the fiscal year and presented to Quality Council.

Courtesy of Tampa General Healthcare, Tampa, Florida.

Exhibit 28–8 Quality Improvement Data Collection and Evaluation Tool

IMPORTANT ASPECT OF CARE: _____ 7. _____

INDICATORS: 1. 4. 8.

    2. 5. 9.

    3. 6. 10.

PATIENT OR MR#	STAFF	1 Y N	2 Y N	3 Y N	4 Y N	5 Y N	6 Y N	7 Y N	8 Y N	9 Y N	10 Y N	Remarks
Total												
Percentage												
Threshold for Eval												
Eval of Data Required												

RECOMMENDATIONS: _____ MORE INFORMATION NEEDED TO EVALUATE

_____ REVIEW AS CALENDARED

_____ RECALENDAR AFTER ACTION PLAN IMPLEMENTED

_____ OTHER: _____

RECOMMENDATION MADE BY: _____

Courtesy of Tampa General Healthcare, Tampa, Florida.

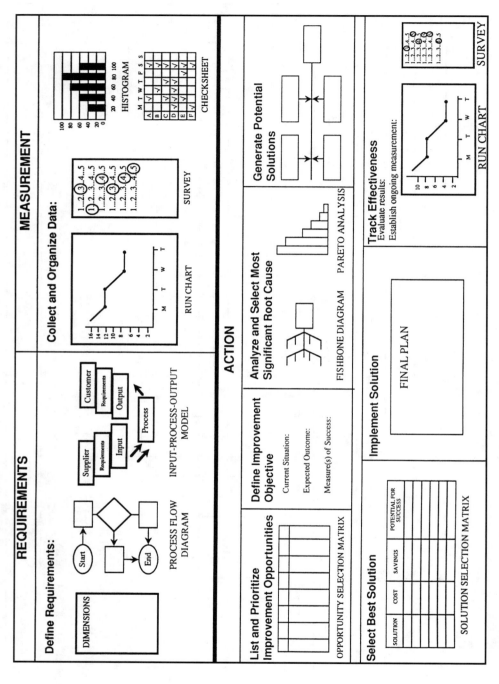

Figure 28–3 Quality leadership process—Storyboard. Courtesy of Tampa General Healthcare, Tampa, Florida.

plinary team's use of the storyboard approach in developing a patient and family teaching protocol and teaching materials for clients with a major depression diagnosis. A sequence of tables, figures, and exhibits illustrates the steps of the storyboard process for the protocol's development (Step 1: define requirements, Table 28–1, Figures 28–4, 28–5, and 28–6; Step 2: collect and organize data, Figures 28–7 and 28–8; Step 3: list and prioritize improvement opportunities, Figure 28–9; Step 4: define improvement objective, Exhibit 28–9; Step 5: analyze and select most significant root cause, Figure 28–10; Step 6: generate potential solutions, Figure 28–11; Step 7: select best solution, Table 28–2; Step 8: implement solution, Table 28–3 and Figure 28–12; and Step 9: track effectiveness, Figures 28–13 and 28–14). The completed protocol (Exhibit 28–10) provides a clear, structured approach to teaching patients and families as well as a multidisciplinary documentation system for patient and family education.

Critical pathways to manage patient care have become popular tools. Many organizations have developed these guidelines to manage the quality and cost outcomes of care processes. There is strong pressure for health care organizations to reduce cost while maintaining quality outcomes. Critical pathways are tools ideally suited to CQI since they outline the cross-departmental processes involved in patient care. They define the sequence of predetermined, interdisciplinary processes or critical events that must occur for a particular patient group or diagnosis to move the patient toward the desired outcomes within a defined period of time.

Another example of QLP in action is a multidisciplinary team's use of the QLP process to develop a critical pathway for patients with major depression (Exhibits 28–11 and 28–12). Exhibit 28–11 shows the predetermined outcomes for a patient with major depression, and

Exhibit 28–12 shows the critical pathway for major depression. Figure 28–15 is an example of a critical pathway for patients and families to use.

The process of evaluating the projected to actual patient care on the critical pathway reveals variances. The analysis of these variances is invaluable in determining why an expected client outcome or clinical quality indicator has not been met. Typical variance categories include the following:

- patient or family
- clinician or health care provider
- institution or system
- community

Variances are collected and analyzed monthly using the Variance Analysis Form (Exhibit 28–13). The case manager documents and reports monthly to quality management using the Case Manager Report (Exhibit 28–14). Evaluating patient outcomes, analyzing variance trends, and evaluating actions taken to correct variances from the critical pathway will provide support to the organization's QI program.

Critical pathways serve as the benchmark for expected patient outcomes. Through the daily monitoring and tracking of a patient's expected progress in achieving critical outcomes on the critical pathway, practitioners can provide ongoing assessment and improvement in the quality of care. With the use of the critical pathway as a benchmark, CQI goals and indicators can be established for each population or diagnosis. Data and CQI reports can be evaluated in the aggregate to determine whether the expected outcomes were achieved by patients. The analysis of data will facilitate identifying opportunities to improve care or to determine the effectiveness of interventions that have been implemented on the critical pathway or identify opportunities for improving care.

Table 28–1 Storyboard Step 1: Define Requirements—*Analysis* by Customer Requirement Dimensions

Requirement Dimension	Physician	Patient/Family	Staff
Performance	Include biological approach Consistent information Updated materials	Immediate information Understandable language Consistent information	Assessment Tools/booklets for guidance
Features	Use handout Booklet or video Management	Personalized materials Complete information Diagnosis, medications, therapies	Convenient materials Handouts, video, booklet
Reliability	Consistency Scientifically validated	Updated information Reinforced by all staff	Simple, easy to read by all Graphics, 5th- to 6th-grade level
Responsiveness	Effective documentation	Information when needed	Individual, educational and groups
Credibility	Educator knows subject matter	Accurate, scientific	Continuity of information
Tangibles	Video, handouts	Booklet, questions, and answers	Standards and protocols Medication-specific handout
Courtesy	Polite, pleasant, unhurried	Friendly, consideration of needs Respect	Receptive to questions, respect
Security	Safety, privacy	Follow-up with physician	Reassurance, safety

Courtesy of Tampa General Healthcare, Tampa, Florida.

REQUIREMENT	DO WE MEET IT?		HOW IMPORTANT IS IT TO US? Least (1) to Most (5)
Get Education Immediately	Yes	(No)	1 2 (3) 4 5
Have Patient/Family Handouts	Yes	(No)	1 2 3 4 (5)
Consistent Information	Yes	(No)	1 2 3 4 (5)
Accurate Information	Yes	(No)	1 2 3 4 (5)
Appropriate Educational Level	Yes	(No)	1 2 3 (4) 5
Interdisciplinary Teaching	(Yes)	No	1 2 (3) 4 5
Standardized Information	Yes	(No)	1 2 3 4 (5)
Minimal Education for All Patients	Yes	(No)	1 2 3 4 (5)
Meaningful for the Patients	(Yes)	No	1 2 3 (4) 5
Flexible Teaching Approaches	(Yes)	No	1 2 3 (4) 5
Answer Patient and Family Questions	(Yes)	No	1 2 3 (4) 5
Trust in Staff and Information	Yes	(No)	1 2 3 4 (5)
Simple Documentation System	Yes	(No)	1 2 3 4 (5)
Courtesy of Staff	Yes	(No)	1 2 3 4 (5)
Treated with Respect	Yes	(No)	1 2 3 4 (5)
Teaching Protocol	Yes	(No)	1 2 (3) 4 5
Staff Training on "How tos" of Education	(Yes)	No	1 2 3 (4) 5
Patient Education Packets	Yes	(No)	1 2 3 4 (5)

Figure 28–4 Storyboard Step 1: Define requirements—*Analysis* by fullfillment and importance. Courtesy of Tampa General Healthcare, Tampa, Florida.

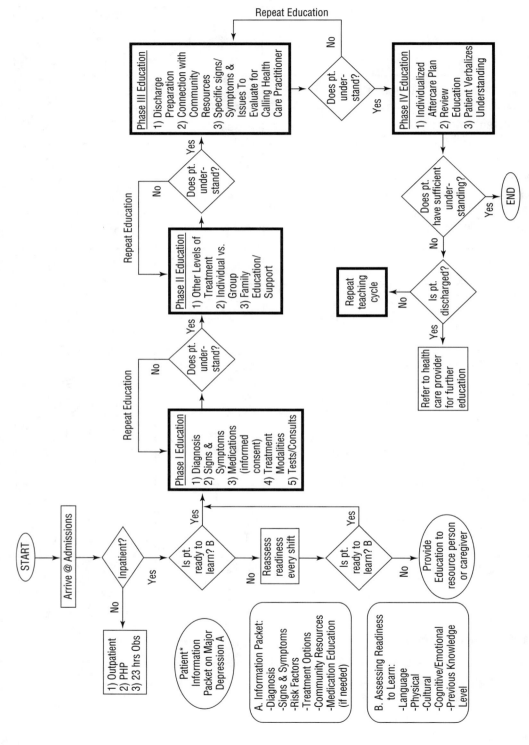

Figure 28–5 Storyboard Step 1: Define requirements—*Flowchart*. Courtesy of Tampa General Healthcare, Tampa, Florida.

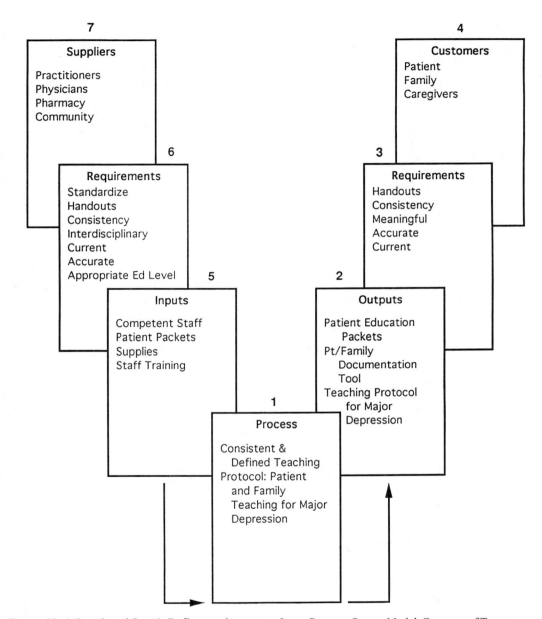

Figure 28–6 Storyboard Step 1: Define requirements—*Input-Process-Output Model*. Courtesy of Tampa General Healthcare, Tampa, Florida.

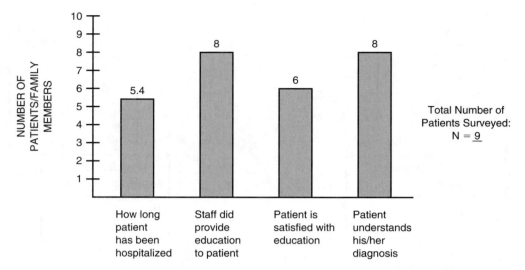

Figure 28–7 Storyboard Step 2: Measurement; Collect and organize data—*Histogram* of patient and family education survey results for major depression cases. Courtesy of Tampa General Healthcare, Tampa, Florida.

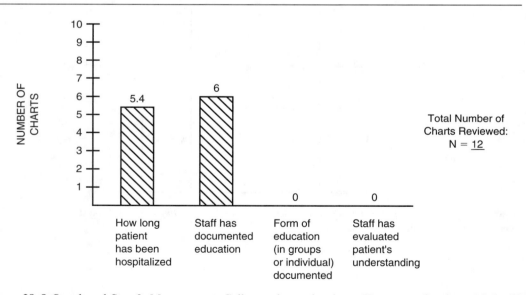

Figure 28–8 Storyboard Step 2: Measurement; Collect and organize data—*Histogram* of patient and family education documentation results for major depression cases. Courtesy of Tampa General Healthcare, Tampa, Florida.

Requirements	Supports Org. Objectives	Valued Added	Can Implement	Is There a Deadline	Est. Cost If Not Done	What Needs To Be Done First
Patient/Family Education Packets/Handouts	YES	YES & NO	YES	NO	May lose customers if we don't do something	2
Simple Interdisciplinary Documentation System	YES	YES & NO	YES	YES 1.5 yrs	Waste staff time, aimless treatment. Survey process	1
Consistent/Accurate/ Standardized Information	YES	YES	YES	YES 1.5 yrs	Patient/family confusion Nonadherence	2
Materials and Education at Appropriate Level	YES	YES	YES	YES 1.5 yrs	Mis-understanding Pretended gains	2
Trained Staff	YES	YES	YES	YES 1.5 yrs	Decreased job satisfaction Improved work environment	3
Courtesy/Respect/Trust	YES	YES	YES & NO	NO	Increased loyalty Parallel process	4

Figure 28–9 Storyboard Step 3: List and prioritize improvement opportunities—*Opportunity selection matrix.* Courtesy of Tampa General Healthcare, Tampa, Florida.

Exhibit 28–9 Storyboard Step 4: Define Improvement Objective—*Improvement Objectives Worksheet*

Current Situation:
- No consistent educational material or outlines for psychiatric diagnoses.
- No designated documentation system for patient and family education.
- Nursing competencies in process, no other competencies in place.

Expected Outcomes:
- Interdisciplinary staff will be competent to provide patient and family education.
- Patient/family education will be delivered in consistent, accurate, and standardized fashion.
- Patient/family education will be provided through individual and group programs using written and psychoeducational materials.
- Patient/family materials will be at the appropriate developmental level and education level.
- Patient/family education will be consistently documented in the medical record through a formalized documentation system.

Measure of Success:
- Quality assessment—indicators for patient/family education
- Patient and family satisfaction/outcome surveys
- Knowledge test
- Staff level of competencies documented

Courtesy of Tampa General Healthcare, Tampa, Florida.

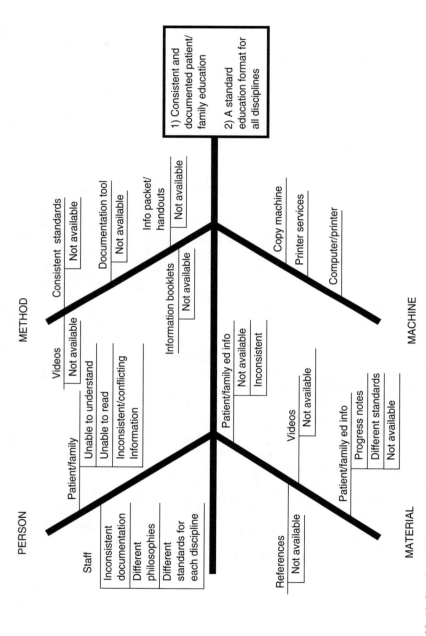

Figure 28–10 Storyboard Step 5: Analyze and select most significant root cause—*Fishbone diagram*. Courtesy of Tampa General Healthcare, Tampa, Florida.

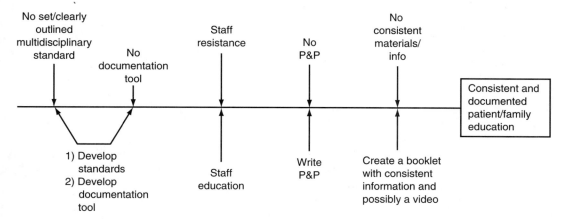

Figure 28–11 Storyboard Step 6: Generate potential solutions—*Force-Field analysis*. Courtesy of Tampa General Healthcare, Tampa, Florida.

Table 28–2 Storyboard Step 7: Select Best Solution—*Solution Selection Matrix*

Possible Solutions	Cost of Implementing	Savings & Gains	Chance of Success	% of Root Cause Removed
1) Create diagnosis-specific booklets	Hrs of staff involved Materials Duplication			
	High	Med	High	High
2) Develop a standard & document-ation tool	Hrs of staff involved Paper cost			
	Med	Med	High	High
3) Educate staff on patient/ family education	Hrs of educator staff time Materials			
	Med	Med	High	High
4) Write P&P on patient/ family education & documentation	Hrs of staff involved Paper cost			
	Low	Med	High	High

Courtesy of Tampa General Healthcare, Tampa, Florida.

Table 28–3 Storyboard Step 8: Implement Solution—*Implementation Plan*

What	Who	When	Expected Outcome
1) Create a booklet on Major Depression	Team	Start within 2 wks	A multidisciplinary patient/family teaching booklet on Major Depression
2) Develop a standard and documentation tool	Team	Complete in 2 wks	A multidisciplinary standard on MD for patient/family education
3) Educate staff on patient/family education with Major Depression	Team CNS Supervisors	Complete in 1.5 months	Trained individuals in patient/family education & documentation
4) Write P&P on patient/family education and documentation	Team P&P Committee	Start by 1 month Complete in 2 months	A P&P on patient/family education and documentation

Courtesy of Tampa General Healthcare, Tampa, Florida.

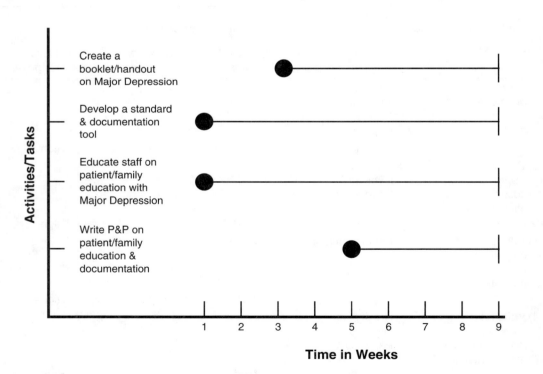

Figure 28–12 Storyboard Step 8: Implement solution—*Gantt chart timeline*. Courtesy of Tampa General Healthcare, Tampa, Florida.

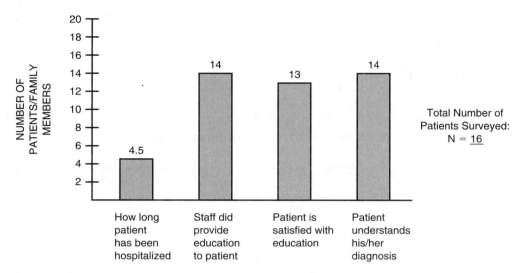

Figure 28–13 Storyboard Step 9: Track effectiveness–*Histogram* of patient and family education postimplementation survey results for major depression cases. Courtesy of Tampa General Healthcare, Tampa, Florida.

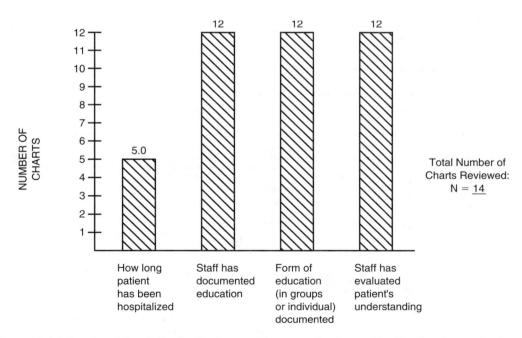

Figure 28–14 Storyboard Step 9: Track effectiveness–*Histogram* of patient and family education postimplementation documentation results for major depression cases. Courtesy of Tampa General Healthcare, Tampa, Florida.

Exhibit 28–10 Completed Teaching Protocol for Major Depression

---

TGH-UNIVERSITY
PSYCHIATRY CENTER

Addressograph

TEACHING PROTOCOL - MAJOR DEPRESSION

OUTCOME STANDARDS TO BE MET PRIOR TO DISCHARGE		DATE/INITIAL	MET	NOT MET
PHYSIOLOGIC:	The patient/family will actively participate in the management of depression to significantly reduce adverse physical disturbances.			
PSYCHOLOGIC:	The patient/family will demonstrate awareness of affective coping management towards depressive illness and therapeutic regimen.			
COGNITIVE:	The patient/family will recognize exacerbation of illness and identify adverse effects of medications and respond appropriately.			

BOOKLET RECEIVED:_____ (Date)

LEARNING NEEDS ASSESSMENT

Identify potential needs for discharge: _____

_____

Identify barriers or enhancers to learning: (knowledge level, physical/sensory limitation, psycho-social status, language)

_____

_____

---

* EVALUATION KEY

S = Successfully meets outcome   N = Needs further instruction   U = Unable to comprehend   * = See Patient Ed Notes

---

Patient/Family Learning Outcomes	Information To Be Presented/ Patient Learning Activities	Teaching Method	Patient	Family	Date/ Time Initial	* Eval Key
1. Verbalizes an awareness of Major Depression as an illness. (All Disciplines)	1. Major Depression is a treatable illness. 2. Major Depression is not a shameful reflection of weakness. (Page 1 and 2)	Handbook Education Group				

Initial	Signature/Title	Initial	Signature/Title

continues

Exhibit 28–10 continued

**TGH-UNIVERSITY
PSYCHIATRY CENTER**

Addressograph

TEACHING PROTOCOL - MAJOR DEPRESSION

Patient/Family Learning Outcomes	Information To Be Presented/ Patient Learning Activities	Teaching Method	Patient	Family	Date/ Time Initial	* Eval Key
2. Verbalizes the causes of Major Depression as a complex interaction among brain chemicals, hormones and external stressors. (All Disciplines)	1. Family history and genetics 2. Bio-chemical and psychological make-up 3. Prolonged stress 4. Stressful life events or traumatic life crises (i.e. loss, unresolved or unexpressed anger, frustration and self-doubt, etc.) (Page 4 and 5)	Handbook Education Group				
3. Verbalizes understanding of the signs and symptoms of Major Depression. (All Disciplines)	1. Depressed mood 2. Loss of interest or pleasure 3. Change in appetite 4. Weight loss or gain 5. Insomnia or hypersomnia 6. Psycho-motor agitation or retardation 7. Fatigue or loss of energy 8. Feelings of worthlessness 9. Impaired concentration 10 Thoughts of death or suicide 11. Feelings of helplessness or hopelessness 12. Unmanageable anxiety (Page 5 and 6)	Handbook Education Group				
4. Verbalizes benefits of treatment for Major Depression. (All Disciplines)	1. Shortens episodes of depression 2. Reduces pain, disability and cost 3. Reduces relapse and recurrence 4. Improves quality of life 5. Healthier life style including exercise and proper nutrition (Page 10 and 11)	Handbook Education Group				
5. Verbalizes treatment options for Major Depression. (All Disciplines)	1. Support group 2. Psycho-therapy 3. Anti-depressant medication 4. ECT 5. Individualized combination of any of the above treatments (Page 9 and 10)	Handbook Education Group				

Initial	Signature/Title	Initial	Signature/Title

continues

Exhibit 28–10 continued

**TGH-UNIVERSITY
PSYCHIATRY CENTER**

Addressograph

TEACHING PROTOCOL - MAJOR DEPRESSION

Patient/Family Learning Outcomes	Information To Be Presented/ Patient Learning Activities	Teaching Method	Patient	Family	Date/ Time Initial	* Eval Key
6. Verbalizes understanding of prescribed antidepressant's name, dosage, purposes and possible side effects. (Pharmacy/MD/Nsg; All Disciplines)	1. Tricyclics—dry mouth, blurred vision, constipation, sedation, drowsiness, weight gain, postural hypotension, cardiac effects, and dizziness. 2. Monoamine Oxidase Inhibitors—note diet restriction. Possible side effects are same as Tricyclics. 3. Serotonin Reuptake Inhibitors—nausea, nervousness, insomnia, sexual dysfunction, and headache. 4. Anxiolytics—dizziness, drowsiness, light-headedness, unsteadiness. 5. Antidepressant medication prescribed: a. b.	Handbook Education Group Medi- cation Group				

7. Verbalizes understanding of purpose for prescribed testing, procedures and consults. (MD/Nsg)	1. Lab levels
	     a. Prescribed medications
	     b. Thyroid Function Test
		Handbook				

	2. Procedures
	     a. Depression Scales
	     b. EKG
	     c. EEG
	     d. Other test as prescribed by physician
		Handbook				

	3. Consults
	     a. Psychological testing
	     b. Medication evaluation consultation
	     c. Medical consultation
	     d. Dietary consultation
	 (Page 14 and 15)
		Handbook				

Initial	Signature/Title	Initial	Signature/Title

continues

Exhibit 28–10 continued

TGH-UNIVERSITY
PSYCHIATRY CENTER

<u>Addressograph</u>

TEACHING PROTOCOL - MAJOR DEPRESSION

Patient/Family Learning Outcomes	Information To Be Presented/ Patient Learning Activities	Teaching Method	Patient	Family	Date/ Time Initial	* Eval Key
8. Verbalizes understanding of community resources for Major Depression. (Case Manager; All Disciplines)	1. Tampa Bay Chapter of the National Depressive and Manic-Depressive Association 2. Hillsborough County Chapter of the National Alliance for the Mentally Ill 3. National Alliance for the Mentally Ill (NAMI) 4. National Foundation for Depressive Illness, Inc. (Page 16 and 17)	Handbook Education Group				
9. Verbalizes expected outcomes of treatment for Major Depression. (All Disciplines)	1. Reduction of symptoms and maladaptive coping responses 2. Restoration of pre-illness level of functioning 3. Improvement in patient's quality of life 4. Prevention of future relapse and recurrence 5. Recognition of need for treatment related to relapse and/or exacerbation of symptoms (Page 17)	Handbook Education Group				

DATE	PATIENT EDUCATION NOTES

Initial	Signature/Title	Initial	Signature/Title

Courtesy of Tampa General Healthcare, Tampa, Florida.

Exhibit 28–11 Predetermined Outcomes for Patients with General Depression

DATE INITIATED:

DIAGNOSIS: Major Depression

Date Stated	Initials	Expected Outcome (Day)	Discip.	Target Date	Date Met
		GAF 0-50 Score (Day 1)	Team		
		BECK Depression Scale Score Moderate/Severe (Day 1)	Team		
		No injury, contracts signed (Day 1)	Nsg		
		With assistance sets goals for Tx (Day 1)	Team		
		Communicates unsafe impulses (Day 1)	Team		
		Communicates feelings to staff (Day 2)	Team		
		Starts Mood Chart/Journal and shares with staff (Day 2)	Team		
		Demonstrates ability to manage destructive impulses (Day 3)	Team		
		Sleeping 3–4 hours each night (Day 3)	Nsg		
		Eating 50% of each meal (Day 3)	Nsg		
		Increase function and concentration while engaged in priorities/goals (Day 3)	Team		
		Recognizes periods of mood relief (Day 3)	Team		
		BECK Depression Scale Score Moderate or below (Day 1)	Team		
		Sleeping 4–5 hours each night (Day 4)	Nsg		
		Eating 75% of each meal (Day 4)	Nsg		
		GAF Score over 50 (Day 5)	Team		
		Sleeping pattern stabilized (Day 5)	Nsg		
		Appetite stabilized (Day 5)	Nsg		
		Verbalizes post discharge safety plan (Day 5)	Team		
		Mood stabilized or improved (Day 5)	Team		

Courtesy of Tampa General Healthcare, Tampa, Florida.

Exhibit 28–12 Critical Pathway for Major Depression

DATE INITIATED:_____

DIAGNOSIS: **MAJOR DEPRESSION**   Expected LOS: 5 Days

MEASUREMENT PHASE	Day 1	Day 2	Day 3	Day 4	Day 5
CONSULTS	- Medical Consult (if needed)				
TESTS	- SMAC (fasting) - CBC, TSH - UA, UDS - Beta HCG (if female) - EKG (if > 40 and not done in last 6 months)	- B12/Folate (if CBC abnormal) - Lab Results on Chart			
INTERVENTIONS	- Initiate Treatment Orders - Evaluate Need for Individual, Family or Marital Therapy	- Order Individual Family or Marital Therapy (if needed)			
MEDICATIONS	- Informed Consent Documented by MD - Monitor Medication Adherence - Monitor Side Effects - Vital Signs (Q____) - Med Education Before 1st Dose By RN/LPN and Documented (if minor family med. ed) - Antidepressant - Program (Circle) Mood A&D Eating Seniors	---------> ---------> - Vital Signs (Q____)	---------> ---------> - V/S (Q____)	---------> ---------> - V/S (Q____) - Antidepressant Effective? **Yes No**	---------> ---------> V/S (Q____)
DIET	- Regular				

ACTIVITY/MILIEU THERAPY	- Patients √s (Circle)
	  1:1 CVO Q15 Q30
	- Orientation Unit/Program
	- Introduction to Groups
	- Explain Pt. Responsibilities
	- Provide Handbook
		- Patient √s (Circle)
		  Q15 Q30
			- Patient √s: Q30
			- Evaluation of Progress & Expected Outcomes by MDT
				--------->
				--------->
					--------->

TEACHING	- Assess Educational Needs - Initiate Teaching Protocol	- Assess Understanding of Teaching Protocol Outcomes	- Review & Reinforce D/C instructions/Follow-up - Reinforce Protocol		- Review Understanding of Patient/Family Education
PSYCHOSOCIAL	- Psychosocial History - Depression Scale - Suicidal Rating - History and Physical (unless within 30 days)	- Mental Status Assess by RN/MD - Depression Scale - Suicidal Rating	--------->	---------> - Depression Scale - Suicidal Rating	--------->
DISCHARGE PLANNING	- Assess D/C Needs - Initiate D/C Plan - Diagnostic Criteria Met		- D/C Plan Complete		- Discharge - PHP/OP Referral (if Applicable)

Addressograph

Initials   Signature

_____   _____

_____   _____

_____   _____

_____   _____

TAMPA GENERAL HEALTHCARE
CRITICAL PATH

Courtesy of Tampa General Healthcare, Tampa, Florida.

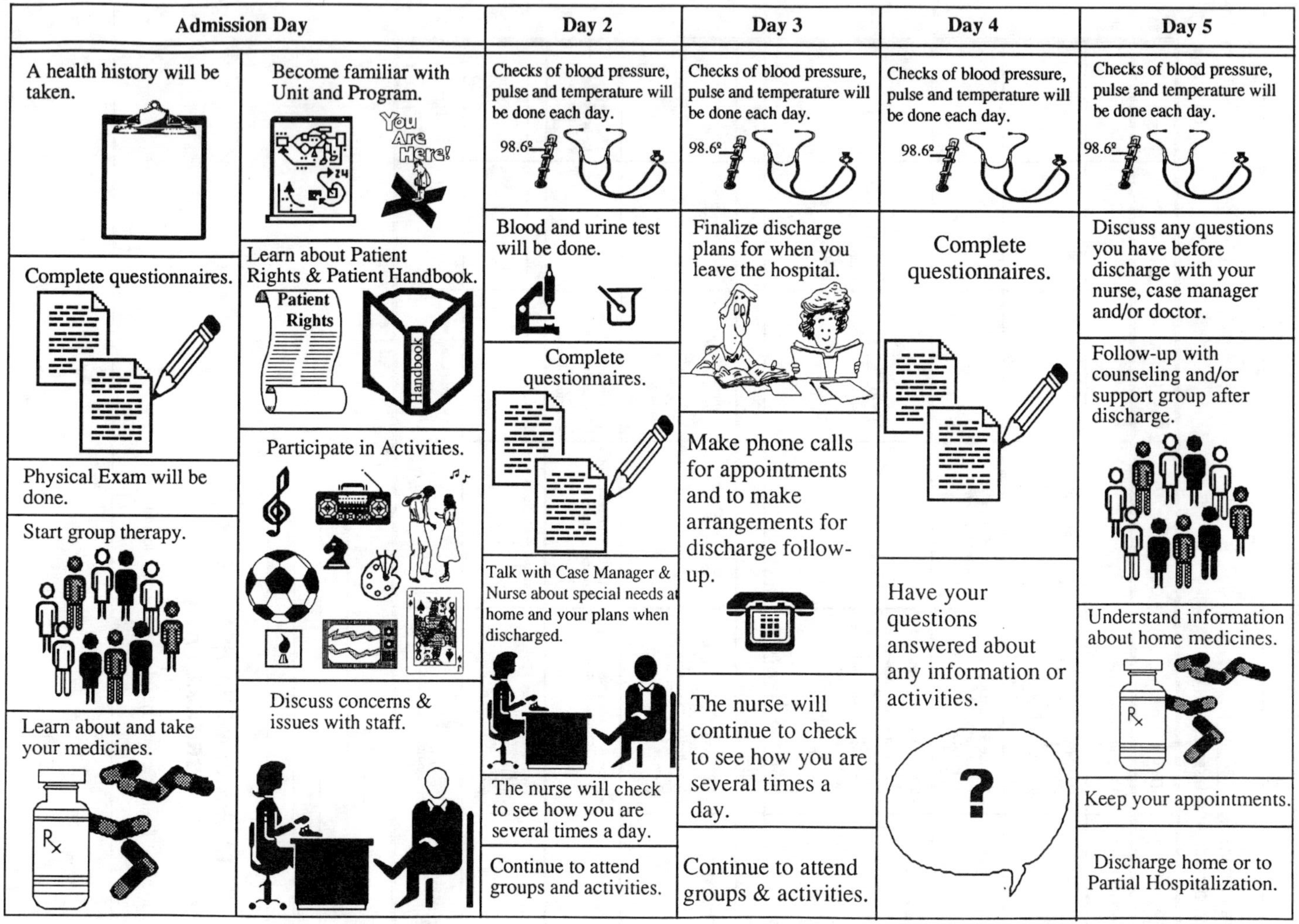

Admission Day	Day 2	Day 3	Day 4	Day 5
A health history will be taken.	Checks of blood pressure, pulse and temperature will be done each day. 98.6°	Checks of blood pressure, pulse and temperature will be done each day. 98.6°	Checks of blood pressure, pulse and temperature will be done each day. 98.6°	Checks of blood pressure, pulse and temperature will be done each day. 98.6°
Become familiar with Unit and Program. You Are Here!	Blood and urine test will be done.	Finalize discharge plans for when you leave the hospital.	Complete questionnaires.	Discuss any questions you have before discharge with your nurse, case manager and/or doctor.
Complete questionnaires.	Complete questionnaires.	Make phone calls for appointments and to make arrangements for discharge follow-up.		Follow-up with counseling and/or support group after discharge.
Learn about Patient Rights & Patient Handbook. Handbook Patient Rights				
Physical Exam will be done.				
Participate in Activities.	Talk with Case Manager & Nurse about special needs at home and your plans when discharged.	The nurse will continue to check to see how you are several times a day.	Have your questions answered about any information or activities. ?	Understand information about home medicines. Rx
Start group therapy.	The nurse will check to see how you are several times a day.			
Discuss concerns & issues with staff.	Continue to attend groups and activities.	Continue to attend groups & activities.		Keep your appointments.
Learn about and take your medicines. Rx				Discharge home or to Partial Hospitalization.

Figure 28–15 Critical pathway for patients' and families' use: Major depression patient treatment plan. Courtesy of George Byron Smith, RN, MSN, Tampa, Florida.

Exhibit 28–13 Variance Analysis Form

Instructions: For use when patient is not progressing according to the times specified on the critical path. Record date variance is noted next to the type of variance that occurred. Retain this form for collection by case manager. Not a part of the permanent record.

Critical Path: Nurse/Case Manager:

NUM.	DATE	TYPE	
1A		PATIENT:	PHYSIOLOGICAL
1B		PATIENT:	EDUCATIONAL/LANGUAGE
1C		PATIENT:	CHOICE
1D		PATIENT:	FAMILY FACTORS
1E		PATIENT:	OTHER (list)
2A		CLINICIAN:	DECISION MAKING
2B		CLINICIAN:	RESPONSE TIME
2C		CLINICIAN:	SKILL PERFORMANCE
2D		CLINICIAN:	OTHER (list)
3A		INSTITUTION:	BED AVAILABILITY
3B		INSTITUTION:	SUPPLIES NOT AVAILABLE
3C		INSTITUTION:	SERVICE NOT AVAILABLE
3D		INSTITUTION:	OTHER (list)
4A		COMMUNITY:	FOLLOW UP CARE
4B		COMMUNITY:	BED NOT AVAILABLE
4C		COMMUNITY:	PAYER ARRANGEMENTS
4D		COMMUNITY:	OTHER (list)
5A			
5B			
5C			

Addressograph

Courtesy of Tampa General Healthcare, Tampa, Florida.

Exhibit 28–14 TGH Case Manager Monthly Summary Report

Case Manager Report:

DRG or ICD-9CM Code Number:

Length of Stay Outcomes	
Average Length of Stay	
Percent Change From Previous Month	**%**
Total Number of Outlier Days	
Cost of Care Outcomes	
Average Cost per Case	
Percent Change From Previous Month	**%**
Additional Savings (attach activity log or other documentation)	**attachment**
Cost of Care Outcomes	
Discharge Disposition of Patients (attach disposition summary form)	**attachment**
Return to Emergency Care Center Within 72 hours of Discharge	
Variances from path (attach variance summary form)	**attachment**
Patient Satisfaction Indicators and Results:	**attachment**
Source: _____ Ask a Patient Tool	
_____ Outcome Assessment & Evaluation Data	

Courtesy of Tampa General Healthcare, Tampa, Florida.

OUTCOMES EVALUATION

Managed care or managed competition have greatly affected mental health services. According to Oss and Bengen-Seltzer (1995), three industry trends have and will continue to revolutionize psychiatric-mental health services:

1. Managed-care organizations are continually experiencing horizontal as well as vertical mergers and acquisitions.
2. Health care providers are being forced to develop new and diverse product lines while traditional inpatient revenue bases erode and consolidations take place all across the country.
3. The traditional roles and sites for providers are changing toward a local community-based health care system.

Amid these turbulent changes, providers of psychiatric-mental health services are required to demonstrate value to consumers, third-party payers, and regulatory agencies.

With the continued health care movement toward deinstitutionalization, the lack of community mental health services, and the decreasing resource dollars to provide care, it is imperative for mental health care providers to examine ways to foster continuity of care across the entire continuum of mental illness and to focus on a wide range of services that demonstrate cost-effective, quality outcomes. Within the current health care environment, it is imperative that psychiatric-mental health service organizations develop objective measures to assess the outcomes and quality of care.

According to Sederer, Dickey, and Hermann (1996), integrating outcome assessment and management into clinical practice will serve the following three functions:

1. to promote the development and adoption of treatment guidelines that can be linked to specific outcomes
2. to produce data that will legitimize and validate the treatment of psychiatric and substance abuse problems
3. to regain public trust with mental health services by offering accountability for outcome management.

Outcome assessment and evaluation will continue to be an important function in psychiatric-mental health care. There will continue to be a demand for service organizations to evaluate and demonstrate their quality of care as well as the need for mental health services. Table 28–4 provides a list of outcomes assessment tools used in psychiatric-mental health services.

Table 28–4 Outcome Evaluation Measurement Tools

Instrument & Author	Measurement	Respondent	Description
Addiction Severity Index— ASI (Mclellan, Luborsky, Cacciola, & Fureman, 1980)	Contributing factors to substance abuse	Interview	Semistructured interview 60–70 minutes 7 domains
Beck Depression Inventory—BDI (Beck, 1961)	Depression	Self-report	21 items 4-point scale
Behavior and Symptom Identification Scale— BASIS-32 (Eisen, 1989)	Psychiatric symptoms and functioning	Self-report	32 items 5 domains Patient's point of view of treatment

continues

Table 28–4 continued

Instrument & Author	Measurement	Respondent	Description
Brief Psychiatric Rating Scale—BPRS (Overeall & Groham, 1962)	Psychiatric symptoms and functioning	Clinician	18 symptom constructs 7-point scale 7 domains
Brief Symptom Inventory—BSI (Derogatis & Melisaratos, 1983)	Psychiatric symptoms	Self-report	53 items Abbreviated version of SCL-90
Child Behavior Checklist—CBCL (Achenbach & Edelbrock, 1981)	Psychiatric symptoms Social competence Academic performance	Parent-teacher	2 versions • ages 2–3 yrs • ages 4–18 yrs
Clinical Global Impression—CGI (Guy, 1976)	Overall improvement	Clinician	3 items: severity, improvement, & efficacy
Consumer Satisfaction Questionnaire (Larsen, 1991)	Patient satisfaction	Self-report	8 items 4-point scale
Eating Disorder Inventory-2 EDI-2 (Garner, 1993)	Psychological symptoms	Self-report	91 items 11 domains 6-point scale
Family Burden Interview Schedule—Short form—FBIS/SF (Tessler, 1994)	Burden of caregivers of adults with severe mental illness	Interview	5 domains
Geriatric Depression Scale (Yesavage, 1983)	Depression	Interview	11 items
Global Assessment of Functioning Scale—GAF (Endicott, 1976)	Psychiatric functioning and daily living skills	Clinician	Single rating 100-point scale
Goal Attainment Scale (Kiresuk & Sherman, 1968)	Individually defined goals	Interview	Behaviorally defined outcomes 5-point scale
Group Health Association of America (GHAA) Consumer Satisfaction Survey (Davies & Ware, 1991)	Patient satisfaction	Self-report	63 items 5-point scale
Hamilton Rating Scale for Anxiety—HRSA (Hamilton, 1960)	Anxiety	Clinician	14 items 4-point scale
Hamilton Rating Scale for Depression—HRSD (Hamilton, 1960)	Depression	Clinician	21 items 4-point scale

continues

Table 28–4 continued

Instrument & Author	Measurement	Respondent	Description
Life Skills Profile—LSP (Parker, 1989)	Function and disability in adults with schizophrenia	Interviewer	39 items 4-point scale 5 domains
MOS Health Status Survey —SF-36 (Ware, 1992)	Global well-being	Self-report	36 items 8 domains
Patient Satisfaction Questionnaire—PSQ III (Hays, Davies, & Ware, 1987)	Patient satisfaction	Self-report	50 items 5-point scale
Psychiatric Outcomes Module: Depression—DOM (Smith, 1992)	Treatment, outcomes, client characteristics in adults with depression	Interviewer Medical Record Self-report	4 domains or subscales
Psychiatric Outcomes Module: Substance Abuse—SAOM (Smith, 1995)	Treatment, outcomes, prognostic characteristics in adults with substance abuse	Self-report Medical record	3 domains or subscales
Quality of Life Review— QOLI (Lehman, 1982)	Quality of life	Interviewer	153 items 8 life domains
Rapid Disability Rating Scale (Linn, 1982)	Functional status and daily living skills	Clinician	18 items 4-point scale
Speilberger State Trait Anxiety Scale—STAI (Speilberger, 1970)	Anxiety	Self-report	20 items 4-point scale
Symptom Checklist-90-Revised—SCL-90-R (Derogatis, 1993)	Psychiatric symptoms	Self-report	90 items 5-point scale 9 domains, 3 global scores
Service Satisfaction Scale-30 —SSS-30 (Greenfield, 1994)	Patient satisfaction	Self-report	30 items
Treatment Services Review— TSR (Mclellan, Alterman, Luborsky, & Cacciola, 1992)	Service provision	Self-report	87 items 7 domains
Yale Brown Obsessive Compulsive Scale (Goodman, 1989)	Obsessive-compulsive disorders	Self-report	10 items 5-point scale

In summary, the QI program for psychiatric-mental health services at TGH is composed of

- the organization-wide QI plan
- the department-specific QI plan

- a QLP or multidisciplinary team approach to improving quality that includes developing services, programs, and products (teaching protocols, critical paths)
- an outcomes evaluation program

REFERENCES

Baxter Healthcare Corporation. (1991). *Meeting customer requirements: Participant guide.* Tampa, FL: Author.

National Committee for Quality Assurance. (1996). *1997 draft standards for accreditation of managed care organizations.* Washington, DC: Author.

Sederer, L.I., Dickey, B., & Hermann, R.C. (1996). The imperative of outcomes assessment in psychiatry. In L.I. Sederer & B. Dickey (Eds.). *Outcomes assessment in clinical practice.* Baltimore: Williams & Wilkins.

SELECTED READING

American Psychiatric Association. (1996). *Practice guidelines.* Washington, DC: Author.

Burdick, M., Stuart, G., & Lewis, L. (1994). Measuring nursing outcomes in a psychiatric setting. *Issues in Mental Health Nursing, 15*(2), 137–148.

Coalition of Psychiatric Nursing Organizations. (1994). *Statement on psychiatric-mental health nursing practice and standards of psychiatric-mental clinical nursing practice.* Washington, DC: American Nurses Publishing.

McDowell, I., & Newell, C. (1987). *Measuring health: A guide to rating scales and questionnaires.* New York: Oxford University Press.

Meisenheimer, C.G. (1992). Assuring quality in psychiatry. In *Improving quality: A guide to effective programs,* pp. 471–495. Gaithersburg, MD: Aspen.

Sederer, L.I., & Dickey, B. (Eds.). (1996). *Outcomes assessment in clinical practice.* Baltimore: Williams & Wilkins.

Spath, P. (1982). *Clinical paths: Tools for outcomes measurements.* Chicago: American Hospital Publishing.

Wilken, D., Hallam, L., & Doggett, M. (1992). *Measures of need and outcomes from primary health care.* New York: Oxford University Press.

CHAPTER 29

Improving Quality in Public Health

Judy Crouch-Smolarek and Susan K. Kratz

CHAPTER OBJECTIVES

After completing this chapter, the reader will be able to

- identify numerous programs and activities intended to promote optimal health to individuals and communities by public health practitioners
- discuss in detail a quality improvement process designed to ensure the implementation and effectiveness of an immunization program

As in other states, Public Health in Wisconsin is modeled after National Public Health Standards and is an organized set of activities aimed at promoting optimal health for individuals; protecting communities, families, and individuals from communicable disease and potential environmental health hazards; and preventing or controlling chronic and acute illness.

The official public health department is the focal point for the delivery of public health services. Local public health agencies (LPHAs) work under the direction of and in partnership with the Wisconsin State Division of Health (SDOH), Bureau of Public Health, in implementing public health programs (Figures 29–1 and 29–2). There are also many other voluntary health and social service agencies whose work requires coordination with the local public health department. Such relationships enhance a public health delivery system. It is the re-

sponsibility of the local health department to ensure that all available health resources are being used effectively and efficiently for the purpose of maintaining or improving the public's health in the community as a whole.

To accomplish this purpose, certain basic public health services are provided by city and county health departments statewide:

1. *Communicable Disease Control:* to eliminate all vaccine-preventable communicable diseases and reduce the incidence of other communicable diseases.
2. *Environmental Health:* to protect the community by minimizing health risks from food and water consumption, sewage, and other human health hazards.
3. *Maternal and Child Health:* to ensure safe and satisfying birth and birth outcomes and to provide each child with a conducive environment for growth and development.
4. *Family Health:* to assist families to make health decisions, take actions, and adopt practices promoting health.
5. *Health Education:* to promote citizens' use of preventive health services, practices, and facilities appropriately and their understanding of and participation in decision making concerning their care.
6. *Chronic Disease Control:* to prevent or delay the onset and reduce the morbidity

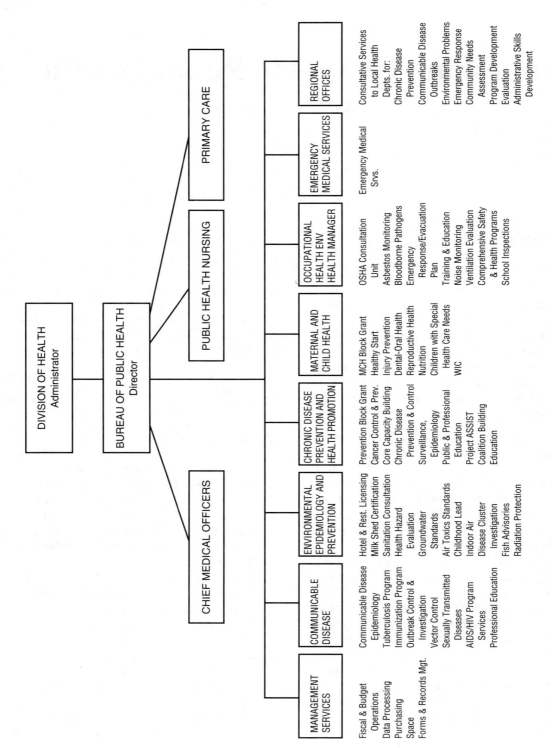

Figure 29–1 State division of health organizational structure. *Source:* Reprinted from the Wisconsin Department of Health and Family Services, Bureau of Public Health.

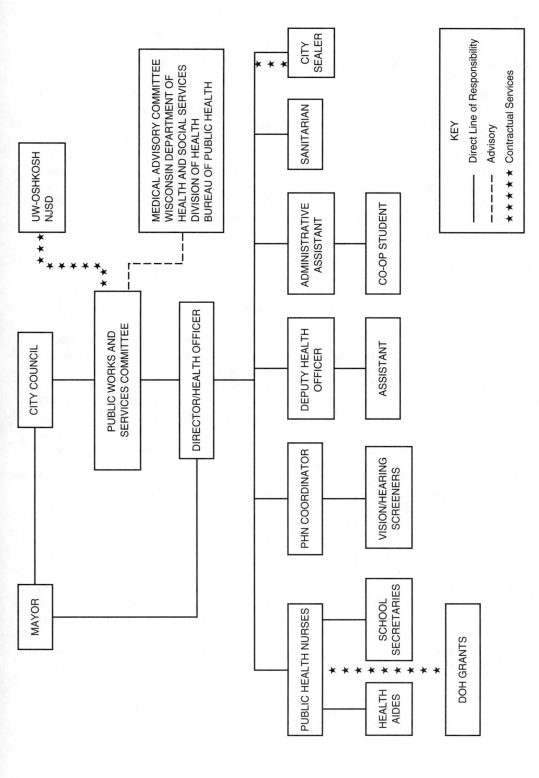

Figure 29–2 Neenah Department of Public Health organizational structure. *Source:* Reprinted from the City of Neenah Department of Public Health, 1996.

and mortality of chronic disease and disability.

7. *School Health:* to ensure that the school population is provided a healthful environment in which to work and study, together with needed preventive health services and health instruction.

8. *Elderly Health:* to promote and sustain a high level of health and well-being among the elderly.

9. *Home Health Services:* to provide personal and supportive care services to the sick and disabled, enabling them to continue living at home rather than in a health care institution.

Improving the quality of the Public Health delivery system takes many forms. An effective quality improvement program uses (1) goals and objectives, (2) written standards, (3) policies and procedures, (4) action plans, and (5) consultation and audit reports, which assist in evaluating the success of the program. While improving the quality of patient care is the intention of all providers of these numerous and varied programs, for purposes of this chapter, we have chosen to focus on one segment of public health programming, the Immunization Program, which is part of the Communicable Disease Section of the Bureau, to illustrate the ways that the SDOH and LPHAs work together to implement quality improvement measures.

The goals and objectives of the Immunization Program (Exhibit 29–1) were taken from *Healthier People in Wisconsin: A Public Health Agenda for the Year 2000* (Wisconsin Department of Health and Social Services, 1990, pp. 28–32) and are based on the national objectives *Healthy People 2000: National Health Promotion and Disease Prevention Objectives* (U.S. Public Health Service, 1990, pp. 511–514, 519, 521–524). The similarity between the state and national objectives allows us to use the state standard for purposes of this chapter. The objectives and implementation steps used for this project are not all-inclusive of the Communicable Disease Section's broader goal of preventing

vaccine-preventable diseases. Rather, they are specific to the parameters of the Immunization Action Plan (IAP) grant.

The Immunization Program provides guidelines for LPHA immunization clinics. The SDOH's policy and procedure manual (1996) and the recommendations of the Advisory Committee on Immunization Practices (Wisconsin Department of Health and Social Services, 1992) are required for use by LPHAs for full utilization of state vaccine and full implementation of immunization programs. The U.S. Public Health Service's *Standards for Pediatric Immunization Practices* (1993) are quality improvement guidelines that assist us in reaching our goals and can be used to evaluate our services (see Exhibit 29–2). These standards are recommended by the National Vaccine Advisory Committee and endorsed by the American Academy of Pediatrics, the American Nurses' Association, the Association of Maternal and Child Health Programs, and the National Association of Pediatric Nurse Associates and Practitioners.

Exhibits 29–3 and 29–4 are sample policy and procedure statements for LPHAs to ensure delivery of high-quality immunization programs to all clients; ensure safe, competent clinic practices; and ensure consistent utilization of state standards.

Our State IAP Work Plan (Exhibit 29–5) details required and recommended action steps that LPHAs should follow to enhance immunization efforts, with the goal of achieving a 90% immunization level in children 24 to 35 months of age by each antigen by the end of calendar year 1996 and a composite level of 90% by the year 2000. As the exhibit shows, the SDOH uses this work plan to monitor LPHAs' progress on the action steps to record anticipated completion dates.

Another tool that the SDOH uses to monitor LPHAs is the IAP Project Consultation Report (Exhibit 29–6), which tracks LPHA expenditures under the IAP grant, notes any budget variance, and makes recommendations on any budget revisions.

Exhibit 29–1 State of Wisconsin Immunization Program: Goal, Objectives, and Implementation Steps

Goal: To reduce the incidence of vaccine-preventable diseases by achieving an optimally immunized population.

Objective 1: By 2000, no indigenous cases of measles will occur.

Objective 3: By 2000, the annual reported incidence of meningitis caused by *Haemophilus influenzae* type b (Hib) among persons less than 3 years of age will be less than 27 cases per 100,000 population.

Objective 4: By 2000, the annual reported incidence of pertussis among persons less than 5 years of age will be less than 8 cases per 100,000 population.

Objective 5: By 2000, at least 90% of all children will have completed their primary vaccinations against measles, mumps, rubella, polio, diphtheria, pertussis, tetanus, and *Haemophilus influenzae* type b by their second birthday.

Measurement: Data collected from kindergarten immunization records during the 1987–88 school year showed only 56% of children had completed their primary vaccinations (excluding Hib vaccination) by their second birthday.

Commentary: The schedule for routine childhood immunization recommends completion of primary doses at 18 months of age. Targeting completion by 24 months of age allows for the unavoidable delays that occur due to illness, scheduling conflicts, finances, and other factors. Currently, the 90% completion level is not reached in Wisconsin until age 4 years. Furthermore, the completion percentage at age 2 is declining. Tardy immunization in the first 2 years of life is clearly due to failure to follow through with all recommended vaccination visits on time, rather than failure to start the schedule on time. Among 1987–88 kindergartners, 87% had their first vaccination, recommended at 2 months of age, before 4 months of age. However, only 37% had their fourth DTP, recommended at 18 months, before 20 months.

Objective 6: By 2000, 95% of children attending licensed day care centers and 98% of school children in kindergarten through grade 12 will have completed the doses of vaccines specified for their age or grade by administrative rule (HSS 144).

Objective 14: By 2000, at least 50% of persons in populations designated as targets by the ACIP will be immunized within 5 years of licensure of new vaccines recommended for widespread use.

Implementation Steps

A. In conjunction with private health care providers, day care centers, and schools, the State Division of Health (SDOH) should continue to conduct and disseminate the results of annual surveys of childhood immunization levels.

F. Health professional groups, local public health agencies (LPHAs), and SDOH should promote the use of immunization tracking and recall among private health care providers in conjunction with computerized billing systems. LPHAs should establish and/or maintain immunization tracking and recall systems.

S. Health professional groups and SDOH should regularly disseminate recommendations for vaccine use to health care providers through mailings and hospital inservice programs, and health professional groups should incorporate more immunization information in their continuing medical education activities.

T. LPHAs and private health care providers should regularly inform the public of recommendations for vaccine use. Special emphasis should be placed on educating parents of children receiving vaccinations recommended at 15 months of age to return at 18 months.

W. By 1992, SDOH, in cooperation with health professional groups, should develop and recommend methods for maintaining staff awareness of the need to evaluate patient immunization status during routine medical visits, and identifying and notifying patients who are candidates for immunization due to their health status, e.g., age or chronic illness.

Source: Reprinted from *Healthier People in Wisconsin: A Public Health Agenda for the Year 2000,* 1990, Wisconsin Department of Health and Family Services, Division of Health.

Exhibit 29–2 Standards for Pediatric Immunization Practices

Standard 1:	Immunization services are readily available.
Standard 2:	There are no barriers or unnecessary prerequisites to the receipt of vaccines.
Standard 3:	Immunization services are available free or for a minimal fee.
Standard 4:	Providers utilize all clinical encounters to screen and, when indicated, immunize children.
Standard 5:	Providers educate parents and guardians about immunization in general terms.
Standard 6:	Providers question parents or guardians about contraindications and, before immunizing a child, inform them in specific terms about the risks and benefits of the immunizations their child is to receive.
Standard 7:	Providers follow only true contraindications.
Standard 8:	Providers administer simultaneously all vaccine doses for which a child is eligible at the time of each visit.
Standard 9:	Providers use accurate and complete recording procedures.
Standard 10:	Providers co-schedule immunization appointments in conjunction with appointments for other child health services.
Standard 11:	Providers report adverse events following immunization promptly, accurately, and completely.
Standard 12:	Providers operate a tracking system.
Standard 13:	Providers adhere to appropriate procedures for vaccine management.
Standard 14:	Providers conduct semi-annual audits to assess immunization coverage levels and to review immunization records in the patient populations they serve.
Standard 15:	Providers maintain up to date, easily retrievable medical protocols at all locations where vaccines are administered.
Standard 16:	Providers operate with patient-oriented and community-based approaches.
Standard 17:	Vaccines are administered by properly trained individuals.
Standard 18:	Providers receive ongoing education and training on current immunization recommendations.

Source: Reprinted from the United States Department of Health and Human Services, Public Health Service, Centers for Disease Control and Prevention, 1993.

Still another tool is the Wisconsin Public Health Agency/Clinic Audit (1996) form (Exhibit 29–7), which facilitates on-site review of clinic flow, staffing levels, equipment, barriers to immunization, emergency procedures, data-processing systems for tracking and notification of noncompliant clients, and other LPHA procedures and characteristics.

LPHAs have varying ways to fulfill the goals of the work plan. Computerized tracking systems assist them in notifying parents of children who are behind schedule for their age at regular intervals. Personal phone contacts, home visits, and postcards are ways in which clients are notified of their need for return visits for timely immunization. Data-processing equipment assists LPHAs in collecting, maintaining, and analyzing immunization data for age-specific, population-based compliance levels within their communities. For high-risk populations—that is, low-income, single-parent, or culturally diverse families—special outreach measures are implemented, such as home visits and WIC (Women, Infants, and Children) clinic site education and immunization. These measures ensure that existing barriers, such as phone access, transportation, and time limitations, are kept to a minimum. The local health officer monitors the acute and communicable disease reports for data that reflect the incidence of vaccine-preventable diseases (i.e., measles, pertussis, polio, and diphtheria) in his or her jurisdiction. These data assist the health officer in further determining demographics relative to diseases reported, emerging community needs, and overall program effectiveness.

Exhibit 29–3 General Protocols (Policies and Procedures) for Public Health Clinics

1. An immunization program established by the local public health agency (LPHA) shall be supervised (sponsored) by a physician who shall sign immunization program orders (medical authorization) for the administration of vaccines. The orders per ss. 140.05 (16) (fm) shall be in accordance with the written protocols (policies and procedures) issued by the Department of Health and Social Services (DHSS), Division of Health, Bureau of Public Health, Immunization Program (IP). A copy of the protocols and orders shall be available at each vaccine delivery site.

2. The immunization program orders shall be supplemented as needed with the recommendations of the United States Public Health Service (USPHS) Immunization Practices Advisory Committee (ACIP). Please note that the vaccine manufacturers' package inserts are acceptable sources of information about vaccine storage, reconstitution, and administration; but they should not be used for determining contraindications or recommendations.

3. Clinics shall be conducted at times and places selected to ensure convenient access and ample opportunity for clients to stay on schedule.

4. Clinic staffing, in the absence of an on-site physician, shall consist of at least one registered professional nurse in charge of the clinic and at least one other adult acting as an aide to the nurse. All persons working in the clinic shall receive an orientation to immunization protocols, procedures, and emergency care.

5. Administration of vaccines in the absence of a physician shall be done in accordance with ss. 441 and 448, and shall be done only by the following persons who have demonstrated competence and have been specifically instructed in vaccines and their administration and in emergency procedures:

   5.1. A physician's assistant;

   5.2. A registered nurse;

   5.3. A licensed practical nurse and/or student nurse under the direct supervision of an RN;

   5.4. A jet-injector operator (non-licensed state of Wisconsin employee) specifically trained in this technique under the direct supervision of an RN or MD.

6. The emergency medical service (EMS) located in the clinic's geographical area shall be used as needed. The name and telephone number of the service must be in the possession of personnel staffing each clinic and clearly posted. An on-site telephone shall be readily available to the staff.

7. Clinic staff should be given the opportunity to wash their hands. If soap, running water, and disposable towels are not available, agencies can provide waterless soaps as an adequate substitute in the immunization setting.

8. Clinic staff shall review the health history of each individual to be vaccinated to ensure no contraindications listed in the most current "Vaccine Information Pamphlet(s)" or "Important Information" form(s) exist to the vaccine(s) being requested.

9. The client's private physician shall be consulted for each individual who has a condition that necessitates special caution due to the potential for an adverse event (e.g., stable neurologic condition or HIV infection). Care should be taken to ensure persons are not denied vaccines when no contraindications exist.

10. Individuals for whom a vaccine in contraindicated shall be referred to their private physician for appropriate immunization.

11. A vaccination requested by a private physician on referral, which is contraindicated per these protocols, shall not be administered; and the physician shall be informed accordingly.

continues

Exhibit 29–3 continued

12. The most current "Important Information" form(s) or "Vaccine Information Pamphlet(s)" shall be provided to each individual to be immunized or to the authorized person making the request for a minor. The signatures should be obtained at the same time the vaccine is to be administered. The information portion of the forms or pamphlets shall be made available to the client and the signed acknowledgment retained for at least 10 years.

13. A permanent medical record listing the name of the vaccine recipient along with the following information for each vaccination shall be maintained: type, manufacturer, and lot number of vaccine, date vaccine was administered, and name and title of person administering the vaccine. This record may be the signed portion of the "Vaccine Information Pamphlet" or "Important Information" form provided the above required information appears on the form.

14. For each vaccine administered, the individual shall be provided with a personal immunization record or have their existing record updated.

15. The agency shall maintain a record of each client's immunization history in a file system designed to alert the agency of children overdue for a vaccination and in need of follow-up.

16. A "Monthly Vaccine Report" (DOH 4451) shall be filed with the IP by the 5th of each month.

17. All adverse events that occur after a vaccination shall be reported to the IP on form DOH 9058 ("Vaccine Adverse Events Reporting System"-VAERS).

18. Home administration of vaccines consistent with LPHA policy may be done in selected instances.

19. All vaccines provided to LPHA gratis by the IP shall be administered without charge for the cost of the vaccine. Any agency charging an administration fee or requesting a donation must display in a prominent location the charging "NOTICE" that is available through the IP.

20. No child medically eligible for a vaccine may be denied vaccine at any vaccination site assisted by state or federal grant funds. If a child is denied publicly purchased vaccine for other than a valid medical reason, the DHSS would be in violation of the federal guidelines and vaccine could be withheld from not only the local agency but the state of Wisconsin as well.

21. LPHAs are requested to terminate any requirements that have been imposed upon children before they can receive vaccines (e.g., physician referral, physical examination before receiving vaccines, residency, income guidelines, and immunizations only by appointment).

Source: Reprinted from the Wisconsin Department of Health and Family Services, Bureau of Public Health.

Exhibit 29–4 Immunization Schedule for Use by Local Health Departments Based on USPHS and American Academy of Pediatrics (AAP) Recommendations

ROUTINE IMMUNIZATIONS STARTED DURING INFANCY (<15 MONTHS OF AGE)

Age[1]	*Immunizing Agents*	*Options*	
		One	*Two*
Birth (before Hospital discharge)		Hep B[3]	
2 months	DTP/Hib[2], OPV	Hep B	Hep B[3]
4 months	DTP/Hib, OPV		Hep B
6 months	DTP/Hib, OPV		
6–18 months		Hep B[4]	Hep B[4]
12–15 months	DTP/Hib[5] (DTaP, Hib)[6], MMR		
At school entrance (4 thru 6 yrs.)	DtaP[7], OPV[8], MMR[9]		
At 10-year intervals thereafter	Td		
Note: 7–11 months	If Hib conjugate vaccine has not been given earlier, a total of 3 doses are recommended; the first 2 doses should be given 2 months apart followed by a booster after 12 months of age, at least 2 months after the second dose.		
Note: 12–14 months	If Hib conjugate vaccine has not been given earlier, a total of 2 doses are recommended; the first dose should be given and repeated 2 months later.		
Note: 15–60 months	If Hib conjugate vaccine has not been given earlier, 1 dose should be given.		

IMMUNIZATIONS STARTED AGES 15 MONTHS THROUGH 6 YEARS

Timing	*Immunizing Agents*
First visit	DTP/Hib[2,10], OPV, MMR
2 months after first visit	DTP, OPV, Hep B
2 months after second visit	DTP, OPV, Hep B
6 to 12 months after third visit	DTaP, Hep B
At school entrance (4 thru 6 yrs.)	DTaP[7], OPV[8], MMR[9]
At 10-year intervals thereafter	Td

IMMUNIZATIONS STARTED AGES 7 YEARS AND OLDER

Timing	*Immunizing Agents*
First visit	Td, OPV[11], MMR[12,13], Hep B[14]
2 months after first visit	Td, OPV, MMR[9], Hep B
6–12 months after second visit	Td, OPV, Hep B
At 10-year intervals thereafter	Td

Note: Influenza and pneumococcal polysaccharide vaccines are recommended for persons ≥ 65 years.
[1]These recommended ages should not be construed as absolute, i.e., 2 months can be 6–10 weeks, etc.
[2]DTP/Hib = combined DTP + Hib. Separate doses of DTP and Hib conjugate vaccine administered at different sites can be substituted for DTP/Hib. Ideally, children who have started their series prior to 15 months of age with one conjugate vaccine should continue the primary series with vaccine produced by that same manufacturer. However, any combination of Hib conjugate vaccine licensed for use among infants may be used to complete the primary series.

continues

Exhibit 29–4 continued

[3]A. *Low Risk:* Infants whose mothers are HBsAg− should receive the first dose of Hepatitis B (Hep B) vaccine at birth (or 1–2 months of age), the second dose 1–2 months after the 1st dose, and the third at 6–18 months of age. Longer intervals between the last two doses result in higher final titers of anti-HBs.

B. *High Risk:* Infants whose mothers are HBsAg+ should receive the first dose of Hepatitis B (Hep B) within 12 hours of birth along with HBIG, the second dose 1 month later, and the third at 6 months of age.

C. *Risk Unknown:* Infants whose mothers' HBsAg test results are unknown should receive the first dose of Hep B vaccine within 12 hours of birth. If the mother is later found to be HBsAg+, the infant should receive HBIG ASAP (within 7 days of birth) and should follow the schedule described above in [3]B. If the mother is found to be HBsAg−, the infant should follow the schedule described above in [3]A.

[4]For low risk children, the Department recommends administering the Hep B#3 at the 12–15 month visit. If vaccine is to be deferred so as not to administer 3 injections (i.e., DTP/Hib, Hep B, and MMR) in one visit, the DTP/Hib can be rescheduled.

[5]At least 6 months must elapse between the administration of DTP#3 and DTP#4.

[6]A separate dose of DTaP and Hib administered at different sites should be substituted for the DTP/Hib combined vaccine if the child is 15 months of age or older.

[7]If DTP #4 (or DTaP) was administered after the 4th birthday, a 5th DTaP is not indicated.

[8]If OPV #3 was administered after the 4th birthday, a 4th OPV is not indicated.

[9]For the 1994–95 school year, children in all grades except 5th and 11th will be required to demonstrate having received 2 doses of MMR administered after the first birthday and separated by no less than 30 days. For the 95–96 school year and thereafter, all children in all grades will be required to demonstrate having received 2 doses of MMR after the first birthday.

[10]Hib is restricted for use in children less than 5 years of age.

[11]OPV is not routinely given to persons 18 years of age or older.

[12] Measles and rubella vaccines are indicated for persons born during or after 1957. When 2 doses of MMR are to be administered, they must be spaced less than 30 days apart.

[13]Rubella vaccine is particularly recommended for females through 45 years of age.

[14]Hepatitis B vaccine is recommended for adolescents and adults who are in selected high-risk groups (see ACIP recommendations). It is routinely available from the Division of Health through public clinics for all children who are 18 years of age or younger. In addition, it is available for any household or sexual contact of a HBsAg carrier.

Source: Reprinted from the Wisconsin Department of Health and Family Services, Bureau of Public Health.

Exhibit 29–5 Immunization Action Plan (IAP) Work Plan

IAP Grant Recipient (LHD):   Regional Office:

Immunization Program Representative: Date of Visit:

Action Steps	Ongoing or Anticipated Completion Date	Progress on Action Steps
I. Immunization Record Storage System:		
Required:		
____ Establish immunization record system capable of identifying clients who are actively seeking immunization services.		
____ Record storage system will identify children that are behind schedule for recommended immunizations.		
Recommended:		
____ Establish computerized immunization record storage system capable of meeting requirements listed above.		
Planned or Possible Enhancements:		
II. Tracking and Recall Activity		
Required:		
____ Establish system to recall clients who are more than two months behind for recommended immunizations.		
____ Notify parents of children identified as being behind schedule using either e-mail, phone, personal contact or a combination of these efforts.		
Recommended:		
____ Establish computerized system capable of meeting above requirements.		
Planned or Possible Enhancements:		

continues

Exhibit 29–5 continued

Action Steps	Ongoing or Anticipated Completion Date	Progress on Action Steps
III. Service Delivery Required:		
Annually assess clinic staffing patterns and timing of operations to ensure that services are conducive to clients' needs.		
Assess need for alternative clinic hours to meet the needs of working families.		
Consult, at least twice yearly, with WIC, Health Check, and other infant and child health services to ensure effective delivery of all immunization services to their clients.		
Determine and address the need for special outreach clinics for high-risk populations.		
Ensure adequate staff with recent training in aspects of vaccine delivery and the provisions of health services to diverse cultural populations.		
Assess and remove barriers to client's accessing immunization services, e.g., administration charges, missed opportunities, etc.		
Recommended:		
Work with private medical community to ensure that immunization services are available to all children in service area.		
Consider making vouchers or free passes for immunizations available to programs serving low-income families.		
Planned or Possible Enhancements:		
IV. Outreach and Education Requirements:		
Devise methods to provide assistance to clients experiencing difficulty in obtaining an up-to-date record of previous immunizations.		
Identify transportation needs of clients and establish or identify method(s) to ensure needed services are available.		
Develop and implement strategies for reaching the target population with immunization information and education that meets the diverse cultural needs of the population served.		

continues

_____ Devise methods to assist day care center providers in ensuring that children in their centers are up-to-date for all recommended immunizations.

_____ Contact the local medical community to establish their interest on exchanging client's immunization records.

Recommended:

_____ Develop a community coalition to identify and enlist the assistance of persons and/or organizations with a direct line to the target populations.

_____ Provide positive incentives to parents to complete immunizations on schedule.

_____ Identify community resources that can enhance immunization efforts.

_____ Identify methods to sustain enhanced programs in absence of grant sponsorship.

Planned or Possible Enhancements:

V. Coordination with WIC

Required:

_____ Establish and maintain regular contact between local WIC Project, LHD director(s) and State Regional Office Immunization Program and WIC Program Representatives to ensure access to immunization services for all WIC participants.

_____ Provide training as needed to WIC Project staff in regard to the recommended immunization schedule.

_____ Assist local WIC Project(s) in devising methods to bring WIC participants up-to-date with recommended immunizations.

Exhibit 29–5 continued

Action Steps	Ongoing or Anticipated Completion Date	Progress on Action Steps
Recommended: _____ Provide coupons to WIC participants (available from the Immunization Program) for free administration of immunizations at LHD. Planned or Possible Enhancements: _VI. Evaluation:_ Required: _____ Conduct annual assessments per instructions from the Immunization Program, of the immunization records of two-year-old children served by the agency to determine the completion of the primary immunization series (by August 1). Recommended: _____ Conduct annual retrospective immunization record assessment of kindergarten children in service area. _____ Conduct annual audit of two-year-old children's immunization records using public and private provider data.		

continues

Exhibit 29–5 continued

1996 Immunization Action Plan Budget

LHD Burnett County

Personnel Services	% of Time Budgeted	Hourly Rate/Hours Per Week	Number of Weeks Budgeted	Annual Costs
Total				
Agency Operations				
Total				
Consultant and Contractual Costs				
Total				
Supplies and Equipment				
Total				
Grand Total (1–4 Above)				

Source: Reprinted from the Wisconsin Department of Health and Family Services, Bureau of Public Health.

Exhibit 29–6 Immunization Action Plan (IAP) Project Consultation Report

Immunization Program Representative: Regional Office: 　SE　S　N　W　NE	Date of Visit: _____/_____/_____	Grant Review Period: From_____/_____/_____/ To_____/_____/_____/ [_] Midyear　[_] Final　[_] Other

Agency Information		
Agency Name:	Agency Address:	
Grant Contact Person(s):	Phone Number: (　　)_____	Grant Award Amount [__]　$16,089 [__]　Other_____

Fiscal Review

1.　Estimated Expenditures As of Review Date　$_____

2.　Estimated Percent of Total Grant　　　　_____%

3.　Noted Budget Variance　　　　　　[__] Yes [__] No

If yes, please detail

_____

_____

_____

4.　Budget Revision Requested　　　　　　[__] Yes [__] No

5.　Budget Revision Granted　　　　　　　[__] Yes [__] No

From Which Budget Area: [__] Salary/Fringe　　　　[__] Agency Ops
　　　　　　　　　　[__] Consultant Contractual [__] Supplies and Equipment

Budget Revision Detail/Budget Recommendations

_____

_____

_____

Source: Reprinted from the Wisconsin Department of Health and Family Services, Bureau of Public Health.

Exhibit 29–7 Wisconsin Public Health Agency/Clinic Audit Form

REVIEW DATE: _____

COUNTY:_____   AGENCY NAME:_____

ADDRESS: _____   TEL NO:_____

CITY:_____   REGION: _____   REVIEWER:_____

DIRECTOR: _____   HEALTH OFFICER: _____

Director of Nursing:_____

Medical Advisor(s): _____

CENSUS: _____   AGENCY SERVICE AREA: A=COUNTY   B=CITY   C=COUNTY & CITY
                       O = OTHER:

OF PHYSICIANS SEEING PEDIATRIC PATIENTS: _____   # IMMUNIZING: _____

AGENCY STAFF
      ACTUAL # of: NURSES:_____   AIDES: _____   CLERKS:_____   OTHER:_____
      FTE's: NURSES:_____   AIDES: _____   CLERKS:_____   OTHER:_____

DOES AGENCY REQUIRE STAFF TO BE PROTECTED AGAINST: METHOD OF PROOF:_____

	NURSE	AIDES	CLERKS	OTHER	TITER	SHOT	HX
MEASLES	Y/N	Y/N	Y/N	Y/N	Y/N	Y/N	Y/N
RUBELLA	Y/N	Y/N	Y/N	Y/N	Y/N	Y/N	Y/N
HEP B	Y/N	Y/N	Y/N	Y/N	Y/N	Y/N	Y/N

DOES AGENCY PROVIDE INFLUENZA VACCINE ANNUALLY: Y/N   # OF DOSES: _____
IF   YES,   TO   WHOM: STAFF: Y/N   CITIZENS: Y/N   COUNTY/CITY   EMPLOYEES: Y/N

DOES AGENCY PROVIDE PNEUMOCOCCAL VACCINE: Y/N   # OF DOSES: _____

AGENCY: HEALTH CK PROV SITE: Y/N   PRIVATE PROVIDERS: Y/N
           COMM HEALTH: Y/N   IMMUNIZATION ONLY: Y/N   WELLCHILD (MCH):   Y/N
           CONNECTED w/WIC: Y/N   OTHER:_____

SCHED APPOINT ONLY: Y/N   SCHED APPOINT AND WALK-INS: Y/N
OPEN CLINIC, NO APPOINT: Y/N   NO SCHED CLINIC, IMM ON REQUEST: Y/N

AUDIT SITE: PRIMARY IMMUNIZATION SITE: Y/N   VACCINE STORAGE SITE: Y/N
           SATELLITE SITE: Y/N   TOTAL SATELLITES: _____

COMPUTER IN USE: Y/N   Type: _____
Used for Immunization Tracking/Recall?   Y/N   Program? _____

CLINIC TIMES: DAILY: Y/N   WEEKLY: Y/N   BIWEEKLY: Y/N   MONTHLY: Y/N
OTHER TIMES: _____   TOTAL HOURS PER MONTH: _____

CHARGES?:   Y/N   PER DOSE: $ _____   PER VISIT: $ _____
DONATION?: Y/N   AMT HIGHEST FEE: $ _____   SLIDING FEE: $ _____
DISCLAIMER POSTED?:   Y/N   RANGE: $ _____

STATE POLICY AND PROCEDURES   MANUAL AVAILABLE?:   Y/N   CURRENT?:   Y/N
                                   EPINET AVAILABLE?:   Y/N   CURRENT?:   Y/N
                                   ACIP AVAILABLE?:   Y/N

Last date P & P was signed: _____

continues

Exhibit 29–7 continued

AGENCY NAME: _____   REVIEW DATE: _____

DOES THE AGENCY MAINTAIN AN ACTIVE RELATIONSHIP WITH HOSPITALS, NURSING HOMES, UNIVERSITIES, DAY CARE CENTERS, AND SCHOOLS FOR:

DISEASE REPORTING: Y/N   DISEASE FOLLOW-UP: Y/N   OUTBREAK CONTROL: Y/N

IMPORTANT INFORMATION FORMS (IIF):

SUPPLY OF IIFs: DTP: _____   MMR: _____   OPV: _____   HIB: _____   HB: _____

IS THE CURRENT IMP INFO FOR EACH ANTIGEN BEING USED: Y/N

ARE FORMS USED CORRECT FOR THE ANTIGEN GIVEN: Y/N

ARE FORMS COMPLETE, BOTH PERSONNEL AND CLINIC USE AREAS: Y/N

IS A NEW FORM USED FOR EACH DOSE: Y/N

IS ADVERSE EVENTS TELEPHONE NUMBER PROVIDED TO PARENT: Y/N

IS THERE A METHOD OF STORAGE?: Y/N CLINIC RECORD: Y/N

OTHER: Y/N   NAME: Y/N

IS STORAGE PERMANENT?: Y/N

DOES THE CLINIC USE LOCALLY GENERATED INFORMATIONAL CHECK SHEETS ALONG WITH THE IMP. INFOR. FORMS (IF SO PLEASE ATTACH A COPY): Y/N

VACCINE:

LOCATION OF VACCINE: IS ROOM SECURE: Y/N   LOCKED: Y/N

ARE NEEDLES IN A SECURED (LOCKED) LOCATION: Y/N

IS A COPY OF VAC STORAGE/HANDLING RECOMMENDATION POSTED ON DOOR: Y/N

IS THERE A WORKING TEMPERATURE CHART RECORDER IN REFRIGERATOR: Y/N

    IF NO, IS THERE A THERMOMETER IN REFRIGERATOR?: Y/N
    HOW OFTEN IS IT CHECKED: D = DAILY   W = WEEKLY   N= NOT AT ALL
    IS TEMP WITHIN LIMITS (35–46 F.): Y/N

DOES THE PERSON RESPONSIBLE SIGN AND DATE A CHECKLIST: Y/N

IS THERE AN ALARM SYSTEM: Y/N

IS VACCINE APPROPRIATELY STORED IN THE REFRIGERATOR: Y/N

IS ICE IN THE FREEZER WITH THE POLIO VACCINE: Y/N

DOES LIABILITY INSURANCE COVER VACCINE LOSS: Y/N

IS AN INVENTORY OF VACCINE KEPT BY AN EXPIRATION DATE: Y/N

IS SHORT-DATED VACCINE USED FIRST: Y/N

WILL ALL VACCINE BE USED PRIOR TO EXPIRATION DATE: Y/N

HOW ARE EXPIRED VACCINES DISPOSED OF: R = RETURNED TO DOH   D = DISPOSED LOCALLY

HOW OFTEN ARE THE FOLLOWING IN-SERVICED ON VACCINE HANDLING & STORAGE:

STAFF: E = NEW EMPLOYEE ONLY   F = FORMAL   I = INFORMAL   N = NOT DONE

MAINTENANCE PERSONNEL: E = NEW EMPLOYEE ONLY   F = FORMAL   I = INFORMAL

    N = NOT DONE

continues

Exhibit 29–7 continued

AGENCY NAME: _____   REVIEW DATE: _____

ARE THERE WRITTEN EMERGENCY PROCEDURES TO USE IN EVENT OF POWER FAILURES, INCLUDING MAINTENANCE STAFF & EMERGENCY PHONE NUMBERS?: Y/N

IS COLD CHAIN MAINTAINED FOR VACCINES TRANSPORTED TO AND USED IN SATELLITE CLINICS?: Y/N

ARE PREVIOUS DOSES ADMINISTERED BY ANOTHER HEALTH CARE PROVIDER NOTED BY DATE ON THE CHILD'S CHART: Y/N

HOW IS THE INFO VERIFIED: PARENT RECALL: Y/N   RECORD CARD: Y/N
                       CONTACT WITH PREVIOUS PROVIDER?: Y/N   OTHER?: Y/N

HOW MANY ANTIGENS WILL BE GIVEN PER VISIT: (#) _____

ARE EMERGENCY PROCEDURES WRITTEN, SIGNED, AND POSTED IN THE CLINIC: Y/N

DOES THE CLINIC HAVE A RECALL PROGRAM: Y/N

    IF YES, IS IT USED AS A REMINDER FOR ALL CLIENTS: Y/N

    FOR MISSED APPOINTMENTS: Y/N OR, FOR CHILDREN NOT UP-TO-DATE: Y/N

    METHOD: MAIL: Y/N   PHONE: Y/N   OTHER: _____

    ARE RETURN CARDS PROVIDED: Y/N

ARE PERSONAL IMMUNIZATION RECORD CARDS GIVEN EACH CLIENT: Y/N

DOES THE AGENCY USE THE WISCONSIN STANDARD CARD: Y/N OR THEIR OWN: Y/N

DOES THE AGENCY TELL PARENTS TO REPORT AN ADVERSE EVENT: Y/N

ARE ALL FEMALES ELIGIBLE FOR MMR: Y/N

ARE FEMALES ADVISED ABOUT WARNINGS OF NOT BECOMING PREGNANT FOR 3 MONTHS POST IMMUNIZATION: Y/N

ARE CHILDREN OF PREGNANT FEMALES GIVEN MMR: Y/N

ARE WIC AND AGENCY COOPERATING ON A PROGRAM TO IMMUNIZE WIC CLIENTS: Y/N

    IMMUNIZATION OFFERED ON-SITE: Y/N   OFF-SITE: Y/N

    EDUCATION ONLY: Y/N   REFERRAL MADE: Y/N

DOES THE CLINIC SEPARATE INACTIVE FILES FROM ACTIVE FILES: Y/N

DOES THE STAFF CONDUCT ASSESSMENTS OF IMMUNIZATION RECORDS OF CHILDREN 15–24 MONTHS OF AGE?

                # OF CHILDREN CHECKED (AT LEAST 25): _____

                # UP-TO-DATE: _____   PERCENTAGE: _____

continues

Exhibit 29–7 continued

AGENCY NAME: _____   REVIEW DATE: _____

CLINIC OPERATION OBSERVATIONS:

IS CLINIC IN OPERATION?: Y/N (IF NO, CURSOR JUMPS TO END OF FORM)

IF YES, ANSWER THE FOLLOWING BASED ON OBSERVATION:

Clinic Site Observed: _____   Date: _____

ARE VACCINES ADMINISTERED BY APPROPRIATE ROUTES: Y/N

WHAT LENGTH OF NEEDLE IS USED FOR: (Choose one response 5/8″, 1″, 1 & 1/2″)

   DTP: _____   MMR: _____   HIB: _____   HB: _____   Influenza: _____

ARE CLIENTS OFFERED MULTIPLE ANTIGENS: Y/N   MAX. NUMBER/VISIT: _____

IS MMR VACCINE PROTECTED FROM LIGHT?: Y/N

KEPT IN COLD ENVIRONMENT PRIOR TO ADMINISTRATION?: Y/N

MIXED AHEAD OF TIME?: Y/N

IS THAWED POLIO VACCINE MARKED AS TO LENGTH OF TIME THAWED AND NUMBER OF THAWS?: Y/N

DO CLIENTS HAVE OPPORTUNITY TO ASK QUESTIONS: Y/N

DO CLIENTS HAVE AMPLE TIME TO READ THE IMPORTANT INFO FORMS: Y/N

ARE CLIENTS REQUESTED TO REPORT ADVERSE EVENTS: Y/N

ARE CLIENTS QUERIED AS TO THE POSSIBLE CONTRAINDICATIONS: Y/N

IS THE CLINIC FLOW APPROPRIATE: Y/N

WERE IMPROVEMENTS DISCUSSED WITH THE CLINIC DIRECTOR: Y/N

WERE CLIENTS GIVEN A RECORD OF THEIR IMMUNIZATIONS AND A RETURN APPOINTMENT?: Y/N

LIST OF IMMUNIZATION BARRIERS TO LOOK FOR:

PHYSICAL EXAM REQUIRED: Y/N

ONLY BY APPOINTMENT (IDEAL APPT WITH OPEN CLINIC): Y/N

TEMPERATURE REQUIRED TO BE TAKEN: Y/N

WRITTEN PHYSICIAN ORDER REQUIRED FOR EACH CHILD: Y/N

REFERRAL REQUIRED FROM PRIMARY CARE PROVIDER: Y/N

ENROLLMENT IN WELL-BABY: Y/N

continues

Exhibit 29–7 continued

AGENCY NAME: _____   REVIEW DATE: _____

ROUTINE EXCESSIVE WAIT (i.e., MORE THAN 30 MINUTES): Y/N

REFUSE SIMULTANEOUS ADMINISTRATION OF VACCINES: Y/N

FAILURE TO SCREEN FOR IMMUNIZATION WHEN OTHER SERVICES PROVIDED: Y/N

APPOINTMENTS NOT COORDINATED WITH OTHER SERVICES: Y/N

INVALID CONTRAINDICATIONS: Y/N

INADEQUATE LOCATION—PARKING, BUS: Y/N

INADEQUATE HOURS OF OPERATION: Y/N

INADEQUATE STAFFING: Y/N

LITTLE OR NO TRACKING OF CLIENTS: Y/N

CLINIC EXPERIENCE NOT CONDUCIVE TO CLIENT'S RETURN: Y/N

RESIDENCE REQUIREMENT: Y/N

REMARKS: _____

WAS A COPY OF THIS REPORT LEFT WITH THE DIRECTOR?: Y/N

END OF FORMS

Source: Reprinted from the Wisconsin Department of Health and Family Services, Bureau of Public Health.

Clearly, the mechanisms are in place for implementation and close monitoring of immunization programs in LPHAs in the state of Wisconsin. We believe the features highlighted in this chapter demonstrate the many ways in which quality improvement measures are integrated throughout the local and state immunization record. Certainly, plans for the future include continuing this ongoing surveillance, improving and strengthening our networks in the public and private sectors, building our databases to reflect immunization levels of all populations, identifying and removing any and all barriers to immunization, and, finally, increasing our compliance levels to reflect state and national goals. It is our hope that by the year 2000, this can and will be done.

REFERENCES

U.S. Public Health Service. (1990). *Healthy people 2000: National health promotion and disease prevention objectives.* (DHHS 91-50213). Washington, DC: U.S. Government Printing Office.

U.S. Public Health Service. (1993). *Standards for pediatric immunization practices.* Washington, DC: U.S. Government Printing Office.

Wisconsin Department of Health and Social Services, Division of Health. (1990). *Healthier people in Wisconsin: A public health agenda for the year 2000.*

Wisconsin Department of Health and Social Services, Division of Health. (1992). *Recommendations of the Immunization Practices Advisory Committee (ACIP).*

Wisconsin Department of Health and Social Services, Division of Health. (1996). *Immunization protocols, policies & procedures for immunization programs.*

## CHAPTER 30

Improving Quality in Rehabilitation

Adrianne E. Avillion

CHAPTER OBJECTIVES

After completing this chapter, the reader will be able to

- describe the three major factors influencing quality improvement in rehabilitation
- discuss the essential components of a quality improvement program
- identify clinical indicators dependent on interdisciplinary collaboration to promote a seamless delivery system of patient care

Rehabilitation is the process of helping persons to achieve or regain their maximum state of wellness. Successful rehabilitation depends upon health care professionals' knowledge of the environments from which patients come and of the environments to which patients must return. Of equal importance is the ability to assist patients to make necessary adaptations as they re-enter communities primarily designed for able-bodied people.

Improving quality in rehabilitation is influenced by three major factors (Avillion & Mirgon, 1989). The first is the length of stay. The average acute care patient spends about 5 days in the hospital. A rehabilitation patient may spend from several weeks (e.g., for an orthopaedic injury) to over a month (e.g., for a spinal cord or traumatic brain injury). Although not currently governed by diagnosis-related groups (DRGs), rehabilitation specialists are actively engaged in measuring lengths

of stay according to various functional independence scales and researching rehabilitation outcomes based on such objective measurements. These activities are the precursors of proposed DRGs for rehabilitation. Appropriate rehabilitation quality improvement actions emphasize evaluating the effectiveness of various rehabilitation programs (e.g., stroke or spinal cord injury) implemented within specific lengths of stay.

The second factor is the continual interaction among interdisciplinary health care professionals as they work with the patient to provide care and achieve wellness. Rehabilitation quality improvement measures impact health care from the perspective that rehabilitation specialists work as a team to ensure desired patient outcomes. Rehabilitation quality improvement is team driven as opposed to discipline driven.

Finally, the need for patient/family involvement in the plan of care cannot be overemphasized. Indeed, the patient is the most critical member of the rehabilitation team. The rehabilitation patient has usually experienced an injury or illness that may necessitate permanent lifestyle changes. Without well-documented monitoring of patient/family education, desired rehabilitation outcomes cannot be achieved.

The current health care environment demands a "seamless" provision of care, including not only acute and rehabilitation services but home health and preventive measures as well. To provide this spectrum of care, hospitals are merging, and health care corporations are forming to include inpatient, outpatient, preventive, and home health operations. Rehabilitation specialists cannot afford to isolate themselves from other aspects of care. They must be aware of what happened to the patient prior to the need for rehabilitation interventions and what will happen after discharge. Rehabilitation quality concerns must now reflect a knowledge of the entire range of health care services and cannot be limited in scope to a particular specialty or service. The design of rehabilitation quality improvement plans must incorporate the concerns of a "seamless" health care environment. In part, these concerns are generated from the process of customer identification and meeting the needs of these customers.

CUSTOMER SERVICE IN REHABILITATION: AN EVOLVING ISSUE

There has been a huge amount of time devoted to customer identification recently in the health care arena. Physicians, patients, families, third-party payers, equipment vendors, and staff, to name a few, have all been heralded as customers. Entire workshops and seminars have been devoted to both customer identification and how to "treat" these customers so that they utilize a particular health care entity. However, organizations are destined to self-destruct unless they provide quality health care that produces *measurably significant* patient outcomes. Customers demand and expect quality care. Stating that one offers quality care is viewed as redundant by most health care consumers. What needs to be stated is the proven track record of services offered. This can best be done by an effective quality improvement program.

In rehabilitation, customer service is an evolving issue. Until recently, rehabilitation specialists often worked in organizations devoted primarily to the practice of physical rehabilitation. These specialists interacted with community and acute health care workers as colleagues but were not usually part of the same parent organization. However, as a result of the trend toward mergers and seamless health care, rehabilitation specialists must now plan, implement, and evaluate their clinical programs as part of a multicare delivery system. The rehabilitation component of care may be provided from within a corporation that provides all levels of care from preventative through and including community health.

Rehabilitation customer expectations include all of these levels of care. These expectations change as rapidly as health care technology changes, making the health care providers' lives challenging, to say the least. A climate of constant change is now the norm, not the exception. This means that to meet customer expectations of quality care, rehabilitation specialists must consult their customers regularly and often (Leebov & Ersoz, 1991).

One of the best measures of customer satisfaction and of the effectiveness of an organization's rehabilitation programs is a sound quality improvement program. Although the Joint Commission on Accreditation of Healthcare Organizations (Joint Commission, 1996) no longer mandates specifics of written quality improvement plans or the structures within which quality improvement is implemented, an organized written plan is still an essential component of any quality improvement program. This plan must clearly delineate accountability and what actions are taken to continually improve care and correct any deficiencies.

Exhibit 30–1 describes a sample rehabilitation quality improvement plan. Such plans should now incorporate the concept that rehabilitation specialists must include facets of preventive, acute, and home health care as part of their program delivery. The sample plan depicted in Exhibit 30–1 is written from the perspective of a rehabilitation facility that is part of a network offering the entire spectrum of health care services.

Exhibit 30–1 Sample Quality Improvement Plan

Purpose: To monitor, evaluate, and improve the quality and appropriateness of patient care and rehabilitation services from within a network that provides a seamless network of health care from preventative measures through and including community health.

Objectives:

1. to involve all personnel, via a systematic, ongoing process, in the timely identification and resolution of actual/potential problems that influence patient care, rehabilitation services, and successful community reintegration.
2. to establish indicators for the analysis of patient care services and program effectiveness.
3. to identify strengths and areas for improvement in patient care, rehabilitation practice, and collaboration among the practitioners from the various levels of health care services.
4. to recommend corrective action for problem resolution and for the improvement of program effectiveness.
5. to analyze the effectiveness of corrective action.

Responsibility

The Board of Directors of the _____ Rehabilitation Hospital, in conjunction with the Board of Directors of _____ Healthcare Corporation, retains overall responsibility and authority for the quality and appropriateness of patient care delivery. The board has delegated the responsibility for implementing the hospital quality improvement plan to the chief executive officer in conjunction with the Medical Executive Committee.

The chief executive officer, in conjunction with the Medical Executive Committee, delegates the responsibility for the development, implementation, and evaluation of quality improvement to the director of quality management services. The director of quality management services has the authority to organize and establish a committee to analyze trends, assist with the evaluation of quality improvement services, make recommendations for improvement, and to act as a liaison among the various _____ Healthcare Corporation facilities to enhance the quality of services for all levels of corporate care. The committee receives and reviews quarterly reports from all departments/services of _____ Rehabilitation Hospital to facilitate the coordination of the quality improvement process.

Scope of Services

_____ Rehabilitation Hospital's quality improvement activities may be categorized according to the hospital's rehabilitation specialty programs: spinal cord injury, stroke, traumatic brain injury, and outpatient services. Each clinical program director (physician) and each program specialty manager is responsible for the development, implementation, and evaluation of quality improvement activities in his or her area. The plan is based on interdisciplinary evaluations of patient care as well as indicators that require peer review.

Important Aspects of Care

Identification of important aspects of care is based on a comparison of actual rehabilitation practice to the standards of rehabilitation practice as established by _____ Rehabilitation Hospital and _____ Healthcare Corporation. These standards are based on external standards of government, accrediting, and professional organizations, including but not limited to Joint Commission standards, Commission on Accreditation of Rehabilitation Facilities (CARF) standards, licensure requirements, and health department requirements.

continues

Exhibit 30–1 continued

The quality improvement plan is a systematic, ongoing process that involves
1. the review of results and recommendations of all quality improvement activities
2. the assessment of problem identification, action taken, and evaluation of all quality improvement interventions
3. organized review and approval of all departmental and clinical program quality improvement plans
4. the review of _____ Rehabilitation Hospital's interface with other corporate entities to provide a seamless provision of health care

Identification of Indicators and Threshold Establishment

Utilizing appropriate standards, indicators are established with thresholds set at the ideal level. Indicators will measure the achievement of program objectives, be reviewed and revised as necessary, and correlate with corporate goals and objectives.

Data Collection

Sources of data collection and problem identification include but are not limited to
- reviews of functional measurement scale outcomes
- adverse occurrence reports
- program outcomes
- corporate clinical outcomes
- accreditation surveys
- infection control reports
- patient satisfaction surveys
- evaluations from education programs
- program evaluation results
- employee performance evaluations
- medical records

Evaluation and Actions To Improve Care

Results of monitoring are analyzed and evaluated, and actions to resolve problems and improve program outcomes are taken. Actions are clearly identified and include time frames for completion, accountability for implementation, authority to carry out actions, and a system for evaluation of the effectiveness of actions taken.

Communication

The findings of all quality improvement activities are discussed at the Quality Improvement Committee, which consists of representatives from all hospital departments, programs, and services. Results are channeled to the board of directors of both the _____ Rehabilitation Hospital and the _____ Healthcare Corporation via the chief executive officer and the medical executive committee.

_____
Chief Executive Officer   Date

_____
Director, Quality Management Services

EXAMPLES OF CLINICAL INDICATORS

The interdisciplinary focus of clinical indicators is assumed. However, contemporary rehabilitation specialists must expand their definition of interdisciplinary collaboration to include their corporate colleagues in preventive, acute, and community health care. Thus indicators must be written from this expanded perspective.

Examples of clinical indicators for a spinal injury program might include the following items

- Percentage of spinal-cord-injured patients who return home independent in activities of daily living within 6 weeks of admission. Successful outcomes depend not only on inpatient care but on how well the outpatient and community health staff are involved in the team planning process. It does little good to achieve independence in the inpatient setting if function is significantly lost post discharge.
- Percentage of patients who maintain skin integrity post discharge from rehabilitation. This indicator would be monitored by staff from inpatient, outpatient, and community corporate components. A breakdown in skin integrity might have a number of possible causes, including problems with the patient education provided in the inpatient setting, lack of outpatient follow-up, and/or problems in the community setting. Appropriate monitoring and evaluative actions necessitate the collaboration of team members from various settings, not just rehabilitation.
- Percentage of patients who maintain bladder integrity and stay free of urinary tract problems during hospitalization and post discharge. Again, community health and outpatient staff must be active team members to promote a seamless provision of care.

The results from these and other clinical indicators must be analyzed and an effective action plan formulated for improvement.

EVALUATION ACTIONS

To be successful, an evaluation plan must clearly identify actions to be taken for problem resolution, a time frame for implementation, and the persons responsible for plan implementation. Additionally, the evaluation plan must determine how team members from the various levels of care will work together for an improvement in patient outcomes.

For example, a decrease in a stroke patient's ability to be mobile post discharge requires investigation of a number of factors. Is patient education in any of the settings an issue? Have there been changes in the patient's home or community setting, or were certain facets of these environments overlooked when planning for community reintegration? How can this patient be helped to regain lost function? What measures can be taken to decrease the chances of such problems occurring with other stroke patients? What format has been developed to establish a care planning process that involves team members from all levels of care?

It is not necessary (although it is ideal) to have all team members at the same location to hold an effective team meeting. Conference calls and computer technology offer just two of many ways to communicate. To survive, rehabilitation specialists must learn to be creative and proactive when expanding their concepts of "team." Also, the team members must avoid "we-they" phenomena such as attempting to blame staff from other care delivery levels for an inadequate patient outcome.

Evaluation strategies should also include expanding the definition of rehabilitation to include prevention. Preventive programs should be planned and indicators developed that measure a decrease in the number of spinal cord injuries in a given geographic area or a decrease in the severity or incidence of cardiovascular disease. Such programs may decrease the inpatient revenue but could effectively increase the revenue from patient education programs in the community and home health arena.

Data illustrating that a health care corporation has decreased the cost of illness and injury are more likely to justify third-party reimbursement for patient education, including both preventive strategies and postdischarge follow-up. Data showing such innovative success strategies (especially those showing innovative ways of expanding team collaboration) may also be the foundation for grants, publications, and public speaking events. Those rehabilitation specialists who survive and thrive in the current turbulent health care arena will be those who develop clinical programs that improve patient outcomes while helping to decrease hospitalization costs. Quality management strategies must be implemented that help to achieve both of these items.

It is all very well to discuss issues that must be approved and probably mandated at an administrative or even a corporate level. But how can the staff who must develop and implement these innovative programs be persuaded that this is the way not only to facilitate quality patient care but to enhance their job security as well? A health care system that delivers seamless care with proven patient outcomes is more likely to survive as an employer well into the next century. Staff deserve and need education to be part of this expanded rehabilitation team.

STAFF EDUCATION

According to Leebov and Scott (1994), patient satisfaction is a function of service quality even more than clinical quality. An organization must acknowledge the customers' definition of quality and strive to achieve such quality on the customers' terms. Most staff have, by now, received some type of training on quality improvement and rehabilitation. It is essential that staff, as part of their continuing education, be taught about these evolving issues in quality management.

The changing scope of rehabilitation practice and the expanded definition of the rehabilitation team must be part of any quality improvement training. All levels of staff need to be able to apply quality improvement to the "new" rehabilitation practice arena. Unless adequate training takes place, the organization's quality service efforts stand a good chance of failing.

It is important to note that the classroom setting alone is an inadequate means of education. Staff will view such training efforts as purely theoretical and as having no application to the "real" world, the world of patient care. Staff must be shown how to apply their training for the achievement of desired patient outcomes.

It is up to management to set the stage for effective quality improvement efforts. This means that administration and management must also receive training. Education is not for isolated groups of staff but for all employees whose work will be measured by the effectiveness of its quality outcomes.

CONCLUSION

Rehabilitation quality improvement activities must be implemented within a network of seamless health care services, from preventive care through successful community reintegration. The definition of the rehabilitation team must now include practitioners representing all levels of care.

Quality improvement strategies must be designed to measure the effectiveness of a team effort in all settings. Education regarding the "new" rehabilitation quality improvement must be provided for all levels of staff. Such knowledge must then be applied to improve patient services so that measurable gains can be documented.

REFERENCES

Avillion, A.E., & Mirgon, B.B. (1989). *Quality assurance in rehabilitation nursing: A practical guide*. Gaithersburg, MD: Aspen.

Joint Commission on Accreditation of Healthcare Organizations. (1996). *Accreditation manual for hospitals*. Oakbrook Terrace, IL: Author.

Leebov, W.L., & Ersoz, C.J. (1991). *The health care manager's guide to continuous quality improvement*. Chicago: American Hospital Association.

Leebov, W.L., & Scott, G. (1994). *Service quality improvement: The customer satisfaction strategy for health care*. Chicago: American Hospital Association.

CHAPTER 31

Improving Quality in Subacute Care

Kathleen M. Griffin and Debra J. Gillett

After completing this chapter, the reader will be able to

- define characteristics of the subacute level of care
- describe the various requirements of state and federal governments as well as voluntary accrediting agencies for demonstrating continuous quality improvement in subacute care
- identify numerous structural elements necessary to improve quality in subacute care facilities
- distinguish process and outcome criteria for improving quality of patient care
- design a patient satisfaction survey for a patient receiving subacute care

Subacute care is a level of care between the acute hospital and the skilled nursing facility levels of care. Subacute care has emerged as an important and growing industry because it serves as a cost-effective alternative to acute hospital care for many patients. Although the vast majority of patients in a subacute care unit are elderly, new medical technologies have increased survival rates of infants born with severe anomalies and have sustained life for patients of all ages with disease and trauma. As a result, pediatric through geriatric patients with a variety of diseases and disorders are served in subacute care units.

DEFINITIONS

Two definitions are commonly accepted throughout the industry. The National Subacute Care Association (NSCA, 1994) defines *subacute care* as follows:

> Subacute care is a comprehensive and cost-effective inpatient program for patients who have had an acute event as a result of an illness, injury, or exacerbation of a disease process; have a determined course of treatment; and do not require intensive diagnostic and/or invasive procedures. The severity of the patient's condition requires physician direction; intensive nursing care and significant utilization of ancillaries; and, an outcomes-focused interdisciplinary approach utilizing a professional team to deliver complex clinical interventions (medical and/or rehabilitation). Typically short-term, the subacute level of care is utilized as an inpatient alternative to an acute care hospital admission or as an alternative to continued hospitalization.

The NSCA discusses subacute care in terms of the following characteristics:

- *Comprehensiveness*—Subacute care programs are designed to provide the full range of necessary medical, rehabilitation, and professional services required to provide efficient and effective care for the specific medical conditions treated within a program.

- *Cost-effectiveness*—Subacute programs are designed to maximize value to patients and payer sources through the delivery of necessary, appropriate care with optimal outcomes in the lowest cost setting.
- *Outcome orientation*—Subacute programs are designed to achieve quantifiable, measurable outcomes such as, but not necessarily limited to, functional restoration, clinical stabilization, avoidance of medical complications or exacerbation of a disease process, and discharge to the patient's least restrictive living environment.
- *Professional staffing*—Subacute interventions, because of their duration, complexity, and intensity, are provided under the direction of a physician. An interdisciplinary team provides a coordinated program of care. The team may include physicians, nurses, therapists, social workers, psychologists, pharmacists, dietitians, case managers, discharge planners, and other professionals.
- *Program description*—Programs are organized around patient populations with related treatment or service needs that result in common goals, measures of outcomes, treatment plans, and resources delivered at similar levels of intensity. Subacute programs may include medical rehabilitation and respiratory, nutritional, cardiac, oncological, and wound care programs. Levels of intensity for specific disciplines will vary from program to program but will generally range from 3.5 to 8 nursing hours per patient day, up to 5 hours per patient day for therapy, as well as appropriate use of nutritional, laboratory, pharmacy, radiology, and other ancillary services.
- *Site of care*—The site of care is not a distinguishing characteristic of subacute care. Subacute programs can be delivered in a variety of settings, including acute

hospitals, specialty hospitals, free-standing skilled nursing facilities, hospital-based skilled nursing units, outpatient ambulatory centers, residential living facilities, and home health settings. Most existing subacute programs are inpatient programs serving as an alternative to prolonged acute hospitalization. However, given the existence of a broad range of treatment and cost alternatives to acute hospitalization, site of care should not be a limiting factor in the delivery of subacute services. Distinctions among subacute services should be focused on program differences, not settings.

- *Continuum of care*—Subacute care is essential to the development of a complete continuum of care. Subacute programs are necessary components of vertically integrated health care systems.

The definition prepared by the Joint Commission on Accreditation of Healthcare Organizations (Joint Commission, 1994) has many of the same elements as the NSCA definition:

> Subacute care is comprehensive inpatient care designed for someone who has an acute illness, injury, or exacerbation of a disease process. It is goal-oriented treatment rendered immediately after, or instead of, acute hospitalization to treat one or more specific active complex medical conditions or to administer one or more technically complex treatments, in the context of a person's underlying long-term conditions and overall situation.

> Generally, the individual's condition is such that the care does not depend heavily on high-tech monitoring or complex diagnostic procedures. Subacute care requires the coordinated services of an interdisciplinary team including physicians, nurses, and other relevant professional disci-

plines, who are trained and knowledgeable to assess and manage these specific conditions and perform the necessary procedures. Subacute care is given as part of a specifically defined program, regardless of the site.

Subacute care is generally more intensive than traditional nursing facility care and less than acute care. It requires frequent (daily to weekly) recurrent patient assessment and review of the clinical course and treatment plan for a limited (several days to several months) time period, until the condition is stabilized or a predetermined treatment course is completed.

SUBACUTE PATIENTS: TYPES AND ACUITY LEVELS

Subacute patients have a range of acuity levels and exhibit a wide variety of diseases and disorders. Typically, subacute care units attempt to group patients with similar needs by program. Examples of subacute patient types and programs are

- Medically complex/postsurgical patients may require the following types of care:
  1. active treatment of disease under direction of physician (administering IV medications, epidural medications, continuous infusion pumps, hyperdermiclysis; monitoring/evaluating signs and symptoms of condition change; teaching care to patient and/or significant others; providing respiratory therapy and care; performing hemodialysis and peritoneal dialysis, evaluating effective intervention through laboratory values and signs and symptoms)
  2. postsurgical care (managing and evaluating drains and tubes; complex dressing changes; evaluating and assessing changes in wounds)
  3. nutrition management (enteral and parenteral feedings; monitoring the effect of intervention and therapeutic diets through weight, tissue turgor, wound healing, and laboratory values)
- Wound management patients may require complex treatment and dressing procedures; whirlpool treatment and debridement; electrical stimulation specialty beds and pressure-reducing devices; frequent laboratory evaluation; teaching of care to the patient and/or significant others; and ongoing assessment of the effective treatment by changes in wound status.
- Cardiopulmonary patients may have been hospitalized because of congestive heart failure or suspected myocardial infarction. These patients typically are deconditioned as both cause and effect of acute treatment, possibly exacerbated by their stay in the intensive care unit (ICU) or their course of treatment, resulting in malnourishment, weakness, frailty, and poor physical stamina. Patients also may have complicating comorbidities requiring that the subacute services be provided in an environment that allows immediate access to the high-technology equipment and services of the acute hospital.
- Respiratory patients for subacute care often have respiratory infections, pneumonias, or chronic obstructive pulmonary disease (COPD) with medical complications. Respiratory care patients may be ventilator dependent and admitted to the subacute unit for ventilator weaning.
- Oncology patients admitted to a subacute unit typically require care for the following types of symptom management:
  1. pain management (infusing and titrating analgesia; evaluating pain and effect of analgesia; managing side effects of analgesia)
  2. nutrition management (counteracting nausea/vomiting/dehydration through IV hydration, antiemetic administration, and enteral feedings/total par-

enteral nutrition; evaluating nutrition and interventions' effectiveness)

3. management of mucositis (monitoring and treating pain; administering analgesia, antibiotics, and antacids; managing nutrition)

4. management of neutropenia (infusing IV antibiotics; administering GCSF/ neurogen; providing a protective environment; managing fever symptoms; neutropenic diet; services for deconditioned states; restorative nursing services; therapy services)

Intensive monitoring of the disease process and/or the response to treatment may be required through laboratory evaluation and medication adjustment. Finally, active treatment may be required for these patients, including the administration of chemotherapeutic agents via continuous infusion pumps, epidural infusions, and administration of blood products and IV gamma globulin.

SUBACUTE CARE CATEGORIES

Four categories of subacute care as shown in Exhibit 31–1 have been recognized. Typically, subacute units in hospitals and specialty hospitals providing subacute care focus on transitional subacute care, whereas free-standing nursing facilities tend to provide general subacute and chronic subacute care. These categories of subacute care can be operationally defined in terms of acuity of nursing care and length of stay.

Transitional subacute care can be described as short stay (5 to 30 days) with nursing levels at 5.5 to 8 hours per patient day. Transitional subacute facilities and units are utilized by payers, providers, and physicians for patients who require regular medical care and monitoring; highly skilled and intensive nursing care; an integrated program of therapies, both rehabilitative and respiratory; and extensive utilization of pharmaceutical and laboratory services. This type of subacute care unit or facility serves as a hospital step-down entity and results in a significant reduction of acute hospital days. Transitional subacute facilities and units have a variety of physician program directors or consultants, a dedicated staff of acute or critical care nurses, 24-hour respiratory therapy, and 7-day-per-week rehabilitation therapies.

Clinically, patients in transitional subacute units may require cardiac management following heart attacks or cardiac surgical procedures; pulmonary management and ventilator weaning programs; wound management for burns or multiple Stage III and IV decubiti or following vascular or other surgeries; oncology recovery, including chemotherapy and radiation therapy; rehabilitation for cerebrovascular accidents (CVAs) or for complications following orthopaedic surgery; or care for medically complex conditions combined with diabetes, digestive disorders, or renal disorders/failure.

General subacute care is short stay (10 to 40 days) and is most often utilized for patients who require medical care and monitoring at least weekly, short-term nursing care at a level of approximately 3.5 to 5 hours per patient day, and rehabilitative therapies that may extend from 1 to 3 hours per patient day. A significant number of patients in general subacute units are patients who may require subacute rehabilitation, or wound management IV therapies for septic conditions, without significant other medical complications. Although there is some overlap in the clinical programs with the transitional subacute units and facilities, the key difference is the acuity level of the patients. A sizable number of patients in the general subacute units are Medicare beneficiaries because younger patients at these acuity levels tend to be cared for by home health services.

The goal of transitional and general subacute units is to manage the patient's recovery or rehabilitation in a cost-effective manner and to discharge the patient home, or in some cases, to a less expensive level of care such as long-term care or assisted living.

Chronic subacute care units manage patients with little hope of ultimate recovery and functional independence, such as chronic ventila-

Exhibit 31–1 Subacute Care Categories

PATIENT LENGTH OF STAY — SHORT → LONG

NURSING INTENSITY — HIGH → LOW

TRANSITIONAL SUBACUTE
⟹ 5 to 30 days
⟹ Step down from hospital in hospital-based nursing unit/facility or free-standing units
⟹ High-intensity medical
⟹ Nursing at 5.5 to 6.5 hours per patient day
⟹ Medically complex; acute rehab; cardiopulmonary
⟹ High ancillaries
⟹ Rehabilitation
⟹ Respiratory therapy
⟹ Discharged home

LONG-TERM TRANSITIONAL SUBACUTE
⟹ 60 to 90 days +
⟹ Long-term care acute hospitals
⟹ High-intensity medical
⟹ Nursing at 6.5 to 9 hours per patient day
⟹ Medically complex; ventilator dependent
⟹ High ancillaries
⟹ Minimal rehabilitation
⟹ Respiratory therapy
⟹ Expire, home, or long-term care

GENERAL SUBACUTE
⟹ 10 to 40 days
⟹ Higher level than skilled nursing facility, usually nursing facility units
⟹ Low- to moderate-intensity medical
⟹ Nursing at 3.5 to 5 hours per patient day
⟹ Subacute rehab; wound management, IV therapies
⟹ Low ancillaries
⟹ Rehabilitation
⟹ Discharged home or to long-term care

CHRONIC SUBACUTE
⟹ 60 to 90 days +
⟹ Higher level than skilled nursing facility; may be in nursing facility units or long-term care acute hospital
⟹ Low- to moderate-intensity medical
⟹ Nursing at 3.5 to 5 hours per patient day
⟹ Ventilator dependent, comatose, terminal
⟹ Low ancillaries
⟹ Respiratory therapy
⟹ Expire, home, or long-term care

tor-dependent patients, long-term comatose patients, and patients with progressive neurological disease. Typically, these patients require nursing staffing at the level of the general subacute unit (3.5 to 5 hours per patient day), medical monitoring biweekly to monthly, and restorative therapies usually provided by nursing staff with guidance from rehabilitation therapists. Either these patients will eventually be stabilized so that they can be discharged home or cared for in a long-term care facility or they may expire. Their average length of stay is 60 to 90 days.

Long-term transitional subacute care facilities most often are licensed as hospitals rather than as nursing facilities and are exempt from the Prospective Payment System (PPS) as long-term care hospitals with average lengths of stay of 25 days or more. Typically, these facilities provide care for acute ventilator-dependent or very medically complex patients. At a hospital, attending physicians visit the patients daily. Nursing staff tends to be primarily RNs, and nursing hours per patient day may range between 6.5 and 9, depending on the types and acuity levels of patients.

SUBACUTE PROVIDERS

Although subacute care may be provided in hospital swing beds and rehabilitation hospitals, the most common subacute providers are long-term care hospitals, hospital-based subacute skilled nursing units, and free-standing nursing facility subacute units.

Long-Term Care Hospitals

Long-term care hospitals may qualify for an exemption from the hospital PPS if the average length of stay for patients is 25 days or more (42 CFR § 412.23). Licensed as a hospital, long-term care or specialty hospitals generally focus on the long-term transitional subacute category. The primary reasons for the focus are related to the regulations that patients in a long-term care hospital must require a hospital

level of care (as opposed to a subacute skilled nursing level) and that the average length of stay for patients must be 25 days or more in order for the facility to qualify for the PPS exemption as a long-term care hospital.

Hospital-Based Subacute Skilled Nursing Units

Acute hospitals throughout the nation have been involved in creating seamless care continuums in order to provide the highest quality care for patients in the most cost-effective manner. For many acute hospitals, the continuum-of-care strategy includes conversion of empty acute hospital beds to skilled nursing facility beds in order to create subacute units. Some states, such as Florida, have recognized the differences in the patient types and acuity levels in hospital-based subacute skilled nursing units as opposed to subacute units in free-standing nursing facilities. Patients in hospital-based subacute skilled nursing facility units often have higher acuity levels, shorter stays, and a higher rate of discharge home than patients in subacute units in free-standing nursing facilities (Panel for the Study, 1995).

To utilize the hospital-based skilled nursing facility subacute unit effectively as an interim step between the medical/surgical floor and home, these units tend to provide primarily the transitional subacute category of care. Acute hospitals with high volumes of orthopaedic and neurological patients also may provide general subacute care, with an emphasis on a short-term orthopaedic or neurological rehabilitation.

Free-standing Nursing Facility Subacute Units

Subacute units in free-standing nursing facilities most often provide general subacute care or chronic subacute care. Because the beds already are licensed as nursing facility beds, the free-standing nursing facility does not have to "convert" beds as does the acute hospital. Instead, the free-standing nursing facility typically dedicates a separate nursing unit to subacute care, often with a separate medical director from the remainder of the facility, a dedicated clinical staff, and clinical protocols and programs that address the needs of the subacute patient.

QUALITY IMPROVEMENT IN SUBACUTE CARE UNITS

As health care providers and payers consolidate and integrate, access to subacute levels of care tends to be a critical factor in the successful management of health care costs. Minimizing costs without compromising quality, however, requires certain fundamental structures and operating systems within the subacute care unit. As in the rest of the health care industry, subacute providers are aggressively seeking ways to measure, predict, and ensure consistency of outcomes. However, like the rest of the health care industry, subacute care is in its infancy in developing statistically valid outcome measurement systems. Therefore subacute providers typically rely on quality improvement methodologies that involve structural and process criteria and, when possible, measurable outcomes.

Structural criteria include the quality implications of the subacute facility's or unit's physical plant, staff-to-patient ratios, staff competencies, equipment, ancillary services infrastructure, and the like. Process criteria are associated with the quality implications of the systems and procedures in the subacute facility or unit, such as the admissions and patient assessment procedures, patient care and treatment protocols, patient and family education systems, utilization management, and discharge planning operations. Outcomes deal with mortality, morbidity, patient satisfaction, and rehospitalization. In other words, outcomes center on what many people regard as subacute care's "bottom line."

SUBACUTE ACCREDITATION

Both the Joint Commission and the Commission on Accreditation of Rehabilitation Facilities (CARF) have developed accreditation programs for subacute care that attempt to focus on structure, process, and outcome. Since January 1995, the Joint Commission has been accrediting subacute care programs utilizing the Accreditation Protocol for Subacute Programs (Joint Commission, 1996b). The subacute protocol incorporates the following 11 major sections:

- Patient Rights and Responsibilities
- Admissions
- Patient Assessment and Evaluation
- Patient Care
- Continuity of Care
- Leadership
- Human Resources Management
- Information Management
- Quality Assessment and Improvement
- Plant, Technology, and Safety Management
- Infection Control

The protocol for the accreditation of subacute care programs uses existing standards that appear in both the *Comprehensive Accreditation Manual for Hospitals* (Joint Commission, 1995) and the *Accreditation Manual for Long-Term Care* (Joint Commission, 1996a), which have been tailored by new interpretations and a new survey process to emphasize the needs of subacute patients.

CARF is the national accrediting agency that establishes standards for organizations serving persons with disabilities. Since July 1995, CARF has surveyed comprehensive inpatient medical rehabilitation programs according to one of three categories of standards (CARF, 1994). Category I is reserved for acute rehabilitation programs within facilities licensed as hospitals. Categories II and III are reserved for subacute rehabilitation. Category II accreditation is available for subacute rehabilitation programs located in facilities licensed as hospitals, hospital-based skilled nursing facilities, or free-standing skilled nursing facilities. Individuals served in subacute programs eligible for Category II accreditation have outcomes that focus on returning home or advancing to another level of rehabilitation care. The Category III designation is for subacute rehabilitation programs in facilities licensed as hospital-based skilled nursing facilities or freestanding skilled nursing facilities. Patients served in programs eligible for Category III accreditation have expected outcomes of returning to the community with or without support (e.g., home, assisted living).

REGULATORY OVERSIGHT

Both specialty hospital and skilled nursing facility subacute providers are subject to certain regulations at the federal and state level that define to a limited degree structural and process criteria believed to be related to quality care. Facilities must meet state licensure requirements, as well as regulations for Medicaid and Medicare reimbursement if the facility chooses to be certified as a Medicaid or Medicare provider. Subacute care provided in skilled nursing facility units also is subject to federal requirements, defined primarily in regulations related to 1987 OBRA (Omnibus Budget Reconciliation Act) legislation (42 CFR § 483.1–483.75).

Most subacute providers, however, have developed quality improvement procedures that go beyond regulatory requirements. Whether or not the subacute unit or facility chooses to apply for accreditation by the Joint Commission or CARF, certain structural, process, and outcome criteria can be utilized to improve quality in subacute units.

STRUCTURAL QUALITY IMPROVEMENT IN SUBACUTE CARE UNITS

Subacute care units must be perceived as an attractive alternative to a continued stay in an acute hospital. As a result, subacute units in hospitals should be housed in areas comparable to the most attractive acute care units. Subacute units in nursing facilities often have a separate entrance to minimize the comingling of short-stay, homebound subacute patients with long-term care residents in the nursing facility.

Other structural areas that may be important for quality improvement in a subacute unit include the following areas.

Nursing Station

In long-term care facilities, nursing stations tend to be of inadequate size for a subacute unit. The subacute patients have higher acuity levels than long-term care residents and thus require significantly more clinical procedures. As a result, there are more staff involved in charting at the nursing station. Daily to weekly visits by physicians, nurse practitioners, and/or physician assistants require that there be a separate charting area with access to telephones. The intravenous and intramuscular medication requirements of the subacute patient population result in a need for medications and nutrition rooms that are significantly larger than those typically found in a nursing facility.

Respiratory Therapy

Respiratory therapy services are important components of most subacute care programs. Subacute units that include specialized respiratory care or ventilator management programs or cardiopulmonary management programs usually provide respiratory therapy services on a 24-hour basis. There should be an appropriate area for respiratory therapy cleaning and charting, preferably near the subacute unit's nursing station.

Rehabilitation

The vast majority of subacute patients require physical therapy, occupational therapy, and/or speech-language pathology services as well as recreational therapy. The patient acuity levels and short stays of subacute patients support the need for a rehabilitation therapy area of at least 15 square feet for each hour of therapy provided. The ideal location for the therapy area is in or adjacent to the subacute unit. To prepare the patient for home, the therapy area should have a training kitchen and training bathroom.

Isolation

A separate patient isolation room should be available on the subacute care unit, preferably with reversed air flow. A good rule of thumb is that there should be one isolation room for each 10 patients on a subacute care unit.

Furniture and Equipment

Electric beds, support mattresses and pads, and adequate lighting are essential equipment in a subacute unit. Frequently, clinical procedures are performed at bedside. The physician, nurse, or therapist must have adequate space and lighting to perform the procedures safely and accurately with a minimum amount of disruption to the patient. This goal also requires that there be adequate space on the subacute unit or adjacent to the subacute unit for storage of supplies and equipment.

Staffing

Subacute units typically have dedicated clinical staffs. In hospitals, the dedicated clinical staffs are necessary due to the specialized knowledge needed to comply with regulatory requirements for operating as a skilled nursing facility subacute unit within the hospital.

In free-standing nursing facilities, patients in subacute units require significantly more nursing procedures than do long-term care residents. Whereas the nursing emphasis for long-term care residents is both clinical and psy-chosocial, the primary needs of subacute patients tend to be clinical. Most subacute units in nursing facilities employ a dedicated staff of nurses with recent acute hospital experience, who have proven competencies in providing high-acuity nursing clinical procedures.

Medical Director

Usually, the subacute unit's medical director has a specialty that is consistent with the major programs offered in the subacute unit. Subacute unit medical directors often are internists, pulmonologists, and cardiologists. However, a subacute unit with a major emphasis in rehabilitation may have a physiatrist medical director.

Moreover, subacute units tend to have medical consultants who oversee the quality of the individual programs offered in the subacute unit. For example, an oncologist may assist in the development of admission criteria, clinical protocols, outcome measurements, and discharge criteria for patients in an oncology management or oncology rehabilitation program.

The subacute medical director or subacute medical consultants may serve as attending physicians for patients whose attending physicians opt not to follow the patient in the subacute unit.

The medical director's job description should clearly define responsibilities, including compliance with regulatory requirements for a skilled nursing facility subacute unit, (e.g., psychotropic medications and restraint reduction).

Nursing

Nursing staffing in subacute units ranges from 3.5 direct nursing hours per patient day to 8 direct nursing hours per patient day. Typically, however, general subacute care units provide 3.5 to 5 direct nursing hours per patient day with at least 40% of the nursing staff as RNs or licensed practical nurses (LPNs).

Transitional subacute care units provide between 5.5 and 6.5 nursing hours per patient day, and at least 50% of the nursing staff are licensed nurses. RN coverage is essential 24 hours per day, 7 days a week.

Subacute units should have initial and annual nursing competency assessments, which focus on nursing procedures required for high-acuity patients such as those found in subacute units. The nursing continuing education program, then, should be based on the results of the subacute competency assessment. A sample of a subacute nursing competency assessment instrument is shown in Exhibit 31–2.

Specialized subacute programs may require that nursing staff be certified to provide certain services or specialized care, such as ACLS, chemotherapy, rehabilitation, or oncology nurse certification.

Social Services

The majority of patients in transitional and general subacute care units are discharged home. With an average length of stay for subacute patients of under 30 days, social workers are important team members in subacute units.

Hospitals with subacute units may elect to have the social services performed by case management or discharge planning staff from the hospital. Nursing facilities also may share social workers with the long-term care or other specialty units within the nursing facility. However, a good rule of thumb is that there should be at least one dedicated social worker per 30 subacute patients. If the social worker is also responsible for discharge planning and placement, one social worker for 15 patients is appropriate.

Ancillary Services

Nearly all subacute patients require physical rehabilitation. The rehabilitation services should be provided throughout the day, 7 days per week.

Although nursing facilities may share recreational therapists or activities personnel with the long-term care components of the facility, usually subacute skilled nursing facility units in hospitals employ a dedicated recreational therapist to provide the activities program required by federal regulation.

A majority of subacute patients require active nutrition management by registered dietitians as an integral component of their recovery or rehabilitation program. Although most subacute patients require weekly or semiweekly oversight by a registered dietitian, those patients with specific enteral or parenteral nutrition programs need more frequent interventions. Although daily access to registered dietitians is essential, the ratio of registered dietitians to subacute patients will depend on the types of patients and their needs within a specific subacute unit.

Another key clinical staff member in the subacute unit is the pharmacist. The acuity levels of subacute patients are consistent with use of pharmaceuticals to a degree commonly found during the latter days of acute hospitalization, as opposed to the less intensive pharmaceutical utilization found in typical nursing facilities. Pharmacy consultation must be accessible at all times for monitoring of drug regimens and drug interactions.

PROCESS CRITERIA FOR QUALITY IMPROVEMENT IN SUBACUTE UNITS

Whereas structural criteria focus on whether the building blocks for a quality subacute unit are in place, process criteria address whether the operations, systems, and procedures are actually implemented in a manner consistent with professional expectations or standards. Process criteria for improving quality in subacute units may be divided into six areas:

- admissions
- assessment and care planning
- clinical procedures and protocols
- interdisciplinary patient management
- patient and family education
- utilization management/quality improvement programs

Exhibit 31–2 Sample Pages from a Subacute Care RN/LPN Competency Skills Inventory

Nursing Skills	Can Perform w/o Training	Training Needed	N/A	Date Due	Person Responsible for Training	Date Completed (w/Signature of Instructor)
ADMISSION/ DISCHARGE TRANSFER						
• Admits Patient						
• Transfers Patient						
• Discharges Patient						
CAN UTILIZE THESE FORMS						
• Assessment Flow Sheet						
• I & O Sheet						
ASSESSMENT PROCEDURE						
• Minimum Data Set						
• Use of RAPS						
• Patient Care Plan Process						
SUPERVISION OF STAFF						
CHANGE OF SHIFT REPORTS						
WEIGHING PATIENTS						
• Bedscales						
• Chairscales						
• Standing scales						
• Hoyer scale						
EMERGENCY EQUIPMENT						
• Crash cart						
• Airway						
• Ambu bag						
• Backboard						
• CPR/ACLS						
• Code ____						
• Suction machine						
SUCTIONING						
• Nasal/Pharyngeal						
• Endotracheal						
TUBE FEEDING						
• Use of pumps						
• Administering medications via tube						
• Hanging of bags, syringes						
• G-tube care						
• J-tube care						
• N/G tube care						

Admissions

Because subacute units may be composed of specialty hospital beds or skilled nursing facility beds, patient admissions must comply with appropriate regulations governing hospitals and/or nursing facilities respectively. Other commonly accepted indicators of quality for admissions include the ability to admit a patient within 24 hours of the referral, assuming that the patient meets admission criteria. This degree of responsiveness requires that clearly defined and understood procedures are in place for referral tracking, clinical preadmission assessments, financial verification, attending physician communications, and interfacility or interunit transportation. Although long-term care facilities will have bed turnovers averaging between 1 and 2 years, subacute units within those facilities typically will turn over beds 1.25 to 1.5 times per month. Subacute unit beds within hospitals will have more frequent turnover, between 2 and 3 times per month.

To best ensure seamless health care delivery for the patient, medications, special equipment and supplies that were utilized during the patient's acute hospital stay should be immediately available to the patient upon admission to the subacute unit.

Assessment and Care Planning

The assessment process should be designed to ensure that each patient receives a comprehensive assessment that determines both the patient's capacity to perform daily life functions and any significant impairments. Ideally, the assessment should involve both the patient and his or her family. The interdisciplinary care team should conduct the assessment, which should be initiated within 24 hours and completed within 48 hours of admission. Interdisciplinary team members in a subacute unit are listed in Exhibit 31–3.

The care management and coordination function frequently is performed by a designated case manager. The case manager may be

Exhibit 31–3 Subacute Interdisciplinary Team Members

Medical director
Medical staff and consulting staff
    Physician
    Physician assistants
    Nurse practitioners
Nursing staff
    Registered nurses
    Licensed practical nurses
    Nurse assistants/aides
Physical therapy staff
    Physical therapists
    Licensed physical therapy assistants
    Therapy aides or rehabilitation technicians
Occupational therapy staff
    Occupational therapists
    Certified occupational therapy assistants
    Therapy aides or rehabilitation technicians
Speech-language pathologists
Respiratory therapists
Therapeutic recreation specialists
Registered dietitians
Social workers
Pharmacists

an active caregiver member of the interdisciplinary team or may be a separate position. Case management responsibilities in the subacute care units are shown in Exhibit 31-4.

An interim plan of care should be developed as soon as possible after admission, but at least within the first 24 hours. The more comprehensive interdisciplinary plan of care developed following the assessment procedures should be developed within 72 hours after completion of the assessment. The care plan should include at least the following:

- identified patient needs
- patient and family goals that are objective, realistic, understandable, measurable, and achievable

Exhibit 31–4 Case Management Responsibilities in Subacute Care Units

Prior to Admission
- Conducts clinical and financial preadmission assessment
- Procures necessary equipment and supplies prior to patient transfer
- Notifies direct care providers (nurses, therapists, physician) of the admission and care needs prior to arrival
- Secures necessary authorizations from third-party payers

During Patient Stay in Subacute Unit
- Verifies that required services are provided as prescribed on a timely basis
- Addresses care needs. Interacts with patient and family and caregivers to address care and discharge needs
- Arranges for necessary consultations and treatments
- Arranges for transportation to/from appointments
- Monitors patient progress toward discharge goals

Discharge Planning
- Establishes discharge needs
- Assists patient and family in procuring community services
- Arranges for home equipment and home health services
- Assists with transportation arrangements
- Follows up on patient status post discharge

- procedures that will be used to meet the goals
- interdisciplinary team members who will be involved in the care of the patient
- frequency with which services will be provided
- expected date or dates for achievement of goals
- discharge plan

Clinical Procedures and Protocols

To achieve consistent, predictable outcomes, clinical procedures and protocols must be standardized for groups of patients with similar disease or disability characteristics. Critical pathways for subacute care are in the very early stages of development. However, process quality improvement requires that the clinical team utilize consistent clinical procedures and protocols in the subacute unit. At a minimum, clinical procedures and protocols should be available for the clinical areas noted in Exhibit 31–5.

Interdisciplinary Patient Management

Communication among the interdisciplinary team members is enhanced by regularly scheduled team conferences. Most subacute units schedule weekly interdisciplinary team conferences to review the progress of patients in the subacute unit. Other units have daily rounds that center on key issues for a subset of patients within the subacute unit. Regardless of the particular methodology used for team conferences, the important quality indicator is that they be held on a regular basis and be documented with signatures of all interdisciplinary team members present at the conference. Whenever possible, patients and families should be invited to the care conferences or rounds and be actively involved in the goal setting and discharge planning for the patient.

Discharge planning begins at admission to the subacute unit. Home visits by rehabilitation therapists and/or nurses should occur as part of the initial patient assessment to ensure that the

Exhibit 31–5 Clinical Procedures and Protocols in Subacute Units

- ✔ Initial Assessment
- ✔ Ongoing Assessment
- ✔ Responses to Complications
- ✔ Adverse Reactions
- ✔ Physician Communications
- ✔ Peripheral IV Therapy
- ✔ Central IV Therapy
- ✔ Intraspinal/Subcutaneous Therapy
- ✔ Infusion Therapy
- ✔ Respiratory Therapy
- ✔ Cardiovascular Therapy
- ✔ Wound and Strain Therapy
- ✔ CAPD Therapy
- ✔ Rehabilitation
- ✔ General Nursing Procedures (i.e., blood glucose monitoring, applying elastic bandages to amputated extremities, triangular sling, care of leg urinary drainage bag, bladder irrigation, colostomy and ileostomy care, hypoglycemia and hypo/hyperthermia management)

care plan and care management include realistic goals for the patient who is expected to return home.

Patient and Family Education

Subacute patients should be trained in self-care as appropriate for their status, and self-care as part of the recovery and rehabilitation process should be emphasized, along with support and assistance from the members of the patient's family or significant others. Because the vast majority of subacute patients return home, involvement of the patient's family or significant other should begin upon admission and continue throughout the patient's stay in the subacute unit.

Utilization Management/Quality Improvement Program

Each subacute program should have in place specific procedures for ensuring that the pa-

tient receives the right care at the right time in the right place at the right cost and with the right outcome. Quality improvement procedures include ongoing monitoring and evaluation, focusing on high-volume and high-risk areas first. When problems have been identified, the remediation of the problem should be monitored to ensure that there is effective resolution and that there is no recurrence of the problem at a later time.

OUTCOME QUALITY IMPROVEMENT MEASUREMENTS FOR SUBACUTE UNITS

Outcomes management is a top priority for most health care providers today. Outcomes management might be defined as the process of looking at the results of subacute care to determine what works best and then implementing the best practices. CARF (1994) defined outcomes evaluation as a systematic procedure for monitoring the effectiveness and efficiency with which results are achieved as well as customer satisfaction following termination of services. An outcomes measurement procedure should allow a systematic evaluation of the efforts of subacute care in terms of the operation, provision of services, appropriateness and effectiveness of services, efficiency of the system, and adequacy of serving the needs of the patient (Forer, 1995).

Considerations

Most subacute patients have a combination of medical care needs and rehabilitation needs. An outcome measurement system for subacute care, therefore, must include an evaluation of medical improvement, functional improvement, and quality of life. Outcome measurements in subacute care traditionally have focused on either clinical benchmarks or financial benchmarks. Clinical benchmarks might be health status, level of function, ability to manage activities of daily living, absence of clinical adverse events, length of treatment, and discharge disposition. Financial benchmarks are used to measure results as they relate to the cost of caring for the patient. Financial benchmarks may include

- length of stay
- total costs of subacute stay
- resource utilization during the subacute stay
- cost per patient day
- total days of care required

According to Forer (1995), the clinical outcomes indicators that should be considered in evaluating subacute care are

- diagnosis/impairment-specific measures
- severity/acuity indices
- medical outcomes
- discharge destination
- program interruptions (e.g., transfers back to acute care)
- medical complications (comorbid and concurrent)
- patient/family satisfaction
- follow-up status (medical, functional, future health care use and costs)
- health-related quality of life (perception of wellness)
- return to previous lifestyle

Today, most subacute providers use informal outcome measurements as opposed to standardized instruments. Whether formal or informal, outcome measurement systems in subacute care should have adequate validity and reliability and should be sensitive to small increments of patient improvement or change.

Outcome Measurement Instruments

Five types of instruments have been used to measure outcomes in subacute units:

- Functional Independence Measure (FIM)
- Medical Outcome Scales
- Resource Utilization Group system (RUGs)
- selected elements from the Minimum Data Set (MDS)
- patient satisfaction measures

Information on each of these instruments is summarized in Table 31–1.

Functional Independence Measure

The Functional Independence Measure (FIM) is reported to be the most widely used system in the world for documenting the severity of patient disability and the outcomes of medical rehabilitation (U.B. Foundation, 1994). Two assessment tools are available: the Functional Independence Measure for Adults (Adult FIM) and the Functional Independence Measure for Children (WeeFIM).

The Adult FIM is used for patients who are teens and adults. The WeeFIM is useful for children 6 months to 7 years, and older. The Adult FIM centers on patient disabilities, whereas the WeeFIM provides an assessment of functional abilities within a developmental context. A seven-level ordinal scale ranging from *least independent* to *most independent* is used to measure self-care, sphincter control, mobility, communication, psychosocial adjustment, and cognitive function. Exhibit 31–6 shows the categories that are assessed with the FIM. The FIM is used by the interdisciplinary care team. The initial FIM assessment occurs as part of the admission assessment. The tool is administered at least once more prior to discharge and it is expected that the tool will once again be used as a follow-up measure for discharged patients 60 to 90 days after discharge.

Medical Outcomes Scales

The Medical Outcomes Scales were developed to assess the status of subacute patients with regard to comorbid disease, pain, respiratory problems, wounds, nutrition, and infection. The instruments were designed to obtain data at the time that treatment is initiated and again when treatment is discontinued. Scoring is on a 5-point scale (Formations in Health Care, 1995).

Resource Utilization Group System

The Resource Utilization Group System (RUGs) is a 44-group classification system used by the Health Care Financing Administration (HCFA) for nursing facility residents

Table 31–1 Outcome Measurement Instruments

Category	Functional Independence Measure (FIM)	Medical Outcome System (MOS)	Resource Utilization Group System (RUGs)	Minimum Data Set (MDS)	Patient Satisfaction
Initial development	1983	1992	1989	1987	1970s–80s
Available to public	1988	1995 (May)	1993	1990	1980s–90s
Patient type	Acute and subacute medical rehabilitation	Subacute medically complex	Chronic subacute and long-term care	Chronic subacute and long-term care	Acute, subacute, and long-term care
Purpose	Assess function/severity of disability Measure outcomes of medical rehabilitation	Measure outcomes of medical treatment	Classify homogeneous groupings for: • prospective payment • quality monitoring	Standardized assessment of resident functions	Assess customer satisfaction
Setting	Acute or comprehensive rehab Subacute rehab	Subacute care: nursing home and hospital	Long-term care	Long-term care	All environments
Size of database	>800,000	Pilot studies: 618	Multi-state long-term care population	30 nursing facilities in 6 states	Varied; innumerable
Impairment/service/program type	Stroke Pulmonary Cardiac Debility Amputation Brain dysfunction Arthritis Orthopaedic conditions Neuromuscular disorders Spinal cord dysfunction Pain syndromes Major multiple trauma Congenital deformities Other disabling impairments	Respiratory Wounds Pain Nutrition Infection	Rehabilitation (special) Extensive services Special care Clinically complex Impaired cognition Behavior problems Physical functions (reduced)	All types	All types
Focus area	Self-care/ADL Sphincter control Transfers/mobility Locomotion Communication Social cognition	Medical acuity status Respiratory indicators Wound indicators Pain indicators Nutrition indicators Infection indicators	Hierarchy of resident types (MDS driven) Resident functionality (ADLs) Additional problems/services required: • Number of extensive therapies • Sad mood (depressed) • Nursing rehabilitation	ADLs Nutritional status Presence of ulcers Use of medications Use of restraints Incontinence Behavior	Service/treatments Staff encountered Procedures explained Courteous treatment Recommend/return Discharge planning
Score/Measurement Style		Score 5 levels, check (✔) and "fill in" the blank	ADL scores 1–5, 4 levels of rehab, count of services	Four ordinal levels	Score/level 1–5 (most common)
Desired Outcomes	Maximize functional independence. Maximize return to community. Maximize LOS efficiency. Maximize charge efficiency.	Attain optimal health. Minimize use of health care resources.	Maximize reimbursement. Monitor quality.	Obtain baseline data on each admission from which to measure improvement or decline of the resident.	Increase customer satisfaction. Improve patient services. Establish performance standards. Document job performance differences. Build employee morale.

Exhibit 31–6 Functional Independence Measure (FIM): Categories for Assessment

---

MOTOR ITEMS

Self-Care
1. Eating
2. Grooming
3. Bathing
4. Dressing—upper body
5. Dressing—lower body
6. Toileting

Sphincter Control
7. Bladder management
8. Bowel management

Transfers
9. Bed, chair, wheelchair
10. Toilet
11. Tub or shower

Locomotion
12. Walk/wheelchair
13. Stairs

COGNITIVE ITEMS

Communication
14. Comprehension
15. Expression

Social Cognition
16. Social interaction
17. Problem solving
18. Memory

(Hiller, 1992). The data used to design the classification system include measures of resident characteristics and staff care time.

Nursing home residents are classified into one of the mutually exclusive RUGs groups. Placement into a group follows sequential evaluation of partitioning logic on three levels. Residents in each of the RUGs groups are expected to used similar quantities and patterns of resources.

Residents are first assigned to a RUGs group on the basis of three dimensions:

1. hierarchy of major resident types
2. resident functionality as measured by activities of daily living

3. additional problems or services required by the resident

The hierarchy of major resident types has seven categories:

1. rehabilitation
2. extensive services
3. special care
4. clinically complex
5. impaired cognition
6. behavior problems
7. physical functions (reduced)

Resident functionality is measured through four activities of daily living:

1. bed mobility
2. eating
3. transfer
4. toilet use

A final assessment involves additional problems or services, including the number of extensive therapies required, a depressed or sad mood, and a requirement for nursing rehabilitation. Because the instrument was designed for long-term care residents, if it is to be used as an outcome measurement tool, it is likely to be most useful for chronic subacute care patients. To be useful as an outcome measurement tool, it should be used to assess the patient on admission, when there is any significant change in condition, and prior to discharge.

Minimum Data Set

Although the Minimum Data Set (MDS) is best known as a tool to monitor changes in nursing home residents over time, portions of the instrument may be used as an outcome measurement system (Burke, Feldman, Schneider, Foley, & Fries, 1992). The MDS uses a 4-point ordinal scale for rating physical functioning, cognitive patterns, communication/hearing patterns, activities of daily living, self-performance items, continence, weight variances, types and stages of decubitis ulcers, and chemical or physical restraint utilization. Any of these may be selected to measure the baseline for potential improvement in the patient's condition throughout the subacute stay.

The MDS was designed for measuring changes in nursing home residents. As a result, if it is to be used as an outcome measurement tool for subacute care, it will be most appropriately used for the chronic subacute care patient who has an average length of stay of 60 to 90 days in the subacute unit.

Patient Satisfaction Measures

Subacute providers frequently use their own proprietary instruments to measure patient satisfaction. Typically, patients and their families are asked to complete a patient satisfaction measurement tool upon discharge or 30 to 60 days after discharge from the subacute unit. Areas to be measured may include the following:

- services/treatment
- staff encountered
- procedures explained
- courtesy treatment
- recommend the unit to others or return if necessary
- discharge planning

Scoring systems vary among proprietary instruments, although many use a 5-point scale that allows the patients and families to rate their degree of satisfaction with the particular category of service. An example of a patient satisfaction form for a Subacute Wound Management Program is included in Exhibit 31–7.

QUALITY IMPROVEMENT SUCCESS STRATEGIES

Quality improvement in subacute units occurs because there is staff buy-in to and commitment to the effort and to the results of the effort. Forer (1994) suggested that strategies having the most success are

- involving staff in care decisions
- studying the outcomes data available
- comparing to regional and national averages
- improving outcomes data management
- providing training on how to use outcomes evaluation effectively to improve performance
- providing narrative executive summaries of results
- identifying the benchmark facilities and programs
- developing critical pathways
- implementing case management
- reengineering the delivery process to ensure that the best possible outcomes are achieved at the lowest possible cost

Exhibit 31–7 Sample Patient Satisfaction Form

Subacute Care
Wound Management Program

Patient Satisfaction Survey Cover Letter

(LETTERHEAD)

(DATE)

Dear (NAME OF PATIENT):

We would like to take this opportunity to thank you for choosing (NAME OF FACILITY)'s Wound Management Program.

In order to help us provide the highest quality of care, we would like your opinion regarding your stay in (NAME OF FACILITY)'s Wound Management Program. Please complete the enclosed questionnaire at your earliest convenience. All information will be kept confidential. You are encouraged to express your candid opinions.

Please return the completed questionnaire in the enclosed postage paid envelope. Thank you.

Sincerely yours,

(NAME)
Program Director

Enclosure

---

continues

Exhibit 31–7 continued

Subacute Care

Subacute Wound Management
Patient Satisfaction Survey

Read each item carefully and *CIRCLE* the one answer that is best for you.

SA - Strongly Agree   **N** - Neutral   **SD** - Strongly Disagree
A - Agree   **D** - Disagree   **NA** - Not Applicable

PROGRAM AWARENESS

1. I was involved with setting my program goals.	SA	A	N	D	SD	NA
2. I felt the activities were designed to help me achieve my program goals.	SA	A	N	D	SD	NA
3. During my stay, I had sufficient opportunity to discuss my plans and make arrangements for my discharge.	SA	A	N	D	SD	NA
4. I was aware of the various team members who were responsible for my treatment during my rehabilitation:						
• Physician	SA	A	N	D	SD	NA
• Nurse	SA	A	N	D	SD	NA
• Nursing Assistant	SA	A	N	D	SD	NA
• Enterostomal Therapy Nurse	SA	A	N	D	SD	NA
• Diabetic Nurse Educator	SA	A	N	D	SD	NA
• Physical Therapist	SA	A	N	D	SD	NA
• Social Worker	SA	A	N	D	SD	NA
• Dietitian	SA	A	N	D	SD	NA

5. By the time I was discharged, I had been sufficiently instructed in how to carry out my program at home. (Please rate areas applicable to you.)

	SA	A	N	D	SD	NA
• Medication knowledge	SA	A	N	D	SD	NA
• Diet instruction	SA	A	N	D	SD	NA
• Personal care (skin, bowel, or bladder programs)	SA	A	N	D	SD	NA
• Therapy home programs	SA	A	N	D	SD	NA
• Special equipment	SA	A	N	D	SD	NA

6. On a scale of 1 through 5, 1 being lowest and 5 being highest, please rate your degree of confidence in the following staff's ability to work with you in meeting your goals.

	SA	1	2	3	4	5
	SA	1	2	3	4	5
• Physician						
• Nurse						
• Nursing Assistant						
• Enterostomal Therapy Nurse						
• Diabetic Nurse Educator						
• Physical Therapist						
• Social Worker						
• Dietitian						

HUMAN RELATIONS

	SA	A	N	D	SD	NA
7. During my program my right to privacy was respected.	SA	A	N	D	SD	NA
8. I felt the staff aided me in my adjustment to my disability.	SA	A	N	D	SD	NA
9. The staff was empathetic and understanding of me and my personal needs.	SA	A	N	D	SD	NA

continues

Exhibit 31–7 continued

10. Please check the appropriate illness for which you were treated in the rehabilitation program

     ❑ Pressure of decubitus ulcer   ❑ Post-surgical wound

     ❑ Burn   ❑ Other (please specify) _____

Comments: _____

_____

_____

Thank you for taking the time to complete this questionnaire. Your confidential responses and comments will help us in making modifications to our program to better serve future patients at the Wound Management Program.

Source: Reprinted with permission from *Subacute Wound Management Manual,* © 1996 Griffin Management, Inc.

CONCLUSION

Subacute providers are strongly motivated today to engage in quality improvement activities, particularly outcomes evaluation. Not only are patients, families, and referral sources demanding high-quality care, but also payers, both managed care organizations and government payers, have begun questioning the value of payment for subacute care without measurable outcomes. Subacute providers must demonstrate that their involvement in the continuum of care results in reducing or at least containing the cost of care and in optimizing the functional status of patients. There is a definite need to demonstrate clearly the cost-effectiveness, quality, and outcomes of subacute programs; and then to use this information to improve programs and services and to position subacute units as essential components of integrated health care systems.

REFERENCES

Burke, R., Feldman, G., Schneider, D., Foley, W., & Fries, B. (1992). *Multistate nursing home case-mix and quality demonstration, description of the Resource Utilization Group, Version III (RUG III) System.* The Circle, University of Michigan, Ann Arbor, and Rensselaer Polytechnic Institutes, New York.

Commission on Accreditation of Rehabilitation Facilities. (1994). *Standards manual for organizations serving people with disabilities.* Tucson, AZ: Author.

Forer, S. (1994, November). Quality and outcomes management. *LTC Update,* 2–3.

Forer, S. (1995, June/July). Outcomes evaluation and subacute care. *Rehab Management,* 138–140, 164.

Formations in Health Care, Inc. (1995). *Medical outcome system.* Chicago: Author.

Hiller, R. (1992). *MDS Plus/RUG III.* Paper presented at the Ohio Health Care Association Fall Conference.

Joint Commission on Accreditation of Healthcare Organizations. (1994). *Digest: Subacute care protocol.* Oakbrook Terrace, IL: Author.

Joint Commission on Accreditation of Healthcare Organizations. (1995). *Comprehensive accreditation manual for hospitals.* Oakbrook Terrace, IL: Author.

Joint Commission on Accreditation of Healthcare Organizations. (1996a). *Accreditation manual for long-term care.* Oakbrook Terrace, IL: Author.

Joint Commission on Accreditation of Healthcare Organizations. (1996b). *1996 accreditation protocol for subacute programs.* Oakbrook Terrace, IL: Author.

National Subacute Care Association. (1994). *Definition of subacute care.* Bethesda, MD: Author.

Panel for the Study of Skilled Nursing Care. (1995). *A comparison of hospital-based skilled nursing units and freestanding nursing homes in Florida.* Tallahassee, FL: Agency for Health Care Administrators.

U.B. Foundation, Inc. (1994). *Getting started with the Uniform Data System for Medical Rehabilitation.* Buffalo, NY: Uniform Data System.

## CHAPTER 32

Improving Quality Care: Developing Partnerships between Integrated Systems and the Community

Marjorie D. Weiss

CHAPTER OBJECTIVES

After completing this chapter, the reader will be able to

- relate the process of a hospital partnering with other community systems, such as judicial organizations, governments, health care organizations, schools, churches, and industry to measure and improve the health status and quality of life for a community
- delineate the development of four coalitions to continue defining a shared community vision, evaluating needs, and improving the quality of health for the community

---

Success in improving the health status and quality of life for a community requires measurement of the community's health via key community indicators. These indicators help to define priorities, document successes, and detect trends. Developing community indicators requires a thorough assessment of the community: health patterns in the population, subpopulations at risk, and the concurrence of selected conditions or events affecting the health of the community. Community health is a reflection of the ability of the community to care for its members with appropriate utilization of resources and elimination of redundancy among community systems (judicial, government, health care, schools, churches, employers, and other community agencies). To establish community indicators, one must ask: What are the issues in the community? What capacity does the community have for addressing these issues? What is important to the community?

The Partnership Project was formed in January 1995 to assess the human and health needs of the Fox Cities community and to develop collaborative approaches to community problem solving. The Fox Cities is the third largest urban area in Wisconsin, with a population of over 200,000.

The Steering Committee included representatives from industry, local government, human services providers (including Winnebago and Outagamie counties), health care organizations, the media, the community foundation, and the local United Way. The Partnership Project sought to measure knowledge, attitudes, perceptions, and behaviors within political, social, economic, cultural, health, and human service delivery systems (see Exhibit 32–1).

The Partnership Project had three phases:

- *I. Data Collection (January 1995 through November 1995).* Quantitative data were gathered from state and local agencies and analyzed. Qualitative data were gathered

Exhibit 32–1 Mission Statement and Goals of the Partnership Project

---

Mission
The Partnership Project's Mission is to improve our community's ability to respond to the community's basic human needs: physical, mental, and economic.

Goal #1
Identify the basic human needs in our community: physical, mental, and economic.

Goal #2
Identify existing resources that address the needs in our community.

Goal #3
Develop strategies, working within an agreed-upon action plan, that will produce tangible results for our community.

Goal #4
Ensure an evaluation process that measures action plan results.

---

via opinion surveys targeted at key community leaders, random households, and service providers. A Health Status Survey tool was sent to a random sample of community members to assess health status perceptions of the community. The purpose of data collection was to define the major needs of the community and to assess the community's array of resources addressing these needs.

- *II. Priority Setting/Planning (December 1995 through March 1996).* Using detailed analyses to identify community need priorities, the Partnership Project worked collaboratively with service providers and community organizations to develop an agreed-upon action plan for matching community needs with community capacities.

- *III. Implementation/Follow-up (April 1996 and beyond).* Implementation of the action plan, measuring change, and seeking feedback from the community will continue, on the basis of the community indicators developed during the Partnership Project.

This report focuses on the quality improvement tools and strategies used during the phases of the Partnership Project.

PHASE I: DATA COLLECTION

Prior to initiating data collection, the Steering Committee developed a mission statement and goals for the Partnership Project. The definition of *community* was based on geography and included all of the Fox Valley: Northern Calumet, Outagamie, and Northern Winnebago counties. Southern Winnebago County had begun a similar process about 6 months prior to the start of the Partnership Project. Toward the middle of Phase II, it was agreed that the Partnership Project and Winnebagoland Focus would investigate joint recommendations to the communities they represented. Both data collection and provider service delivery areas overlap significantly. Although the goals of the Partnership Project and Winnebagoland Focus were similar, the strategy for follow-up action following the initial assessment of the community varied slightly.

The Partnership Project Steering Committee members divided into three subgroups—Data Collection Committee, Process Committee, and Communications Committee—each with defined responsibilities. Once the mission and goals were clarified, the Data Collection

Committee (composed of Steering Committee members, public health nurses, and a research expert from one of the local universities) began meeting. Both quantitative and qualitative data sources were considered.

Quantitative data

Quantitative data were obtained from approximately 280 sources, including those listed in Exhibit 32–2. Many of these quantitative reports came from state departments, and results were reported on a "county" level. A resource person compiled the information by topic, and members of the Data Collection Committee reviewed the information for relevance to the project. Relevant statistics were abstracted and computerized by the project manager and the Data Collection Committee chair. Personnel from the Wisconsin Division of Health were instrumental in providing many of the statistical reports.

Qualitative data

Qualitative data were obtained via four survey instruments. A *key informant survey* was administered to 772 key community leaders. This survey tool asked for a rating of the unmet needs in the community. It also collected demographic information on the respondent. The

---

Exhibit 32–2 Examples of Quantitative Data Sources

Morbidity Statistics
Mortality Statistics
Natality Statistics
Department of Transportation Statistics
Economic Indicators
Search Institute Studies
Annual Surveys
Health and Human Services Statistics
Disability Statistics
Employment Statistics

---

second survey tool was a *household survey*. This survey was administered to a random sampling of households in the geographic area determined to be "the community" for the Partnership Project (with geographic distribution evenly distributed to each census tract). Of the 4,914 household surveys mailed, 960 were returned and tabulated. A *health status survey* was mailed to 4,914 different households using the same selection method. Response rate was 1,232. The fourth survey tool used was a *survey mailed to health and human service providers* (including religious organizations) in the community. Of the 550 programs that received a survey, 250 responded. Additional information about service providers was gathered through the local United Way's Information and Referral Service. The first three tools described were mailed surveys that were scannable documents. Increased printing costs were offset by compilation efficiency. The fourth instrument required hand keying for data entry. Information from the key informant survey, household survey, and provider survey were all entered into "Compass" software for analysis. Key community indicators were developed.

Survey respondents identified many community strengths: traditional values, a strong economy and full employment, quality schools and educational resources, opportunities to experience the arts, cultural events/activities and recreational activities, and quality health care. Survey respondents also identified some community weaknesses: increasing crime, gangs, use of drugs, youth problems, poor traffic management, local government, and high taxes.

Results from the quantitative data—the key informant, household, and health status surveys—were formatted into a Progress Report to the community. The Progress Report identified points at which the quantitative and qualitative data converged and conflicted. For example, although many responses from the perceptual surveys indicated growing awareness and concern about violence in the community, in reality the number of violent crimes was much lower than for most urban areas in the state. Another disparity noted was the contrast between low unemployment rates (2.9%) in August 1995, as compared to 3.1% for the state and 5.6% for the nation, and the percentage of people spending more of their income on basics, such as housing. Changing demographics indicated a decline in household size and an increase in single-parent households with an escalating demand for affordable, adequate housing. Previous community studies had highlighted family dysfunction, the rise of single-headed households, propensity of women to earn less, the need for parenting skills/training, lack of support for families, pressure on family units, and lack of parent interaction with schools as community concerns.

Community concerns about unsupervised youth focused on lack of before- and after-school child care, infant care, and respite care. Unhealthy habits, including overuse of alcohol and tobacco use, seemed to be linked to community mortality rates. As with state rates, the major causes of death in the community were heart disease, cancer, stroke, chronic lung disease, pneumonia/influenza, injuries, diabetes, infections, and suicide.

"Coping with change" was identified as an emerging theme: as the community had grown and become more diverse, it had sought to address newly discovered problems through studies and the creation of service programs or agencies. This method of addressing community problems had led to the creation of many organizations that appeared to duplicate the activities of others, and the result seemed to be confusion among the public. Fragmentation of services and lack of clear-cut directions for cooperation were identified by service providers as barriers to collaborative efforts.

In addition to "Coping with change," the Progress Report also delineated four other themes that were emerging from the data: (1) families, (2) youth, (3) community health, and (4) prosperity/disparity.

Community volunteers willing to help with Phase II were identified at a community presentation of the Progress Report organized by the communication team. A half-day prioritization session was used to organize the recommendations generated from the study groups. The final report to the community included a brief description of the quantitative and qualitative data, identification of community needs/issues, a recommended action plan, and key community indicators to serve as outcomes measures.

PHASE II: PRIORITY SETTING/PLANNING

The Steering Committee members used half-day, facilitated sessions to identify key issues. The Process Committee helped to facilitate Phase II by identifying community resources to facilitate the work of the Steering Committee. Using a situation analysis methodology, committee members evaluated identified issues as to seriousness, urgency, and timeliness. Output from this meeting helped to shape the agenda for six study groups on (1) families, (2) youth, (3) domestic violence, (4) substance use/abuse, (5) housing, and (6) utilizing preventive care. The tool used to structure the study groups is provided in Exhibit 32–3.

Steering Committee members not involved in facilitation of the study groups met to discuss "Coping with Change—Coordination and Collaboration." In a 4-hour facilitated session, the study groups (composed of providers, consumers, and community representatives) further defined and prioritized four key community issues, assessed the ability of the community to address the issues, and recommended actions to address these issues more effectively (Exhibit 32–4). The study group sessions took place over a 2-week time period and were facilitated by Steering Committee members who had worked together to delineate a common agenda and format. The agenda for the study groups included

Exhibit 32–3 Partnership Project Study Groups Agenda

WHAT	HOW	TIME
INTRODUCTION	• Review expected meeting outcomes, agenda, and ground rules • Participant introductions—name, role with issue	30 min.
IDENTIFY ISSUES WITHIN THE TOPIC	• List issues associated with the topic • Separate and clarify issues	20 min.
IDENTIFY PRIORITY ISSUES	• Rate or rank issues to identify top priority, using a benchmark • Discuss; agree	30 min.
DESCRIBE DESIRED PERFORMANCE	• Form small groups for each of the top 3 priority issues & answer the following questions: • What would we like to accomplish with this issue? • What's the Vision?	30 min.
BREAK	BREAK	10 min.
IDENTIFY STRENGTHS AND BARRIERS	• Each small group lists strengths and barriers of community in dealing with the issues considering: – experience and expertise with the issue – community operating practices associated with decision making, information sharing, coordination, cooperation	20 min.
DEVELOP RECOMMENDATIONS	• Small groups review vision, strengths, and barriers and identify strategies for effectively addressing the priority issues	45 min.
PRESENT FINDINGS	• Reconvene. Small groups report to full group.	45 min.
NEXT STEPS	• Indicate actions that will be taken to communicate this information to Partnership Project and community. • Evaluate the meeting • Adjourn	10 min.

Courtesy of Partnership Project, Fox Cities, Wisconsin.

a focus on coordination of services and community collaboration. The reports and recommendations were then presented to the Steering Committee. In a facilitated half-day session, the Steering Committee prioritized the recommendations from the study group sessions.

Phase II ended with a report to the community that included a review of the quantitative and qualitative data, a recommended action plan, and key community indicators to be used for outcome measurement. A partial listing of the key community indicators is included in Exhibit 32–5. The key findings listed in

Exhibit 32–4 Key Community Issues

Effective Families Urgent Issues

Need for parenting education and development of skills for nurturing

Need for supervised care of dependent family members: child care, respite care, special-needs care

Need for community support of all families, including nontraditional families

Need for more youth recreation alternatives

Personal Safety Urgent Issues

Need for knowledge of and access to resources for those affected by domestic violence

Environments that accept and support violence lead to a continued pattern of violence

Need for personal safety for community youth

Need for community knowledge about violence to address fears/myths

Affordable, Adequate Housing Urgent Issues

Need for coordinated regional planning and regulation of housing

Fears and myths present barriers to providing adequate housing in the Fox Cities

Shortage of affordable, adequate housing in Fox Cities

Community Health Urgent Issues

Need to decrease barriers to preventive care

Culture that accepts use/abuse of alcohol, drugs, and tobacco

Adolescent sexual behavior related to issues such as unplanned pregnancies, substance use/abuse, sexually transmitted diseases

Potential decreases in funding of prevention and treatment requiring cooperation and coordination of services

Exhibit 32–5 Partnership Project Community Indicators (Partial List)

Children and Families
Child abuse/neglect reports/1,000
Youth in foster homes or rate/1,000 children
Certified/licensed child day care slots

Community Public Safety
Juvenile arrests/1,000 children
Secure detention/1,000 children

Economy/Employment/Financial Hardship/Housing
Unemployment rate
AFDC cases/1,000 residents
Percentage of substandard dwellings

Education
Percentage of high school completion rate

Community Health
Child mental health inpatient discharges/1,000
Avg. mental health length of stay
Child AODA discharges/1,000 children
AODA hospital days of stay
Accidental deaths/1,000
Suicide rate
Low-birth-weight baby rate
Infant mortalities
First trimester prenatal care
Teen pregnancy rate/1,000 live births
Motor vehicle deaths
Alcohol use/last 30 days
Cigarette use/2 weeks
Incidence of infectious disease by county: rates per 1,000 population
Immunization compliance
Major causes of death

Natural Environment
Days of impaired air quality
Percentage of homes with excessive radon
Potential for asbestos—percentage of homes built before 1950

Courtesy of Partnership Project, Fox Cities, Wisconsin.

Exhibit 32–6 supported the "Coping with Change" theme identified from the data.

The Partnership Project recommended the formation of four coalitions of service providers, funders, and citizens to address the most urgent issues raised during the current community needs assessment process. These coalitions (Figure 32–1) were self-supporting and independent entities linked to the Partnership Project Steering Committee through scheduled reporting sessions. The coalitions were responsible for maintaining data, establishing benchmarks, planning and implementing actions addressing the key community issues, and communicating with the Partnership and the community. The Fox Cities Community Partnership continues to be responsible for defining a shared community vision, evaluating needs, measuring progress toward community goals, and providing a structure for coordination and reports to the community.

PHASE III: IMPLEMENTATION

The Partnership Project realized that in the past, as the community had grown, it had sought to address new or newly discovered problems through studies and the creation of service programs or agencies, public and private. This method led to duplication of services and confusion by the public as to where services could be obtained. Newer models for cooperation and collaboration in service delivery needed to be developed. A model for addressing an identified community need in a collaborative and coordinated fashion was developed.

The action plan included a recommendation to work with the Winnebagoland Focus (a group with a similar purpose and plan in the southern part of Winnebago County) to identify common action plan items and implement them. The Partnership Project also evaluated its process. The Partnership Project is now in

---

Exhibit 32–6 Key Findings

Community human service organizations are providing high-quality assistance and support for community residents.

Human needs are complex and multifaceted and require flexible, insightful solutions.

We have a great need for improved systems of communication, coordination, funding, and human service planning throughout our community.

There exists a need for people to accept responsibility to take action.

Families lie at the heart of our ability to respond to human needs in our community.

Fragmentation and duplication of services have resulted from focused attention to single-issue problems vs. outcomes-based solutions to interconnecting issues.

We need solutions that emphasize cooperation and communication between service providers and those in need of service.

Multiple governmental and agency service areas often provide invisible barriers to service delivery for people in need.

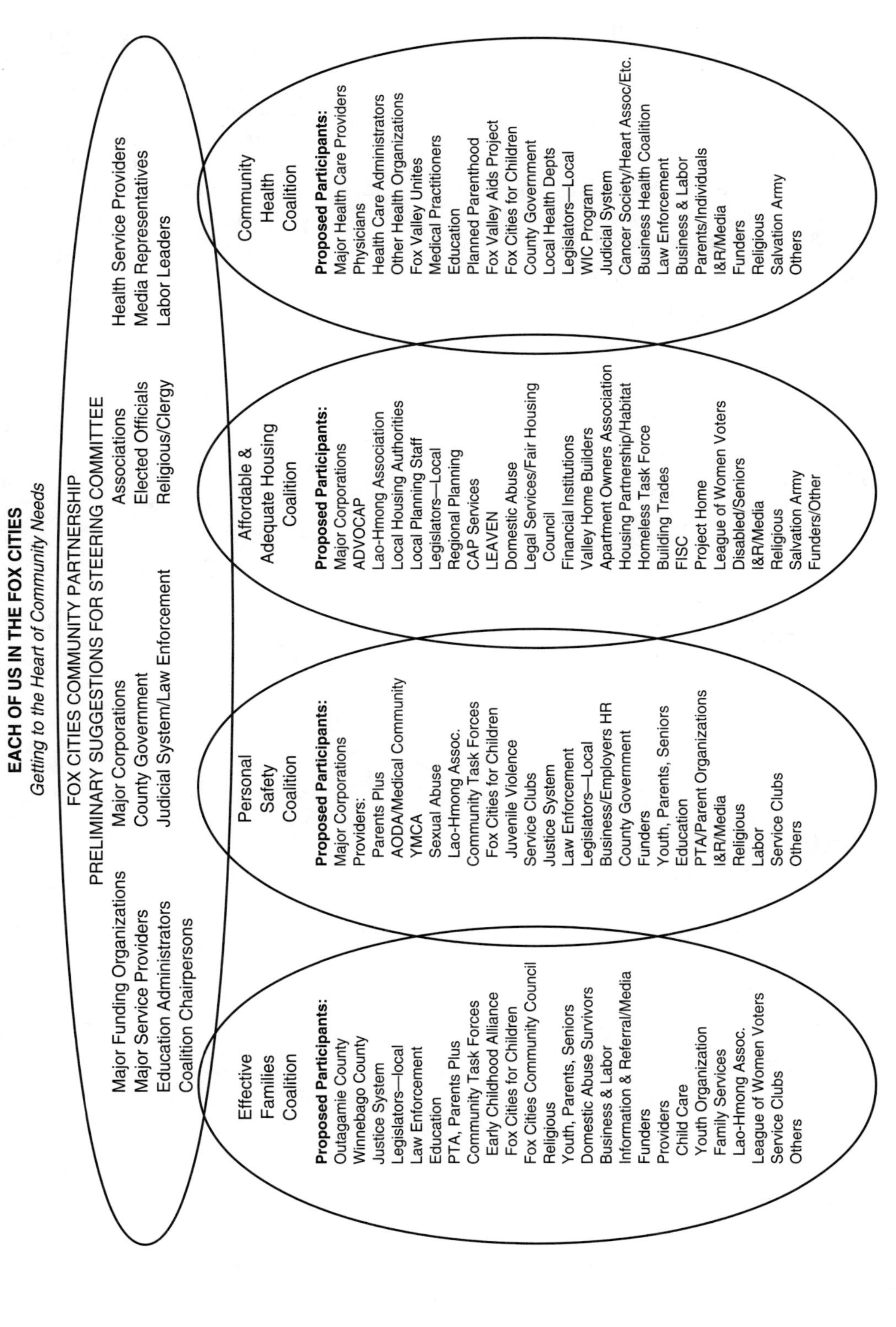

EACH OF US IN THE FOX CITIES
Getting to the Heart of Community Needs

FOX CITIES COMMUNITY PARTNERSHIP
PRELIMINARY SUGGESTIONS FOR STEERING COMMITTEE

Major Funding Organizations   Major Corporations   Associations   Health Service Providers
Major Service Providers   County Government   Elected Officials   Media Representatives
Education Administrators   Judicial System/Law Enforcement   Religious/Clergy   Labor Leaders
Coalition Chairpersons

Effective Families Coalition

Proposed Participants:
Outagamie County
Winnebago County
Justice System
Legislators—local
Law Enforcement
Education
PTA, Parents Plus
Community Task Forces
Early Childhood Alliance
Fox Cities for Children
Fox Cities Community Council
Religious
Youth, Parents, Seniors
Domestic Abuse Survivors
Business & Labor
Information & Referral/Media
Funders
Providers
Child Care
Youth Organization
Family Services
Lao-Hmong Assoc.
League of Women Voters
Service Clubs
Others

Personal Safety Coalition

Proposed Participants:
Major Corporations
Providers:
Parents Plus
AODA/Medical Community
YMCA
Sexual Abuse
Lao-Hmong Assoc.
Community Task Forces
Fox Cities for Children
Juvenile Violence
Service Clubs
Justice System
Law Enforcement
Legislators—Local
Business/Employers HR
County Government
Funders
Youth, Parents, Seniors
Education
PTA/Parent Organizations
I&R/Media
Religious
Labor
Service Clubs
Others

Affordable & Adequate Housing Coalition

Proposed Participants:
Major Corporations
ADVOCAP
Lao-Hmong Association
Local Housing Authorities
Local Planning Staff
Legislators—Local
Regional Planning
CAP Services
LEAVEN
Domestic Abuse
Legal Services/Fair Housing Council
Financial Institutions
Valley Home Builders
Apartment Owners Association
Housing Partnership/Habitat
Homeless Task Force
Building Trades
FISC
Project Home
League of Women Voters
Disabled/Seniors
I&R/Media
Religious
Salvation Army
Funders/Other

Community Health Coalition

Proposed Participants:
Major Health Care Providers
Physicians
Health Care Administrators
Other Health Organizations
Fox Valley Unites
Medical Practitioners
Education
Planned Parenthood
Fox Valley Aids Project
Fox Cities for Children
County Government
Local Health Depts
Legislators—Local
WIC Program
Judicial System
Cancer Society/Heart Assoc/Etc.
Business Health Coalition
Law Enforcement
Business & Labor
Parents/Individuals
I&R/Media
Funders
Religious
Salvation Army
Others

Figure 32–1 Diagram of partnership project coalitions. Courtesy of Partnership Project, Fox Cities, Wisconsin.

the Plan–Do–Check–Act phase of a quality improvement process.

CONCLUSION

The initial phases of the Partnership Project were successful for a number of reasons. First, the team included representation from key stakeholders. Second, the mission and goals were identified early and used frequently to keep the team on task. Third, both quantitative and qualitative data were used as the basis for action planning. Fourth, appropriate quality tools/methods were used to facilitate decision making. Fifth, key community indicators were developed to serve as a means of assessing progress.

Glossary

AAHP: See **American Association of Health Plans (AAHP).**

AAPCC: See **Adjusted Average Per Capita Cost (AAPCC).**

Abstract: Summary of a patient's medical data that provides a basis for classifying the patient according to treatment, diagnosis, age, discharge status, or any of an extensive number of patient attributes.

Acceptability: From the recipient's perception, the degree to which the provided service meets or exceeds the health care need and expectations.

Accessibility: Degree of ease with which the individual or the population can obtain the need when they need it; relates to admittance to the various segments of the health care delivery system in a timely and appropriate fashion.

Accountability: Condition of being responsible for providing a reckoning to the persons who gave the authority to act (the public, a review committee of peers, an employer); the obligation to disclose, in adequate detail and form, appropriate data surrounding an activity or venture (i.e., report cards for professionals/ organizations).

Accreditation: Acknowledgment by an official, independent review agency (e.g., Joint Commission; National League for Nursing; National Committee for Quality Assurance) that the institution or individual meets some predetermined standard of practice; required for third-party reimbursement, training of professionals, etc.

ACR: See **Adjusted Community Rate (ACR).**

Activity: Action that is intended to cause change.

Actual Practice Data: Entries in patients' medical records and other agency records of diagnostic and therapeutic care rendered, including observations; physical, laboratory, and radiology findings; assessment modes; and patient responses.

Actuarial Assumptions: Assumptions an actuary uses in calculating the expected costs/revenues of a health care insurance plan (e.g., utilization rates, age, sex, enrollee mix, cost of services).

Acuity: A measurement of patient severity of illness and usage of resources.

Adequacy: Degree to which the total needs, or the portion of the total need that is specified in the program objectives, are met.

Adjusted Average Per Capita Cost (AAPCC): Used by HCFA to estimate the amount of money it costs to care for Medicare recipients under fee-for-service Medicare in a given area; Medicare risk contract reimbursement based on 95% of the AAPCC on a 5-year rolling average for a county or parish; the 122 actuarial stratifications include factors of age, sex, Medicaid eligibility, institutional status, presence of end-stage renal disease, and whether a person has both Part A and Part B of Medicare.

Adjusted Community Rate/Rating (ACR): A type of rate setting that adjusts for key variables within patient groups; mandated by HCFA as the Medicare projection tool to be used by HMOs and CMPs performing Medicare risk.

Adult Day Care: Geriatric care services directed toward multiple lower cost options for seniors, to include a mix of nursing care, therapy services, group day settings, rehabilitation, and home health care services.

Affordability: Degree to which the service has a monetary cost that is within reasonable reach of the population served.

Agency for Health Care Policy and Research (AHCPR): Created as part of OBRA by Congress in December 1989 (successor to National Center for Health Services Research and Health Care Technology Assessment); Mission: to generate and disseminate information that improves the delivery of health care; Agenda addressing: Patient outcomes research; clinical practice guidelines (19 guidelines as of 1/97); Consumer choice; Quality, cost, and access; Health care delivery; Technology assessments; and Data standards and health information systems development.

Aggregate: To combine standardized data and information; to treat as a whole; a collective body.

Aggregate Data Indicator: A performance measure that quantifies a process or an outcome related to many cases, as opposed to individual cases/events.

AHCPR: See **Agency for Health Care Policy and Research (AHCPR).**

Algorithm: Series of exact, finite steps for addressing a specific problem, with each step dependent on the previous step.

Alpha Testing: First phase of field testing of indicators/standards.

American Association of Health Plans (AAHP): Created with the merger of Group Health Association of America, Inc. (GHAA) and American Managed (Medical) Care and Review Association (AMCRA) in February 1996; trade association serving nearly 1,000 HMOs, PPOs, and other managed-care organizations; representing nearly 100 million enrollees in America.

Appropriateness: Degree of importance and priority of the objectives that are specified for a particular service when compared with other possible objectives for the particular service or other services; the degree to which accurate care is provided, given current knowledge base and available resources.

APR: See **Average Payment Rate (APR).**

Aspects of Care/Service: Key functions, procedures, treatments, processes, or other activities that affect patient care; selection prioritized by experts, organization resources, and importance to patients. Activities or processes that are identified as high-volume, high-risk to the patient (through omission or commission), high-cost, and/or problem prone for patients or providers.

AS-SCORE Index: Severity-of-illness classification system based on five factors: the age of the patient, the systems involved in the illness, the stage of the disease, complications, and the patient's response to therapy (acronym derived from the first letter(s) of each factor).

Assess: To measure, appraise, estimate, or judge the characteristics, qualities, or attributes of a problem, issue, or condition. Approaches to quality assessment include standards-based evaluation, case-based review, and statistical profiling.

Assure: To make sure and give confidence or trust; to guarantee.

Audit (Study): To examine the record of transactions and attest to the excellence of these activities.

(Audit) Study Sample: Selected groups of patients whose care is reviewed in an (audit) study and is therefore considered representative of the care provided to other patients covered by the (audit) study topic.

(Audit) Study Topic: Subject of an (audit) study; may be a diagnosis, problem, surgical procedure, or critical process of care.

Average Payment Rate (APR): Amount HCFA could pay an HMO or CMP for services to Medicare recipients under a risk contract.

Benchmarking: Continuous process of comparing product/service best practices with internal or external competitors; current status of service/process; a point of reference or standard by which others may be measured and continually improved.

Beta Testing: Second phase of field testing of indicators/standards.

Board Certified: A physician or other health professional who has passed an exam from a medical specialty board and is thereby certified to provide care within that specialty.

Brainstorming: Group process technique to help participants suggest ideas in a creative manner through an interactive sequential process; large collection of ideas without regard to validity or judgment (free-form approach).

Capability (Process Capability): A statistical measure of the inherent process variability for a given characteristic, i.e., the standard deviation or a multiple of the standard deviation.

Capital Costs: Costs associated with facilities and equipment, including depreciation and interest expenses.

Capitation: Method of prepaying for health services (rather than on actual cost of separate episodes of care) in which an individual or institutional provider is paid a fixed, per capita amount for each person served without regard to the actual number or nature of services provided to each person (*pmpm*—per member per month).

Care: Actions taken to fulfill responsibility for the positive well-being of persons.

Caregiver: Individual (professional, spouse, family member, or significant other) responsible for assisting the patient's return to maximal functioning.

Caring and Respect: In reference to care providers, attitudes evidenced by facilitation of clients' involvement in their own care decisions and provision of services in a manner that is sensitive and responsive to clients' needs and expectations, including individual differences.

Carve out: A category of health care not covered as a benefit within the contract (thus carved out of the pricing structure), usually an area of high cost or requiring special expertise, such as behavioral, subacute, podiatry, chiropractic, X-ray, or transplants, that is not subject to discretionary utilization and not included within the capitation rate.

Case-Based Review: Review of individual medical records to judge acceptable quality of care delivered.

Case Management: Coordination of treatments or services provided by an organization, including referrals to appropriate community resources and liaisons with other individuals to meet the ongoing identified needs of the patient, to ensure implementation of the plan of care or services, and to avoid unnecessary duplication and over- and underutilization of resources; correct utilization of services based on the patient's need.

Case Mix: Categories of patients (diagnoses/conditions, volume, severity of illness, utilization of resources) treated by an agency, which represent the complexity of the organization's caseload.

Center of Excellence: Health care institution that has been credentialed and, through clinical expertise and capital equipment improvements, has proven ability to provide a major resource-intensive procedure, such as organ or bone marrow transplant, open heart surgery, high-risk obstetrics, or neonatal intensive care, in a more effective and efficient manner than possible anywhere else in a defined region; centers of excellence are listed in the Federal Register.

Certificate of Authority (COA): The state-issued operating license for an HMO.

Certificate of Need (CON): Certificate of approval issued by a governmental agency to an organization that proposes to construct or modify a health care facility, incur a major capital expenditure, or offer a new or different health service.

Certification: Method of payment for health services in which an agency identifies that an individual or organization has met predetermined standards specified by that profession/agency.

CHAMPUS: See **Civilian Health and Medical Program of the Uniformed Services (CHAMPUS).**

CHAP: See **Community Health Accreditation Program (CHAP) of National League for Nursing.**

Charges: Prices assigned to units of health service; may not be related to the actual costs of providing the services. See **MAC.**

CHIN: See **Community Health Integrated Network (CHIN).**

Civilian Health and Medical Program of the Uniformed Services (CHAMPUS): A federal program providing military dependents, and certain others, supplementary civilian-sector hospital and medical services beyond those available in military treatment facilities; basically indemnity insurance coverage (TRICARE Standard).

Claims Data: Information derived from providers' claims to third-party payers.

Clinical Path: Pertaining to actions (actual observations and treatment or process) by health care practitioners.

Clinical Practice Guideline: A process standard that outlines the care, outcomes, time frames, and responsible person(s) for specific patient diagnosis.

Clinical (Practice) Privileges: Authorization by the governing body to provide specific patient care and treatment services in the organization, within well-defined limits, based on an individual's license, education, training, experience, competence, and judgment.

Closed Panel: Managed care plan that contracts with physicians on an exclusive basis for services, not allowing members to access physicians outside of the limited panel of providers for routine care.

CMP: See **Competitive Medical Plan (CMP).**

COA: See **Certificate of Authority (COA).**

COB: See **Coordination of Benefits (COB).**

COBRA: See **Consolidated Omnibus Budget Reconciliation Act of 1985 (COBRA).**

Coinsurance: Form of cost sharing; a general set of financing arrangements whereby the insured must personally pay to receive care at the point of consumption (i.e., upon initiation or during provision of care). A provision in a member's coverage that limits the amount of coverage by the plan to a certain percentage (commonly 80%); additional costs are incurred by the member.

Common Cause Variance: See **Variance.**

Community Health Accreditation Program (CHAP) of National League for Nursing: (Standards for Home Health Care Organizations and Community Health Organizations). HCFA-deemed status for home health agencies accredited by CHAP to participate in Medicare program.

Community Health Integrated Network (CHIN): The collaborative formation of previously independent hospitals, provider networks, or integrated delivery systems in order to provide network HMO-type health care coverage within a given community.

Comorbidity: Preexisting condition that will, because of its presence with a specific principal diagnosis, cause an increase in length of stay by at least 1 day in approximately 75% of cases; disease or condition present at same time as the principal disease or condition.

Competitive Medical Plan (CMP): A federal designation that allows a health plan to obtain eligibility to receive a Medicare risk contract without having to obtain qualification as an HMO.

Compliance: To act in accordance with stated requirements (i.e., preestablished standards); composed of those controllable patient, staff, and system factors that affect performance.

Complication: Condition that arises during the hospital stay that prolongs the length of stay by at least 1 day in approximately 75% of cases.

Complication Rate: Proportion of cases in an audit study whose charts show that medical and/or nursing complications occurred during hospitalization.

CON: See **Certificate of Need (CON).**

Concurrent Monitor: Device that allows continual or frequent monitoring of a procedure, policy, person, or department to ensure that action taken to resolve problems disclosed by retrospective audit is having its desired effect or to identify problems that require further investigation.

Concurrent Review: Monitoring activity that occurs during the provision of services; PRO activity that includes two related mechanisms—admission certification and continued-stay review; certifies the necessity, appropriateness, and quality of services during a hospital episode.

Concurrent Study (Review): Type of patient/medical care evaluation study performed while a patient is still hospitalized; involves process or intermediate outcome criteria and continuous data collection. Allows for alteration of process during hospitalization.

Conditions of Participation (COP): Standards that must be met by an agency in order for it to become a certified provider eligible to receive Medicare and Medicaid funds.

Conformance: Fitting into a set of rules/expectations; an affirmative indication or judgment that a product or service has met the requirement of the relevant specifications, contract, or regulation; absence of defects.

Consolidated Omnibus Budget Reconciliation Act of 1985 (COBRA): A federal law requiring employers to offer continuation benefits to specified workers and families when employment has been terminated; also requires every hospital that participates in Medicare and has an emergency role to treat any patient in an emergency condition or in active labor, whether or not covered by Medicare and regardless of ability to pay.

Continued-Stay Review: Hospital or HMO UR activities to certify the need for a patient's added length of stay.

Continuing Education: Education beyond initial professional preparation that is relevant to the type of patient care delivered in the organization, that provides current knowledge relevant to an individual's field of practice, and that is related to findings from quality assessment and improvement activities.

Continuity: Course or procession; the continuous, orderly, harmonious, forward-moving arrangement of persons or things. In delivery of health care, continuity is the sequence of events in the delivery of care, the coordination among different segments of the system, and the integrated action among members of the team.

Continuous Quality Improvement (CQI): Approach to quality management that builds upon traditional quality assurance methods by emphasizing the organization and systems; focuses on "process" rather than the individual; recognizes both internal and external "customers"; promotes the need for objective data, using statistical process control tools, to analyze and improve processes. Implies that a process and its service/outcome are never optimized (core of TQM philosophy). "If it ain't broke, make it better" on the basis of understanding and control of variation. CQI and quality assurance are not synonymous; they enjoy a symbiotic relationship.

Continuum of Care: Concept that health care providers maintain consistent patient treatment and service regardless of health care setting; a spectrum of health care options, ranging from limited care needs through tertiary care, to provide the appropriate expertise for the patient without providing a more expensive setting than necessary.

Control Chart: See **Statistical Quality Control Techniques.**

Control Limits: Expected upper and lower limits (thresholds) of common-cause variation (not specification or tolerance limits), based on past performance and national regulatory standards. The limits are used as criteria for signaling the need for action or for judging whether a set of data does or does not indicate a state of statistical control.

Coordination of Benefits (COB): Agreement that prevents double payment for services when a subscriber has coverage from two or more sources; National Association of Insurance Commissioners developed language/ order for primary and secondary payment sources.

COP: See **Conditions of Participation (COP).**

Copayment: That portion of a claim or medical expense that a member must pay.

COQ: See **Costs of Quality (COQ).**

Costs: Actual expenses incurred in the provision of services or goods.

Costs of Quality (COQ): Concept defined by Juran in the 1950s: costs incurred due to bad quality within a given process; the price of doing it wrong (not conforming to requirements); the price of inspecting.

Council: The group of individuals assigned accountability for a specific ongoing function within the organization (e.g., Quality Council).

CPT-4: *Current Procedural Terminology*, fourth edition—a set of five-digit codes that apply to medical services delivered; used for billing by professionals.

CQI: See **Continuous Quality Improvement (CQI).**

Credentialing: The review process by a hospital or insurer to approve a provider; a careful review of documents, medical license, evidence of malpractice insurance, and educational background of professional providers.

Criteria: Objective, predetermined elements of health care, the presence, absence, and completeness of which indicate the quality and appropriateness of an aspect of care; substantiated by policies and procedures, rules and regulations, current knowledge, and/or generally accepted standards.

Criteria, Empirical: Criteria derived from actual practice.

Criteria, Essential: Research-based criteria that are predictive of specific outcomes.

Criteria, Implicit: Subjective, internal opinions that "peer" evaluators use in defining good practice.

Criteria Mapping: Process evaluation method to assess clinical decision making based on the presence or absence of certain signs, symptoms, and patient needs.

Criteria, Normative: Opinions of experts as to what constitutes good care.

Criterion: Standard, model, norm, test, or rule used in comparisons; an indicator that represents a desired level of patient care used for the purpose of screening large numbers of patient records to determine the quality of care provided. In study methods, a criterion consists of an element (minimum essential evidence of an aspect of care), a standard (desired occurrence or nonoccurrence of the element, expressed as a percentage), and an exception (acceptable reasons or circumstances that account for the absence [or presence] of an element in a patient's record).

Criterion, Outcome: Desired results in terms of maintenance or changes in health status.

Criterion, Process: Elements of appropriate clinical management.

Criterion, Structural: Desired hospital and health care organization and resources for the provision of care.

Critical Management: Elements of care attached to complication criteria whose presence in a chart tends to demonstrate that known preventive measures were taken or that the occurrence of the complication was recognized and that appropriate responsive measures were taken.

Critical Path: Various steps involved in a work process; required tasks to accomplish an objective or meet a goal.

Critical Process: A process that is high volume, high risk, problem prone, and high cost; important to the patient or provider.

Cross-Department/Function/Service/Organization Study: Monitoring/evaluation review in which representatives from two or more departments, functions, or services ("teams") develop criteria and analyze variations from predetermined criteria pertinent to the respective areas.

Cultural Change: In total quality management (TQM) philosophy, a paradigm shift from traditional management by results to "top-down" total quality management; organizational culture characterized by a shared vision, values, and leadership, empowered employees, openness to feedback and data, and cooperation/collaboration among organizational units as they work to improve processes; reflects beliefs and behaviors inherent in individuals/organization.

Customer: The receiver or beneficiary of an output of a workgroup process (products, services, or information); it is possible to be both a customer of one process and a supplier of another. (Sometimes interchangeable with *consumer, client, patient, or resident.*)

Customer-Driven Organization: Recognition of (based on) customer/supplier relationships.

Customers, External: Patients, physicians, business community, insurers, contract employees, etc.

Customers, Internal: Employees; all individuals employed by an organization involved in producing the product/service.

Data: The collection of facts, materials, or items (measurements or statistics) used as a basis for discussion and decision making.

Data Accuracy: Degree to which data required by indicators are free of errors.

Data Completeness: Degree to which data required by indicators exist and are available for use.

Data Pattern: Identifiable grouping or distribution of data characteristics relative to a data set that may trigger further investigation of the event monitored by a process or outcome indicator.

Data Retrieval: Gathering of patient care or professional practice information from medical records and other sources.

Data Trend: A movement or general direction forming a data pattern on a run chart or control chart that rises or falls in a series of points; becomes a concern when the points exceed predetermined upper or lower limits.

Database: An organized collection of data in a standardized format, typically stored in a computer system so that any particular item or set of items can be extracted or organized as needed.

Deductible: The minimum threshold payment that must be made by the enrollee each year before the plan begins to make payments on a shared or total basis; a common cost-sharing arrangement of traditional indemnity insurers in which a policy holder must pay a set amount toward covered services before the insurer is required to pay claims.

Deficiency: Determination by the auditor/committee that a given variation from an audit criterion is, in fact, a sign of substandard performance by the institution/individuals responsible for care; a deviation from preestablished standards/criteria.

Deployment Chart: A graphic representation of the flow of a process and which people or groups are involved at each step. Charts show the major steps of a process along with which person or group is the center of the activity for that step.

Diagnosis-Related Groups (DRGs): Classification scheme that categorizes patients who are medically related with respect to diagnoses, presence of a surgical procedure, age, sex, and presence or absence of significant comorbidities or complications and who are statistically similar in their length of stay; form of prospective reimbursement system (PRS) used by HCFA for Medicare recipients, as well as some states and private health plans for contracting purposes since October 1, 1983.

Dimensions of Performance: Characteristics of organizational performance that are related to organizations' "doing the right thing well the first time."

Discharge Planning: Process of assessing needs and obtaining or coordinating appropriate resources for patients as they move through the health care system in preparation for leaving an organization.

Discharge Summary: Written record including (1) the date and reason for discharge, (2) the status of problems identified on admission and subsequently, (3) the overall status of the patient, and (4) a summary of the care and services provided.

Disease State Management Measures: Indicators of the health plan's success in treating the entirety of a disease across the continuum of care (related to the family of outcome measures that treat the disease as opposed to managing health); may include measures for major diagnostic categories (e.g., hypertension, diabetes), primary care (e.g., patient satisfaction, utilization of preventive services, illness episodes per 1,000), specialty care (e.g., diagnostic or therapeutic guidance compliance, diagnosis-specific health status scores), acute care episodes (e.g., average length of stay per major DRG categories, surgeries per 1,000, readmission rates), or rehab and recovery (pa-

tient compliance, DRG-specific health status scores).

DME: See **Durable Medical Equipment (DME).**

Documentation: The information recorded as a result of data collection, planning, interventions provided, and evaluation.

Documentation Variation: Variation so designated because documentation is absent, insufficient, or too ambiguous to determine whether actual practice conformed to a criterion.

DRGs: See **Diagnosis-Related Groups (DRGs).**

Dual Choice: Employees' option of joining an HMO, or an indemnity insurance plan, as a basic entitlement.

Dual Eligible: A beneficiary who is eligible for Medicare and Medicaid.

Durable Medical Equipment (DME): Equipment that can endure repeated use without being subject to disposal after one-time use (e.g., insulin pumps, wheelchairs).

Effectiveness: Degree to which specified objectives are attained as a result of activities; level of benefit to patients when care is provided appropriately; the degree to which the care/intervention is provided in the correct manner, given the current state of knowledge, to achieve the desired/projected outcome(s) for the patient.

Efficacy: Probability of benefit to patients in a defined population from a medical technology or interpretation applied for a given problem under ideal conditions/circumstances; the degree to which the care/intervention used for the patient has been shown to accomplish the desired/projected outcome(s).

Efficiency: Cost of resources—money, effort, and waste used to attain specified objectives; the ratio of the outcomes (results of care/intervention) for a patient to the resources used to deliver the care.

Employee Retirement Income Security Act of 1974 (ERISA): A federal law that mandates reporting and disclosure requirements for group life and health plans, with relevant guidance on the sponsorship, administration, and servicing of plans, some claims processing, and appeals regulations.

Empowerment: Employee involvement and motivation; the assignment of ownership of a process to an employee; enabling employees to assume authority over their practice without undue interference.

EMR: Electronic medical record.

Enrollment Area: The area specified by an HMO in which an individual must reside in order to be eligible for plan coverage.

EPO: See **Exclusive Provider Organization (EPO).**

ERISA: See **Employee Retirement Income Security Act of 1974 (ERISA).**

Evaluation: Determination of the outcome achieved by an activity (or activities) designed to attain a valued objective; mechanisms by which a program/service will be monitored, including quality assessment, customer satisfaction, and research; assessment of quality and/or appropriateness of care, service, continuity, and resources, based on measurement against criteria, or preestablished levels of performance (thresholds, benchmarks).

Evaluation Study: Systematic, in-depth appraisal of care accomplished by using predetermined structure, process, or outcome criteria and a wide variety of data collection techniques, such as interviewing, observation, reviewing of patient records, and performing of patient satisfaction surveys.

Exception: Clearly defined reason, instance, or circumstance that, if documented in the patient record, accounts for the absence (or presence) of the element in the record, or alternate secondary evidence that is acceptable to the reviewer.

Exclusive Provider Organization (EPO): Form of CMP; similar to an HMO in that it uses primary physicians as gatekeepers, often capitates providers, has a limited provider panel, uses an authorization system, etc.; generally regulated under insurance statutes rather than HMO regulations.

Expert: Individual who has appropriate knowledge and experience pertinent to a given need.

Facilitator: Expert serving as a process guide, teacher, and consultant in connecting the work to the knowledge necessary for improvement (e.g., team facilitator).

Feedback: Information (data) communicated to an individual (or individuals); the return to a point of origin of evaluative or corrective information about an action or process; the return to the input of a part of the output of a system or process.

Fee-for-service: Method of payment under which providers are paid for each service performed.

Fishbone Diagram: See **Statistical Quality Control Techniques.**

Flowchart: See **Statistical Quality Control Techniques.**

Focused Review: Concentrated review, usually by an accrediting body, of key or important areas of care (high-volume or high-risk events, or events with a history of associated problems); time frame individually determined by topic being studied.

FOCUS-PDCA Cycle: Sometimes referred to as the Deming or Shewhart cycle. Strategy that helps build knowledge of process, customer, and small-scale improvement, using the scientific method; improvements are planned, tried, and checked to see if they deserve to be implemented or abandoned. Acronym meaning: *F*ind a process to improve, *O*rganize a team that knows the process, *C*larify current knowledge of the process, *U*nderstand sources of process variation, *S*elect the process improvement, *P*lan the improvement, *D*ata collection and analysis. *C*heck and study the results, *A*ct to hold the gain and to improve the process.

Follow-up: Deliberate action taken to ensure the continuing resolution of a problem (issue).

Force-Field Analysis: Technique matching the driving forces and the restraining forces to help in thinking about the influence of these factors in determining the best course of action.

Fraud & Abuse Legislation: Federal laws that include the original Social Security Act against making false benefit claims or statements (1965); the criminal and felony treatment of kickback schemes (1977); civil penalties against providers submitting improper claims for Medicare and Medicaid (1981), with yet broader restrictions in 1987.

Function (Key): Goal-directed interrelated series of processes believed to have a significant effect on the probability of desired patient outcomes. A high-risk function exposes patients to a greater chance of adverse occurrences if not performed effectively and/or appropriately or is inherently risky due to patient characteristics or newness of services. A high-volume function is performed frequently or affects large numbers of patients. A problem-prone function has historically created problems for the patient, organization, and/or professional.

Gatekeeper: A term sometimes used to refer to a Primary Care Physician (PCP/NP) or, in some settings, to a nurse practitioner, because of their responsibility for referring members to hospitals, HMOs, and other health care settings.

Generic Algorithm: Mathematical procedure developed to approximate the impact that a patient's procedures and secondary diagnoses could have on the costs of hospitalization; discriminates among the variety of diagnoses and procedures and provides for all possible combinations encountered in patient populations.

Generic Screen: Review and display of patient care using criteria that apply equally to all patients, regardless of sources of, or persons responsible for, care ordered or provided.

Goal: The desired, measurable end results toward which activities/resources are directed.

Governance Model: A visual portrayal of the type of governance style being used by the health care organization's leadership.

Governing Board: Group of individuals who are responsible for adopting written governing policies (e.g., bylaws, mission/vision statement) detailing services to be provided and management of the agency, and who oversee the quality of care provided to patients by employed staff and individuals under contract.

Grievance Procedure: Process by which an individual may file complaints and seek remedies from an offending individual/organization; may include board reviews or outside arbitrators.

Guidelines: Descriptive tools that are standardized specifications for care developed by a formal process that incorporates the best scientific evidence with expert opinion; usually pertain to practitioner practice for "typical" patient in the "typical" situation. Accepted synonyms: *clinical standards, practices, parameters, protocols*.

Health Care Financing Administration (HCFA): Federal agency overseeing all aspects of health financing for Medicare and the Office of Prepaid Health Care.

Health Care Quality Improvement Act of 1986 (HCQIA): A federal law addressing peer review and credentialing activity that seeks to improve the quality of care; the act grants immunity that prevents quality-related functions and programs from falling under state and federal antitrust laws.

Health Care Reform Act of 1996: Enacted 7/1/96 (effective 1/1/97); includes $8-million-per-year grant program to ensure, through quality and accountability measures, that ending its 14-year history of setting prospective reimbursement rates for hospitals will not erode access to or outcomes of health care. Creates a 30-member task force on health care quality improvement and information systems; has a broader mandate than the existing Task Force on Guidelines and Medical Technology;

funds collaborative community-based efforts to measure and improve health status.

Health Maintenance Organization (HMO): Prepaid medical insurance based on an ambulatory care-preventive medicine model; provides health care for a preset amount of money on a per-member per-month basis. Three basic organizational types: (1) staff—each practitioner is employed by the HMO; (2) group practice—involves different specialties practicing as a group; and (3) independent practice association (IPA)—independent physicians in private practice who contract with HMO to provide care to members within their private office setting.

Health Plan Data Information Set (HEDIS): A group of performance measures that gives employers objective information with which to evaluate health plans and hold them accountable; used by National Committee for Quality Assurance (NCQA) for HMOs, etc.

HEDIS: See **Health Plan Data Information Set (HEDIS).**

High Risk: An important process, procedure, or activity that exposes a patient to potentially undesirable outcomes if not carried out effectively or appropriately; has implications for financial security (e.g., malpractice, suing) of an organization.

High Volume: A process, procedure, or activity that is performed frequently or affects large numbers of patients.

Histogram: See **Statistical Quality Control Techniques.**

HMO: See **Health Maintenance Organization (HMO).**

Home Health Care: That component of comprehensive health care in which services are provided to individuals and families in their residences for the purpose of promoting, maintaining, or restoring health or minimizing the effects of illness and disability. Services appropriate to the needs of the individual patient and family are planned and coordinated by a home health care agency using employed staff or through contractual agreements.

ICD-9-CM: *International/National Classification of Diseases*, ninth edition, *Code Manual*. Classification of disease by diagnosis, codified into four-digit numbers; frequently used for billing purposes.

IDS: See **Integrated Delivery System (IDS)/Integrated Health Care System.**

Incident Report: Formal reporting mechanism through which exceptional occurrences taking place within an organization are identified.

Indemnity: The insurance protection against injury or loss of health.

Independent Practitioner Organization (IPO): Similar to an IPA; physicians contract with a variety of health care plans for a variety of services (health care, utilization review, etc.). A mixed-model IPO is a managed-care plan with both closed- and open-panel delivery systems.

Indicator: Measure of specific, measurable, objective events, occurrences, facets of treatment, etc. May be a structure (i.e., a resource), process (i.e., measures an event or activity performed directly or indirectly for patients), or outcome of care (i.e., a process or patient health status) measure. Used to monitor and evaluate the quality and appropriateness of important governance, management, clinical, and support functions that affect patient outcomes; professionally developed, clinically valid, and reliable aspect of the health care process, clinical event, complication, or outcome for which data can be collected and compared with criteria related to the indicator. Two types of indicators are (1) *rate-based*—assess events for which a certain proportion of the events that occur represent expected care; significant trends/patterns in data require ongoing investigation (e.g., medication errors, nosocomial infections, inadequate staffing, patient falls, equipment failure); and (2) *sentinel event*—assess "serious," predictable events that require further investigation for each occurrence. Threshold always set at 0%.

Indicator Reliability: Degree to which indicator accurately and completely identifies indicator occurrences from among all cases at risk of being an indicator occurrence.

Indicator Validity: Degree to which indicator identifies events that merit further review.

Integrated Delivery System (IDS)/Integrated Health Care System: A health care system that provides all types and levels of health care services within the same health plan, including primary, secondary, tertiary, community, and home care. *Horizontal integration*: the formation of health entities that contain multiple groupings of similar care components along the continuum of care, with financial incentives for alignment into the larger group (e.g., multiple hospitals, long-term care, home care). *Vertical integration*: the connecting of dissimilar or other than horizontal entities (e.g., HMO, hospitals, physician practices).

IPA: Independent practice association; see **Health Maintenance Organization (HMO).**

IPO: See **Independent Practitioner Organization (IPO).**

Joint Commission on Accreditation of Healthcare Organizations (Joint Commission): Founded in 1951, a private, not-for-profit organization dedicated to improving the quality of patient care in hospitals, long-term care, ambulatory care, mental health, home care, home medical equipment, hospice, laboratory, pharmacy, managed care, preferred provider organizations, behavioral health care, and other organized delivery services through standards setting, survey evaluation, accreditation decision making, and education.

Justification: Category of criteria that evaluates the appropriateness of medical intervention; also a clinically supportive reason that renders acceptable a record from audit criteria, thereby permitting the record to pass committee review and eliminating it from further study.

Kaizen: Japanese concept—a continual improvement process involving everyone in a personal quest for excellence; reflects Deming's focus (see **Quality Improvement Gurus**).

Key Functions: Functions having the greatest effect on the quality of care the patient ultimately receives: *patient-focused functions*, including (1) patient rights and organizational ethics, (2) patient assessment, (3) care of patients, (4) education, and (5) continuum of care, and *organizational functions*, including (1) performance improvements; (2) leadership; (3) management of the environment of care; (4) management of human resources; (5) management of management; and (6) surveillance, prevention, and control of infection. Structures within functions include governance, management, medical staff, and nursing.

Levels of Care/Staging: Outcome-oriented evaluation method to determine the severity of medical problems or functional limitations at time of admission.

Licensed Independent Practitioner: Individual permitted by law and an organization to provide patient care services without direction or supervision, within the scope of his or her license and in accordance with individually granted clinical privileges.

Licensure: Process by which an agency of the state government grants permission to individuals accountable for the practice of a profession and prohibits all others from legally practicing. Home health care agency or nursing home licensure is the process by which a state recognizes and authorizes an agency to operate. The agency must meet minimum operational standards (varying in each state) and comply with the state's certificate of need (CON), in states where applicable.

MAC: Maximum allowable charge.

Managed Care: A method of delivering and paying for health care through a system of networks of providers. Managed care seeks to ensure the quality and contain the cost of comprehensive medical care. Managed-care plans include HMOs, PPOs, EPOs, point-of-service plans, and similar coordinated care networks.

Managed Competition: A system that provides for universal coverage, with employer's contribution of a fixed sum for the employee's plan of choice and with transferable coverage between jobs; designed to discourage unnecessary utilization by the client; allows for selection of care plans offering the most competitive rates; concept drafted by the "Jackson Hole Group."

Management Information System (MIS): Computer hardware and software that provide the data gathering and manipulation support for a program/organization.

Management Services Organization (MSO): A legal entity that offers practice management and administrative support to physicians or that purchases physician practices and obtains payer contracts as a physician hospital organization.

Maximization: Intentional manipulation of data to optimize reimbursement.

MCE: See **Medical Care Evaluation (MCE).**

MCO: Managed-care organization.

Measurable: Being objectively quantifiable or assessable by the use of standard measuring devices.

Measure: Device for gauging the quantity and quality of some dimension of performance of a function or process.

Measurement: The systematic process of data collection, about a single event or repeated over time; the process of quantifying the amount, degree, capacity, or dimensions of something.

Measurement Validity: Absence of random and/or systematic measurement error.

Medicaid (Title XIX): Amendment to the Social Security Act, passed in 1965; government program of health insurance for the eligible aged (65 and over) and disabled; financed by both the state and federal governments.

Medical Care Evaluation (MCE): Process of studying the effectiveness and efficiency of medical care delivered to patients, resulting in recommendations for change beneficial to patients, staff, facility, and community; required by governmental bodies.

Medical Record: Permanent document recording an individual's health care; includes patient identification, diagnoses, care needs, plans, outcomes, and other data required by external and internal review bodies; does not include data collected for quality assurance purposes.

Medicare (Title XVIII): Government program of health insurance for the eligible aged (65 and over) and disabled; financed by the federal government; authorized in 1965 to cover costs of hospitalization, medical care, and some related services. Part A is hospital insurance (inpatient), and Part B is supplementary medical insurance; covers outpatient and physician costs; operated by HCFA; amendment to the Social Security Act (Medicare Preservation Act of 1995: plan to preserve, protect, and strengthen Medicare and maintain its solvency in the face of projected bankruptcy by 2002).

Minutes: Record of business introduced, transactions and reports made, conclusions reached, and recommendations made by officers, committees, and others involved in quality issues. Copies of reports filed in the quality assurance committee report book should indicate page number in minutes.

MIS: See **Management Information System.**

Mission: The overall purpose (business) in which an organization is engaged; reflects values and beliefs of organization.

Monitoring: Planned, systematic, and ongoing collection, compilation, and organization of data about an indicator of the quality and/or appropriateness of an important aspect of care, and the comparison of those data to a preestablished level of performance to determine the need for improvement.

Morbidity: The prevalence and rate of disease for a given population within a stated region.

Mortality: Death rate; the prevalence of death at each age based on previous actual experience for a given population or persons within a particular region.

MSO: See **Management Services Organization.**

Multidisciplinary Study: Type of patient/medical care evaluation study in which representatives of two or more professional disciplines develop criteria and analyze variations from criteria pertinent to their respective disciplines.

Multivote (Multiple Voting): A group decision-making technique designed to reduce a lengthy list to one of manageable size.

National Committee for Quality Assurance (NCQA): An independent, private-sector group formed in 1979 to review care quality and other procedures of HMOs and similar types of managed care plans to render an accreditation.

Nominal Group Technique: A structured group decision process used to arrive at consensus. Provides a way for everyone in a group to have an equal voice in the group's choice. Useful technique when all or some group members are new to each other, when some members may dominate others, when highly controversial issues are discussed, or when a team is stuck in disagreement.

Objective: Measurable, realistic activity that is performed to achieve a goal.

OBRA: See **Omnibus Budget Reconciliation Act of 1985 (OBRA).**

Occurrence Screen: Screen used for concurrent identification of signal events that warrant review, either as individual events or in the aggregate.

Omnibus Budget Reconciliation Act of 1985 (OBRA): Portions of this act created Quality Review Organizations (QROs) and empowered QROs and peer review organizations

(PROs) to monitor quality of care for Medicare recipients.

Outcome: Product (results) of one or more processes (e.g., complications, adverse events, and short- and longer-term results of care and service); the degree to which outputs meet the needs and expectations of the customer.

Outcome Audit: Review of end result of care.

Outliers: Patients displaying atypical characteristics relative to other patients in a DRG.

Patterns of Care: Overall statistical performance profile of the clinical behavior of all persons involved in the care of the patients in a study or of the institution as a whole.

PCP: See **Primary Care Physician (PCP).**

PDCA Cycle: See **Plan–Do–Check–Act (PDCA) Cycle.**

Peer: An equal. In delivery of care, peers are those who are involved together in goal-directed care transactions with a very specific patient population and who thereby have a high degree of expertness.

Peer Review: Review of colleagues by colleagues of the quality and efficiency of services ordered and/or performed; focuses on improving practice.

Peer Review Organization (PRO): Successor of PSRO (Professional Standards Review Organization); effective November 15, 1984; agency having contract with organizations for utilization review functions; to monitor quality of medically appropriate and necessary services and review validity of diagnosis and procedures and appropriateness of admission and discharge; current primary functions: health partnerships—development of cooperative quality enhancing projects for Medicare patients.

Per Diem Reimbursement: Payment based on a set rate per day rather than on charges; may vary by service or be uniform regardless of intensity of services.

Performance: The execution of an activity or pattern of behavior; the application of inherent and/or learned capabilities to complete a process according to prescribed specifications or standards.

Performance-Based Quality-of-Care Evaluation: System employing guidelines and standards that provide the basis for describing an appropriate and effective course of action, and performance indicators that determine whether the course of action was followed and its effect on patient outcomes.

Performance Review: Review of individual's objective characteristics as well as the contributions made to the organization's quality improvement efforts; an activity that involves collecting performance data, comparing actual results with projected behaviors to determine variance, and designing an improvement plan with designated time frames.

PERT: See **Program Evaluation and Review Technique (PERT).**

Philosophy: Values and beliefs of an organization regarding customer service, staff performance, and governance.

Plan–Do–Check–Act Cycle: Sometimes referred to as the Deming or Shewhart cycle; the scientific methodology in which improvements are planned, tried, and checked to see if they deserve to be implemented or abandoned. See **FOCUS-PDCA Cycle.**

Plan of Treatment (POT): Proposed plan of care for the patient written by the attending physician or written by a nurse and countersigned by a physician; includes a description of the types of services to be provided, the frequency and duration of treatment, the diagnosis, any functional limitations, medications and diet, needed medical supplies, and the expected outcome of treatment.

Policy: A structure standard that defines the service, practice, and governance rules of an organization; creates a legal threat to the customer, employee, or organization when not heeded.

POT: See **Plan of Treatment (POT).**

PPO: See **Preferred Provider Organization (PPO).**

PPS: See **Prospective Payment System (PPS).**

Practice Guidelines: Descriptive tool or standardized specification(s) for care of the typical patient in a typical situation; developed by experts using scientific evidence of effectiveness; a written process standard for symptom/disease management for client care to improve the quality of clinical and consumer decision making, reduce cost using appropriate treatment interventions. *ANA*: "includes assessment and diagnosis, planning, intervention, evaluation and outcome," *Joint Commission*: "a descriptive tool or standardized specification(s) for the care of the 'typical' patient in the 'typical' situation." *AHCPR*: "a systematically developed statement to assist practitioner and patient decisions about appropriate health care for specific clinical circumstances."

Preferred Provider Organization (PPO): Organization with discounted "fee for services" contract between employers and providers; a health plan in which a member's health care services are completely paid for if obtained from one of a select group of "preferred" providers chosen by the plan or are partially paid if obtained from an unaffiliated provider.

Primary Care: Focuses on the prevention and early detection of health problems through regular physicals, blood pressure tests, immunizations, mammograms, and similar procedures.

Primary Care Physician (PCP): A physician who provides, arranges, authorizes, coordinates, and monitors the care of HMO members. Primary care physicians are usually internists, family practitioners, or pediatricians. Member chooses a PCP.

PRO: See **Peer Review Organization (PRO).**

Problem: Deviation from accepted standard of patient care or professional practice.

Problem-Focused Approach: Activities designed to eliminate or reduce problems with patient care or professional practice.

Procedure: A series of specified behaviors for the completion of a specific task or activity.

Process: Series of ordered steps to a desired outcome; manner in which service will be delivered; activities and interactions that act upon an "input" from a "supplier" to produce an "output" for a "customer"; activities carried out by health care professionals in their care for patients (e.g., assessment, treatment planning, test ordering and interpretation, medication administration, performance of invasive procedures, and discharge planning); whole or totality of the service; includes the outcomes, activities, continuity, resources, and population dimensions of the service.

Process Audit: Evaluation based on process measures; conducted during hospitalization.

Process Capability: The measured built-in reproducibility of the outcome of a process.

Productivity: The process of yielding favorable, desirable, or useful results.

Professional Advisory Board: Group of individuals (physician, nurse, and appropriate representatives from other professional disciplines who are neither owners nor employers of the organization) who periodically review an organization's services, including the quality of care provided and received, and make recommendations to the governing board concerning them.

Professional Standards Review Organization (PSRO): Organization created by 1972 amendments to the Social Security Act, designed to involve local health professionals in the ongoing review and evaluation of health care services covered by Medicare, Medicaid, and maternal/child health (MCH) programs. The legislation (Public Law 92-603) was based on the concepts that health professionals are the most appropriate individuals to evaluate the quality of medical services and that effective peer review at the local level is the soundest method for ensuring the appropriate use of health care resources and facilities. Predecessor of PRO.

Profile Analysis: Retrospective reviews through which aggregate patient care data are compiled to analyze the patterns of health care services and lengths of stay.

Program Evaluation and Review Technique (PERT): Chart that aids in the reduction of overall project time by showing which things can be done simultaneously and enabling a reduction of delays between things that are done sequentially.

Prospective Payment System (PPS): Established by Title VI of the Social Security Amendments of 1983 and developed and implemented by HCFA to pay health care facilities for Medicare patients.

Prospective Review: Monitoring and evaluating the necessity for hospitalization or a service prior to admission to determine if it is medically necessary and at the appropriate level of care.

Provider: Health care professional or organization that provides health care services to patients.

PSRO: See **Professional Standards Review Organization (PSRO).**

QA: See **Quality Assurance (QA).**

QI: Quality improvement. See **Continuous Quality Improvement (CQI).**

QM: See **Quality Management (QM).**

Quality: Distinguishing characteristics that determine the value, rank, or degree of excellence or expectation; the totality of features and characteristics of a health care process that bear on its ability to satisfy stated or implied needs; a process or outcome that consistently conforms to requirements, meets expectations, and maximizes value or utility for the customer. For the customer: getting what you were expecting and more; for the supplier: getting it right the first time, every time. *Joint Com-*

mission: "the degree to which patient care services increase the probability of desired patient outcomes and reduce the probability of undesired outcomes given the current state of knowledge."

Quality Assessment: Measurement of the level of quality at some point in time; monitoring, data collection, and making a judgment regarding adequacy with no effort to change or improve. Not synonymous with quality assurance.

Quality Assurance (QA): Distinguishing characteristics that determine the value or degree of excellence and the mechanisms to efficiently and effectively monitor and improve patient care provided by competent professionals with appropriate resources; the quantitative and qualitative measurement of the quality of existing processes and systems. QA builds quality into the design of new products and services.

Quality Control: Retrospective inspection; comparing a random sample of a product with a predetermined acceptable threshold for defects using statistical measures; originally used in the manufacturing industry with inspection of equipment.

Quality Function Deployment: A system that identifies the needs of the customer and gets that information to all the right people so that the organization can effectively meet the customer's most important needs.

Quality Improvement (QI): See **Continuous Quality Improvement.**

Quality Improvement "Gurus": Individuals responsible for designing, refining, and popularizing TQM (CQI, QI). *Dr. W. Edwards Deming*—introduced to Japan, post W.W. II, 14 principles (Obligations to Management): (1) create constancy of purpose for improvement of product and service; (2) adopt the new philosophy (cultural change); (3) cease dependence on mass inspection; (4) end the practice of awarding business on price tag alone; (5) improve constantly and forever the system of production and service; (6) institute training; (7) institute leadership; develop performance measures; (8) drive out fear; (9) break down barriers between departments and staff; (10) eliminate goals, slogans, exhortations, and targets for the work force; (11) eliminate numerical quotas; (12) institute massive training in statistical techniques; (13) institute a vigorous program of education and training; and (14) establish "teams" to accomplish the transformation. *Dr. Walter Shewhart*—introduced quality control chart based on the principles of statistical techniques and a model of linked quarter circles: Plan, Do, Check, Act. *Dr. Joseph Juran* introduced error-tree performance philosophy and "fitness for use" as a central theme for quality improvement, in which the customer defines/dictates what is "fit for using." *Dr. Kaoru Ishikawa*—introduced "cause-and-effect" diagram; *Philip Crosby*—introduced "art of corporate wellness," zero-free defects, and a positive approach that the employee knows there is a right way and will do the right thing. *Dr. E.A. Codman*—introduced QI to medicine in 1912. *Dr. Avedis Donabedian*—introduced structure, process, and outcome model. *Dr. Donald Berwick,* a pediatrician and health services researcher at Harvard Community Health Plan, led the National Demonstration Project (NDP) in 1987, with Dr. Paul Batalden, a pediatrician and currently with Dartmouth-Hitchcock Medical Center, Hanover, New Hampshire and A. Blanton Godfrey, Vice President of the Juran Institute.

Quality Management (QM): The process by which people and other resources are mobilized to achieve quality goals. See **Total Quality Management (TQM).**

Quality of Care: Degree to which services increase the probability of desired patient outcomes and reduce the probability of undesired outcomes, given the current state of knowledge. Determined by nine components: accessibility, appropriateness, continuity, effectiveness, efficacy, efficiency, patient perspectives issues, safety of care environment, and timeliness of care. Quality is customer's perception (reality) of the product/service and the supplier's knowledge of customer requirements, variation between customers, and applicable standards of practice.

Randomization: Distribution of items (individuals) such that all have an equal chance for selection in proportion to their frequency or occurrence within the population under study.

Rate-Based Review: Program of review by an external body of charges for health care, for the purpose of controlling or containing the rise in cost of care; the external body may be a hospital association, a third-party payer, or the government.

Reengineering: "The fundamental rethinking and radical redesign of business processes to achieve dramatic improvements in critical, contemporary measures of performance, such as cost, quality, service, and speed" (Hammer & Champy, 1993). Reengineering is not about fixing processes; it is about starting all over from scratch.

Reimbursement, Cost-Based: Amount of payment based on the costs to the provider of delivering the service (i.e., full cost, full cost plus an additional percentage, allowable cost, or a fraction of costs).

Reimbursement, Prospective: Payment method set prior to rendering services; based on expected classes and volumes of patients (e.g., DRGs, HMOs); capitation; involves some financial risk for organization.

Reimbursement, Retrospective: Payment to providers by a third-party carrier for costs or charges actually incurred by subscribers in a previous time period.

Reliability: The ability of an indicator to identify accurately the targeted events across multiple organizations; reproducibility of findings.

Report Cards: NCQA comparative reports on a core set of HEDIS measures. Consumer-supplied comparative data regarding the quality of a health plan performance. Surveys conducted by the NCQA, HCFA, the Federal Employee Health Benefits Program (Washington, DC), Foundation for Accountability (FAACT, Portland, OR), national and regional large employers, purchaser coalitions, state and local agencies, and health plans themselves are attempting to capture "value," as perceived by the consumer, of care provided over time by measuring health status and health outcomes.

Requirement: The customers' needs and expectations for a particular product or service; implies a certain necessity or condition for a current or existing situation.

Resource Based Relative Value Scale (RBRVS): A system used initially by Medicare, but with spin-off influence on other sectors, to assess more properly the skill and resource relationships to specific CPT codes, thereby dictating reimbursement levels.

Resources: Human and material means that provide assistance and support to an organization/individual.

Restudy: Subsequent complete new study of a topic previously audited to assess the impact/improvement of the initial study's corrective measures on the problems identified.

Retrospective Review: Review of care/professional practice after it has been provided; permits analysis of data gathered over time, involving large number of "cases"; examines deviations and patterns over time that may not be evident in the single-case review.

Return on Investment (ROI): The institution's financial investment in TQM as compared to the financial benefits realized; at some point, the financial investment in TQM plateaus, and the financial benefits achieved continue to escalate.

Review: Formal, prospective, concurrent, or retrospective critical examinations with a view to improvement.

Review Committee: Any professional group/department/service charged with the responsibility for assessing the quality and/or utilization of medical and health care being provided.

Review Criteria: The written policies, decision rules, medical protocols, or guides used by the utilization review organization to determine certification (i.e., appropriateness evaluation protocol [AEP] and intensity-of-service, severity-of-illness, discharge, and appropriateness screens).

Risk Management (RM): The controlling of those circumstances/events of health care that pose a threat to the safety and comfort of patients, which simultaneously protects an organization and its financial assets from liability (e.g., losses associated with patient, employee, or visitor injuries; property loss/damage). Speculative risks are associated with patient care (e.g., procedures and treatments, medications, research) intended to have positive outcomes; pure risks are associated with probability of loss and depletion of financial resources. Both are key focuses of RM.

RM: See **Risk Management (RM).**

ROI: See **Return on Investment (ROI).**

Root Cause: The original reason for not meeting requirements within a process; when removed, the nonconformance or defect will be eliminated.

Safety of Care: Degree to which the care environment is free from hazard or danger; a judgment of the acceptability of risk in a specified situation; the degree to which the risk of an intervention and the risk in the care environment are reduced for the patient and others, including the health care provider.

Sample: Data units or cases in a study; should be sufficient enough in number to ensure validity.

Satisfaction: The customer's evaluation of the value of the service provided; perception is reality for the individual.

Scope of Care/Service: Activities/range of care provided by an organization, department, or service, including conditions treated, managed, or prevented; treatments provided; procedures used; patient populations served; times and locations where care or services are provided, by various disciplines and specialties for various patients; and key governance, managerial, clinical, and support functions. The delineation of the scope of care or service is the basis for identifying the important aspects of care (practice) service or governance on which monitoring and evaluation are focused.

Screening: Method by which charts in a study that conform to explicit, predetermined criteria are excused from further scrutiny. Charts that conform are said to have "passed through the screen"; nonconforming charts are "screened out" for individual attention.

Sentinel Event: See **Indicator.**

Service-Oriented Strategy: Course of action employed by an organization that promotes the example of the customer always coming first.

Severity of Illness: Acuity of patient's condition from clinical evaluation and evidence; usually determined by classification systems that evaluate, measure, and rank.

Shared Leadership: An organizational culture characterized by a shared vision, empowered employees; cooperation/collaboration among and between organizational units and services as "teams" work to improve processes; receptivity to feedback and data; and optimization of the organizational whole rather than its individual parts.

Standard: Any established measure of extent, quantity, quality, or value; an agreed-upon or expected level of performance; the expression of the range of acceptable variations from a norm or criterion.

Standard Deviation: A measure of the dispersion of a frequency distribution that is the square root of the variance; a quantification (positive or negative) of the variability of indicator rates about their mean.

Standard of Governance: A written value statement that defines the rules, actions, and conditions that direct organizational functions.

Standard of Practice: A written value statement that defines the rules, actions, or conditions that direct the maintenance of professional status and credibility.

Standards, Outcome: Identify the results of the performance or nonperformance of a function or activity.

Standards, Process: Identify activities that should or should not be done by governance, management, clinical, and support personnel, such as patient assessment and planning, treatments and procedures, and policy development.

Standards, Structural: Identify the type, number, and characteristics of the resources (manpower and technology) of an organization.

Statistical Control: A process is considered to be in a state of statistical control if the variations among the observed sampling result from what can be attributed to a constant system of chance causes; a state in which the results of measuring a process fall consistently within the target parameters but without an obvious trend or pattern.

Statistical Quality Control (SQC): The application of statistics for the control of a process or system.

Statistical Quality Control Techniques: Tools used to measure common- and special-cause variations in a process and/or outcome. Using large databases (e.g., claims databases, interventions), statistics provide tools for setting up procedures for assembling data, recording them properly, and classifying them so that individual facts may be integrated into like-charactered groups. Provides the ability to order groups into one kind of hierarchy or another and extract any knowledge, generalizations, or conclusions that may be justifiably drawn from them. In addition to Brainstorming (see **Brainstorming**) and nominal group technique (see **Nominal Group Technique**), some examples of tools are

- **Cause-and-Effect Diagram (Fishbone Diagram; Ishikawa Diagram):** Graph used during situation analysis to explore and display all the factors that may influence or contribute to a given outcome. Effect is the desired outcome; cause(s) form the "spines" of the diagram. Common variables include materials, machines, methods, management, and manpower.

- **Control Chart:** Ongoing record of the results of periodic monitoring of a process and/or outcomes; display of data in the order that they occur with statistically determined upper and lower limits of expected common cause variation; used to indicate special causes of process variation, to monitor a process for maintenance, and to determine if process changes have had the desired effect.

- **Flowchart:** Graphic display using standardized symbols illustrating in detail all the steps within a process, including yes/no branches; used to identify customer/supplier relationships in a process, to verify or form an appropriate team, to create common understanding of the process flow, and to establish current "best method" of performing the process by identifying redundancy, unnecessary complexity, and inefficiency in a process.

- **Frequency Distribution:** A tally of measurements that shows the number of times each measurement is included in the tally; help determine whether chance causes alone exist (normal distribution curve) or whether an assignable cause (variation) is present.

- **Histogram:** Frequency distribution put into block form showing a process during a specific given period of time.

- **Pareto Chart:** Bar graph used to display the relative importance of data by highlighting the vital few in contrast to the many others. Used to analyze the decision matrix of a process.

- **Scatter Diagram:** Graphic display of positive, negative, or no relationship between two characteristics; determines cause(s) for process problems and illustrates what happens to one variable when another variable changes.

Statistical Thinking: Data-driven method for decision making and benchmarking, based primarily on an understanding of process variation and small-scale pilot studies.

Storyboarding: Technique used to organize, prioritize, and place ideas into categories for further action; midway point between brainstorming and nominal group technique; use of cards to arrange data.

Stratification: Method of collecting and arranging data to reveal underlying patterns in data; characteristics that may lead to variation in process to verify existence of pattern.

Structure: Arrangement and functional union of the related parts in a combination that forms a whole. For audit purposes, may include number, mix, qualifications, and organization of staff, equipment, material, facilities, and financial resources.

Supplier: Individuals or entities that furnish input to a process. An individual may be both a supplier and a recipient (e.g., person, department, organization, educational institution may provide a service and receive from others).

System: Collection of processes that work in concert to produce a desired outcome; composed of input, throughput, output, and feedback.

Target: A statistically derived mean that serves as the aim, benchmark, objective, or point for control of a process; the border between performance and nonconformance.

Targeted Review: Review process that focuses on specific diagnoses, services, organizations, or group of practitioners, rather than on all services provided or proposed to be provided.

Team, Quality Improvement: Individuals (cross-department/functions/services) knowledgeable about a particular aspect of care or service and commissioned to improve a process that has been identified as requiring at-tention (also called *[natural] work groups* and *quality action teams*).

Team Building: Act of bringing together a cross section of individuals who are related to the process in question. Occurs in four stages: (1) *forming*—initial phase of becoming comfortable with team members; (2) *storming*—determining actions to take; (3) *norming*—beginning support stage; no more competition; significant time and energy spent on project at hand; and (4) *performing*—group becomes cohesive; there is unity of purpose; group works effectively to accomplish task.

TEFRA: Tax Equity and Fiscal Responsibility Act. Passed in 1982; placed a cap on Medicare reimbursement for hospital services.

Test Site: Health care organization in which an indicator or indicators undergo alpha (initial review) and/or beta testing to measure their reliability and validity.

Threshold: Predetermined important single clinical event or preestablished level of performance for a practitioner, department, or organization related to a specific indicator of the quality and/or appropriateness of an important aspect of care. Failure to achieve threshold may trigger an intensified review of a specific component of patient care or practice to determine why threshold was not reached or crossed. The term *benchmark* is currently used by business and health care to indicate ongoing process of measuring products, services, and practices (see **Benchmarking**).

Timeliness of Care: Degree to which care/intervention is provided to patients when it is most beneficial to the patient.

Top Management: Anyone who can make a decision that affects patient care, policy, or budget.

Total Quality Management (TQM): Management system fostering continuously improving performance at every level of every function by focusing on maximization of customer satisfaction. Requires a commitment to an organized, systematic, collaborative, and pervasive quality program with dedicated resources. Requires rigorous process flow and techniques for statistical analysis (quality control), evaluation of all ongoing activities, methods for managing large data sets (integrated computer systems—MIS), and recognition and application of underlying psychosocial principles affecting individuals and groups within an organization. Assumes that most problems are not the result of administrative or clinical professionals' errors, but the inability of the structure (system) to perform adequately. Focus is on process, not individuals.

TQM: See **Total Quality Management (TQM).**

Tracers: A process and outcome evaluation method best suited to evaluate care provided to a group of patients by an agency rather than an individual professional. Tracers measure how the components of a system work together to affect health status.

Trending: Evaluation of data collected over a period of time for the purpose of identifying patterns or changes.

Triage: Sorting or classifying patients in accordance with the nature or degree of injuries/illness.

UCR: See **Usual, Customary, and Reasonable Reimbursement (UCR).**

UR: See **Utilization Review (UR).**

Usual, Customary, and Reasonable Reimbursement (UCR): A method of profiling prevailing fees in an area and reimbursing providers on the basis of that profile.

Utilization Review (UR): Formal, prospective, concurrent, or retrospective critical examination of necessity, efficiency, and appropriateness of use (over-, under-, or optimum use) of resources and segments of the health care system; includes review of the appropriateness of admissions, length of stay, discharge practices, and services ordered and provided on a preadmission, concurrent, or retrospective basis. Guidelines for concurrent review and general

administrative procedures were collaboratively developed by the American Hospital Association (AHA), the American Managed Care and Review Association (AMCRA), the American Medical Association (AMA), the Blue Cross and Blue Shield Association (BCBSA), and the Health Insurance Association of America (HIAA) in October 1990. The Utilization Review Accreditation Commission (URAC) formed in 1990 to refine national utilization review standards developed by the Tennessee Health Relations Group, referred to AMCRA.

Validity: Ability to measure what is purported to be measured; a measure of the extent to which an observed situation reflects the real situation.

Validity, External: Measure of the extent to which study results can be generalized beyond the study sample.

Validity, Face: Degree to which indicator and hypothesized relationships make sense to the informed user.

Validity, Internal: Measure of the extent to which study results reflect the true relationship of a risk factor (i.e., treatment or technology) to the outcome of interest in study subjects.

Variation: Anything that causes a process to deviate from acceptable standards. Sources of variation in a patient care process include materials, machines, methods, manpower, and management. There are two types of variation: (1) *special-cause variation*, assignable to a specific cause(s) and arises because of special circumstances; instability in a process results in outcomes that would not be predictable by chance alone; these variations signify that something out of the ordinary is occurring in the process; an extrasystematic cause is affecting the process; random causes tend to cluster by place, person, and time; and (2) *common-cause variation*, due to the process itself and produced by interactions of variables of that process.

REFERENCES

Hammer, M., & Champy, J. (1993). *Reengineering the corporation: A manifesto for business revolution.* New York: Harper Business.

Joint Commission on the Accreditation of Healthcare Organizations. (1990). *Primer on indicator development and application.* Oakbrook Terrace, IL: Author.

Selected Bibliography

BOOKS AND ARTICLES

Allen, H., & Rogers, W. (1996). Consumer surveys of health plan performance: A comparison of content and approach and a look to the future. *The Joint Commission Journal on Quality Improvement, 22*(12), 775–794.

Arnold, K. (1994). *The manager's guide to ISO 9000.* New York: The Free Press.

Aspen Health Law Center. (1996). *Physician organizations and medical staff: Contracts, rights and liabilities.* Gaithersburg, MD: Aspen.

Avillion, A., & Mirgon, B. (1989). *Quality assurance in rehabilitation nursing: A practical guide.* Gaithersburg, MD: Aspen.

Barber, N. (1996). *Quality assessment for healthcare: A Baldrige-based handbook.* Milwaukee, WI: American Society for Quality Control.

Belasco, J. (1990). *Teaching the elephant to dance: Empowering change in your organization.* New York: Crown Publishers.

Berwick, D. (1989). Sounding board: Continuous improvement as an ideal in health care. *New England Journal of Medicine, 320*(1), 53–56.

Berwick, D., Godfrey, A., & Roessner, J. (1990). *Curing health care: New strategies for quality improvement.* San Francisco: Jossey-Bass.

Blumenthal, D., & Scheck, A. (Eds.). (1995). *Improving clinical practice: Total quality management and the physician.* San Francisco: Jossey-Bass.

Bulau, J. (1990). *Quality assurance: Policies and procedures for ambulatory health care.* Gaithersburg, MD: Aspen.

Bonstingl, J. (1996). (2nd ed.). *Schools of quality: An introduction to total quality management in education.* Alexandria, VA: Association for Supervision and Curriculum Development.

Caldwell, C. (1995). *Mentoring strategic change in health care: An action guide.* Milwaukee, WI: American Society for Quality Control.

Carey, R., & Lloyd, R. (1995). *Measuring quality improvement in health care: A guide to statistical process control applications.* New York: Quality Resources.

Center for Health Care Economics. (1994). *The nation's health care bill: Who bears the burden?* Walthman, MA: Author.

Codman, E.A. (1914). The products of a hospital. *Surgical Gynecological Obstetrics, 118*, 491–496.

Cornesky, R. (1993). *The quality professor: Implementing TQM in the classroom.* Madison, WI: Magna Publications.

Crosby, P. (1979). *Quality is free: The art of making quality certain.* New York: New American Library.

Crosby, P. (1988). *The eternally successful organization: The art of corporate wellness.* New York: McGraw-Hill.

Crosby, P. (1992). *Completeness: Quality for the 21st century.* New York: Dutton.

Deming, W. (1982). *Quality productivity and competitive position.* Cambridge: MIT Center for Advanced Engineering Study.

Deming, W. (1989). *Out of crises.* Cambridge: MIT Center for Advanced Engineering Study.

Donabedian, A. (1980). *Explorations in quality assessment and monitoring: The definition of quality and approaches to its assessment.* Vol. 1. Ann Arbor: Health Administration Press.

Donabedian, A. (1982). *Explorations in quality assessment and monitoring: The criteria and standards of quality.* Vol. 2. Ann Arbor: Health Administration Press.

Donabedian, A. (1988). The quality of care: How can it be defined? *Journal of the American Medical Association, 260*, 1743–1748.

Donabedian, A., Wheeler, J., & Wyszewianski, L. (1982). Quality, cost and health: An integrative model. *Medical Care, 20,* 975–992.

Feigenbaum, A. (1983). *Total quality control.* 3rd ed. New York: McGraw-Hill.

Finkleman, A. (1990). *Quality assurance for psychiatric nursing.* Gaithersburg, MD: Aspen.

Gaucher, E., & Coffey, R. (1993). *Total quality in health-care: From theory to practice.* San Francisco: Jossey-Bass.

Gitlow, H., Gitlow, S., Oppenheimer, A., & Oppenheimer, R. (1989). *Tools and methods for the improvement of quality.* Homewood, IL: Richard D. Irwin.

Goldfield, N., & Nash, D. (Eds.). (1989). *Providing quality care: The challenge to clinicians.* Philadelphia: American College of Physicians.

Goonan, J. (1995). *The Juran prescription: Clinical quality management.* San Francisco: Jossey-Bass.

Graham, N. (1995). *Quality in health care: Theory, application, and evolution.* Gaithersburg, MD: Aspen.

Harrington, M. (1992) *Quality of care: Issues and challenges in the 90s: A literature review.* Ottawa, Ontario: Canadian Medical Association.

Health Care Quality Improvement Act of 1986, 42 U.S.C. 11101 et seq. (1986).

Hiam, A. (1992). *Closing the quality gap: Lessons from America's leading companies.* Englewood Cliffs, NJ: Prentice-Hall.

Imai, M. (1986). *Kaizen: The key to Japanese competitive success.* New York: Random House.

Ishikawa, K. (1985). *What is total quality control? The Japanese way.* Englewood Cliffs, NJ: Prentice-Hall.

Jablonski, J. (1991). *Implementing total quality management: An overview.* San Diego: Pfeiffer & Co.

Juran, J. (1988). *Juran on planning for quality.* New York: Free Press.

Juran, J. (1989). *Juran on leadership for quality: An executive handbook.* New York: Free Press.

Juran, J., & Gryna, F. (1988). *Juran's quality control handbook.* (4th ed.). Milwaukee, WI: American Society for Quality Control.

Katz, J., & Green, E. (1997). *Managing quality: A guide to system-wide performance management in health care.* (2nd ed.). St. Louis, MO: Mosby-Year Book.

Kazandjian, V. (1995). *The epidemiology of quality.* Gaithersburg, MD: Aspen.

Koch, M., & Fairly, T. (1993). *Integrated quality management: The key to improving nursing care quality.* St. Louis, MO: Mosby-Year Book.

Larrabee, J. (1996). Emerging model of quality. *Image: Journal of Nursing Scholarship, 28*(4), 353–358.

Lewin, V.H.I., Inc. (1995). *The states and private sector: Leading health care reform states as payers: Managed care for Medicaid populations.* (94SW0027): The National Institute for Health Care Management, Washington, DC.

Lohr, K. (Ed.). (1990). *Institute of Medicine & Medicare: A strategy for quality assurance.* Vols. 1, 2. Washington, DC: National Academy Press.

McLaughlin, C., & Kaluzny, A. (Eds.). (1994). *Continuous quality improvement in health care: Theory, implementation, and applications.* Gaithersburg, MD: Aspen.

Meisenheimer, C. (1989). *Quality assurance for home health care.* Gaithersburg, MD: Aspen.

Morton, R., Hebel, J., & McCarter, R. (1990). *A study guide to epidemiology and biostatistics.* 2nd ed. Gaithersburg, MD: Aspen.

Naisbitt, J. (1994). *Global paradox.* New York: William Morrow.

O'Neil, E. (1993). *Health professions education for the future: Schools in service to the nations.* San Francisco: Pew Health Profession Commission.

Orlikoff, J. (1990). *Quality from the top: Working with governing boards to assure quality care.* Chicago: Precept Press.

Palmer, R., Donabedian, A., & Povar, G. (1991). *Striving for quality in health care: An inquiry into policy and practice.* Ann Arbor: Health Administration Press.

Pew Health Professions Commission. (1991). *Healthy America: Practitioners for 2005.* Dunham, NC: Author.

Schmele, J. (Ed.). (1996). *Quality management in nursing and health care.* Albany, NY: Delmar Publishers.

Schroeder, P. (Ed.). (1991). *The encyclopedia of nursing care quality.* Vols. I, II & III. Gaithersburg, MD: Aspen.

Schroeder, P. (Ed.). *Improving quality and performance: Concepts, programs, and techniques.* St. Louis, MO: Mosby-Year Book.

Scholtes, P. (1990). *The team handbook.* Madison, WI: Joiner Associates.

Sholtes, P. (1995). Teams in the age of systems. *Quality Progress, 28*(12), 51–59.

Senge, P. (1990). *The fifth discipline: The art and practice of the learning organization.* New York: Doubleday/Currency.

Senge, P., Roberts, C., Ross, R., Smith, B., & Kleiner, A. (1994). *The fifth discipline fieldbook.* New York: Doubleday.

Shewhart, W. (1980 [1931]). *Economic control of quality of manufactured product.* Milwaukee, WI: American Society of Quality Control.

Shewhart, W. (1986). *Statistical methods from the viewpoint of quality control.* Dover.

Vincenzino, J. (1994). Developments in health care costs: An update. *Bulletin Metropolitan Insurance Companies*, 75(1), 30–35.

United States Department of Commerce. (1997). *1997 Application guidelines: Malcolm Baldrige National Quality Award*. Gaithersburg, MD: National Institute of Standards and Technology.

U.S. Department of Health and Human Services. (1992). *Patient outcomes research: Examining the effectiveness of nursing practice*. (NIH Publication No. 93-3411). Rockville, MD: Author.

Walton, M. (1990). *Deming management at work*. New York: The Putnam Publishing Group.

Youngberg, B. (1990). *Quality & risk management in health care: An information service*. Gaithersburg, MD: Aspen.

SELECTED QUALITY-RELATED PUBLICATIONS

Abstracts of Clinical Guidelines
Joint Commission on Accreditation of Healthcare
  Organizations
One Renaissance Blvd.
Oakbrook Terrace, IL 60181
(630) 792-5000

American Journal of Medical Quality
Williams & Wilkins
428 East Preston St.
Baltimore, MD 21202
(800) 638-5198

Business & Health
Medical Economics Publishing
5 Paragon Dr.
Montvale, NJ 07645
(800) 526-4870

Case Management Advisor
American Health Consultants, Inc.
P.O. Box 740059
Atlanta, GA 30374
(800) 688-2421

Clinical Performance and Quality Health Care
SLACK Incorporated
6900 Grove Rd.
Thorofare, NJ 08086
(609) 848-1000

CQI Quality Chronicle
SSM Health Care System
477 N. Lindbergh Blvd.
St. Louis, MO 63141
(314) 994-7800

Health Systems Leader
Bader & Associates, Inc.
P.O. Box 2106
Rockville, MD 20847-2106
(301) 468-1610

Health Technology Trends
ECRI
5200 Butler Pike
Plymouth Meeting, PA 19462
(215) 825-6000

Healthcare Demand Management
National Health Information, LLC
4343 Shallowford Rd.
Bldg. B, Suite 8B
Marietta, GA 30062
(800) 597-6300

Healthcare Quality Abstracts
COR Healthcare Resources
P.O. Box 40959
Santa Barbara, CA 93140-0959
(805) 564-2146

Healthcare QI Training Report
COR Healthcare Resources
P.O. Box 40959
Santa Barbara, CA 93140-0959
(805) 564-2177

Homecare Quality Management
American Health Consultants, Inc.
3525 Piedmont Road
Building Six, Suite 400
Atlanta, GA 30305
(404) 262-7436

Hospital Benchmarks
American Health Consultants, Inc.
P.O. Box 740059
Atlanta, GA 30374
(800) 688-2421

Inside Health Law
Aspen Publishers, Inc.
7201 McKinney Circle
Frederick, MD 21704
(800) 638-8437

Joint Commission Perspectives
Joint Commission on Accreditation of Healthcare
    Organizations
One Renaissance Blvd.
Oakbrook Terrace, IL 60181
(630) 792-5000

Journal for Healthcare Quality
National Association for Healthcare Quality
5700 Old Orchard R., First Floor
Skokie, IL 60077
(708) 966-9392

Journal of Nursing Administration
Lippincott-Raven Publishers
227 East Washington Square
Philadelphia, PA 19106
(215) 238-4200

Journal of Nursing Care Quality
Aspen Publishers, Inc.
7201 McKinney Circle
Frederick, MD 21704
(800) 638-8437

Long-Term Care Quality
American Health Consultants, Inc.
3525 Piedmont Road
Building Six, Suite 400
Atlanta, GA 30305
(404) 262-7436

Managed Care Quality
American Health Consultants, Inc.
P.O. Box 740059
Atlanta, GA 30374
(800) 688-2421

Managed Care Quarterly
Aspen Publishers, Inc.
7201 McKinney Circle
Frederick, MD 21704
(800) 638-8437

Modern Healthcare
740 Rush St.
Chicago, IL 60611
(800) 678-9595

Nursing Management
S-N Publications
103 North Second St., Suite 200
Dundee, IL 60118
(708) 426-6100

Outcomes Measurement & Management
The Zitter Group
90 New Montgomery, Suite 820
San Francisco, CA 94105
(415) 495-2450

Patient-Focused Care
American Health Consultants, Inc.
P.O. Box 740059
Atlanta, GA 30374
(800) 688-2421

Patient Satisfaction Management
American Health Consultants, Inc.
3525 Piedmont Road
Building Six, Suite 400
Atlanta, GA 30305
(404) 262-7436

QI/TQM
American Health Consultants, Inc.
P.O. Box 740059
Atlanta, GA 30374
(800) 688-2421

QRC Advisor
Aspen Publishers, Inc.
7201 McKinney Circle
Frederick, MD 21704
(800) 638-8437

Quality Management in Health Care
Aspen Publishers, Inc.
7201 McKinney Circle
Frederick, MD 21704
(800) 638-8437

Quality Management Update
Faulkner & Gray's Healthcare Information Center
Eleven Penn Plaza
New York, NY 10001
(212) 967-7060

The Quality Letter for Healthcare Leaders
Capitol Publications, Inc.
1101 King St., Suite 444
Alexandria, VA 22314
(800) 655-5597

Report on Medical Guidelines & Outcomes
    Research
Capitol Publications
1101 King St., Suite 444
Alexandria, VA 22314
(800) 655-5597

Subacute Care Management
American Health Consultants, Inc.
3525 Piedmont Road
Building Six, Suite 400
Atlanta, GA 30305
(404) 262-7436

The Joint Commission Journal on Quality
    Improvement
Mosby-Year Book, Inc.
11830 Westline Industrial Dr.
St. Louis, MO 63146
(800) 453-4351

Trends in Integrated Health Care
Aspen Publishers, Inc.
7201 McKinney Circle
Frederick, MD 21704
(800) 638-8437

QUALITY-RELATED INTERNET SITES

American Society for Quality Control
http://www.asqc.org.

Aspen Publishers, Inc.
http://www.aspenpub.com

American Health Consultants
http://www.ahcpub.com

Agency for Health Care Policy and Research
http://www.ahcpr.gov

Deming Electronic Network
http://deming.eng.clemson.edu/

Healthcare Quality Assessment Page
http://www.qserve.com/hcass/

Hospital Web
http://neuro-www.mgh.harvard.edu/hospitalweb.nclk

Joint Commission on Accreditation of Healthcare
  Organizations
http://www.jcaho.org

Malcolm Baldrige Award
http://www. NIST.gov/quality_program

National Committee for Quality Assurance (NCQA)
http://www.ncqa.org

On-line quality resource list
http://pages.prodigy.com/J/O/N/john/onlineqlist.html

Quality Resources Online
http://www.quality.org/qc/

Peer Review Organizations (quality improvement issues)
http://www.aqaf.com/pro/prolist2.html

Total Quality Management Page
http://akao.larc.nasa.gov/dfc.qtec.html

REFERENCES

American Health Consultants. (1996). Fire up your Internet link, enhance QI work. *QI/TQM*, *6*(10), 122–124.

Leeuwen, D., & Marks, L. (1996). Using the Internet for professional development. *Journal for Healthcare Quality, 18*(3), 22–23.

Index